Your Essential Revision Guide

MRCOG PART ONE

Your Essential Revision Guide

MRCOG PART ONE

The official companion to the
Royal College of Obstetricians and
Gynaecologists revision course

Edited by
Alison Fiander and Baskaran Thilaganathan

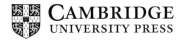

CAMBRIDGE
UNIVERSITY PRESS

CAMBRIDGE
UNIVERSITY PRESS

Registered names

The use of registered names, trademarks, etc. in this publication does not imply, even in the absence of a specific statement, that such names are exempt from the relevant laws and regulations and therefore free for general use.

Product liability

Drugs and their doses are mentioned in this text. While every effort has been made to ensure the accuracy of the information contained within this publication, neither the authors nor the publishers can accept liability for errors or omissions. The final responsibility for delivery of the correct dose remains with the physician prescribing and administering the drug. In every individual case the respective user must check current indications and accuracy by consulting other pharmaceutical literature and following the guidelines laid down by the manufacturers of specific products and the relevant authorities in the country in which they are practising.

The rights of the authors to be identified as Authors of this work have been asserted by them in accordance with the Copyright, Designs and Patents Act, 1988.

A machine-readable catalogue record for this publication is available from the British Library [www.bl.uk/catalogue/listings.html]

Library of Congress Cataloging-in-Publication Data
Your essential revision guide : MRCOG part one : the official companion to the Royal College of Obstetricians and Gynaecologists revision course / edited by Alison Fiander, Baskaran Thilaganathan. – 2.
        p. ; cm.
MRCOG part one : the official companion to the Royal College of Obstetricians and Gynaecologists revision course
Includes bibliographical references and index.
ISBN 978-1-107-66713-6 (paperback)
I. Fiander, Alison, editor. II. Thilaganathan, Baskaran, editor. III. Royal College of Obstetricians and Gynaecologists (Great Britain). IV. Title: MRCOG part one : the official companion to the Royal College of Obstetricians and Gynaecologists revision course.
[DNLM: 1. Obstetrics–Examination Questions. 2. Gynecology–Examination Questions. WQ 18.2]
RG111
618.10076–dc 3   2015032438

ISBN 978-1-107-66713-6

Published by the RCOG Press at the
Royal College of Obstetricians and Gynaecologists
27 Sussex Place, Regent's Park
London NW1 4RG

Registered Charity No. 213280

RCOG Press Editor: Fiona Courtenay-Thompson

Artwork by Oxford Designers & Illustrators
(David Morris, Elaine Leggett and Sue Aldridge)

Index: Cath Topliff MSocInd(Adv)

Printed in the United Kingdom by Clays, St Ives plc.

Contents

About the authors

Nazar N Amso PhD FRCOG FHEA
Obstetrics and Gynaecology, Cardiff University School of Medicine, Cardiff, UK

Gul Bano MD FRCP
Senior Lecturer in Clinical Endocrinology, St George's Hospital NHS Trust, London, UK

Rosemary Bland PhD
Honorary Associate Professor, Warwick Medical School, The University of Warwick, and University Hospitals Coventry and Warwickshire NHS Trust, Coventry, UK

Mary Board MA DPhil(Oxon)
Biochemistry Lecturer, St Hilda's College, University of Oxford, Oxford, UK

Annette Briley MSc
Consultant Midwife /Clinical Trials Manager, King's Health Partners, Division of Women's Health, St Thomas' Hospital, London, UK

Fiona Broughton Pipkin MA DPhil FRCOG (ad eundem)
Professor Emeritus of Perinatal Physiology, University Department of Obstetrics and Gynaecology, City Hospital, Nottingham, UK

Daniel Brudney MRCP(UK)
Specialty Registrar, Department of Microbiology, Royal Free Hospital, London, UK

Sharon Cookson PhD
Formerly Postdoctoral Research Assistant, University of Oxford, Nuffield Department of Obstetrics and Gynaecology, John Radcliffe Hospital, Oxford, UK

Arri Coomarasamy MBChB MD FRCOG
Professor of Gynaecology and Director of Tommy's National Centre for Miscarriage Research, Institute of Metabolism and Systems Research, University of Birmingham, UK; Consultant Gynaecologist and Sub-specialist in Reproductive Medicine and Surgery, Birmingham Women's Hospital, UK

Rohan D'Souza MD MSC MRCOG FCPS DNB DGO DFP
Maternal–Fetal Medicine Physician, Mount Sinai Hospital, Toronto, Canada; Assistant Professor, Obstetrics and Gynaecology, University of Toronto

Prathiba M De Silva BSc (Hons) MBBS AICSM
Academic Foundation Doctor, West Midlands Deanery, UK; Honorary Research Fellow, Birmingham Women's Hospital and University of Birmingham, UK

Alison Fiander DM, MSC FRCOG
Clinical Lead RCOG Leading Safe Choices Programme, and Honorary Chair Obstetrics and Gynaecology, Cardiff University, Cardiff, UK

Raji Ganesan MBBS Cest Med Ed FRCPath
Consultant in Histopathology, Department of Cellular Pathology, Birmingham Women's NHS Foundation Trust, Edgbaston, Birmingham, UK

Phillip E Hay FRCP
Reader in HIV/Genitourinary Medicine, Department of Genitourinary Medicine, St George's, University of London, London, UK

Kevin Hayes MRCOG
Consultant and Senior Lecturer, St George's, University of London, London, UK

Mark Heining FRCA
Consultant in Anaesthesia, Nottingham University Hospitals NHS Trust, Nottingham, UK

Des Holden PhD MRCOG
Medical Director, Surrey and Sussex Healthcare NHS Trust, Redhill, Surrey and Medical Director, Kent, Surrey and Sussex Academic Health Science Network

Susan Hopkins FRCPI MScEpi
Consultant in Infectious Diseases, Department of Microbiology, Royal Free Hospital, London, UK

Malcolm Johnston MRCS FRCR
Consultant Radiologist, Brighton and Sussex University Hospitals and Western Sussex Hospitals and Senior Lecturer and Lead for Radiology Education at Brighton and Sussex Medical School, Brighton, UK

Asma Khalil MRCOG
Senior Research Fellow in Feto-Maternal Medicine, University College London, UK

Diana Lawrence-Watt PhD
Emeritus Professor of Human Anatomy, Brighton and Sussex Medical School, Brighton, Sussex, UK

Maryann Lumsden MBBS MD FRCOG
Professor of Medical Education and Gynaecology, School of Medicine, University of Glasgow, Glasgow, UK

Fiona Lyall MBA PhD
Professor of Maternal and Fetal Health, School of Medicine, University of Glasgow, Yorkhill Hospitals, Glasgow, UK

Michael Marsh MD FRCOG
Consultant in Obstetrics and Gynaecology, King's College Hospital, London, UK; Honorary Senior Lecturer, King's College School of Medicine, London, UK; Honorary Senior Lecturer, Institute of Psychiatry, London, UK

Helen Mason PhD
Senior Lecturer, Basic Medical Sciences Division, Faculty of Medicine and Biomedical Sciences, St George's, University of London, London, UK

Anthony E Michael PhD, FRSB
Reader in Reproductive Biology and Director of Taught Programmes, School of Biological and Chemical Sciences, Queen Mary, University of London, London, UK

Julia Montgomery FRCOG, MA
Senior Educational Research Fellow, Honorary Clinical Lecturer, Brighton and Sussex Medical School and Consultant Obstetrician and Gynaecologist, Brighton and Sussex University Hospitals Trust, Brighton, UK

Vivek Nama MD MRCOG
Consultant Gyn Oncologist, Croydon University Hospital, London, UK

Aris T Papageorghiou MRCOG
Consultant in Fetal Medicine and Obstetrics, Fetal Medicine Unit, Department of Obstetrics and Gynaecology, St George's Hospital NHS Trust, London, UK

Neil Pugh PhD F InstP
Chair and Consultant Physicist, School of Medicine, Cardiff University, Cardiff, UK

Shwetha Ramachandrappa PhD
Specialist Registrar in Clinical Genetics, South West Thames Regional Genetics Service, Department of Genetics, St George's Hospital NHS Trust, London, UK

Philip Rice FRCPath
Department of Microbiology, Norfolk and Norwich
University Hospitals NHS Foundation Trust, UK

Ian Sargent PhD
Emeritus Professor of Reproductive Science, University
of Oxford, Nuffield Department of Obstetrics and
Gynaecology, John Radcliffe Hospital, Oxford, UK

Ram Sharma PhD
Lecturer, Centre for Learning Anatomical Sciences,
Division of Medical Education, School of Medicine,
University of Southampton, Southampton General
Hospital, Southampton, UK

Andrew H Shennan MD FRCOG
Professor of Obstetrics, Maternal and Fetal Research
Unit, Division of Women's Health, King's College
London, UK

Andrew Sizer MPH MD PhD MRCOG DFSRH PGCert
Consultant in Reproductive Medicine and
Surgery, Clinical Director for Gynaecology, Royal
Shrewsbury Hospital, Shrewsbury, UK; Senior
Lecturer, Keele University School of Medicine,
Keele, UK

Katrina Tatton-Brown MD
Consultant in Clinical Genetics, South West
Thames Regional Genetics Service, Department
of Genetics, St George's Hospital NHS Trust,
London, UK

Baskaran Thilaganathan MD FRCOG
Director, Fetal Medicine Unit, Department of Obstetrics
and Gynaecology, St George's Hospital NHS Trust,
London, UK

Acknowledgements

We thank Jan Sharp, senior medical artist in Cardiff for her anatomical diagrams in chapters 2, 3 and 4. We would also like to acknowledge the help of Chris Chivers of the RCOG Examination Department.

Abbreviations used in the book

^{125}I	iodine-125
^{131}I	iodine-131
^{137}Cs	caesium-137
^{177}Lu	lutetium-177
^{192}Ir	iridium-192
^{192}Ir	iridium-192
2,3-DPG	2,3-diphosphoglycerate
5α-DHT	5α-dihydrotestosterone
^{90}Y	yttrium-90
β-hCG	beta-human chorionic gonadotrophin
θ	scattering angle
ρ	density of a material
ABPA	allergic bronchopulmonary aspergillosis
ACE	angiotensin-converting enzyme
aCGH	array comparative genomic hybridisation
ACTH	adrenocorticotrophic hormone
ADA	American Diabetes Association
ADH	antidiuretic hormone
ADP	adenosine diphosphate
AFP	alpha fetoprotein
ALT	alanine transaminase
AMP	adenosine monophosphate
ANP	atrial natriuretic peptide
AP	accessory proteins
APC	adenomatous polyposis coli
APC	antigen-presenting cell
APECED	autoimmune polyendocrinopathy, candidiasis and ectodermal dystrophy
APS	autoimmune polyendocrinopathy syndrome
APUD	amine precursor uptake and decarboxylation
ASD	atrial septal defect
ATD	antithyroid drugs
ATM	ataxia telangiectasia mutated

ATP	adenosine triphosphate
AVP	arginine vasopressin
AVSD	atriventricular septal defect
B cell	bursa-equivalent cell
BAC	bacterial artificial chromosome
BHIVA	British HIV Association
BMD	bone mineral density
B-mode ultrasound	brightness mode ultrasound
BMUS	British Medical Ultrasound Society
bNOS	brain nitric oxide synthase
BSO	bilateral salpingo-oophorectomy
BSO	bilateral salpingo-oophorectomy
c	(in the context of ultrasound) speed of a sound wave
C	carbon atom
CaBP	Ca^{2+}-binding protein
CAH	congenital adrenal hyperplasia
CaMK	Ca^{2+}/calmodulin-dependent kinase
cAMP	cyclic adenosine monophosphate
CaSR	Ca^{2+}-sensing receptor
CCA	common carotid artery
CCR	chemokine C-C motif receptor
CDI	*Clostridium difficile* infection
CDK2	cyclin-dependent kinase 2
cDNA	complementary DNA
CEMACH	Confidential Enquiry into Maternal and Child Health
CEMD	Confidential Enquiry into Maternal Deaths
cffDNA	cell-free fetal DNA
CGH	comparative genomic hybridisation
CGIN	cervical glandular intraepithelial neoplasia
cGMP	cyclic guanosine monophosphate
CHD	coronary heart disease
CI	clearance interval

CID cytomegalic inclusion disease
CIN cervical intraepithelial neoplasia
CMACE Centre for Maternal and Child Enquiries
CMI carbimazole
CMV cytomegalovirus
CNS central nervous system
CO carbon monoxide
CoA coenzyme A
COPD chronic obstructive pulmonary disease
COX cyclooxygenase
CRH corticotrophin-releasing hormone
CRH-BP corticotrophin-releasing hormone binding protein
CRP C-reactive protein
CRT conformal radiotherapy
CT computed tomography
CTG cardiotocograph(y)
CVS chorionic villus sampling
CYP cytochrome P450
CYP11A1 cholesterol side chain cleavage enzyme
CYP17A steroid 17α-hydroxylase
CYP19 aromatase
DC dendritic cell
DCC defective in sister chromatid cohesion
DCT distal convoluted tubule
DDAVP desmopressin
DEET N,N-diethyl-m-toluamide
dex dexamethasone
DEXA dual energy X-ray absorptiometry
DHA docosahexaenoic acid
DHEA dehydroepiandrosterone
DHEAS dehydroepiandrosterone sulphate
DOPA dihydroxyphenylalanine
DPPC dipalmitoylphosphatidylcholine
E_1 estrone
E_2 17-beta-estradiol
E_3 estriol
EASD European Association for the Study of Diabetes
EBM evidence-based medicine
EBV Epstein–Barr virus
ECG electrocardiogram
EDTA ethylenediaminetetraacetic acid
EFSUMB European Federation of Societies for Ultrasound in Medicine and Biology
EIA enzyme immunoassay

EIC endometrial intraepithelial carcinoma
eNOS endothelial nitric oxide synthase
EPO erythropoietin
ER endoplasmic reticulum
ERPC evacuation of retained products of conception
ESBL extended-spectrum beta-lactamase
ESR erythrocyte rate
ESRD end-stage renal disease
Fab antigen-binding fragment
FAD flavin adenine dinucleotide
$FADH_2$ reduced form of flavin adenine dinucleotide
FBM fetal breathing movement
Fc crystallisable fragment
f_d Doppler frequency shift
FDA Food and Drug Administration
FDG flurodeoxyglucose
FHR fetal heart rate
FISH fluorescence in situ hybridisation
FSH follicle-stimulating hormone
ft frequency of a transmitted signal
G protein guanine-nucleotide-binding protein
G (in DNA and RNA sequences) guanine
G0 quiescent state
G1 gap 1
G2 gap 2
GABA γ-aminobutyric acid
GBS group B streptococci
GCV ganciclovir
GDM gestational diabetes mellitus
GDP guanosine diphosphate
GH growth hormone
GHRH growth-hormone-releasing hormone
GI gastrointestinal
Gi inhibitory G protein
GLP glucagon-like peptide
GLUT3 glucose transporter type 3
GM-CSF granulocyte–macrophage colony-stimulating factor
GnRH gonadotrophin-releasing hormone
GRA glucocorticoid-remediable aldosteronism
Gs protein stimulatory G protein
GTP guanosine triphosphate
Gy gray
H0 null hypothesis
H_2CO_3 carbonic acid

H_2O_2 hydrogen peroxide
$H_2PO_4^-$ dihydrogen phosphate
HbA_{1c} glycated haemoglobin
HbF fetal haemoglobin
hCG human chorionic gonadotrophin
HCl hydrochloric acid
HCO_3^- bicarbonate ion
HDL high-density lipoprotein
HFEA Human Fertilisation and Embryology Authority
HLA human leucocyte antigen
HNPCC hereditary nonpolyposis colon cancer
HPG hypothalamo–pituitary–gonadal
HPL human placental lactogen
HPO_4^{2-} hydrogen phosphate
HPV human papilloma virus
HRT hormone replacement therapy
HSD hydroxysteroid dehydrogenase
HSG hysterosalpingogram
HSL hormone-sensitive lipase
HSP heat shock protein
HSV herpes simplex virus
HTN hypertension
HyCoSy hystero-contrast-salpingography
IACR International Association of Cancer Registries
ICA internal carotid artery
ICAM intercellular cell adhesion molecule
ICSI intracytoplasmic sperm injection
IDBP intracellular vitamin-D-binding protein
IFN interferon
Ig immunoglobulin
IGF insulin-like growth factor
IL interleukin
ILT immunoglobulin-like transcript
IMRT intensity-modulated radiation therapy
inh inhibin
iNOS inducible nitric oxide synthase
IP infundibulopelvic
IP_3 inositol trisphosphate
IP_4 inositol tetrakisphosphate
IUCD intrauterine contraceptive device
IUGR intrauterine growth restriction
IVC inferior vena cava
IVF *in vitro* fertilisation
IVIg intravenous immunoglobulin

K dissociation constant
KIR killer cell immunoglobulin-like receptor
KOH potassium hydroxide
KTP potassium titanyl phosphate
KUB X-ray kidney, ureter and bladder X-ray
LDL low-density lipoprotein
Leu leucine
LGV lymphogranuloma venereum
LH luteinising hormone
LMP last menstrual period
LTV long-term variability
MALDI matrix-assisted laser desorption/ionisation
MAO monoamine oxidase
MAP mitogen-activated protein
MB mamillary bodies
MELAS mitochondrial encephalomyopathy with lactic acidosis and stroke-like episodes
MEN multiple endocrine neoplasia
MERFF myoclonic epilepsy with ragged red fibres
Met methionine
MHC major histocompatibility complex
MHRA Medicines and Healthcare products Regulatory Agency
MIBG metaiodobenzylguanidine
MIC major histocompatibility complex
MLCK myosin light chain kinase
MLPA multiplex ligation-dependent probe amplification
MMI methimazole
M-mode ultrasound movement mode ultrasound
MMR maternal mortality ratio
MMR measles, mumps and rubella
MRI magnetic resonance imaging
mRNA messenger RNA
MRSA methicillin-resistant *Staphylococcus aureus*
mVDR membrane-bound vitamin D receptor
NAAT nucleic acid amplification test
NAD^+ oxidised form of nicotinamide adenine dinucleotide
NADH reduced form of nicotinamide adenine dinucleotide
$NADP^+$ oxidised form of nicotinamide adenine dinucleotide phosphate
NADPH reduced form of nicotinamide adenine dinucleotide phosphate

NaHCO$_3$	sodium bicarbonate	PKC	protein kinase C
NCAM	neural cell adhesion molecule	PLC	phospholipase C
Nd:YAG	neodymium-doped yttrium aluminium garnet	PMCA	plasma membrane Ca^{2+}-ATPase
NF	neurofibromatosis	PNMR	perinatal mortality rate
NH$_4^+$	ammonium ion	PO_2	partial pressure of oxygen
NICE	National Institute for Health and Care Excellence	PO$_3^{4-}$	phosphate ion
		POF	premature ovarian failure
NK	natural killer	Pol II	polymerase II
NNRTI	nonnucleoside reverse transcriptase inhibitor	POMC	pro-opiomelanocortin
		PPAR	proliferator-activated receptor
NO	nitric oxide	PPNG	pelicillinase-producing *Neisseria gonorrhoeae*
NPT2	inorganic phosphate cotransporter type II		
NRTI	nucleoside reverse transcriptase inhibitor	PPT	postpartum thyroiditis
NSAID	nonsteroidal anti-inflammatory drug	PRA	plasma renin activity
NT	nuchal translucency	PRF	prolactin-releasing factor
O$_2$	oxygen	PRL	prolactin
OC	optic chiasm	PSA	prostate-specific antigen
OGTT	oral glucose tolerance test	PTH	parathyroid hormone
OH–	hydroxyl ion	PTHR	parathyroid hormone receptor
OPG	osteoprotegerin	PTHrP	parathyroid-hormone-related peptide
OXY	oxytocin	PTU	propylthiouracil
P (encircled)	phosphate group	PUL	pregnancy of unknown location
PAC	plasma aldosterone concentration	PUV	pregnancy of 'uncertain viability'
PAPP-A	pregnancy-associated plasma protein A	PVN	paraventricular nucleus
PAS	periodic acid–Schiff stain	QF-PCR	quantitative fluorescence polymerase chain reaction
PCO_2	partial pressure of carbon dioxide		
PCOS	polycystic ovarian syndrome	RBC	red blood cell
PCR	polymerase chain reaction	RCC	Rathke cleft cyst
PDH	pyruvate dehydrogenase	RCT	randomised controlled trial
PECAM	platelet endothelial cell adhesion molecule	ROC	receiver operating characteristic
PGD	pre-implantation genetic diagnosis	RPR	rapid plasma reagin
PGD	prostaglandin D	rRNA	ribosomal RNA
PGE	prostaglandin E	RXR	retinoid X receptor
PGF$_{2\alpha}$	prostaglandin F$_{2\alpha}$	s or SD	standard deviation
PGH	prostaglandin H	s^2	variance
PGI	prostaglandin I	SBA	single best answer
PGI$_2$	prostacyclin	SCH	subclinical hypothyroidism
pH value	negative logarithm to the base 10 of the H+ concentration	SDS	sodium dodecyl sulphate
		SE	standard error
pheH	phenylalanine hydroxylase	SEM	skin, eye and mouth
Pi	inorganic phosphate	SEM	standard error of the mean
PID	pelvic inflammatory disease	SHBG	sex hormone-binding globulin
PIP$_2$	phosphatidyl bisphosphate	SNHL	sensori-neural hearing loss
pK value	negative logarithm to the base 10 of the dissociation constant K	SO	supraoptic nucleus
		SPA	spiral artery
		spp.	two or more species

ssp. subspecies
StAR steroidogenic acute regulator
STBM syncytiotrophoblast microparticle
STI sexually transmitted infection
STR short tandem repeat
STV short-term variability
Sv sievert
T cell thymus-derived cell
T (in DNA sequences) thymine
t (in the context of pulsed ultrasound) pulse duration
T (in the context of pulsed ultrasound) pulse repetition period
T_3 triiodothyronine
T_4 thyroxine
TAG triacylglycerol
TALH thick ascending loop of Henle
Tc cell cytotoxic T cell
TCA tricarboxylic acid
TCR T cell receptor
TGC time-gain compensation
TGF-β transforming growth factor beta
Th1 cell T helper cell type 1
Th2 cell T helper cell type 2
TIB thermal index in bone
TIC thermal index in the cranium
TIS thermal index in soft tissues
TK tyrosine kinase
TNF-α tumour necrosis factor alpha
TOF time of flight
TPHA *Treponema pallidum* haemoagglutination assay
TPPA *Treponema pallidum* particle agglutination assay
Tr cell regulatory T cell
TRAP tartrate-resistant acid phosphatase
TRH thyrotrophin-releasing hormone
tRNA transfer RNA
TRPV5 epithelial Ca^{2+} channel 1
TRPV6 epithelial Ca^{2+} channel 2
TSH thyroid-stimulating hormone
TTPA *Treponema pallidum* particle agglutination
TZDs thiazolidinediones
U (in RNA sequences) uracil
uE_3 unconjugated estradiol
uNK uterine natural killer cell

UPD uniparental disomy
US ultrasound
USS ultrasound scan
v velocity of a moving object
VaIN vaginal intraepithelial neoplasia
VCAM vascular cell adhesion molecule
VDR vitamin D receptor
VDRL venereal disease research laboratory
VEGF vascular endothelial growth factor
VHL von Hippel-Lindau
VIN vulvar intraepithelial neoplasia
VIP vasoactive intestinal peptide
VLDL very-low-density lipoprotein
VSD ventricular septal defect
VZIG varicella zoster immune globulin
VZV varicella zoster virus
WBC white blood cell
WHO World Health Organization
Z acoustic impedance

Organisms

B. burgdorferi	Borrellia burgdorferi
B. hermsii	Borrellia hermsii
B. pseudomallei	Burkholderia pseudomallei
B. recurrentis	Borrellia recurrentis
C. albicans	Candida albicans
C. difficile	Clostridium difficile
C. diphtheriae	Corynebacterium diphtheriae
C. glabrata	Candida glabrata
C. krusei	Candida krusei
C. pneumoniae	Chlamydia pneumoniae
C. psittaci	Chlamydia psittaci
C. tetani	Clostridium tetani
C. trachomatis	Chlamydia trachomatis
C. tropicalis	Candida tropicalis
E. coli	Escherichia coli
E. faecalis	Enterococcus faecalis
E. faecium	Enterococcus faecium
G. vaginalis	Gardnerella vaginalis
L. mono-cytogenes	Listeria monocytogenes
L. interrogans	Leptospira interrogans
M. abscessus	Mycobacterium abscessus
M. africanum	Mycobacterium africanum
M. avium	Mycobacterium avium
M. bovis	Mycobacterium bovis
M. chelonae	Mycobacterium chelonae
M. fortuitum	Mycobacterium fortuitum
M. genitalium	Mycoplasma genitalium
M. genitalium	Mycoplasma genitalium
M. hominis	Mycoplasma hominis
M. hominis	Mycoplasma hominis
M. intracellulare	Mycobacterium
M. kansasii	Mycobacterium kansasii
M. leprae	Mycobacterium leprae
M. leprae	Mycobacterium leprae
M. marinum	Mycobacterium marinum
M. microti	Mycobacterium microti
M. pneumoniae	Mycoplasma pneumoniae
M. tuberculosis	Mycobacterium tuberculosis
M. ulcerans	Mycobacterium ulcerans
N. gonorrhoeae	Neisseria gonorrhoeae
N. meningitidis	Neisseria meningitides
P. aeruginosa	Pseudomonas aeruginosa
P. carinii	Pneumocystis carinii
P. falciparum	Plasmodium falciparum
P. malariae	Plasmodium malariae
P. ovale	Plasmodium ovale
P. vivax	Plasmodium vivax
S. agalactiae	Streptococcus agalactiae
S. anginosus	Streptococcus anginosus
S. aureus	Staphylococcus aureus
S. bovis	Streptococcus bovis
S. capitis	Staphylococcus capitis
S. dysgalactiae	Streptococcus dysgalactiae
S. epidermidis	Staphylococcus epidermidis
S. equisimilis	Streptococcus equisimilis
S. haemolyticus	Staphylococcus haemolyticus
S. milleri	Streptococcus milleri
S. mitis	Streptococcus mitis
S. mutans	Streptococcus mutans
S. paratyphi	Salmonella paratyphi
S. pneumoniae	Streptococcus pneumoniae
S. pyogenes	Streptococcus pyogenes
S. saprophyticus	Staphylococcus saprophyticus
T. carateum	Treponema carateum
T. pallidum	Treponema pallidum
T. pallidum	Treponema pallidum
T. vaginalis	Trichomonas vaginalis
T. vaginalis	Trichomonas vaginalis
U. urealyticum	Ureaplasma urealyticum

Introduction

CHAPTER 1

Revision Guide Part 1 MRCOG

Revision Guide Part 1 MRCOG

Andrew Sizer and Mary Ann Lumsden

Attainment of the Membership of the Royal College of Obstetricians and Gynaecologists (MRCOG) is an essential component of specialist training in Obstetrics and Gynaecology in the UK.

From September 2016, the MRCOG examination will be split into three parts. The Part 1 MRCOG examination must be passed before entry into the third year of specialist training (ST3).

The current Part 1 MRCOG syllabus is mapped across 14 domains, of which 12 are science domains, and 2 are clinical domains (see Figure 1.1).

Each domain contains components of the syllabus from one or more of the 19 core modules of the curriculum. The mapping of the syllabus across the curriculum modules and domains can be seen in the Part 1 Blueprinting grid which can be viewed online at https://www.rcog.org.uk/globalassets/documents/careers-and-training/mrcog-exam/part-1/ex-part-1-blueprinting-grid-new.pdf.

Please note that core modules 2, 4 and 19 do not contribute to the Part 1 syllabus and are not examined in the Part 1 examination.

Essentially, the Part 1 MRCOG examination tests knowledge of all aspects of basic science related to clinical Obstetrics and Gynaecology. The clinical domains also test clinical knowledge at the level that would be expected from a competent trainee at ST2 level.

FIGURE 1.1 **The 14 domains of the Part 1 syllabus**

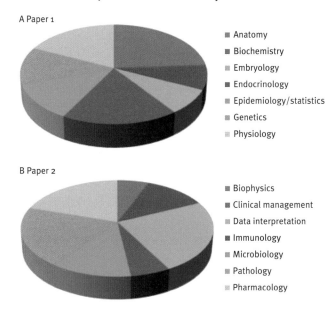

A Paper 1

- Anatomy
- Biochemistry
- Embryology
- Endocrinology
- Epidemiology/statistics
- Genetics
- Physiology

B Paper 2

- Biophysics
- Clinical management
- Data interpretation
- Immunology
- Microbiology
- Pathology
- Pharmacology

TABLE 1.1 **The modules of the RCOG curriculum for specialist training**

1. Clinical skills
2. Teaching, appraisal and assessment
3. Information technology (IT), clinical governance and research
4. Ethics and legal issues
5. Core surgical skills
6. Postoperative care
7. Surgical procedures
8. Antenatal care
9. Maternal medicine
10. Management of labour
11. Management of delivery
12. Postpartum problems
13. Gynaecological problems
14. Subfertility
15. Sexual and reproductive health
16. Early pregnancy care
17. Gynaecological oncology
18. Urogynaecology and pelvic floor problems
19. Developing professionalism

The Part 1 MRCOG examination aims to ask both basic and applied science questions and to keep the questions relevant to the trainee obstetrician and gynaecologist.

Currently, the Part 1 MRCOG examination consists of two papers (see Figure 1.1), each containing 100 Single Best Answer (SBA) questions. 150 minutes are allowed for each paper and there is a break between the two papers on the examination day of approximately one hour.

SBA questions consist of the following components:

1 An introductory stem – clinical or scientific (this component is not necessarily present)
2 A question, sometimes called a 'lead-in' – this should ask a specific question
3 Five options, one of which is the best, or only answer.

The 'single only answer' type of question tends to predominate in science topics whereas the 'single best answer' is more frequent in clinical questions as management is rarely absolutely clear cut.

Correctly constructed SBA questions must pass the 'cover test'. This means that it should be possible to cover up the answer options and still be able to answer the question from the material presented. Application of the cover test is an important part of examination technique since a well-constructed question will have 'distractors' in the answer options. Our advice would be cover the options and try to answer the question; if your proposed answer is in the list of options, then go with that answer since it is more than likely correct.

Ensure that you plan your revision programme properly. It takes at least six months to prepare for the Part 1 examination. Obstetrics and Gynaecology is a vast subject – many would say it's the biggest specialty of all since it requires knowledge of almost all of medicine and surgery in relation to women and pregnancy.

'Practice makes perfect' – it is important to practise the question style to be completely familiar with the format. There are a number of educational resources, both in hard copy and online, that allow extensive practice. However, do not try to memorise questions, A significant proportion of each exam will be new questions and it is also very easy to alter the answer to an SBA question with a very small change in the stem or lead-in. Instead, focus your efforts on understanding, since this is the purpose of the examination – testing your understanding and application of the syllabus.

This book contains the vast majority of the factual knowledge required for the examination, but it is not possible to cover everything and medical knowledge is expanding rapidly, especially in fields such as Genetics and Immunology.

Many of the authors of chapters in this revision guide have taught on the RCOG Part 1 revision course. They are experts in their field and have a clear understanding of the knowledge required for the Part 1 MRCOG examination. We hope you find this guide useful in your exam preparation.

Anatomy

CHAPTER 2

Applied anatomy and imaging of the pelvis, femoral triangle and inguinal canal

Diana Lawrence-Watt, Julia Montgomery and Malcolm Johnston

Over the next three chapters the applied anatomy of the pelvis and its contents will be described, aided by anatomical diagrams and appropriate imaging modalities. The general principles of imaging of the pelvis are discussed below.

Ultrasound

Over the last 20–30 years ultrasound (U/S) has changed practice and become the primary imaging modality in both Obstetrics and Gynaecology.

NORMAL U/S ANATOMY OF THE FEMALE PELVIS

Viewed through a full bladder, the pelvis is a 'bowl' with the pelvic viscera arranged around its walls. The bladder should be full enough to fill the hollow of the pelvis and displace small bowel loops (patients are advised to drink at least 1 litre in the 2 hours prior to examination). The uterus is then straightened relative to the cervix and the broad ligament (ovarian pedicle) pulled taut. The pelvic viscera are therefore at a depth of at least 8 cm, requiring a curvilinear transducer with long focal length.

The vagina The double wall of the vagina is seen, which flattens in the sagittal plane as it progresses cephalad forming the fornices (outpouching) either side of the cervix. The vesicovaginal and vaginorectal septae are not more than 5 mm in thickness.

The pelvic sidewall The pelvic sidewall is lined by the obturator internus, but inferiorly this is indistinguishable on U/S from the pelvic floor (levator ani and coccygeus). The muscles are poorly echogenic. The common iliac vessels are visualised contiguous with these muscles, and the origins of the internal iliac vessels are important landmarks (marking the point of fixation of the ovarian pedicle) as they then pass into the true pelvis and run medial to the obturator internus and lateral to the ovary.

The ureters are very difficult to distinguish on the pelvic sidewall as they run over the internal iliac vessels (posterior to the ovaries) but they are more easily seen as they run medially to enter the trigone of the bladder (the vesico-ureteric junction).

The uterus The position of the uterus varies (being anteverted only with an empty bladder). The cervix is seen to bulge into the vaginal lumen with the cervical canal visualised as an echogenic line of 2–3 mm thickness. The external cervical os may be patulous in the multigravida, and the endocervix may be distended with menstrual blood or congenital cysts. The body of the uterus is ovoid with a distinct point at the cornu. The cavity is seen as an echogenic band with endometrial thickness varying throughout the menstrual cycle.

FIGURE 2.1 **Trans-abdominal midline ultrasound demonstrating the uterus posterior to a full bladder. The uterine myometrium is seen of uniform low echogenicity (muscle density) with the thin bright endometrium demonstrated centrally**

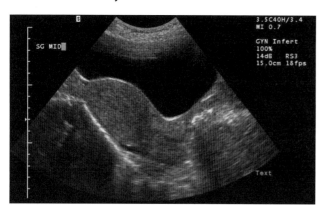

FIGURE 2.2 **Transvaginal U/S demonstrating the uterus. The bright band of the endometrium can be clearly visualised**

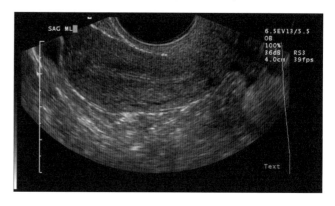

The myometrium is of homogenously poor echogenicity (Figure 2.1).

The ovary The ovary is intraperitoneal, suspended between the lateral pelvic walls by the suspensory ligaments, from the broad ligament by the mesovarium and from the uterus by the ovarian ligament. The ovary is, therefore, free to move between the ovarian fossa on the pelvic sidewall and the pouch of Douglas (rectouterine pouch). The ovary can be elevated out of the true pelvis by an overdistended bladder, pregnancy or a large pelvic mass.

Transabdominal sonography

Transabdominal sonography is now the major technique used in the second and third trimesters of pregnancy (in the second trimester a full bladder may still be required to displace overlying small bowel loops). This technique usually utilises a curvilinear transducer (of frequency 3–5 MHz) although a phased array sector transducer may be useful if access is limited (such as when the fetal head or placenta lie low in the pelvis).

Transvaginal sonography

Transvaginal sonography is now the method of choice for monitoring infertility, differentiating normal and

abnormal first trimester pregnancy and the diagnosis of ectopic pregnancy. Its advantage is the use of a higher frequency transducer giving better resolution images (Figure 2.2).

Magnetic resonance imaging

Magnetic resonance imaging (MRI) techniques obtain images with high soft tissue contrast resolution and the ability to assess anatomy in multiple planes. It is this ability to distinguish tissues of subtly different density that make it the primary technique in the accurate staging of pelvic malignancy.

Sagittal, coronal and axial sections are used. When assessing the uterus, T2-weighted scans display the characteristic zonal anatomy with three distinct areas within the uterine body (Figure 2.3). In a T2 image, fluid and vascular tissue appears bright and the zonal anatomy of the uterus is better defined There is a hyperdense central zone, representing the endometrium, combined with secretions in the uterine cavity, an outer area of intermediate signal from the myometrium, and a low signal junctional zone between, from a layer of compressed myometrium. Changes in size and signal of the three zones occur during the menstrual cycle.

The cervix is visualised on MRI with a hyperintense central zone representing cervical mucus and epithelium, with a low signal outer layer of the fibrostromal wall.

The vagina has a high signal central zone of mucous and epithelium surrounded by a low signal muscular

FIGURE 2.3 **T2 axial MRI scan showing the three zones of the uterus as well as normal ovarian luteal cysts on the left**

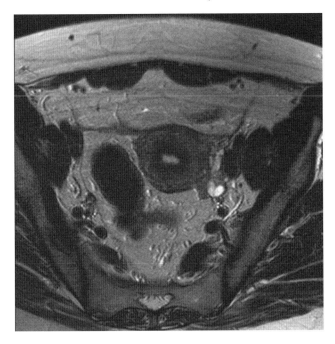

wall. The vagina is divided into three regions: an upper third above the level of the bladder base, a lower third below a line level with the urethra and a middle third between. There is a high signal venous plexus surrounding the cervix and vagina best seen on T2-weighted images.

Computed tomography imaging

Computed tomography (CT) scanning is used with caution, particularly in younger patients, due to the ionising radiation dose, but it is valuable in the primary diagnosis of pelvic tumours, particularly where obesity, previous surgery or an unstable bladder preclude ultrasound imaging. (Note that once a primary diagnosis has been made the accurate staging of the tumour is more accurately achieved with MRI.) Full body scanning is also the primary investigation for the staging of malignant gynaecological tumours. The small bowel is often opacified to distinguish small bowel loops from the ovaries or lymph nodes. A vaginal tampon can be used to define the position and appearance of the vagina and cervix. Cystic masses are usually ovarian

and distinguishable from uterine masses, but not from tubal cystic masses (pyosalpynx).

Bones of the pelvis

The bones of the pelvis form a skeletal ring between the heads of the femurs and the fifth lumbar vertebra. The pelvis consists of the sacrum and right and left hip, or innominate, bones. All three bones allow the pelvis to undertake its role of bearing the weight of the body as well as allowing attachment for the muscles that act upon it. Each hip bone is formed by the fusion of three bones: the ilium, ischium and pubis. These bones unite within the cavity of the acetabulum where the head of the femur articulates. Fusion between the ilium and the pubis takes place at the iliopubic eminence.

GREATER AND LESSER PELVIS

The pelvis itself is arbitrarily divided into two regions, described as the greater pelvis and the lesser pelvis. The greater pelvis is formed by the iliac blades on both sides and by the base of the sacrum posteriorly. The word pelvis translates from its Latin root as basin. However, the lesser pelvis is the region that describes the true 'basin', having an inlet and an outlet as well as the muscular pelvic floor. The pelvic inlet, the boundaries of which are described as the pelvic brim, has obstetric significance in relation to measurements taken in obstetric practice (Figure 2.4A and B). The pelvic brim consists of the promontory and ala of the sacrum posteriorly, the arcuate and pectineal lines laterally and anterolaterally respectively, with the anterior boundary of the inlet being formed of the superior pubic rami, the body of pubis and the pubic symphysis.

PELVIC INLET AND OUTLET

As well as providing the bony elements of the birth canal, the lesser pelvis gives attachments to many ligaments, and to elements of the pelvic floor as well as containing the pelvic viscera. The outlet of the pelvis is formed by four elements of bone: the coccyx posteriorly, the pubic symphysis anteriorly and the two ischial

FIGURE 2.4A **Female bony pelvis**

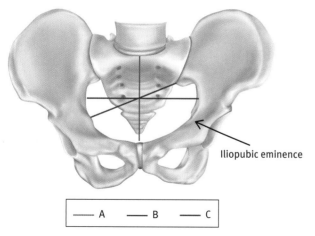

Iliopubic eminence

— A   — B   — C

A Anteroposterior diameter from the midpoint of the sacral promontory to the upper border of the pubic symphysis, usually measured between the third sacral segment and posterior surface of the symphysis
B Transverse diameter measured between two similar points on opposite sides of the pelvic brim
C Oblique diameter measured from the iliopubic eminence to the lowest point of the contralateral sacroiliac joint

> **CLINICAL RELEVANCE**
>
> These anatomical correlates are reflected during labour. The fetal head enters the pelvic inlet positioned with the longer, anteroposterior dimension across the widest and, therefore, transverse diameter of the pelvis. At the pelvic outlet, the fetal head is positioned anteroposteriorly in relation to the pelvic outlet, this being the widest diameter of both head and outlet. The shape of both the pelvic outlet and inlet are, therefore, important considerations in labour, because the cross-sectional shape of the birth canal differs at these anatomical levels.

tuberosities laterally. The strong sacrotuberous ligaments stretch between the sacrum/coccyx and the ischial tuberosities, with the result that the outlet of the pelvis is described as rhomboid in shape. The inlet of the pelvis has a wide, transverse oval opening, whereas the outlet presents a more oval diameter in its anteroposterior relationship.

The shape of the pelvic outlet corresponds to three wide arches, formed by the subpubic arch anteriorly and the two greater sciatic notches posteriorly. Spanning across the posterior region on each side are the sacrotuberous and sacrospinous ligaments, converting the sciatic notches into foramina. These foramina are occupied by muscles and important vessels and nerves. The presence of the sacrotuberous and sacrospinous ligaments and the mobile coccyx ensure that the posterior part of the pelvic outlet is a relatively flexible structure.

PELVIC ARTICULATIONS AND LIGAMENTS

The articulations of the pelvis are the sacroiliac joint, the pubic symphysis and the joint between the sacrum and the mobile coccyx. Although the sacroiliac joint is described as a plane joint with very limited movement,

FIGURE 2.4B **Anteroposterior X-ray of the pelvis demonstrating the bony landmarks of the pelvic brim and the true pelvis**

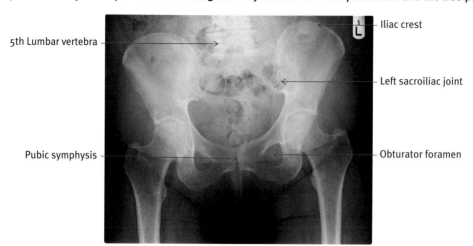

5th Lumbar vertebra

Pubic symphysis

Iliac crest

Left sacroiliac joint

Obturator foramen

the joint surfaces are anything but flat. In fact they interdigitate by a series of depressions and elevations, fitting into each other to restrict movement of the joint and affording it great strength.

The main ligaments of the sacroiliac joint are the ventral sacroiliac ligament, the dorsal sacroiliac ligament and the interosseous ligament. The ventral sacroiliac ligament should not be truly described as a ligament as it is in fact a thickening of the joint capsule.

The dorsal sacroiliac ligament, consisting of quite weak bands of tissue, arises from the intermediate and lateral crests of the sacrum which pass down to the posterior superior iliac spine and the inner lip of the iliac crest. The lower part of this ligament, arising from the third and fourth sacral segments and passing to the posterior superior iliac spine, may form a separate structure termed the long posterior sacroiliac ligament. Some of the fibres of the posterior sacroiliac ligament, when present, may also merge with the sacrotuberous ligament.

The ligament of the sacroiliac joint that deserves most comment is the interosseous ligament, the strongest ligament uniting the hip bones to the sacrum. This interosseous ligament occupies the space between the bony elements at the back of the joint. It is covered by the dorsal sacroiliac ligament, from which it is separated by the dorsal primary rami of the sacral nerves and vessels. Consisting of deep and superficial strata, fibres from the deep layer pass from depressions on the sacrum to depressions on the tuberosity of the ilium. The most notable fibres of the superficial layers frequently form the short posterior iliac ligament which spans between the superior articular process and the lateral crest of the first two segments of the sacrum to the ilium.

The pubic symphysis, forms a secondary cartilaginous joint that unites the two pubic bones via a fibrocartilagenous disc and the superior and arcuate pubic ligaments. The latter is separated from the urogenital diaphragm by an interval, through which the deep vein of the clitoris enters into the pelvis.

PELVIC ARTICULATIONS IN PREGNANCY

In pregnancy, all joints of the pelvis afford a greater degree of movement than in the nonpregnant state. This movement is more pronounced in the sacroiliac joint, which can result in increased strain on the ligaments following pregnancy.

> **CLINICAL RELEVANCE**
>
> While symphysis pubic dysfunction or pelvic girdle pain is common in pregnancy, the actual cause of the pelvic instability is not clear, but probably due to a combination of change in posture due to increasing abdominal mass and hormonal through changes in the pelvic ligaments. In severe cases of pelvic instability there is an associated increase in symphyseal width.

Functional anatomy of the abdominal wall

Supporting and compressing the abdominal contents are the muscles of the anterior abdominal wall, which consist of the external and internal oblique muscles and the transversus and rectus abdominis muscles. The oblique muscles act in compression, their contraction being important in birth when expelling the fetus from the uterus.

EXTERNAL OBLIQUE

The external oblique (Figure 2.5A) arises from the outer surfaces of the lower eight ribs, these fibres interdigitating with fibres of the serratus anterior and the latissimus dorsi muscles. Fibres from the lower two ribs pass vertically down to the anterior part of the iliac crest, whereas fibres from the other ribs pass downwards and medially, becoming aponeurotic level with the tip of the ninth costal cartilage. The fibres of the two external oblique muscles meet in the midline of the body, interdigitating to form the linea alba; a tendinous raphe extending vertically from the xiphoid process to the pubic symphysis. The linea alba is formed of the fibres of all three muscles from each side of the body – the two oblique and the transversus abdominis muscles. It is interrupted by the umbilicus, which transmits the umbilical vessels, the urachus and the vitelline duct during fetal life but closes soon after birth. The median umbilical ligament on the deep surface of the abdominal wall represents the remnants of the urachus. The medial umbilical ligaments represent the remnants of the umbilical arteries. The umbilical vein regresses to give rise to the ligamentum

FIGURE 2.5A **The external oblique**

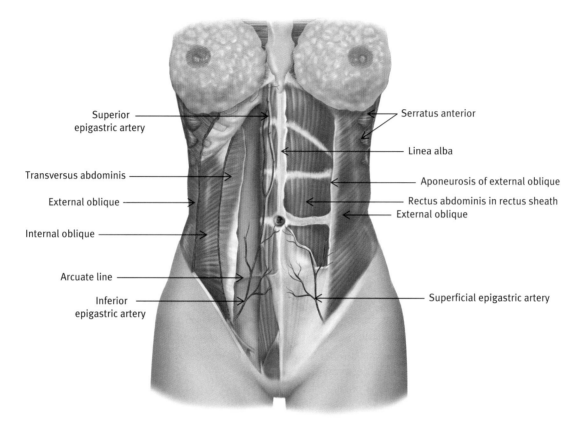

Superior epigastric artery

Serratus anterior

Linea alba

Transversus abdominis

Aponeurosis of external oblique

External oblique

Rectus abdominis in rectus sheath

External oblique

Internal oblique

Arcuate line

Inferior epigastric artery

Superficial epigastric artery

teres, which ascends from the umbilicus to the liver between the two layers of the falciform ligament. The lateral umbilical ligament, discussed below, is a fold of peritoneum encasing the inferior epigastric vessels (see Figure 2.7, below).

The lower fibres of the aponeurosis of external oblique, which stretches from the anterior superior iliac spine to the pubic tubercle, is thickened and folded in on itself to form the inguinal ligament. This infolding forms the floor of the inguinal canal.

From the medial end of the inguinal ligament, fibres pass backwards and medially to the pectineal line to constitute the lacunar ligament. The base of this ligament forms the medial boundary of the femoral ring.

INTERNAL OBLIQUE

The thinner internal oblique muscle arises from the lumbar fascia, the lateral part of the inguinal ligament

and the anterior part of the iliac crest. Posterior fibres ascend vertically to the lower ribs, where they are continuous with fibres of the external intercostal muscles. Fibres arising from the iliac crest pass upwards and medially and meet in the midline, contributing to the linea alba. Fibres from the inguinal ligament arch downwards and medially, crossing over the round ligament and become aponeurotic. These fibres insert behind the round ligament to the pubic crest and medial part of the pectineal line, together with similar fibres from the transversus abdominis, thus constituting the falx inguinalis or conjoint tendon.

The falx inguinalis lies behind the superficial inguinal ring of the inguinal canal to strengthen an otherwise weak point in the abdominal wall. Medially the falx is continuous with the anterior wall of the rectus sheath. Occasionally it may be continuous laterally with a band of aponeurotic fibres, the interfoveolar ligament, which extends from the lower border of the transversus abdominis to the superior ramus of the pubis. This band gives additional strength to the falx inguinalis.

TRANSVERSUS ABDOMINIS

Arising from the same origin as internal oblique, but deep to the oblique muscle, are the fibres of transversus abdominis. Fibres of transversus abdominis are oriented horizontally across the abdomen to meet in the midline in the linea alba (Figure 2.5A). The aponeuroses in the upper approximately fourth-fifths of the muscle pass behind the rectus abdominis, while the fibres of the lower part, those arising from the inguinal ligament and iliac crest, lie in front of rectus abdominis. Additionally, fibres from the transversus muscle originate from the inner aspect of the lower six costal cartilages and interdigitate with the muscular fibres of the diaphragm.

As with the internal oblique muscle, the fibres that take origin from the inguinal ligament pass downwards and medially over the round ligament and contribute to the conjoint tendon, which inserts behind the round ligament to the pubic crest and pectineal line. The rectus abdominis originates from the crest and tubercle of the pubis and broadens as it ascends to insert on the costal cartilages of the fifth, sixth and seventh ribs.

RECTI MUSCLES

The two recti muscles are separated from each other by the linea alba and both present three transverse tendinous intersections, one related to the level of the xiphoid process, one at the umbilicus and one midway between the xiphoid process and the umbilicus. The recti muscles each lie within the rectus sheath, formed by the aponeurosis of the two oblique muscles and the transversus. As the aponeurosis of the internal oblique on each side approaches the lateral border of the rectus it divides into two laminae, one passing deep to the rectus and the other superficial to the muscle. The aponeurosis of the transversus abdominis lies posterior to rectus, and that of the external oblique lies anterior to it. Hence the anterior wall of the rectus sheath is formed of the aponeurosis of the external oblique plus half the thickness of the internal oblique. The posterior wall is formed by half the thickness of the internal oblique aponeurosis and the aponeurosis of the transversus

abdominis. Medial to the rectus muscles the layers from each side reunite with each other to form the linea alba (Figure 2.5A).

This is the arrangement of the rectus sheath from midway between the pubic symphysis and umbilicus to the superior part of the muscle. Below this point all three aponeuroses pass over the rectus muscles, resulting in a deficiency of the posterior wall of the sheath below this point, where it is formed only by the transversalis fascia, which lies deep to the transversus abdominis. The difference in the thickness of the posterior wall of the sheath above and below the division of the internal oblique aponeurosis is evidenced by the presence of the arcuate line, which is the point where the transversus abdominis and half the thickness of the internal oblique aponeurosis pass deep to the rectus muscles. The arcuate line is also the point where the inferior epigastric vessels gain access to the rectus sheath. The transversalis fascia is thin and interposed between the transversus abdominis and the parietal layer of peritoneum. The arrangement of the flat muscles of the abdominal wall and the rectus sheath can seen in axial CT sections (Figure 2.5B).

Inferior epigastric vessels

The inferior epigastric artery arises from the external iliac artery superior to the inguinal ligament (Figure 2.6). Inclining medially as it ascends, the inferior epigastric artery skirts the medial margin of the deep inguinal ring before passing through the transversalis fascia. Above the umbilicus the inferior epigastric artery forms an anastomosis with the superior epigastric artery, one of the terminal branches of the internal thoracic artery, which also enters the rectus sheath from above, and lies between the rectus muscle and the posterior wall of the rectus sheath. The inferior epigastric artery also forms an anastomosis with branches of the lower posterior intercostal arteries.

Both superior and inferior epigastric arteries perforate the recti muscles to supply the muscle itself and continue through the anterior wall of the rectus sheath to supply the skin of the abdomen.

The inferior epigastric artery is accompanied by venae commitantes that unite to form the inferior

FIGURE 2.5B **Transversus abdominis and rectus sheath. Axial CT section taken at the level of the iliac crests demonstrating the internal and external oblique and transversus abdominus muscles laterally and the recti muscles anteriorly surrounded by the rectus sheath (forming the linea alba in the midline)**

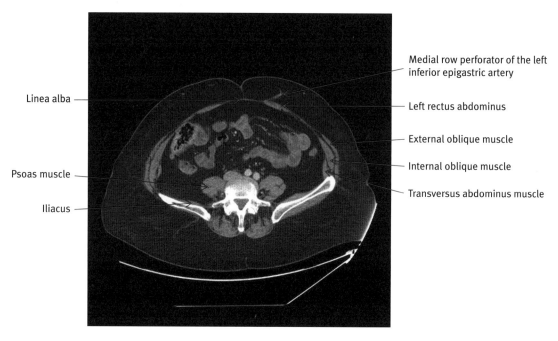

Linea alba

Psoas muscle

Iliacus

Medial row perforator of the left inferior epigastric artery

Left rectus abdominus

External oblique muscle

Internal oblique muscle

Transversus abdominus muscle

FIGURE 2.6 **Axial CT section through the greater pelvis showing the enhanced inferior epigastric arteries immediately deep to both rectus muscles. Common and internal iliac arteries are also enhanced. The image is taken in the arterial phase after administering iodinated intravenous contrast**

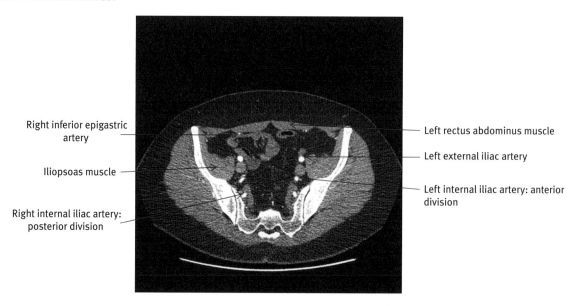

Right inferior epigastric artery

Iliopsoas muscle

Right internal iliac artery: posterior division

Left rectus abdominus muscle

Left external iliac artery

Left internal iliac artery: anterior division

epigastric vein that drains into the external iliac vein just above the inguinal ligament. The inferior epigastric vessels raise a fold of parietal peritoneum and form the landmark of the lateral umbilical ligament on the deep surface of the anterior abdominal wall, lateral to the medial umbilical ligament.

CLINICAL RELEVANCE

It is important to identify the inferior epigastric vessels before inserting the lateral ports at a laparoscopy. Insertion of the port trochar through this vessel will result in major haemorrhage. These vessels are lateral to the medial umbilical ligaments, which are clearly seen at laparoscopy.

CLINICAL RELEVANCE

In caesarean section, the incision through the abdominal wall is made transversely, two finger's breadth above the pubic symphysis. The transverse incision through the skin, subcutaneous fat and rectus sheath is so directed as to prevent cutting across the dermatomes of the anterior abdominal wall, which is innervated by the lower six intercostal nerves travelling in the neurovascular plane between the transversus and the internal oblique. Each intercostal nerve finally enters the rectus sheath, having supplied the muscles of the abdominal wall as well as the area of skin, or dermatome, specific to each nerve. As already noted, the inferior epigastric vessels perforate the rectus muscle to supply the rectus sheath and skin and, thus, care must be taken in achieving haemostasis of these vessels in order to minimise risk of rectus sheath haematomas. A transverse incision appears to result in less scarring as compared with a vertical incision, and is less likely to cause rupture of the rectus muscles and sheath.

Inguinal canal

The inguinal canal (Figure 2.7), situated between the abdominal cavity and the labia majora, is obliquely placed between the deep and superficial inguinal rings and transmits the round ligament of the uterus and the ilioinguinal nerve. The canal is located just superior to the medial half of the inguinal ligament.

The floor of the inguinal canal is formed of the infolded inguinal ligament uniting with the transversalis

fascia, with arching fibres of both transversus abdominis and the internal oblique muscle forming its roof. Contraction of these overarching fibres is increased when there is an increase in intra-abdominal pressure. The anterior wall of the canal is formed of skin, superficial fascia and the external oblique aponeurosis. Muscle fibres of the internal oblique muscle also contribute to the most lateral part of the anterior wall, specifically where it lies opposite the deep inguinal ring. The posterior wall of the canal, formed of transversalis fascia would be exceptionally weak if it were not re-inforced by the conjoint tendon and the reflected part of the inguinal ligament.

The reflected part of the inguinal ligament is an expansion of the lateral crus of the superficial inguinal ring which passes upwards and medially to merge with the rectus sheath, passing behind the external oblique muscle but in front of the conjoint tendon. Both the conjoint tendon and reflected part of the inguinal ligament strengthen the weak part of the abdominal wall caused by the canal, although the oblique orientation of the canal also aids in this strengthening.

DEEP AND SUPERFICIAL INGUINAL RINGS

The deep inguinal ring is formed in the transversalis fascia midway between the anterior superior iliac spine and the pubic symphysis. Transversus abdominis fibres arch over it superiorly and the inferior epigastric vessels are an immediate medial relation to this ring. When intra-abdominal pressure is raised, contraction of internal oblique fibres is increased so that they act as a valve mechanism on the deep inguinal ring, closing it down. The superficial ring is placed above the inguinal ligament, just lateral to the pubic tubercle, and is formed by an opening in the aponeurosis of the external oblique muscle. The margins of this opening are thickened to form the lateral and medial crura of the ring.

ROUND LIGAMENT

The round ligament passes through the transversalis fascia at the deep inguinal ring, although the ring is not visible externally as the fascia at this point forms a covering or sleeve – the internal spermatic fascia – over

FIGURE 2.7 **Femoral sheath and inguinal canal**

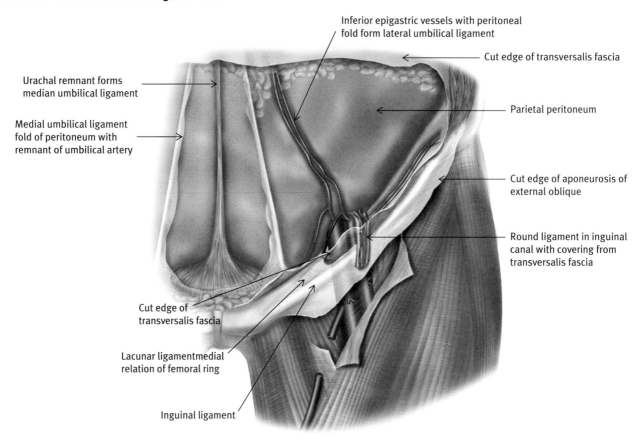

Inferior epigastric vessels with peritoneal fold form lateral umbilical ligament

Cut edge of transversalis fascia

Urachal remnant forms median umbilical ligament

Parietal peritoneum

Medial umbilical ligament fold of peritoneum with remnant of umbilical artery

Cut edge of aponeurosis of external oblique

Round ligament in inguinal canal with covering from transversalis fascia

Cut edge of transversalis fascia

Lacunar ligamentmedial relation of femoral ring

Inguinal ligament

the ligament. As the ligament and internal fascial layer pass through the internal oblique muscle, the round ligament gains another covering from this layer, termed the cremasteric fascia. Even in the female (although more so in the male) this covering contains a few muscle fibres, forming the cremaster muscle. Finally as the round ligament and its gained coverings pass through the external oblique aponeurosis, it is clothed with its outer layer, the external spermatic fascia, derived from this aponeurosis and giving rise to a third layer covering the ligament. Accompanying the round ligament and its coverings through the canal is the ilioinguinal nerve.

ILIOINGUINAL NERVE

From the anterior primary ramus of L1, the ilioinguinal nerve emerges from the lateral border of psoas major,

crosses the quadratus lumborum, perforates transversus abdominis close to the anterior part of the iliac crest and runs in this neurovascular plane until it pierces the internal oblique. At which point, it enters the inguinal canal, emerging through the superficial inguinal ring, to be distributed to skin on the medial aspect of the thigh as well as the skin covering the mons pubis and the related part of the labia majora. In its course it also supplies the fibres of the internal oblique and transversus abdominis muscles, which contribute to the conjoint tendon.

CLINICAL RELEVANCE

Damage to the ilioinguinal nerve weakens the conjoint tendon, potentially inducing the development of a direct hernia.

Femoral triangle

The superficial fascia of the inguinal region is thick and is distinguishable as two separate layers: the superficial layer, which is continuous with the superficial fascia of the abdomen, and the deep layer. Between the two lie the superficial inguinal lymph nodes and the long saphenous vein. The deep layer fuses with the deep fascia of the thigh, the fascia lata, just below the inguinal ligament. The deep layer also contributes to the saphenous opening because it merges with the fascia forming the opening as well as the fascia forming the femoral sheath. The fascia lata is thick both proximally and laterally in the thigh, forming the iliotibial tract. The saphenous opening transmits the great saphenous vein and in this region the fascia lata is divided into two layers.

SUPERFICIAL AND DEEP LAYERS OF THE FASCIA LATA

The superficial layer of the fascia lata is lateral to the saphenous opening and is attached to the entire length of the inguinal ligament, to the anterior superior iliac spine and to the pectineal line of the pubis. It is reflected inferolaterally from the pubic tubercle and forms the falciform margin of the saphenous opening. The deep layer of fascia lata is medial to the saphenous opening, being continuous with the superficial layer at the lower margin of the opening. It continues upward to cover the adductor muscles and, passing behind the femoral sheath, merges with it and ends by attaching to the pectineal line. The superficial layer of the fascia lata is therefore anterior to the femoral sheath, whereas the deep layer is posterior.

FEMORAL SHEATH

The femoral sheath itself is formed by the continuation of the transversalis fascia in front of the femoral vessels and by the fascia covering the iliacus muscle behind these vessels. These two layers terminate by fusing with fascia on the outer layers of the femoral vessels; hence the entire sheath is funnel shaped and wider at its proximal end.

The lateral wall of the femoral sheath is pierced by the femoral branch of the genitofemoral nerve. The medial wall is perforated by the great saphenous vein as it drains into the femoral vein. The femoral sheath lies within the femoral triangle, the boundaries of which are superiorly the inguinal ligament, laterally the medial border of the sartorius and medially the medial border of the adductor longus. The lateral border of the adductor longus contributes to the floor of the femoral triangle, as do the iliacus, the psoas major and the pectineus muscles.

The femoral sheath lies within the femoral triangle and contains, from medial to lateral, the femoral canal, vein and artery. The immediate lateral relation of the sheath is the femoral nerve. The femoral canal contains lymph vessels and deep inguinal lymph nodes. Its proximal opening is the femoral ring, the medial aspect of which is formed by the lacunar ligament. The round ligament of the uterus passes over the femoral vein, just above the femoral ring, as the round ligament enters the deep inguinal ring. Just lateral to this, the inferior epigastric vessels ascend to gain access to the rectus sheath at the level of the arcuate line and travel up the rectus sheath on its posterior wall to anastomose with the superior epigastric vessels. Although the femoral ring allows expansion of the femoral vein, it causes a weak area of the abdominal wall. This area of weakness can result in herniation of abdominal contents through this space – a femoral hernia. As the femoral ring is larger in women, because of the greater width of the female pelvis and smaller femoral vessels relative to the male, femoral hernias are more common in women than men.

Muscles of the pelvis

The musculature of the pelvis (Figure 2.8A and B) is divided into two distinct groups. The first group is formed of the obturator internus and piriformis and clothes the inside of the pelvic walls. The second group, which is of greater relevance to the practice of obstetrics and gynaecology, is formed of the levator ani and the coccygeus and constitutes the pelvic diaphragm or floor.

17

FIGURE 2.8A **Pelvic diaphragm**

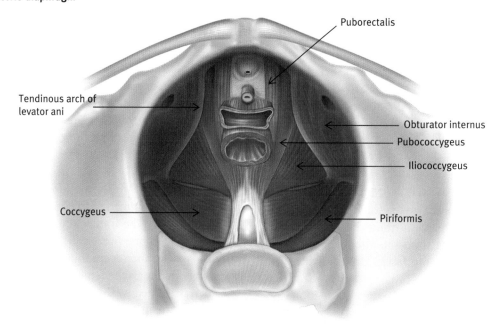

FIGURE 2.8B **Axial images through the ischioanal fossae**

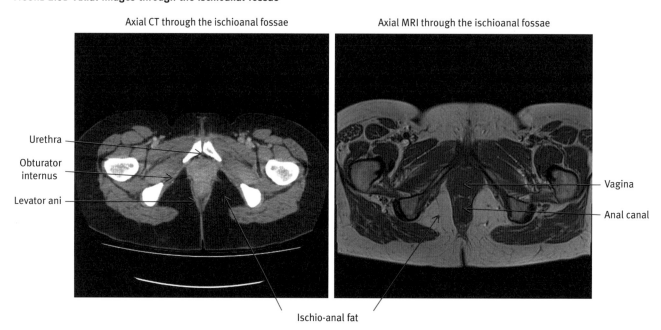

The pelvic diaphragm is covered on both its superior and inferior surface by investing fascia, which is continuous above with the fascia covering the pelvic viscera and below with the fascia of the perineum. The levator ani is attached to two bony points: the inner surface of the pubic bone and the medial aspect of the spine of the ischium. Between these two points, fibres take origin from the fascia overlying the obturator internus.

PUBOVAGINALIS

Fibres of the two levator muscles meet in the median plane. There is variability in the direction of the fibres, giving rise to different named parts of the levator depending on the direction of its fibres. The most anterior fibres originate from the body of the pubis and, passing in an anteroposterior direction to the perineal body (situated in the midline between the urogenital triangle and the anal triangle), pass across the sides of the vagina, forming the pubovaginalis (a supplementary, but significant sphincter of the vagina) before inserting to the anterior surface of the coccyx. Fibres that arise more laterally pass backwards downwards and medially, finally meeting fibres from the opposite side to form the puborectalis. The puborectalis forms a 'sling' of muscle around the junction of the rectum and anus. The fibres of the puborectalis intermingle with the deep fibres of the external anal sphincter and the perineal body.

LEVATOR ANI

Those fibres of the levator ani that lie in an anteroposterior direction give rise to the pubococcygeus part of the muscle. The fibres that arise from the medial aspect of the ischial spines pass from lateral to medial to form the part of levator ani named the iliococcygeus. Between the two bony points that give origin to the levator muscle, the body of the pubis and the ischial spines, fibres arise from the fascia covering the obturator internus. The levator muscle also has a fascial covering, the superior fascia of the pelvic diaphragm, and this contributes to the fascia covering the obturator internus above the levator attachment, giving rise to the structure referred to as the tendinous arch of levator ani. However, some explanation is necessary here, for this structure differs from the tendinous arch of pelvic fascia, which is more medially placed and gives rise to the attachment of the lateral supporting ligament of the urinary bladder The medial borders of the levator muscle meet in a median raphe, although the two sides of the muscle are held apart in the midline by the structures that pass through the diaphragm to exit the pelvis.

COCCYGEUS MUSCLE

Completing the muscular diaphragm of the pelvic floor is the coccygeus, arising from the ischial spine and the deep surface of the sacrospinous ligament to insert to the coccyx and lateral margin of the fifth sacral segment. Both the levator muscle and the coccygeus support the pelvic viscera, with the levator muscle constricting the rectum and vagina. The lower surface of the levator ani is clothed by the inferior fascia of the pelvic diaphragm and forms the medial wall of the ischioanal fossa.

These sections demonstrate the relative position of the rectum and vagina with the adjacent levator ani muscles. The obturator internus muscles are seen lateral to the fat within the ischioanal fossae. The pubic symphysis is seen anteriorly with the urethra immediately posterior.

CLINICAL RELEVANCE

Damage to the pelvic floor muscles occurs during birth. As the pubovaginalis portion of the levator muscle is attached to the perineal body, rupture of the latter can divide the levator muscles and may later predispose to uterovaginal prolapse.

Vessels of the pelvis

The abdominal aorta divides into the right and left common iliac arteries at the level of the verterbral disc between L4 and L5 (Figure 2.9). Owing to the position of the aorta, the right common iliac artery is approximately 1 cm longer than the left and crosses directly in front of L5. Both common iliac arteries are covered in parietal peritoneum, which separates the vessels from the small intestine. Fibres of the superior hypogastric plexus form a meshwork over the common iliac arteries and the psoas lies laterally to each.

Posteriorly, the right common iliac artery is related to the termination of both common iliac veins, which unite to form the inferior vena cava. The left artery is anterolateral to its corresponding vein. Level with the sacroiliac joint, both of the common iliac arteries divide into their internal and external divisions. The external iliac artery continues towards the thigh related to the medial

FIGURE 2.9 **Arteries and veins of the pelvis**

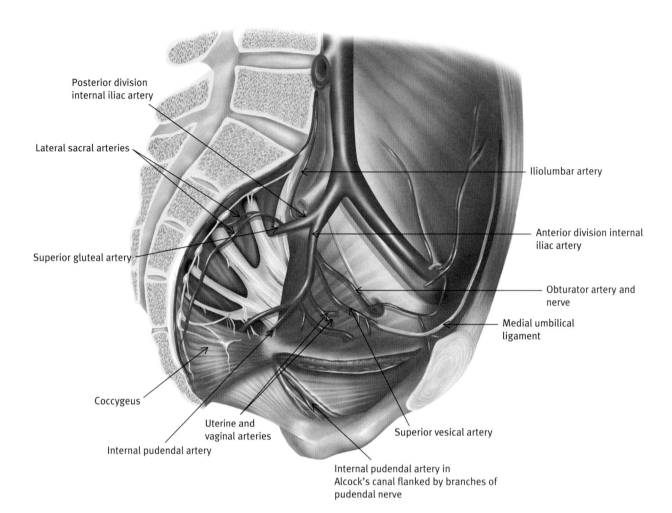

Posterior division
internal iliac artery

Lateral sacral arteries

Superior gluteal artery

Coccygeus

Uterine and
vaginal arteries

Internal pudendal artery

Iliolumbar artery

Anterior division internal
iliac artery

Obturator artery and
nerve

Medial umbilical
ligament

Superior vesical artery

Internal pudendal artery in
Alcock's canal flanked by branches of
pudendal nerve

border of the psoas major, and enters the thigh by passing under the inguinal ligament midway between the pubic symphysis and the anterior superior iliac spine; the mid-inguinal point that lies approximately 1 cm medial to the midpoint of the inguinal ligament.

COURSE OF THE INTERNAL ILIAC ARTERY

At the point of their division into the external and internal arteries, the internal arteries are crossed anteriorly by the ureters as they enter the pelvis. Arising anterior to the sacroiliac joint, the internal iliac arteries continue to the level of the upper margin of the greater sciatic notch, where they divide into anterior and posterior divisions. The posterior division passes through the upper part of the greater sciatic foramen, to divide into its terminal branches of the superior gluteal, lateral sacral and iliolumbar arteries. The anterior division continues into the pelvis to give off numerous branches, taking a course towards the spine of the ischium. Related immediately anterior to this division is the ureter, the ovarian artery and accompanying venae comitantes, the fimbriated end of the uterine tube and the ovary.

The internal iliac veins lie behind the internal iliac arteries. The external iliac veins lie below and medial to the external iliac arteries, with the right external vein positioned posteromedial to the right external artery as the vein continues into the pelvis. The obturator nerve emerges from the medial aspect of psoas major, lying first at the division of the common iliac vessels into their internal and external branches (Figure 2.9) and then on the side wall of the pelvis above the obturator vessels as the nerve and vessels pass through the obturator canal to gain access to the medial compartment of the thigh.

BRANCHES OF THE INTERNAL ILIAC ARTERY

The internal iliac arteries give rise to many branches within the pelvis (Figure 2.9). The original stem of the umbilical artery persists in the adult and crosses the lateral wall of the pelvis on the levator ani muscle. This part of the umbilical artery remains patent and gives rise to one or several superior vesical branches, which supply the superior aspect of the bladder, these vessels also giving branches to supply the distal end of the ureter.

The distal end of the original umbilical artery, having become fibrous, ascends towards the umbilicus and being covered in parietal peritoneum raises a fold of peritoneum on each side of the inner surface of the anterior abdominal wall – the medial umbilical ligament. The obturator artery enters the obturator canal by passing forward on the lateral wall of the pelvis, 2–3 cm below the pelvic brim, to enter the obturator canal. The obturator nerve, which emerges from the medial aspect of the psoas, is an immediate superior relation to the artery as both pass through the canal to leave the pelvis.

UTERINE ARTERY

The uterine artery is the main supply of blood to the uterus although the uterus also receives supply from the ovarian and internal pudendal arteries (see Chapter 3). Branching from the anterior division of the internal iliac artery, the uterine artery courses medially on the fascia overlying the levator muscle, until it reaches the junction with the cervix. In its course it crosses over the ureter as it turns medially, giving some blood supply to the ureter as it does so. The artery then ascends in the broad ligament of the uterus, here its course being very tortuous, until it reaches the junction of the body of the uterus and the uterine tube where it turns laterally and courses in the mesovarium to anastomose with branches of the ovarian artery (Figure 2.10A). Through its course, apart from supplying numerous branches to the uterine muscle, the uterine artery also supplies the cervix, round ligament of the uterus and the vagina through vaginal branches. Blood supply to the vagina usually arises as branches from the uterine artery and descend from the uterine artery supply the mucous membrane of the vagina, as well as supplying the related parts of the bladder and rectum. The vaginal branches, together with uterine branches, contribute to the azygos system of vessels supplying the vagina (see Chapter 3).

> **CLINICAL RELEVANCE**
>
> It is important to know the relationship between the uterine artery and the ureter at the junction with the cervix to prevent accidental ligation of the ureter at this level.

The middle rectal and inferior vesical arteries may arise in common from the internal iliac artery. The middle rectal artery is often elusive, but when present, supplies the muscular wall of the lower part of the rectum. The inferior vesical artery supplies the fundus of the bladder, as well as giving small branches to the distal part of the ureter. The terminal branches of the internal iliac artery are the internal pudendal artery and the inferior gluteal artery, the latter being the larger terminal division. The internal pudendal artery leaves the pelvis through the lower part of the greater sciatic foramen, between coccygeus and piriformis, and winds around the spine of the ischium, sandwiched between the medially placed pudendal nerve and the laterally placed nerve to obturator internus. The internal pudendal artery enters the perineum through the lesser sciatic foramen to enter the pudendal (or Alcock's) canal within the perineum.

PUDENDAL CANAL

Located on the lateral wall of the ischioanal fossa, the fascial sheath of the pudendal canal forms the roof and lateral wall of the fossa. The sheath fuses with the lower part of the obturator fascia, as well as being continuous with the inferior fascia of the pelvic diaphragm and the falciform process of the sacrotuberous ligament (which extends from the ischial tuberosity along the ischial ramus). In the canal, the pudendal artery is accompanied by two veins and the pudendal nerve. The artery lies between the two terminal branches of the pudendal

FIGURE 2.10A **Relationships of uterine artery and lymph vessels and nodes of the pelvis and genitalia**

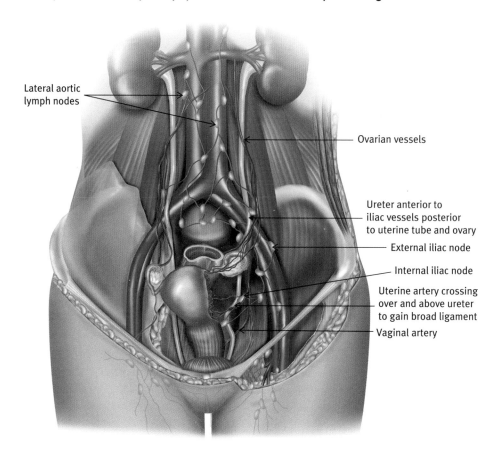

Lateral aortic lymph nodes

Ovarian vessels

Ureter anterior to iliac vessels posterior to uterine tube and ovary

External iliac node

Internal iliac node

Uterine artery crossing over and above ureter to gain broad ligament

Vaginal artery

nerve – the dorsal nerve of the clitoris above and the perineal nerve below – at the anterior end of the canal. The inferior rectal artery branches from the internal pudendal artery at the start of the pudendal canal. Just superior to the ischial tuberosity it emerges from the medial wall of the sheath, crossing the ischioanal fossa to supply the skin and muscles of the anal region. At the anterior end of the pudendal canal, the perineal artery arises from the internal pudendal artery, travelling through the inferior fascial layer of the urogenital dia-phragm to enter the superficial perineal space. The inferior gluteal artery, the larger terminal branch of the internal iliac artery, leaves the pelvis posterior to the internal pudendal artery. The inferior gluteal artery also passes between piriformis and coccygeus via the lower part of the greater sciatic foramen, to supply the gluteal region and structures in the posterior aspect of the thigh.

LYMPHATIC DRAINAGE OF THE PELVIS

As with all other regions of the body, lymph vessels and nodes draining the pelvis are associated with the major regional blood vessels and their branches. Lymph from the pelvis passes to the nodes studded along the internal iliac veins (Figure 2.10A). From here the lymph is carried into the paravertebral or lateral aortic nodes situated on the lateral aspects of the verterbral bodies. These latter nodes receive lymph from the ovaries, kidneys and adrenal glands as well as the muscles of the posterior abdominal wall. From here lymph is carried into the cisterna chyli, positioned posterior to the aorta, at the level of L1–2 and continues from here into the thoracic duct. The internal iliac lymph nodes receive lymph from all of the pelvic viscera and deep perineum, as well as the gluteal region. (For lymphatic drainage of the uterus and vagina see Chapter 4.)

FIGURE 2.10B **Un-subtracted and subtracted angiogram images of the arteries of the pelvis acquired by the injection of iodinated contrast via a catheter positioned in the infra-renal abdominal aorta. The internal iliac origins, as well as the anterior and posterior division branches of the IIA are demonstrated**

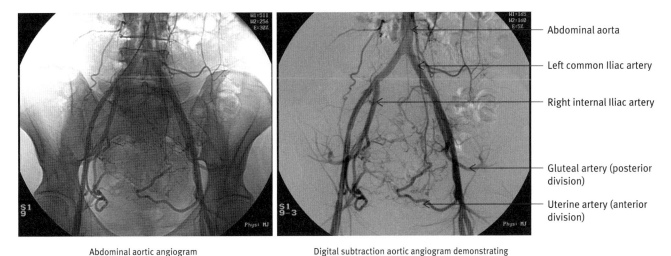

Abdominal aorta

Left common Iliac artery

Right internal Iliac artery

Gluteal artery (posterior division)

Uterine artery (anterior division)

Abdominal aortic angiogram demonstrating the iliac arteries

Digital subtraction aortic angiogram demonstrating the iliac arteries after mask subtraction

FIGURE 2.10C **Selective contrast injection into the internal iliac artery origins shows the anterior division (including the uterine, internal pudendal and vesical arteries) and posterior division (including the superior gluteal and lateral sacral arteries)**

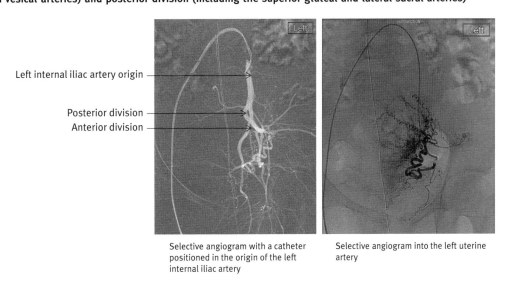

Left internal iliac artery origin

Posterior division
Anterior division

Selective angiogram with a catheter positioned in the origin of the left internal iliac artery

Selective angiogram into the left uterine artery

Innervation of the pelvic region – somatic and autonomic

LUMBAR PLEXUS

Both the lumbar and the sacral plexus contribute to the innervation of the pelvis. The lumbar plexus is formed from the anterior primary rami of T12/L1–L4. The plexus is formed within the substance of psoas major. The lumbar plexus gives rise to both the femoral nerve, through the posterior divisions of L2, 3 and 4, and the obturator nerve from the anterior divisions of these nerve roots. The femoral nerve emerges from the lateral aspect of the psoas major and runs on the iliacus. The nerve runs between psoas major and the iliacus until it reaches the inguinal ligament, where it becomes related to the anterior surface of the iliopsoas as this muscle passes under the inguinal ligament. Superiorly it is therefore separated from the distal end of the external iliac artery and the proximal end of the femoral artery by the psoas but once it enters the thigh it lies immediately lateral to the femoral artery.

The femoral nerve divides into anterior and posterior divisions in the thigh, supplying the muscles and skin in this region. Within the pelvis, the femoral nerve supplies various small branches to the iliacus. From its medial aspect, near the inguinal ligament, it supplies the nerve to the pectineus, which passes behind the femoral sheath and enters the anterior surface of the pectineus.

The obturator nerve emerges from the medial border of the psoas muscle. At the brim of the pelvis it lies behind the common iliac vessels and continues lateral to the internal iliac vessels on the obturator internus, passes above the obturator artery and into the obturator canal above this vessel. The obturator nerve exits the pelvis to supply the adductor muscles and the skin on the medial aspect of the thigh. As the obturator nerve within the pelvis supplies the parietal peritoneum in the vicinity of the ovary, pain arising in this organ may be referred to the medial aspect of the thigh.

The lumbar plexus gives rise to four other nerves: the subcostal, the iliohypogastric, the ilioinguinal (dealt with in relation to the inguinal canal) and the genitofemoral. The subcostal and iliohypogastric nerves both cross the quadratus lumborum, pierce the transversus abdominis and run in the neurovascular plane between transversus abdominis and the internal oblique. They supply the transversus abdominis and the internal oblique and the skin of the lower part of the abdomen. Fibres from L1 and 2 contribute to the genitofemoral nerve. Its fibres initially run through the substance of psoas major but this very slender nerve emerges from the muscle level with L3 or 4 vertebra. It carries on its course, covered in parietal peritoneum, often lateral to the ureter which it crosses posterior to in order to gain this position. Its division into its two terminal branches – the genital and the femoral branches – is quite variable and often the division is high up as it emerges from the substance of psoas. The genital branch crosses the distal part of the external iliac artery to pass through the deep inguinal ring and thereby enter the inguinal canal with the round ligament of the uterus to terminate in the skin of the mons pubis and labia majora. The femoral branch carries on in its course lateral to the external iliac artery. It crosses the deep circumflex iliac artery which has arisen from the external iliac artery opposite the origin of the inferior epigastric artery. By passing deep to the inguinal ligament the femoral branch gains access to the femoral sheath, positioned lateral to the femoral artery. Piercing through the anterior wall of the femoral sheath, and fascia lata, the femoral branch supplies skin overlying the upper region of the femoral triangle.

CLINICAL RELEVANCE

It is important to be aware that damage to the genitofemoral nerve leading to paresthesia over the anterior thigh and groin pain may occur during gynaecological open surgery particularly when using a large Pfannenstiel incision. This damage may occur due to use of deep self-retaining retractors either resting on or causing lateral retraction of the psoas muscles. Damage to the genitofemoral nerve can also occur during retroperitoneal dissection.

SACRAL PLEXUS

Uniting the lumbar plexus to the sacral plexus is the lumbosacral trunk, L4–5. This large trunk, which is related to the medial aspect of psoas, crosses the pelvic brim anterior to the sacroiliac joint and joins the ventral primary ramus of S1. The sacral plexus is formed from the lumbosacral trunk and the anterior primary rami of S1–4. The plexus lies on piriformis, behind the internal iliac vessels, the ureter and the gut. The constituent nerves form into an upper and lower group to exit the greater sciatic foramen and supply the structures of the lower limb. The upper group of nerves, L4–S2 and part of S3, form the sciatic nerve, whereas the lower division of the plexus, mainly S3–4 with a small contribution from S2, forms the pudendal nerve. Within the pelvis, the sacral plexus supplies piriformis and levator ani, the former via the nerve that exits at S1–2 and enters the anterior surface of the muscle and the latter through branches derived from S4.

PUDENDAL NERVE

Of particular note to obstetric anatomy is the pudendal nerve, S2–4. This nerve leaves the pelvis through the greater sciatic foramen, winds around the ischial spine medial to the internal pudendal artery and just deep to the sacrospinous ligament to gain the perineum through the lesser sciatic foramen and enter the pudendal canal to innervate the vulva and perineum. As with the internal pudendal artery, the pudendal nerve gives off the inferior rectal nerve, which crosses the ischioanal fossa to supply the external anal sphincter, the lining of the distal end of the anal canal and the perianal skin. The pudendal nerve further divides into two terminal branches in the perineum – the perineal nerve and the dorsal nerve of the clitoris (discussed further in Chapter 3). The pudendal nerve is important therefore in maintaining sphincter function and, through innervations of the muscles of the region, providing muscular support to the viscera. The positioning of the nerve, deep to the sacrospinous ligament and close to the point of the ischial spine, makes it accessible for a pudendal nerve block to relieve pain during instrumental delivery. The ischial spine and sacrospinous ligament can be palpated vaginally and the pudendal needle is passed through the sacrospinous ligament to the pudendal nerve. The pudendal nerve also supplies sensory branches to the lower part of the vagina through sensory fibres in the inferior rectal nerve and posterior labial branches of the perineal nerve.

SYMPATHETIC AND PARASYMPATHETIC DIVISIONS

Within the pelvis, both sympathetic and parasympathetic divisions of the autonomic nervous system have to be considered. The sympathetic division, being the thoracolumbar outflow, has a contribution from both thoracic and lumbar levels. Thoracic preganglionic sympathetic fibres arise in the thorax and enter the abdomen through the crura of the diaphragm to synapse in the ganglia related to the main aortic branches (Figure 2.11A), particularly the celiac ganglion and the aorticorenal ganglion (Figure 2.11B). In the lumbar region the sympathetic chain consists of four ganglia, which lie on the lateral aspect of the lumbar vertebrae. Sympathetic fibres from this part of the chain are distributed into the pelvis via the superior hypogastric plexus – often erroneously named the presacral nerves (erroneously because they form a meshwork rather than a single nerve).

Superior hypogastric plexus

The superior hypogastric plexus lies anterior to the bifurcation of the aorta (Figure 2.11B). From the plexus, sympathetic fibres are carried into the pelvis as two main trunks – the right and left hypogastric nerves. The plexus also contains parasympathetic fibres, which arise from the pelvic splanchnic nerves (S2–4) (Figure 2.11A and B) and ascend from the inferior hypogastric plexus. However, it is more usual for these parasympathetic fibres to ascend to the left-hand side of the superior hypogastric plexus and cross the branches of the sigmoid and left colic vessel branches, as these parasympathetic branches are distributed along the branches of the inferior mesenteric artery. The hypogastric nerves send sympathetic fibres to the ovarian and ureteric plexuses, the fibres of which originate within the renal and aortic sympathetic plexuses.

Inferior hypogastric plexus

The inferior hypogastric plexus, or pelvic plexus as it is also known, is a continuation of the right and left hypogastric nerves in the pelvis. This plexus is also joined by parasympathetic fibres from the pelvic splanchnic nerves, derived from S2–4 of the sacral plexus. These fibres supply parasympathetic innervation to the pelvic viscera and the hindgut (Figure 2.11A). The inferior hypogastric or pelvic plexus is situated within the fascia surrounding the rectum, with fibres passing from here into the pelvic floor in order to reach the pelvic viscera. Fibres of this plexus lie on either side of the rectum, the cervical and vaginal fornices and the posterior aspect of the bladder. They also send fibres into the broad ligament. The plexus is derived from fibres of the lower three thoracic (T10–12) and upper two lumbar segments (L1–2) of the spinal cord as well as the preganglionic parasympathetic fibres from the pelvic splanchnic nerves.

The fibres of the pelvic/inferior hypogastric plexus that gain access to the broad ligament give rise to the

FIGURE 2.11A **Schema of innervation of female reproductive organs**

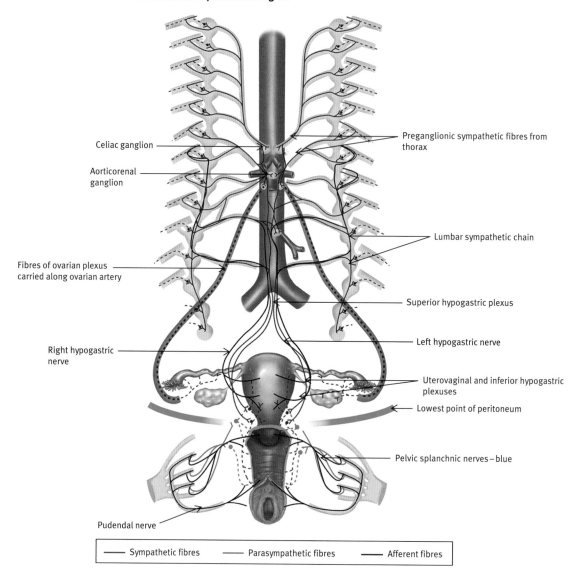

Celiac ganglion

Aorticorenal ganglion

Preganglionic sympathetic fibres from thorax

Lumbar sympathetic chain

Fibres of ovarian plexus carried along ovarian artery

Superior hypogastric plexus

Right hypogastric nerve

Left hypogastric nerve

Uterovaginal and inferior hypogastric plexuses

Lowest point of peritoneum

Pelvic splanchnic nerves – blue

Pudendal nerve

| —— Sympathetic fibres | —— Parasympathetic fibres | —— Afferent fibres |

uterovaginal plexus (Figure 2.11A and B). Some fibres from this part of the plexus travel with both vaginal and uterine arteries, while others pass directly to the cervix. Those travelling with the uterine artery supply the body of the uterus, the upper part of the broad ligament and the uterine tubes and communicate with branches from the ovarian plexus. Fibres travelling with the vaginal arteries are distributed to the walls of the vagina as well as the erectile tissue of the vestibule and the clitoris. While the sympathetic fibres within the inferior

hypogastric/pelvic plexus are responsible for uterine contraction and vasoconstriction and the parasympathetic fibres produce opposing effects, it should be remembered that hormonal regulation of the uterus may alter or even override the effects of the two autonomic divisions. The afferent fibres, which accompany many of the efferent fibres to the viscera, are the sensory components of autonomic function and elicit visceral reflexes. Afferent fibres also include pain fibres and such general visceral afferent fibres are reported to be carried

FIGURE 2.11B **Autonomic nerves and ganglia of the abdomen**

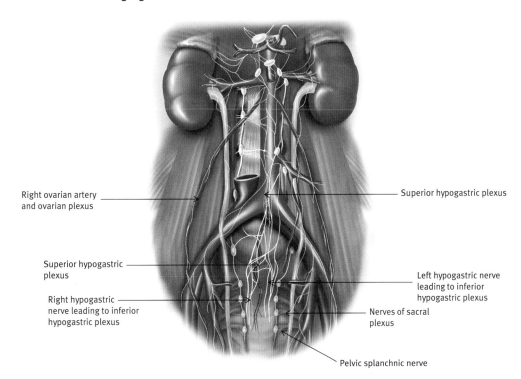

Right ovarian artery and ovarian plexus

Superior hypogastric plexus

Superior hypogastric plexus

Left hypogastric nerve leading to inferior hypogastric plexus

Right hypogastric nerve leading to inferior hypogastric plexus

Nerves of sacral plexus

Pelvic splanchnic nerve

in the pelvic splanchnic nerves. Pain fibres from the body of the uterus pass back to the hypogastric plexus and lumbar splanchnic nerves to the lower thoracic and upper lumbar levels of the spinal cord. Afferent fibres of the cervix and upper part of the vagina, however, pass via the pelvic splanchnic nerves, while afferents from the lower vagina and perineum travel in the pudendal nerves.

Applied anatomy and imaging of the bladder, ureter, urethra, anus and perineum

Diana Lawrence-Watt, Julia Montgomery and Malcolm Johnston

Pelvic viscera

The pelvic viscera within the female are surrounded by visceral peritoneum, resulting in several named spaces anterior and posterior to the various organs. Additionally, folds of fascia or parietal peritoneum are represented by named ligaments that transmit blood vessels and nerves to the pelvic viscera (Figure 3.1).

Urinary bladder

The position of the urinary bladder depends on whether it is full or empty. The empty bladder lies completely within the lesser pelvis, but rises into the abdominal cavity when filled or distended.

The fundus of the bladder is triangular in outline and is related to the anterior wall of the vagina. It is covered in parietal peritoneum that has been reflected from the anterior abdominal wall. The apex of the bladder is directed towards the pubic symphysis. The neck of the bladder lies on the pelvic floor, within the fascia that surrounds the urethra.

The superior surface of the female bladder is not entirely covered in peritoneum as this thin layer of tissue is reflected from it to form the quite shallow vesicouterine pouch (also known as the utero-vesical pouch in obstetric practice). From this pouch, the peritoneum covers the uterus and the posterior fornix of the vagina. The peritoneum is then reflected from the uterus to the middle part of the rectum, where it forms the deep recto-uterine pouch (Figure 3.2).

The relative positions of the urethra, vagina and anus, and more superiorly the positions of the bladder, uterus and sigmoid colon are seen. Note the large intramural fibroid within the fundus of the uterus.

LIGAMENTS OF THE BLADDER

Laterally, the bladder is connected to the pelvic fascia (Figures 3.1, 3.2A). The pelvic fascia is a thickening and condensation of fibrous tissue that forms the lateral true ligaments of the bladder.

Just before the lateral ligaments approach the deep surface of the pubic bone, they diverge to form two thickened bands, one lying more medial to the other. These bands are called the pubovesical ligaments. The medial pubovesical ligament attaches to the inside aspect of the pubic bone, close to the midpoint of the

FIGURE 3.1 **Pelvic viscera**

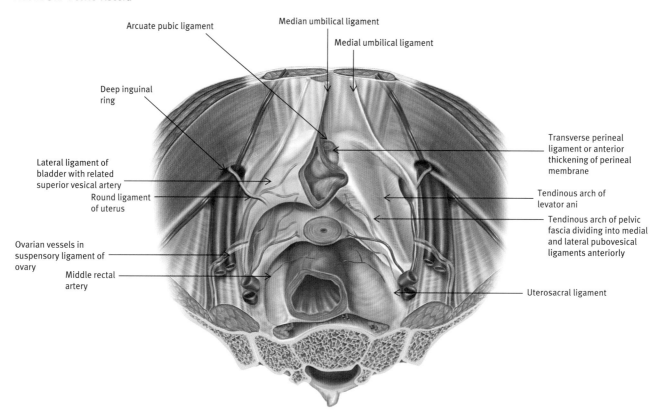

Arcuate pubic ligament

Median umbilical ligament

Medial umbilical ligament

Deep inguinal ring

Lateral ligament of bladder with related superior vesical artery

Round ligament of uterus

Ovarian vessels in suspensory ligament of ovary

Middle rectal artery

Transverse perineal ligament or anterior thickening of perineal membrane

Tendinous arch of levator ani

Tendinous arch of pelvic fascia dividing into medial and lateral pubovesical ligaments anteriorly

Uterosacral ligament

symphysis. From here it passes downwards and backwards to form the floor of the retropubic space. The pubovesical ligaments play a significant role in supporting the bladder neck and in urinary continence.

The apex of the bladder is continuous with the urachus (a fibrous cord covered in a fold of peritoneum), forming the median umbilical ligament and representing the closure of the upper end of the vesicourethral canal present during embryonic development.

MUSCLES AND MEMBRANES OF THE BLADDER

The bladder wall consists of the detrusor muscle. The detrusor muscle is formed of smooth muscle disposed into three layers: outer and inner longitudinal layers, with a middle circular layer interposed between them. The middle layer is relatively thin over most of the bladder but is thickened at the neck of the bladder where it gives rise to the sphincter vesicae around the internal urethral orifice.

Inside the bladder, the mucous membrane is loosely attached to the smooth muscle walls, allowing the membrane to be thrown into folds when the bladder is contracted and to become smooth when the bladder is distended.

On the posterior wall of the bladder lies the trigone (Figure 3.3A). The trigone is derived from the fusion of the distal ends of the two ureters into the posterior wall of the bladder. The ureters, unlike the bladder, are mesodermal in origin and the appearance of the trigone reflects the different developmental origins of the ureters and the bladder. The inferior point of the trigone arises in embryonic development from the fusion of the two mesonephric ducts into the posterior wall of the bladder, these ducts also being of mesodermal origin. The lower point of the trigone in the fully developed bladder is related to the outlet of the urethra at the internal urethral orifice. The mucous membrane covering the trigone is more firmly attached to the underlying muscle. The trigone does not exhibit the

FIGURE 3.2A **Urinary bladder**

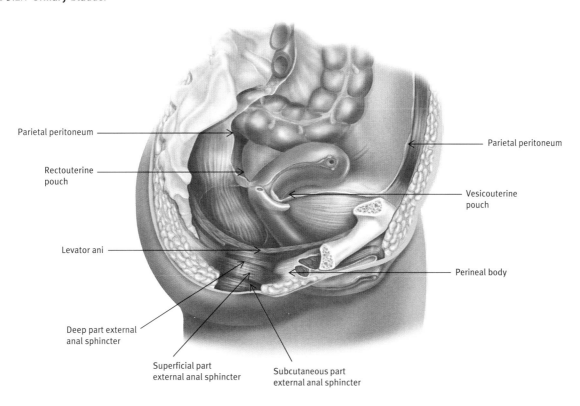

Parietal peritoneum

Parietal peritoneum

Rectouterine pouch

Vesicouterine pouch

Levator ani

Perineal body

Deep part external anal sphincter

Superficial part external anal sphincter

Subcutaneous part external anal sphincter

FIGURE 3.2B **Midsagittal magnetic resonance imaging (MRI) section through pelvis**

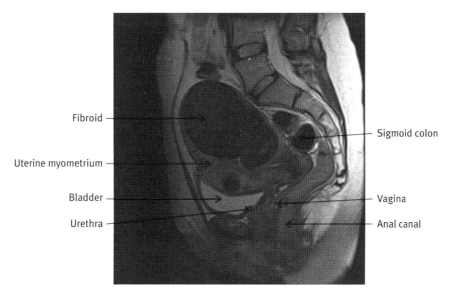

Fibroid

Sigmoid colon

Uterine myometrium

Bladder

Vagina

Urethra

Anal canal

FIGURE 3.3A **Pelvic viscera**

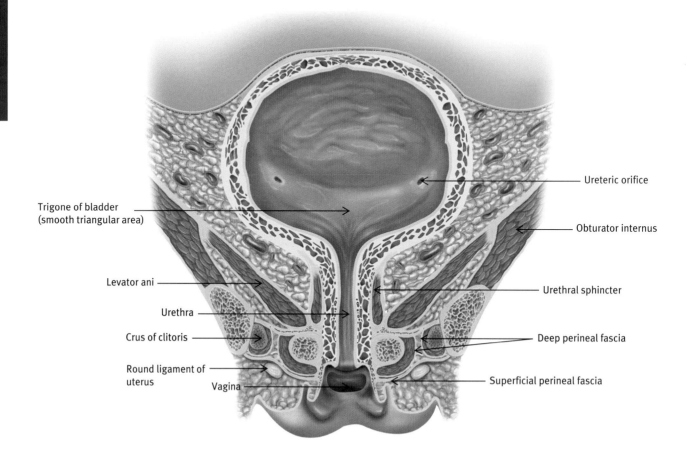

Trigone of bladder
(smooth triangular area)

Levator ani

Urethra

Crus of clitoris

Round ligament of
uterus

Vagina

Ureteric orifice

Obturator internus

Urethral sphincter

Deep perineal fascia

Superficial perineal fascia

folds characteristic of the other regions of the bladder as it does not expand. On an axial computed tomography (CT) section the bladder can be identified anteriorly, deep to the inferior rectus sheath with the uterus invaginating into the posterior wall of the bladder (Figure 3.3B). Behind the uterus the peritoneal reflection of the Pouch of Douglas or recto-uterine pouch can be identified with the rectum situated posterior to the pouch. Contrast is present within the peri-ovarian pelvic veins along the broad ligament.

INNERVATION OF THE BLADDER

The parasympathetic and sympathetic fibres to the bladder are contained within the pelvic plexus. The efferent parasympathetic fibres from the pelvic splanchnic nerves convey motor fibres to the detrusor muscle, but also convey inhibitory fibres to the sphincter vesicae. The urethral sphincter, which forms the urogenital diaphragm (Figure 3.3A), is supplied by the pudendal nerve.

Urethra

The urethra (Figure 3.3A) is a 4–6 cm long muscular tube that runs from the internal urethral orifice of the bladder to the external urethral orifice lying in the vestibule immediately anterior to the opening of the vagina. The two opposing walls of the urethra are in contact with each other at all times, apart from when urine passes through. The urethra itself is firmly attached to the anterior wall of the vagina.

The epithelium of the urethra is thrown into folds. The largest fold of the posterior wall is termed the

FIGURE 3.3B **Axial CT section**

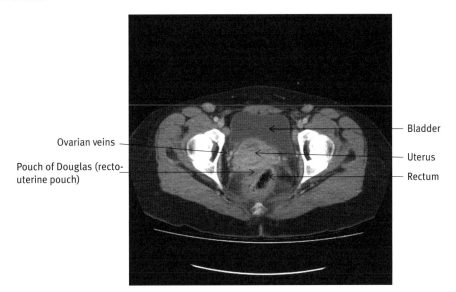

Ovarian veins

Pouch of Douglas (recto-uterine pouch)

Bladder

Uterus

Rectum

urethral crest. Numerous small mucous secreting glands open into the urethra. At the distal end of the urethra on each side, several of these glands cluster together to open into the paraurethral duct. The paraurethral duct runs downwards in the submucosal tissue and opens on the lateral aspect of each side of the external urethral orifice.

MUSCLES, MEMBRANES AND BLOOD SUPPLY

The smooth muscle of the urethra is continuous with the smooth muscle of the bladder. However, in the urethra it is arranged as internal longitudinal and external circular fibres. The circular fibres at the proximal end of the urethra give rise to the sphincter vesicae, or the internal sphincter, whereas those related to the external urethral orifice form sphincter urethrae.

The mucous membrane of the urethra is continuous with that of the bladder. The proximal end of the urethra is composed of transitional epithelium. At a more distal level the urethral epithelium is of a nonkeratinised stratified squamous nature. Below the mucous layer there is a thin layer of erectile tissue containing smooth muscle fibres and elastic connective tissue, as well as a plexus of veins.

Blood supply to the urethra is via the perineal branches of the internal pudendal artery. Blood drains via similar venous branches. The urethra receives autonomic innervation via the pelvic plexus.

CLINICAL RELEVANCE

If rupture of the urethra occurs, urine escapes below the level of the urogenital diaphragm, but deep to the membranous layer of the superficial fascia. However, as both these layers are attached to the ischiopubic rami and are also continuous with each other around the superficial transverse perineal muscles, urine cannot pass laterally or posteriorly. Additionally, urine cannot escape into the lesser pelvis as the opening into this is closed by the perineal membrane. Consequently, the only route the urine can take is via the areolar tissue of the mons pubis and the anterior abdominal wall.

Ureters

Formed in embryonic life from a bud that develops from the distal end of the mesonephric duct, the ureters are approximately 25 cm in length and lie behind the parietal peritoneum.

Each ureter commences at the pelvis of the kidney, descends on the psoas major and crosses in front of the slender genitofemoral nerve. The ovarian arteries and accompanying veins in turn cross anterior to the ureters as they descend towards the pelvis. The ureters enter the pelvis anterior to either the end of the common iliac artery or the proximal end of the internal iliac artery (see Chapter 2, Figure 2.10A), following the lateral wall of the pelvis towards the greater sciatic notch. Level with the ischial spine, the ureters turn medially in the fascia of the pelvic floor to reach the lateral aspect of the bladder. The ureters are crossed superiorly by the uterine vessels as these vessels enter the substance of the broad ligament at the level of the cervix.

At the level of the internal iliac artery, the ovaries are immediately anterior to the ureters. Just above the lateral fornix of the vagina, the ureters pass forwards and are usually described at this point as being placed 2 cm lateral to the supravaginal region of the cervix. Inclining medially, each ureter enters the posterior wall of the bladder, which is related at this point to the anterior aspect of the vagina. However, as the uterus itself is often placed to one side of the median plane, it is often the case that one ureter has a greater relationship to the front of the vagina than the other.

The ureters are described as having three coats: an outer, an inner and an intermediate. At its proximal end, the outer fibrous coat is continuous with the capsule of the kidney and distally merges into the wall of the bladder as the ureters enter the posterior bladder wall. The intermediate muscular coat consists of inner longitudinal and outer circular smooth muscle layers in the upper two-thirds of each ureter. A further outer longitudinal layer of smooth muscle cells is added to this coat in the distal one-third of each ureter (although at this level the inner longitudinal layer of muscle is less well developed). It is important to note that at all levels of the ureters, connective tissue interlaces the smooth muscle and definition of the muscle into distinct layers is not always obvious. The inner mucous coat of each ureter is thrown into longitudinal folds consisting of fibrous and elastic tissue and is covered in a transitional epithelial layer.

The course of the ureter from below the pelviureteric junction to the vesicoureteric junction can be readily demonstrated by axial CT sections through the abdomen and pelvis (Figure 3.4A).

The use of intravenous urogram studies also demonstrates the course of the ureters from the pelviureteric junction to the vesicoureteric junction (Figure 3.4B).

BLOOD SUPPLY AND INNERVATION

Each ureter receives its blood supply through an anastomosis of several arteries. The proximal end is supplied by the renal artery and during its course it also receives supply from the ovarian, common iliac and superior vesical arteries. The nerve supply is through branches from the renal, aortic, presacral and pelvic autonomic plexuses.

Perineum

The perineum overlies the diamond-shaped inferior pelvic aperture (Figure 3.5). The four points of the diamond are the pubic symphysis anteriorly, the coccyx posteriorly and the ischial tuberosities laterally. The region is divided into two triangles by an arbitrary line through the ischial tuberosities. The area anterior to this line is described as the urogenital triangle. The area posterior to this line is described as the anal triangle. The muscles of these two areas are often described separately, but they unite at the perineal body and therefore constitute a single unit.

MUSCLES OF THE PERINEUM

The muscles of the urogenital region are normally described as two groups: superficial and deep. The superficial group of muscles consists of bulbospongiosus, right and left ischiocavernosus and the right and left transverse perineal muscles. The vagina and urethra open on to the surface of the skin of the vestibule, bounded by the labia minora laterally. The labia minora join anterior to the clitoris, thereby defining the anterior boundary of the vestibule.

The deep group of muscles consists of urethral sphincter and the deep transverse perineal muscles. These muscles occupy the deep perineal pouch. Collectively these deep muscles form the structure called the urogenital diaphragm. The urogenital diaphragm, analogous to the pelvic diaphragm, is formed of muscles sandwiched between two layers of fascia. The muscles in this case are the urethral sphincter and the deep transverse perineal muscles. The upper layer of fascia forms the superior fascia of the urogenital diaphragm. The lower layer of fascia is described as the inferior, and

FIGURE 3.4A **(A–D) The ureters. (A) CT section shows the ureter passing inferiorly from the renal pelvis, related to the anterior surface of the psoas major muscle. In (B) and (C) the ureter is seen crossing anterior to the common iliac artery and vein, and in (D) the ureter passes medially towards the vesicoureteric junction on the posterolateral aspect of the bladder**

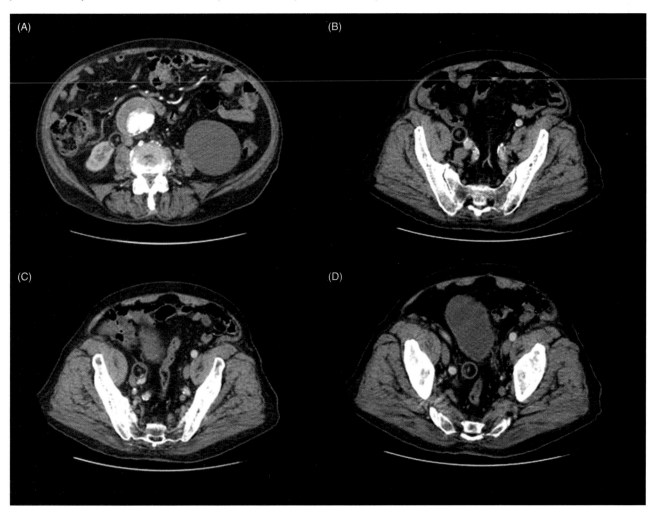

thicker, layer of fascia of the urogenital diaphragm, also called the perineal membrane. The space between the two layers of fascia is the deep perineal pouch. This pouch contains the muscles just described, but also the urethra and urethral glands and various vessels and nerves.

PERINEAL MEMBRANE

The perineal membrane is pierced by the vagina, urethra, blood vessels and nerves. The outer coat of the vagina fuses with the perineal membrane as it passes through (Figure 3.6).

The membrane stretches horizontally across the pubic arch and has a thickened apex. This thickened region is referred to as the transverse perineal ligament. Between this ligament and the arcuate pubic ligament (which spans across the inferior aspect of the pubic symphysis), the deep dorsal vein of the clitoris and the dorsal nerve of the clitoris enter the pelvis to supply the clitoris.

BLOOD SUPPLY TO THE PERINEUM

The main arterial supply to the perineum (Figure 3.7) is via the internal pudendal artery, one of the two terminal

FIGURE 3.4B **In this intravenous urogram study, a complete duplex system is seen on the right with an obstructed lower pole moiety. The position of the bladder (filled with contrast) is seen**

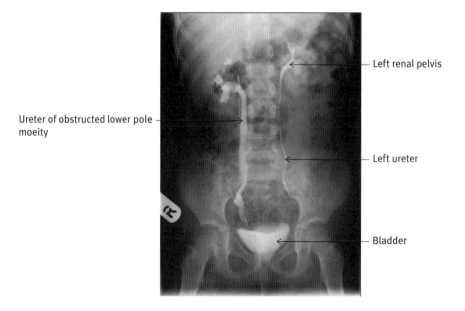

- Left renal pelvis

Ureter of obstructed lower pole moeity

- Left ureter

- Bladder

FIGURE 3.5 **Muscles of the perineum**

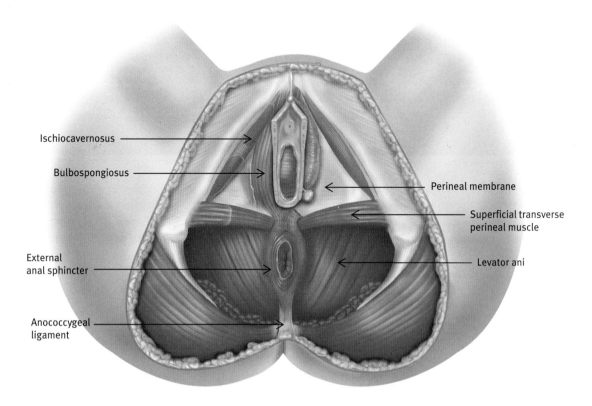

Ischiocavernosus

Bulbospongiosus

Perineal membrane

Superficial transverse perineal muscle

External anal sphincter

Levator ani

Anococcygeal ligament

FIGURE 3.6 **Urethra and surrounding anatomy**

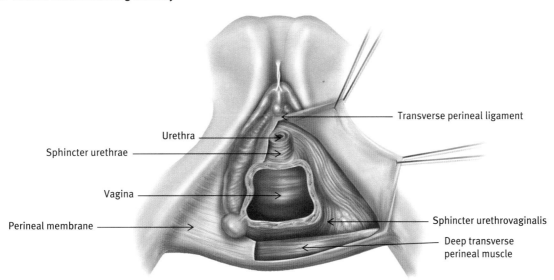

- Transverse perineal ligament
- Urethra
- Sphincter urethrae
- Vagina
- Perineal membrane
- Sphincter urethrovaginalis
- Deep transverse perineal muscle

FIGURE 3.7 **Arteries of the perineum**

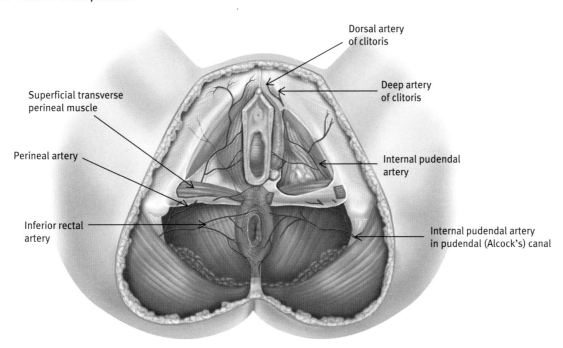

- Dorsal artery of clitoris
- Superficial transverse perineal muscle
- Deep artery of clitoris
- Perineal artery
- Internal pudendal artery
- Inferior rectal artery
- Internal pudendal artery in pudendal (Alcock's) canal

branches of the anterior division of the internal iliac artery. This artery exits the pelvis to enter the gluteal region via the greater sciatic foramen. It winds its way around the ischial spine, accompanied by the medially placed pudendal nerve, to gain entry into the perineum. Here, the artery is confined to the proximal end of the pudendal (or Alcock's) canal, a fascial compartment related to the deep surface of the ischial tuberosity and the ischiopubic ramus. The pudendal canal forms the lateral boundary of the ischioanal fossa, which is bounded medially by the external anal sphincter and the inferior fascia of the pelvic diaphragm.

The roof and lateral wall of the pudendal canal are formed by the lower part of the fascia of obturator internus, extending both upwards to blend with the inferior fascia of the pelvic diaphragm and downwards to become the sacrotuberous ligament. Branches from both the internal pudendal artery and the pudendal nerve escape from the medial aspect of the pudendal canal to supply the region.

The inferior rectal artery leaves the pudendal canal near its proximal end and traverses medially across the ischioanal fossa to supply the anal canal and skin of the region. A more distal branch of the internal pudendal artery is the perineal artery, which branches from the internal pudendal artery near the anterior end of the pudendal canal. The perineal artery supplies branches both deep to and superficial to the perineal membrane, supplying both skin and muscle in this region.

The branches of the perineal artery are as follows: the posterior labial branches, which supply the labia; the artery to the bulb of the vestibule, which supplies the erectile tissue of the bulb of the vestibule; the deep artery of the clitoris, which supplies the corpus cavernosum; and the dorsal artery of the clitoris, which supplies the dorsum, glans and the prepuce of the clitoris.

INNERVATION OF THE PERINEUM

The pudendal nerve supplies similar branches to the internal pudendal artery (Figure 3.8). The inferior rectal nerve supplies the external anal sphincter, the lower part of the anal canal and the perianal skin and accompanies the inferior rectal artery.

The perineal nerve accompanies the perineal artery and divides into posterior labial and muscular branches. The posterior labial branches usually pass superficial to the perineal membrane, but the perineal nerve also supplies branches that pass deep to this membrane. The deep branch of the perineal nerve supplies the ischiocavernosus muscle and gives rise to the dorsal nerve of the clitoris. The dorsal nerve of the clitoris passes deep to the perineal membrane and runs forward to supply the clitoris.

FIGURE 3.8 **Innervation of external genitalia and perineum**

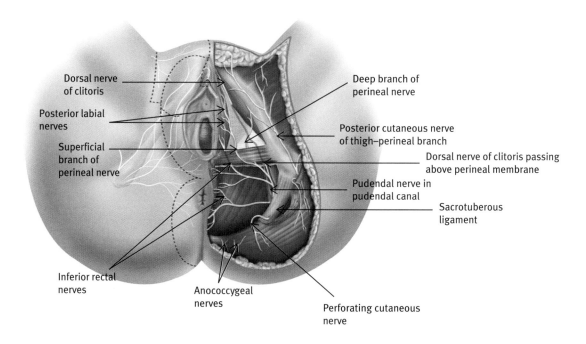

38

Anal region

The boundaries of the anal triangle are the posterior aspect of the perineal membrane and laterally the ischial tuberosities and sacrotuberous ligament. Central to this region is the anal canal, with the ischioanal fossae positioned laterally (Figure 3.9).

The muscles of the urogenital region and the anal region meet in the perineal body. The perineal body is a fibromuscular node between the urogenital region and the anal region where the muscles of the two regions unite to form a functional unit. Fibres of levator ani also contribute to the perineal body.

ANAL CANAL

The anal canal is approximately 3–4 cm long and is surrounded by muscles that act as sphincters to close the canal. The upper part of the anal canal is lined by mucous membrane, which is thrown into longitudinal folds. These folds are termed the anal columns. The anal columns are characterised at their distal end by having anal valves and anal sinuses.

Both internal and external sphincters line the anal canal. The internal anal sphincter surrounds the upper three-quarters of the anal canal and its lower extremity is the white line. The white line is the transition point between the internal anal sphincter and the subcutaneous

FIGURE 3.9 **Muscles of the anal region**

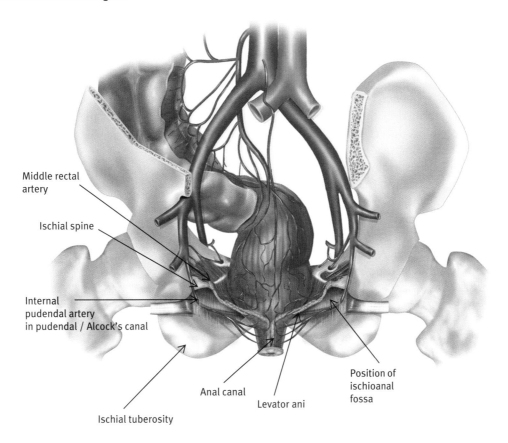

39

FIGURE 3.10 **Anal canal**

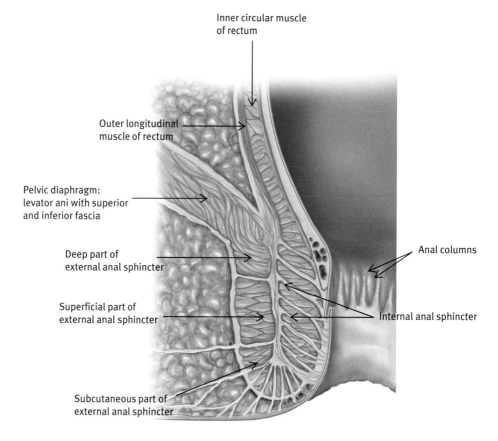

Inner circular muscle
of rectum

Outer longitudinal
muscle of rectum

Pelvic diaphragm:
levator ani with superior
and inferior fascia

Deep part of
external anal sphincter

Superficial part of
external anal sphincter

Subcutaneous part of
external anal sphincter

Anal columns

Internal anal sphincter

part of the external anal sphincter (Figure 3.10). The internal anal sphincter is formed by the circular muscle coat of the rectum becoming thicker at the anorectal junction thus forming the sphincter.

The external anal sphincter surrounds the lower part of the anal canal, overlapping the internal anal sphincter, and is inserted into skin at the lower end of the canal. The external sphincter can be divided into deep, superficial and subcutaneous regions. Deep fibres of the external anal sphincter interdigitate with fibres of the puborectalis, and with the muscles of the deep perineal pouch via the perineal body. Superficial fibres of the external anal sphincter are inserted to the coccyx and contribute fibres to the anococcygeal ligament, a body of fibrous and muscular tissue separating the anus from the coccyx.

The subcutaneous part of the external sphincter is a thin, horizontal band around the distal part of the anal canal. It lies below the internal anal sphincter with some

fibres attaching to the anococcygeal ligament and the perineal body. This part of the sphincter does not have any bony attachments.

> **CLINICAL RELEVANCE**
>
> Perineal tears during childbirth are classified into the following definitions dependent on the anatomy of the perineum and anal region:
>
> First degree: injury to perineal skin only
> Second degree: injury to the perineal muscles but not involving the anal sphincter
> Third degree: injury involving the anal sphincter (3a, less than 50% of the external anal sphincter muscles torn; 3b, more than 50% of the external anal sphincter torn; and 3c when both the external and internal anal sphincter is torn)
> Fourth degree: damage to both external and internal sphincter muscles and anal epithelium

CHAPTER 4

Applied anatomy and imaging of the uterus, vagina, ovaries and breast

Diana Lawrence-Watt, Julia Montgomery and Malcolm Johnston

Uterus

The bulk of the tissue of the uterus is smooth muscle. In the nonpregnant state it weighs approximately 40 g, but in pregnancy its weight increases to approximately 800 g, due to both hypertrophy and hyperplasia of the smooth muscle fibres. In pregnancy, the uterus affords protection for the developing fetus and is also responsible for expulsion of the fetus at term.

While the body of the uterus is composed of smooth muscle fibres, the cervix is composed mainly of dense connective tissue. This connective tissue acts to hold the fetus in the uterus, allowing the smooth muscle of the uterus to stretch and undergo hypertrophy.

> **CLINICAL RELEVANCE**
>
> The junction between the cervix and the uterus undergoes dilation and thinning in pregnancy. This thinner part of the wall is the region that can be incised in caesarean section.

The uterus is entirely located in the lesser pelvis, between the bladder and the rectum (Figure 4.1). The fallopian tubes enter the uterus on either side, at the junction of the fundus and the body.

The uterus is a moveable organ and is held by four ligaments. These are discussed in detail below. In addition to the ligaments, folds of peritoneum form structures related to the uterus, but these folds have a very limited role in holding the uterus in its pelvic location. Anteriorly, the uterovesical fold of peritoneum is reflected on to the upper surface of the bladder from the uterus at the junction of the cervix and uterine body. The rectovaginal fold of peritoneum is reflected on to the surface of the rectum from the posterior fornix of the vagina and forms the floor of the rectouterine pouch. This pouch is bounded anteriorly by the posterior wall of the uterine body, posteriorly by the rectum and laterally by folds of peritoneum passing from the cervix to the posterior walls of the lesser pelvis.

UTEROSACRAL LIGAMENTS

The folds of peritoneum extending posteriorly from the cervix to the walls of the lesser pelvis contain a substantial amount of smooth muscle and fibrous tissue. These folds are attached to the anterior surface of the sacrum and form the true ligaments of the uterus; the uterosacral ligaments (Figure 4.2).

BROAD LIGAMENT

Related to either side of the uterus is the broad ligament, a fold of peritoneum that contains the fallopian tubes,

FIGURE 4.1 **Pelvic viscera and perineum**

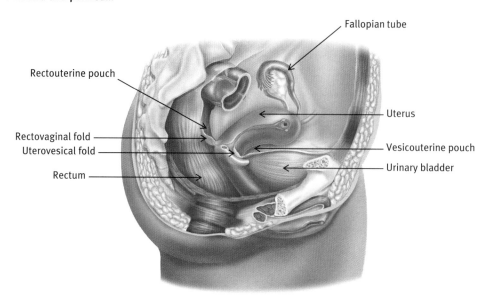

FIGURE 4.2 **Ligaments of the uterus**

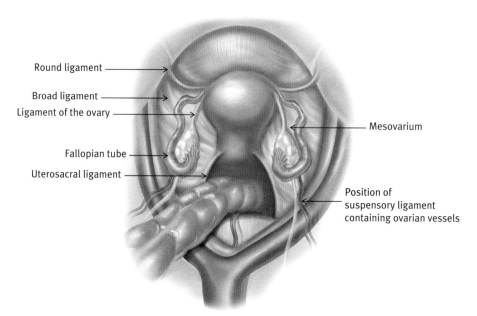

the round ligament of the uterus and the ligament of the ovary.

From the side of the uterus, the broad ligament reaches the lateral wall of the pelvis and results in a septum that interposes between the anterior region of the pelvis containing the bladder and the posterior region of the rectum. The ovary is attached to the posterior layer of the broad ligament via the mesovarium (Figure 4.2).

The suspensory ligament of the ovary is the part of the broad ligament that extends from the infundibulum of the uterine tube and upper pole of the ovary to the lateral wall of the pelvis. The suspensory ligament

FIGURE 4.3 **Uterus and adnexa**

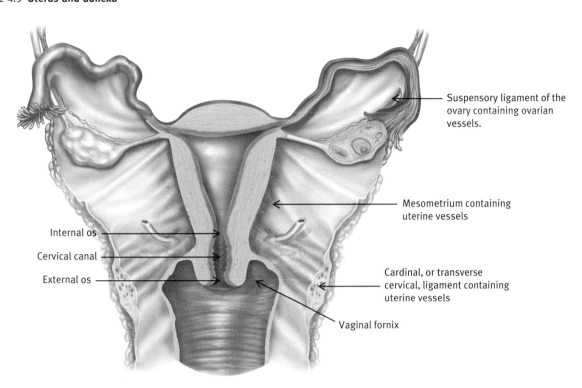

Suspensory ligament of the ovary containing ovarian vessels.

Mesometrium containing uterine vessels

Internal os

Cervical canal

External os

Cardinal, or transverse cervical, ligament containing uterine vessels

Vaginal fornix

contains the ovarian vessels, nerves and lymphatics and continues over the external iliac vessels as a distinct fold. The term mesometrium is used for the part of the broad ligament that extends from the pelvic floor upwards to the ovary and the ligament of the ovary (Figure 4.3).

The uterine artery, a branch of the anterior division of the internal iliac artery, is carried between the layers of the broad ligament. Having crossed above the ureter as it inclines medially to gain the posterior wall of the bladder, the uterine artery passes approximately 1.5 cm lateral to the cervix. The artery then travels superiorly within the substance of the broad ligament to anastomose with branches of the ovarian artery, affording a rich anastomotic supply from both arteries to the uterine tube.

Transverse cervical ligament

From its origin at the internal iliac artery, the uterine artery travels within the substance of the transverse

cervical, or cardinal, ligament (Figure 4.3). This ligament is attached to the lateral aspect of the cervix and the lateral wall of the pelvis and gives considerable support to the uterus. The transverse cervical ligament is one of the ligaments that are instrumental in retaining the position of the uterus within the pelvis. The name here is confusing as it is not truly ligamentous, but rather a condensation of dense connective tissue that has formed around the neurovascular structures extending from the lateral walls of the pelvis to the pelvic viscera. Nevertheless, this 'ligament' is very firmly fused to the fascia surrounding the cervix and upper part of the vagina and passes backwards and upwards to the root of the internal iliac vessels. The transverse cervical ligament supports the cervix and upper vagina, helping to maintain the angle between the axis of the vagina and the anteverted uterus. Inferiorly it is continuous with the superior fascia of the pelvic diaphragm.

Round ligament

The round ligament of the uterus (Figure 4.2) may also play some role in maintaining the uterus in an anteverted position. The round ligament initially courses between the layers of the broad ligament. It then passes through the deep inguinal ring to enter the inguinal canal and end in the tissue of the labia majora, accompanied by the ilioinguinal nerve as it passes through the inguinal canal.

Cervix and vagina

The cervix forms the cylindrical lower one-third of the uterus. The internal os is the communication between the cervix and the uterus. The external os is the communication between the cervix and the vagina (Figure 4.3). The cervix forms a less extensible region around the lower end of the uterus and may give some support to prevent expulsion of the fetus before term.

The cervical mucosa is very different from the endometrium of the uterus, undergoing very little morphological change during the endometrial cycle. During pregnancy, the cervix increases its vascularity and is less rigid than in the nonpregnant state. The mucous secretion of the cervix thickens during pregnancy, serving as a mechanical barrier to infection. In late pregnancy the dense collagen of the cervix loosens owing to uptake of fluid by mucopolysaccahrides. This loosening of the cervix allows the lower section to shorten as the upper section expands.

The vagina is a muscular canal that lies between the cervix and the vestibule and opens on to the perineum. The vaginal part of the cervix continues into the anterior wall of the vagina producing two recesses: the anterior and posterior fornices. The posterior fornix is closely related to the peritoneal cavity and is covered in peritoneum. This peritoneum is reflected on to the rectum, forming the rectouterine pouch (Figure 4.1).

Blood supply and lymphatic drainage of the uterus, cervix and vagina

Although the main blood supply to the uterus is from the uterine arteries, an azygous system of arteries exists to supply the uterus, cervix and vagina with a very rich arterial supply (Figure 4.4). This network of vessels has contributions from the uterine, vaginal and internal pudendal arteries.

Lymph from the uterus mainly passes to the internal iliac nodes. However, there may be some communication with superficial inguinal nodes as lymph vessels may pass via the round ligaments to these nodes. Malignant cells from the uterus can track to the superficial inguinal nodes via such a route.

Fallopian tubes and ovaries

The fallopian tubes and ovaries are situated in the upper margin of the broad ligament (Figure 4.5). Each uterine tube is approximately 10 cm long. The medial end opens into the superior angle of the cavity of the uterus and the lateral end opens into the peritoneal cavity close to the ovary. The lateral end is fimbriated and the fimbriae lead into a funnel-shaped region, or infundibulum, of the tube. The infundibulum in turn leads into the ampulla and then into the isthmus of the tube. The intramural part of the tube passes through the superolateral aspect of the uterine wall to open into the upper part of the uterine cavity.

The ovaries are situated on each side of the uterus, close to the lateral wall of the lesser pelvis. Each one is attached to the posterosuperior aspect of the broad ligament by a short pedicle of peritoneum called the mesovarium. In nulliparous women, the ovary is vertical and has medial and lateral surfaces and tubal and uterine extremities. The ovary sits in a small depression called the ovarian fossa on the lateral wall of the pelvis. Immediate posterior relations to the ovary are the ureter and internal iliac artery with the tubal extremity of the ovary lying close to the external iliac vein (Figure 4.6).

Related to the tubal extremity of the ovary are the fimbriae of the uterine tube and a fold of peritoneum known as the suspensory ligament of the ovary. This suspensory ligament, which contains the ovarian vessels and nerves, passes superiorly over the external iliac vessels. The suspensory ligament of the ovary is the

FIGURE 4.4 **Blood supply to the uterus and ovaries**

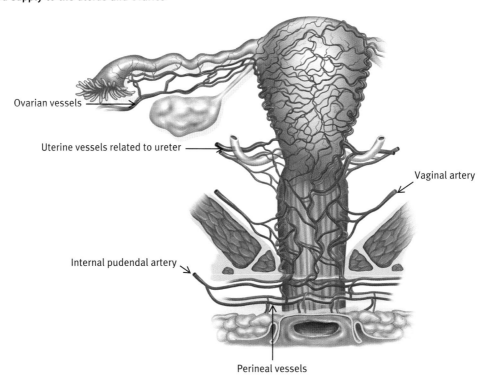

Ovarian vessels

Uterine vessels related to ureter

Vaginal artery

Internal pudendal artery

Perineal vessels

FIGURE 4.5 **Uterus, ovaries and uterine tubes**

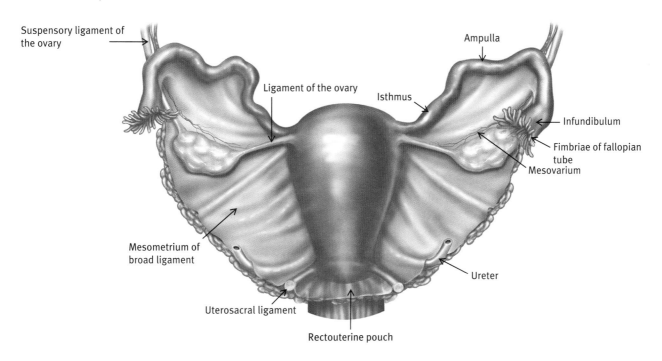

Suspensory ligament of the ovary

Ampulla

Ligament of the ovary

Isthmus

Infundibulum

Fimbriae of fallopian tube

Mesovarium

Mesometrium of broad ligament

Ureter

Uterosacral ligament

Rectouterine pouch

45

FIGURE 4.6 **Neuropathways in parturition**

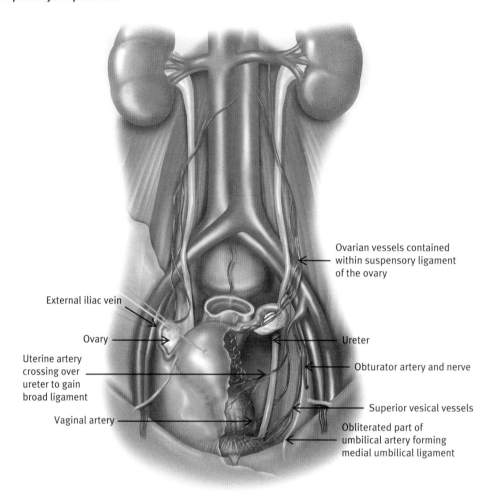

Ovarian vessels contained within suspensory ligament of the ovary

External iliac vein

Ovary

Ureter

Uterine artery crossing over ureter to gain broad ligament

Obturator artery and nerve

Superior vesical vessels

Vaginal artery

Obliterated part of umbilical artery forming medial umbilical ligament

anatomical nomenclature for this structure, whereas in obstetric surgery it is more commonly referred to as the infundibulopelvic or IP ligament. The lateral surface of the ovary is in contact with the parietal peritoneum, which lines the ovarian fossa and separates the ovary from the extraperitoneal tissue and obturator vessels and nerves. The medial surface of the ovary is mainly covered by the uterine tube. The ovarian bursa is the peritoneal recess between the medial aspect of the ovary and the mesosalpinx, the latter being the mesentery of the fallopian tube.

Hysterosalpingograms (HSGs) can be used to visualise the uterus and adnexa using contrast medium (Figure 4.7A and B).

Autonomic nerve supply to the uterus and adnexa

During pregnancy and parturition the neural pathways are of great importance and are highlighted in Figure 4.8 (see Chapter 2 for more detailed discussion of the uterine nerve supply).

Sensory fibres from the uterine body and fundus, drawn in purple on Figure 4.8, travel with sympathetic fibres via both the inferior and superior hypogastric plexuses to thoracic cord levels 11 and 12. The two hypogastric plexuses are continuous with each other via the right and left hypogastric nerves on each side of the body. Sensory fibres from the cervix and upper

FIGURE 4.7 **(A) HSG demonstrates contrast medium within the cervical canal, uterine cavity and both fallopian tubes. (B) Later image from an HSG study now reveals the spillage through the fibrial ends of both fallopian tubes into the peritoneal cavity, thus confirming tubal patency.**

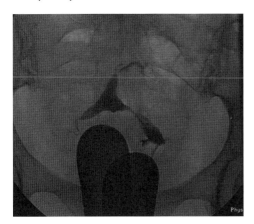

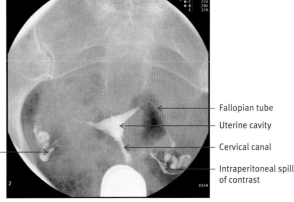

Fimbrial end of right fallopian tube

Fallopian tube

Uterine cavity

Cervical canal

Intraperitoneal spill of contrast

vagina travel via the pelvic splanchnic nerves to S2, 3 and 4. Sensory fibres from the lower vagina and perineum are also distributed to S2, 3 and 4, but via the pudendal nerve.

Motor fibres to the uterine body and fundus are sympathetic in origin, whereas those to the lowest part of the uterus and upper vagina are parasympathetic, travelling via the pelvic splanchnic nerves. Motor fibres to the lower vagina and perineum are somatic fibres, travelling via the pudendal nerve.

Breast

The base of the breast extends from the second rib to the sixth rib and overlies the investing fascia of the pectoralis major muscle. The majority of the tissue of the breast in the nonpregnant state is composed of fat. During pregnancy, the glandular content of the breast increases due to milk production within the lactiferous ducts.

STRUCTURE AND DEVELOPMENT OF THE BREAST

The breast is divided into approximately 20 fat-filled lobules, each of which contains a lactiferous duct. Each lactiferous duct extends in a radial manner towards the nipple, where it opens on to the surface (Figure 4.9). Also opening around the nipple are the areolar glands.

These glands secrete an oily, protective lubricant, particularly during pregnancy and lactation.

The lobules of the breast are separated from each other by fibrous tissue that form suspensory ligaments. These ligaments extend from the deep fascia covering pectoralis major to the dermis of the skin. Additional fibres extend from the connective tissue of the breast to the skin and these may pull on the skin if the organ is swollen with excess tissue fluid. This pulling results in a *peau d'orange* appearance of the skin of the breast.

During puberty, the ducting system of the breast becomes fully established. Alveolar parts of the ducts make their appearance at this time, although during puberty the increase in breast size is attributed to an increase in fat deposition. During pregnancy both the ducts and the alveoli of the glands further develop to produce milk. Following pregnancy the breast returns to its normal pre-pregnant state via a process of apoptosis and the action of macrophages on these tissues. Postmenopause, the breast atrophies further as the suspensory ligaments become less taut due to the withdrawal of estrogens. The breast at this time of life therefore begins to sag.

BLOOD SUPPLY AND LYMPHATIC DRAINAGE OF THE BREAST

The breast is supplied with blood mainly from the lateral thoracic artery, a branch of the axillary artery,

FIGURE 4.8 **Neuropathways**

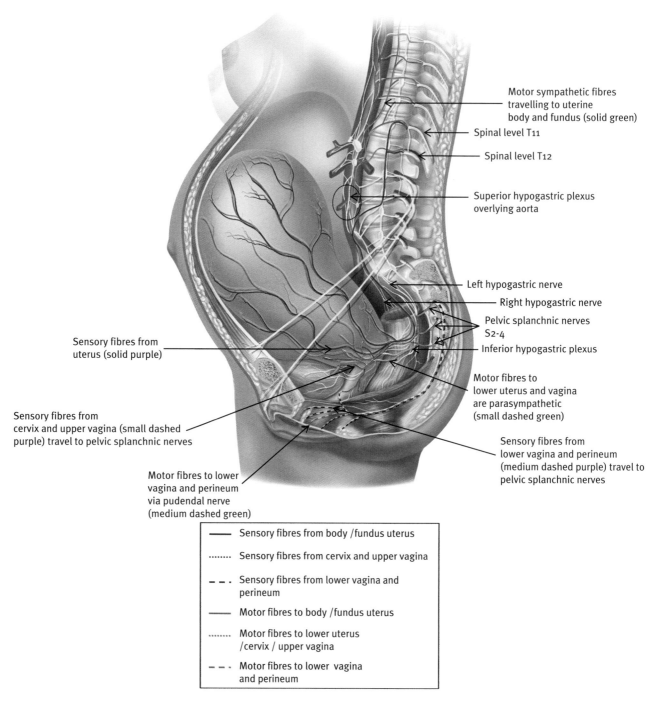

Motor sympathetic fibres travelling to uterine body and fundus (solid green)

Spinal level T11

Spinal level T12

Superior hypogastric plexus overlying aorta

Left hypogastric nerve

Right hypogastric nerve

Pelvic splanchnic nerves S2-4

Inferior hypogastric plexus

Motor fibres to lower uterus and vagina are parasympathetic (small dashed green)

Sensory fibres from uterus (solid purple)

Sensory fibres from cervix and upper vagina (small dashed purple) travel to pelvic splanchnic nerves

Motor fibres to lower vagina and perineum via pudendal nerve (medium dashed green)

Sensory fibres from lower vagina and perineum (medium dashed purple) travel to pelvic splanchnic nerves

——	Sensory fibres from body /fundus uterus
·······	Sensory fibres from cervix and upper vagina
– – ·	Sensory fibres from lower vagina and perineum
——	Motor fibres to body /fundus uterus
·······	Motor fibres to lower uterus /cervix / upper vagina
– – ·	Motor fibres to lower vagina and perineum

through lateral mammary branches. Lateral mammary branches may also arise from lateral cutaneous branches of the posterior intercostal arteries. Medial mammary branches arise from the internal thoracic artery, a branch of the first part of the subclavian artery.

Lymphatic drainage of the breast is extensive, with more than 75% of drainage occurring via the axillary

FIGURE 4.9 **Anterolateral dissection of the breast**

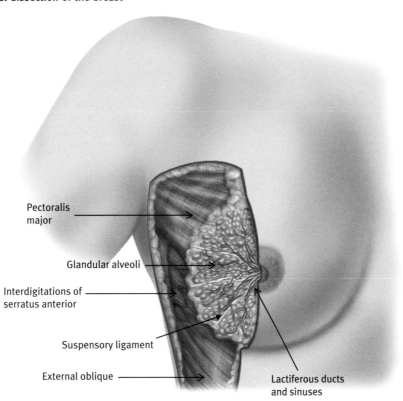

Pectoralis
major

Glandular alveoli

Interdigitations of
serratus anterior

Suspensory ligament

External oblique

Lactiferous ducts
and sinuses

nodes. The various groups of these axillary nodes cluster around the pectoralis minor muscle and the axillary vessels. The remaining drainage is via the para-aortic nodes. Drainage can also occur across the midline and below the diaphragm via interconnecting lymph channels.

Biochemistry

CHAPTER 5

Cell and molecular biology

Fiona Lyall

Structure and function of the cell and its organelles

Two types of cell exist:

- Prokaryotic cells, such as bacteria, have a simple internal organisation and no defined nucleus.
- Eukaryotic cells, which comprise all plant and animal cells, have a more complex internal structure with a clearly defined membrane surrounding the nucleus.

Eukaryotic cells are typically 10–100 micrometres across – about ten times the size of prokaryotic cells. Despite their differences, prokaryotic and eukaryotic cells have certain structures in common and perform many complicated tasks in basically the same way. This chapter focuses on eukaryotic cells.

To maintain their integrity, eukaryotic cells have a plasma membrane that surrounds their watery interior. The plasma membrane consists of a bilayer of phospholipids, with cholesterol embedded within it to make the membrane more rigid. Only plants and fungi have cell walls surrounding the plasma membrane.

The plasma membrane does not only separate the inside of the cell from the outside environment, it also has other functions. For example, protein transporters embedded in it allow transport of water-soluble molecules across the membrane. The plasma membrane also contains receptors that bind circulating signalling molecules and hormones. Activation of receptors through such binding results in the transient reorganisation of certain proteins (the so-called signal transduction

proteins) inside the cell. This in turn leads to a chain of events called cell signalling, which can trigger a variety of processes within the cell.

The majority of eukaryotic cells, including human cells, also contain internal membranes that enclose organelles within the cell (Figure 5.1). Most organelles, the nucleus being one of the exceptions, only have a single membrane. These membranes allow individual organelles to control their own internal ionic composition such that it will differ from that of the cytosol (the area outside the organelles but within the plasma membrane). Thus, the internal structure of the cell is

FIGURE 5.1 **Diagram of a human cell showing major organelles**

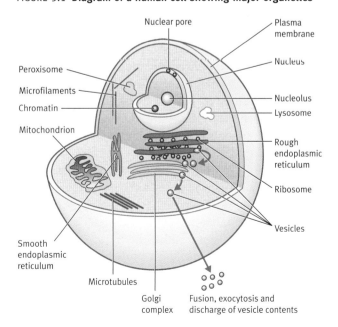

highly organised to support the function of the cell and, ultimately, of the body.

NUCLEUS

The nucleus is the largest organelle. It contains the cell's chromosomes and is the place where almost all DNA replication and RNA synthesis occurs.

The nucleus is separated from the cytoplasm by a double membrane called the nuclear envelope. The nuclear envelope isolates and protects the cell's DNA from various molecules that could accidentally damage its structure or interfere with its processing. Pores in the nuclear membranes regulate the movement of substances between nucleus and cytoplasm. In many cells the outer nuclear membrane is continuous with the rough endoplasmic reticulum.

The nucleus contains a suborganelle called the nucleolus and it is within this suborganelle that most of the cell's ribosomal RNA is synthesised.

ENDOPLASMIC RETICULUM

The endoplasmic reticulum is a network of interconnected internal membranes. There are two varieties: rough and smooth.

The rough endoplasmic reticulum is so called because it has ribosomes attached to its outer surface; the smooth endoplasmic reticulum does not.

The smooth endoplasmic reticulum is the site where synthesis of fatty acids and phospholipids occurs. Many cells have little smooth endoplasmic reticulum but in liver cells it is abundant. Enzymes in the smooth endoplasmic reticulum of liver cells modify and detoxify molecules such as pesticides and carcinogens and exposure to large amounts of such chemicals results in a large increase in endoplasmic reticulum volume in liver cells.

Ribosomes bound to the rough endoplasmic reticulum synthesise organelle and membrane proteins as well as all proteins to be secreted from the cell. Secretory proteins pass through the rough endoplasmic reticulum membrane and accumulate in the inner cavity of the rough endoplasmic reticulum before being transported to their destination. Rough endoplasmic reticulum is particularly abundant in cells that are specialised in the production of secreted proteins such as antibodies

(for example plasma cells) or digestive enzymes (for example pancreatic acinar cells).

Most proteins leave the rough endoplasmic reticulum within minutes after their synthesis in small membrane-bound transport vesicles. These vesicles bud off from the rough endoplasmic reticulum and transport the proteins to the lumen of the Golgi complex.

GOLGI COMPLEX

The Golgi complex is also surrounded by a membrane. Within different regions of the Golgi complex, different enzymes modify secreted proteins and membrane proteins in different ways depending on the structure and ultimate destination of the proteins.

After modification, the proteins are transported out of the Golgi complex in a second set of transport vesicles. Some vesicles will contain proteins destined for the plasma membrane, while others contain proteins for lysosomes or other organelles.

MITOCHONDRIA

Mitochondria are found in nearly all eukaryotic cells, and there are usually several or many in each cell. These organelles burn glucose for fuel in the process of cellular respiration to produce ATP. Essentially, they are the 'power house' of the cell.

Mitochondria have a smooth outer membrane and a convoluted inner membrane, which are separated by an intermembrane space. The convolutions of the inner membrane are called cristae and the space inside the inner membrane is the mitochondrial matrix. As glucose is burned for fuel, a mitochondrion shunts various chemicals back and forth across the inner membrane (from the matrix to the intermembrane space and vice versa).

Mitochondria contain their own DNA, which, in contrast to the nuclear DNA, is inherited through the mother.

LYSOSOMES AND PEROXISOMES

Lysosomes and peroxisomes can be likened to the 'disposal system' of a cell because they remove substances the cell no longer requires, including old organelles.

Lysosomes and peroxisomes are surrounded by a single membrane and are rich in digestive enzymes. For example, lysosomes can contain more than three dozen enzymes for degrading proteins, nucleic acids and polysaccharides. All lysosome enzymes work at acidic pH values; thus, the internal pH value is maintained at around 4.8. The cell would not be able to house such destructive enzymes if they were not contained in a membrane-bound system to protect the rest of the cell.

Many materials degraded by lysosomes are brought into the cell by one of the following processes:

- endocytosis (materials are taken up by invagination of a part of the plasma membrane to form a small membrane-bound vesicle)
- phagocytosis (larger particles such as bacteria are enveloped by the plasma membrane and internalised).

Peroxisomes contain several oxidases that oxidise organic substances. This process generates the toxic molecule hydrogen peroxide (H_2O_2), which is then converted to O_2 and H_2O by the enzyme catalase. The peroxisome is the main organelle for oxidising fatty acids, which are precursors for key synthetic pathways. Toxic molecules in the blood are also cleared by peroxisomes, particularly in liver and kidney cells.

CYTOSOL AND CYTOSKELETON

The cytosol of the cell does not only contain the cell organelles, it also contains the cytoskeleton. The cytoskeleton is made up of three classes of fibres: microtubules (20 nm diameter), microfilaments (7 nm diameter) and intermediate filaments (10 nm diameter). The cytoskeleton gives the cell rigidity and strength, thereby allowing it to maintain its shape, and changes in its organisation underpin a cell's ability to migrate.

Finally, the cytosol also contains many particles such as glycogen-containing granules.

Cell signalling

In multicellular organisms, a complex intercellular communication network exists that coordinates metabolism, differentiation, growth and repair. The term cell signalling refers to the communication between cells by means of signalling molecules. Released by the signalling cell or bound to its surface, signalling molecules produce a response in a target cell that has receptors for that particular signalling molecule. The process of converting an extracellular signal into a response in the target cell is known as signal transduction.

Extracellular signalling by means of secreted molecules can be classified as endocrine, paracrine and autocrine, depending on the distance travelled by the signalling molecule:

- Endocrine signalling involves the release of hormones from endocrine glands; the hormones are then carried in the bloodstream to a distant target site (Figure 5.2A).
- In paracrine signalling the signalling molecule produced by a cell acts only on cells very close to it (Figure 5.2B); neurotransmitters work by paracrine signalling.

FIGURE 5.2 **Extracellular signalling methods**

A Endocrine signalling

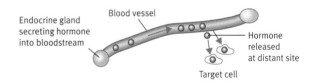

B Paracrine signalling

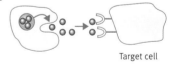

C Autocrine signalling

D Cell signalling via membrane-attached proteins

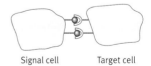

- In autocrine signalling a cell responds to a signalling molecule that it has released itself (Figure 5.2C); many growth factors operate like this and it is commonly seen in tumour growth.

In a fourth method of extracellular signalling, the signalling molecules are membrane-bound proteins that can interact with receptors on adjacent cells (Figure 5.2D).

Most types of animal cell have a characteristic set of high-affinity receptors allowing them to respond to a range of signalling molecules. The effect of some signalling molecules varies depending on the cell type they encounter. For example, acetylcholine increases the contraction of skeletal muscle but decreases the contraction force of heart muscle and thereby the heart rate. Cells can also modulate their response to a particular ligand by altering the number of cell-surface receptors for that ligand.

Some chemical signalling mechanisms are rapid and transient. Examples include insulin secretion in response to raised blood glucose levels and neurotransmission, a process that is even faster than insulin secretion. Some signalling processes are slow in onset and long-lasting such as estradiol production by the ovaries at the onset of puberty.

Many signalling molecules are required just to allow the cell to survive and further signalling molecules are required to enable the cell to proliferate. When deprived of survival signalling molecules, cells may undergo programmed cell death (apoptosis).

SIGNALLING MOLECULES

The binding of ligands to receptors leads to increases or decreases in the concentration of second-messenger molecules such as cyclic adenosine monophosphate (cAMP), cyclic guanosine monophosphate (cGMP), diacylglycerol, inositol trisphosphate (IP_3) and Ca^{2+}. These in turn modify various cell functions.

Inositol trisphosphate and diacylglycerol

IP_3 and diacylglycerol are produced through hydrolysis of inositol phospholipids (phosphoinositides), which are mainly located in the inner half of the plasma membrane. The inositol phospholipid known as phosphatidyl bisphosphate (PIP_2) is the most important member of this class of lipids in terms of cell signalling, even though it accounts for less than 10% of the total inositol lipids and less than 1% of all the phospholipids in the cell membrane. The breakdown of PIP_2 starts with the binding of a signalling molecule to its receptor in the plasma membrane. The activated receptor stimulates a guanine-nucleotide-binding protein (G protein) known as G_q, which in turn activates an inositide-specific phospholipase C called phospholipase C-β. This enzyme cleaves PIP_2 into two products (Figure 5.3):

- IP_3
- diacylglycerol.

These two molecules act as mediators for separate signalling pathways.

IP_3 is small and water-soluble. It diffuses into the cytosol, where it binds to and opens IP_3-gated Ca^{2+} release channels in the endoplasmic reticulum (Figure 5.3) or, in muscle cells, ryanodine receptors in the sarcoplasmic reticulum. In fact, in many cell types both forms of Ca^{2+} receptors are present. To end the Ca^{2+} response, Ca^{2+} is pumped back out of the cytosol and IP_3 is broken down by phosphatases within the cell.

Some of the IP_3 is also phosphorylated to form inositol tetrakisphosphate (IP_4), which may promote the refilling of the intracellular Ca^{2+} stores and/or mediate slower or longer-lived responses within the cell.

Diacylglycerol remains attached to the plasma membrane and has two potential fates. First, it can be cleaved to give arachidonic acid, which can be used as a precursor in the synthesis of eicosanoids. Second, and more importantly, it can act as a second messenger. The initial rise in Ca^{2+} brought about by IP_3 causes an enzyme called protein kinase C (C because it is Ca^{2+}-dependent) to move from the cytosol to the plasma membrane, where it is activated by diacylglycerol (Figure 5.3).

Protein kinase C is a serine/threonine protein kinase that regulates the function of other proteins by phosphorylating their serine and/or threonine residues. In addition, protein kinase C can alter the transcription of specific genes. In one pathway, the enzyme catalyses the

FIGURE 5.3 **Phospholipase C signalling pathway**

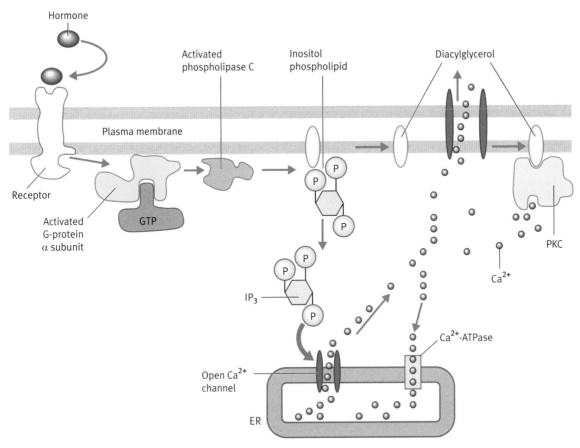

ER = endoplasmic reticulum | GTP = guanosine triphosphate | IP$_3$ = inositol trisphosphate | P = phosphate group | PKC = protein kinase C

phosphorylation of mitogen-activated protein (MAP) kinase, which in turn phosphorylates and activates the transcription factor Elk-1. Together with another protein (the serum response factor), Elk-1 binds to the serum response element, a short DNA sequence in the promoter region of the target gene. This leads to transcription of the gene. In another pathway, activation of protein kinase C results in the release of nuclear factor kappa B, which moves into the nucleus also to activate the transcription of specific genes.

As diacylglycerol is rapidly metabolised, sustained activation of protein kinase C for longer-term responses depends on a second wave of diacylglycerol production. This time, diacylglycerol is released by phospholipase-mediated cleavage of phosphatidylcholine, the major phospholipid in the cell.

Eicosanoids

Eicosanoids are signalling molecules that are continuously made in the plasma membrane of all mammalian tissues. They are synthesised from 20-carbon fatty acid chains (mainly arachidonic acid), which in turn are cleaved from membrane phospholipids by phospholipases. There are four major groups of eicosanoids:

- prostaglandins
- prostacyclins
- thromboxanes
- leucotrienes.

The first three are collectively known as prostanoids. The generation of prostanoids is catalysed by the enzyme prostaglandin H$_2$ synthase, also known as cyclooxygenase

(COX), whereas formation of leucotrienes occurs via a lipoxygenase pathway.

Detailed information on the prostaglandin synthetic pathway is provided in Chapter 6. In the current context, it is important to note that there are two main forms of COX, known as COX-1 and COX-2. These two enzymes have similar functions but are the products of different genes. In general, COX-1 is found in tissues that produce prostaglandins constantly, such as the stomach mucosa, whereas COX-2 is only expressed at sites of inflammation and so is inducible. A third type of COX, COX-3, is formed by alternative splicing of the gene encoding COX-1.

Prostaglandins and leucotrienes are important stimulators of the myometrium during labour (see Chapter 6 for a discussion of the regulation of myometrial contractility). The increase in prostaglandin levels during labour is thought to be caused by induction of COX-2 in fetal membranes. Bacterial products and proinflammatory cytokines can also increase expression of COX-2 and hence prostaglandin synthesis. In addition, high concentrations of prostanoids have been reported during menstruation, in particular in conditions associated with painful menstruation, such as menorrhagia, dysmenorrhoea and endometriosis.

The synthetic pathways of eicosanoids can be targeted by therapeutic drugs. For example, corticosteroid drugs such as cortisone inhibit phospholipase and are used to treat inflammatory conditions such as arthritis. Non-steroidal anti-inflammatory drugs (NSAIDs), including aspirin and ibuprofen, block the first oxidation step of arachidonic acid that is catalysed by COX.

Older NSAIDs such as indometacin inhibit both COX-1 and COX-2. Newer NSAIDs are selective for COX-2. In general, the more COX-2-selective an NSAID is, the better its adverse effect profile. For example, COX-2-selective inhibitors are just as effective in the treatment of menstrual pain as NSAIDs but have fewer gastrointestinal adverse effects.

Aspirin inhibits both COX-1 and COX-2 (it is actually much more active against COX-1 than COX-2; hence its poor adverse effect profile). Unlike most NSAIDs, which are competitive antagonists, aspirin functions by permanently acetylating the active site of the COX enzyme. It can be used at a low dose to inhibit platelet thromboxane synthesis with little effect upon vascular endothelial prostacyclin synthesis. This may be of value in thromboprophylaxis and in the management of pre-eclampsia.

Low doses of aspirin permanently disable platelet COX as the platelets pass through the hepatic portal system. Since the platelet has no nucleus, it cannot synthesise a new supply of COX and so platelet thromboxane synthesis is permanently inhibited. Most of the aspirin is then inactivated within the liver. The small amount of aspirin that then passes into the general circulation may acetylate vascular endothelial COX but, since these cells have a nucleus, they can synthesise a new supply of COX and maintain prostacyclin synthesis.

Nitric oxide and carbon monoxide

Most signalling molecules are hydrophilic molecules but some are small enough to pass straight into the cell where they can directly exert their effects. One such example is the gas nitric oxide (NO). NO is produced from l-arginine by the enzyme NO synthase in the presence of co-factors and O_2; the by-product is l-citrulline. There are three main forms of this enzyme:

- endothelial NO synthase (eNOS)
- inducible NO synthase (iNOS)
- brain NO synthase (bNOS).

These enzyme isoforms are the products of different genes that share about 50–60% sequence homology. Many cells express more than one form of NO synthase.

eNOS was first described in endothelial cells. It is constitutively expressed and is dependent on Ca^{2+} and calmodulin. NO has a very short half-life (5–10 seconds) and is converted to nitrates and nitrites in the blood. Endothelial cells on blood vessels release NO in response to increased shear stress or agents such as acetylcholine. The released NO diffuses to the underlying smooth muscle, where it reacts with iron in the active site of the enzyme guanylate cyclase to produce the intracellular mediator cGMP. The effects of guanylate cyclase are rapid and result in muscle relaxation. Thus, continual release of NO from blood vessels is one of the main mechanisms for keeping blood pressure at its normal level.

In pregnancy, blood pressure falls and it is thought that the associated vasodilation is partly mediated by increased NO release. NO is also important in the regulation of blood flow within the placenta and eNOS is expressed on the entire syncytiotrophoblast surface, just as it is expressed on blood vessels. Placental eNOS is thought to inhibit the aggregation of neutrophils and platelets present in maternal blood in the intervillous space.

The expression of iNOS is induced in response to inflammatory signals such as bacterial cell-wall products, which include lipopolysaccharides and cytokines such as interferon gamma or tumour necrosis factor alpha. It is induced in activated macrophages and neutrophils. NO released from these cells helps them to kill invading microorganisms. The activity of iNOS is independent of Ca^{2+} and calmodulin.

bNOS was first described in the brain. Like eNOS, it is constitutively expressed and is dependent on Ca^{2+} and calmodulin for activity.

NO is released by many types of nerve cell to convey signals to neighbouring cells. For example, NO released by autonomic nerves in the penis causes local blood-vessel dilatation resulting in penile erection. In reproductive biology, NO has also been implicated in the control of myometrial quiescence, in the onset of labour and in cervical ripening, although the evidence for some of these functions is certainly not conclusive.

The effects of NO on blood vessels also explain the efficacy of glyceryl trinitrate in the treatment of angina, for which it has been used for nearly 100 years. Glyceryl trinitrate is converted to NO, which relaxes blood vessels in the heart. Glyceryl trinitrate has also been used in an attempt to prevent preterm labour by relaxing myometrial smooth muscle and to ripen the cervix.

Carbon monoxide (CO) is another gas that stimulates guanylate cyclase. CO is produced by the enzymes haem oxygenase 1 and 2. Haem oxygenase 1 is inducible, while haem oxygenase 2 is constitutively expressed. It is now known that CO, like NO, is important in maintaining vasodilatation in the placenta.

Calcium

Cells maintain low concentrations of free Ca^{2+} (100 nmol/l) despite much higher concentrations in the extracellular fluid (10 mmol/l) and endoplasmic reticulum. Increases in intracellular Ca^{2+} concentrations are one way in which extracellular signals are transmitted across the plasma membrane. When Ca^{2+} channels are transiently opened in the plasma or endoplasmic reticulum membranes, intracellular Ca^{2+} concentrations rise to about 50 micromoles/l and activate Ca^{2+}-responsive proteins in the cell. Resting Ca^{2+} concentrations are kept very low by several means. Ca^{2+}-ATPases in the plasma membrane pump Ca^{2+} out of the cell. Nerve and muscle cells, which use Ca^{2+} to a greater extent for signalling, have an additional Ca^{2+} pump (Na^+,Ca^{2+}-exchanger) in the plasma membrane, which couples Na^+ influx to Ca^{2+} efflux.

In the endoplasmic reticulum, there is yet another Ca^{2+}-ATPase that takes up Ca^{2+} from the cytosol. Mitochondria can also pump Ca^{2+} inside; a low-affinity, high-capacity Ca^{2+} pump in the inner mitochondrial membrane uses the electrochemical gradient generated across the membrane during electron transport in oxidative phosphorylation. This pump only operates when Ca^{2+} levels are extremely high, usually as a consequence of cell damage. Ca^{2+}-binding proteins in the cytoplasm and in the endoplasmic reticulum offer additional Ca^{2+} buffering capacity.

Calmodulin is a Ca^{2+}-binding protein found in all eukaryotic cells. It mediates many Ca^{2+}-regulated processes and undergoes a conformational change when bound to Ca^{2+}. When this happens, the Ca^{2+}–calmodulin complex can bind to various target proteins and alter their activity. Among the Ca^{2+}–calmodulin targets are various enzymes (such as eNOS and bNOS) and membrane transport proteins. Most effects of Ca^{2+}–calmodulin are, however, indirect and are mediated by Ca^{2+}–calmodulin-dependent protein kinases; an example for such an enzyme is myosin light chain kinase, which activates smooth muscle contraction.

Two pathways of Ca^{2+} signalling have been well defined. One is used mainly by excitable cells. When nerve-cell membranes are depolarised by an action potential, voltage-gated Ca^{2+} channels open and Ca^{2+} enters the cell, leading to the secretion of neurotransmitters. In the other pathway, binding of extracellular signalling molecules to cell-surface receptors ultimately leads to the opening of channels in the endoplasmic reticulum and a rise in the intracellular Ca^{2+} concentration.

The opening of these channels is brought about by the intermediate molecule IP_3.

Cyclic adenosine monophosphate

cAMP is synthesised from ATP by the plasma-membrane-bound enzyme adenylate cyclase (also known as adenylyl cyclase) and is rapidly and continually destroyed by cAMP phosphodiesterases. cAMP-mediated phosphory-lation and dephosphorylation can increase or decrease the activity of many different enzymes. The effects of cAMP are mediated via activation of cAMP-dependent protein kinases (also known as protein kinases A).

The cellular response to cAMP varies depending on the cell type. For example, increased cAMP levels in the liver stimulate glycogen breakdown; in adipocytes they stimulate the production of fatty acids and in ovarian cells they induce the formation of estradiol and progesterone.

Cyclic guanosine monophosphate

The synthesis of cGMP is catalysed by guanylate cyclase, which converts guanosine triphosphate (GTP) to cGMP. Membrane-bound guanylate cyclase is activated by peptide hormones such as atrial natriuretic peptide, while soluble guanylate cyclase is activated by NO to stimulate cGMP synthesis.

cGMP relaxes smooth muscle. It also activates protein kinase G enabling it to phosphorylate a number of substrates.

cGMP is degraded by phosphodiesterases. Sildenafil (Viagra®; Pfizer, New York, NY, USA) enhances the vasodilatory effects of cGMP by inhibiting phosphodiesterase 5.

CELL-SURFACE RECEPTORS

Cell-surface receptors belong to one of four major classes. Each will be discussed in detail.

G-protein-coupled receptors

Ligand binding to a G-protein-coupled receptor activates a G protein, which in turn activates a target enzyme that either generates a second messenger or modulates an ion channel. In fact, most G proteins regulate the concentrations of the intracellular signalling molecules cAMP or Ca^{2+} by targeting adenylate cyclase or phospholipase C, respectively.

Receptors linked to G proteins comprise the largest family (over 100 members) of cell-surface receptors. They all have a similar structure consisting of a polypeptide chain that threads back and forth through the plasma membrane seven times.

The G proteins themselves are fully known as trimeric GTP-binding regulatory proteins. They are called trimeric because they are made up of alpha, beta and gamma subunits. The nature of the alpha subunit determines the action of the G protein. For example, stimulatory G proteins (G_s proteins) have an alpha s subunit that activates adenylate cyclase, resulting in the production of cAMP; inhibitory G proteins (G_i proteins) have an alpha i subunit that inhibits adenylate cyclase and thus blocks the production of cAMP; G_q proteins have an alpha q subunit that activates phospholipase C, thereby triggering the production of the second messengers IP_3 and diacylglycerol.

The detailed mechanism of G protein activation is shown in Figure 5.4 using adenylate cyclase activation as an example. The inactive G_s protein is bound to the inside surface of the cell membrane and the alpha unit binds guanosine diphosphate (GDP). When a ligand binds to the receptor, the conformation of the receptor is altered, exposing a binding site for the G_s protein. Assembly of the ligand–receptor–G_s protein complex is brought about by diffusion of the subunits within the membrane and results in the alpha subunit switching its affinity from GDP to GTP.

Binding of GTP instead of GDP causes the dissociation of the alpha subunit from the beta and gamma subunits and this in turn exposes the alpha subunit's binding site for adenylate cyclase. The alpha subunit now binds to and activates adenylate cyclase, resulting in the conversion of ATP to cAMP.

When the ligand dissociates, the receptor returns to its original conformation. The alpha subunit will eventually hydrolyse the attached GTP to GDP by its inherent enzymatic activity, allowing the alpha subunit to reassociate with the beta and gamma subunits so that the system returns to the original inactivated state.

FIGURE 5.4 **G-protein-coupled activation of adenylate cyclase**

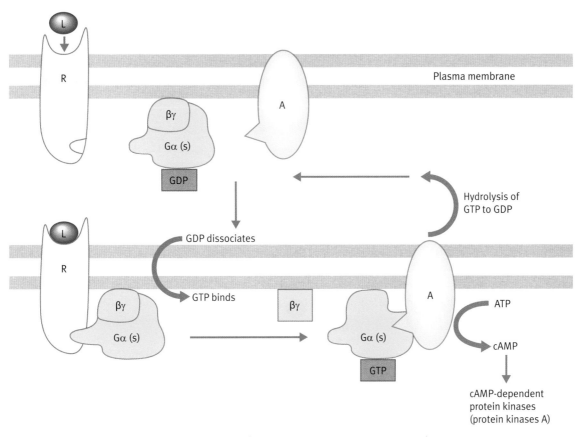

A = adenylate cyclase | βγ = beta and gamma subunits of a G protein | cAMP = cyclic adenosine monophosphate |
Gα (s) = alpha subunit of a stimulatory G protein | GDP = guanosine diphosphate | GTP = guanosine triphosphate |
L = ligand | R = receptor

Many hormones, neurotransmitters and local mediators (for example epinephrine, serotonin and glucagon) signal through G-protein-coupled receptors. In some cases, the same ligand can stimulate or inhibit cAMP production depending on the receptor to which it binds. For example, when adrenaline binds to beta-adrenergic receptors, it activates adenylate cyclase; by contrast, binding to alpha-2-adrenergic receptors inhibits the enzyme. This is because beta-adrenergic and alpha-2-adrenergic receptors are coupled to different G proteins, the former to G_s and the latter to G_i.

Several bacterial toxins also act via G-protein-coupled receptors. Cholera toxin is an enzyme that alters the alpha subunit of G_s so that it can no longer hydrolyse GTP. The constitutive stimulation of adenylate cyclase results in the prolonged production of cAMP in intestinal epithelial cells, causing a large efflux of Na^+ and

H_2O and leading to the symptoms of severe diarrhoea that are characteristic of cholera.

Pertussis toxin (produced by the bacterium *Bordetella pertussis*, which colonises the respiratory tract and causes whooping cough) alters the alpha i subunit to prevent its interaction with G-protein-coupled receptors, so that the subunit cannot inhibit adenylate cyclase. This increases cAMP concentration and thus affects normal cellular signalling. It is not known whether this contributes to the cough itself but it does facilitate adherence to the tracheal epithelium.

Ion channel receptors

Ligand binding to an ion channel receptor changes the conformation of the receptor (Figure 5.5 A). This allows specific ions to flow through the receptor, thus altering

FIGURE 5.5 **Cell-surface receptors**

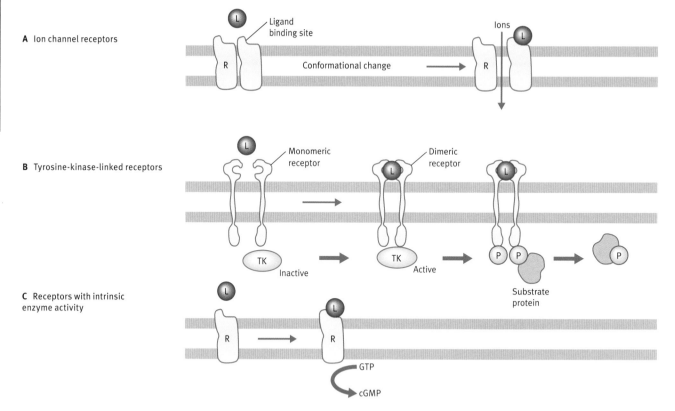

cGMP = cyclic guanosine monophosphate | GTP = guanosine triphosphate | L = ligand | P = phosphate group | R = receptor | TK = tyrosine kinase

the electric potential across the membrane. An example of this type of receptor is the acetylcholine receptors at nerve–muscle junctions.

Tyrosine-kinase-linked receptors

Ligand binding to a tyrosine-kinase-linked receptor results in the formation of a receptor dimer from two monomeric receptors (Figure 5.5B). The cytosolic portion of the dimeric transmembrane receptor then binds to, and activates, the cytosolic enzyme tyrosine kinase. The activated tyrosine kinase in turn phosphorylates tyrosine residues in the receptor. As a result, substrate proteins that bind to the phosphotyrosine residues are phosphorylated.

Tyrosine-kinase-linked receptors are also known as the superfamily of cytokine receptors, with ligands including erythropoietin and the interferons.

Receptors with intrinsic enzyme activity

The fourth group of cell-surface receptors are those that have their own intrinsic enzyme activity in their cytosolic domain (Figure 5.5C). Again, ligand binding tends to induce dimerisation of the receptor. One example is the enzyme guanylate cyclase, which generates the second messenger cGMP. Another example is receptors with intrinsic tyrosine kinase activity. The latter example includes some receptors for growth factors, such as nerve growth factor and platelet-derived growth factor, and the receptor for insulin.

An important downstream signalling molecule that is activated through receptor tyrosine kinases is the GTP-binding protein Ras. Ras belongs to the same superfamily of intracellular switch proteins as does the alpha subunit of G proteins. However, while the alpha subunit acts as part of a trimeric protein, Ras is a monomeric

GTPase. Activation of Ras induces a kinase cascade that ends in the activation of MAP kinase. This serine/threonine kinase can enter the nucleus, where it phosphorylates many proteins including transcription factors.

Cell–cell adhesion

In multicellular organisms, many cells have the ability to connect with each other tightly for the purpose of communication. A number of integral membrane proteins called cell adhesion molecules enable cells to adhere to each other and to the extracellular matrix. We will see later that cells are also able to interact with each other and communicate locally via specialised cell junctions.

The major classes of cell adhesion molecules are cadherins, immunoglobulins, selectins and integrins.

CADHERINS

Cadherins cause adhesion via homophilic (self–self) binding to other cadherins in a Ca^{2+}-dependent manner. Cadherins hold cells together, enable the segregation of cell collectives into discrete tissues during development, maintain tissue integrity and are expressed in a temporal and spatial manner during embryonic development. Most cadherins function as transmembrane linker proteins, with the cytoplasmic domain interacting with the cytoskeleton (actin and intermediate filaments) of the cells they join together.

IMMUNOGLOBULIN-LIKE MOLECULES

Immunoglobulin-like adhesion molecules comprise a large group of molecules that are generated from a comparably small number of genes by alternative splicing. Collectively, they have both homophilic and heterophilic binding properties. The best-studied members of this group are the neural cell adhesion molecules (NCAMs), which are expressed predominantly in nervous tissue, and the intercellular cell adhesion molecules (ICAMs) 1, 2 and 3. This family also includes platelet endothelial cell adhesion molecule 1 (PECAM-1) and vascular cell adhesion molecule 1 (VCAM-1).

INTEGRINS

Integrins are a diverse and large group of heterodimeric glycoproteins. The two subunits, alpha and beta, both participate in binding. Integrins participate in cell–cell adhesion and facilitate communication between the cytoskeleton and the extracellular matrix, allowing each to influence the orientation and structure of the other. Events such as clustering of integrins activate a number of intracellular signalling pathways.

Some integrins exist in active and inactive states. For example, a group of integrins responsible for the binding of white blood cells to the endothelium are normally inactive, allowing the leucocytes to circulate freely. In response to inflammatory mediators, these integrins become activated and mediate a process termed extravasation or diapedesis (Figure 5.6). Defects in the expression of certain integrins can result in diseases characterised by abnormal inflammatory responses.

SELECTINS

The selectins (E-, P- and L-selectin) are primarily expressed by leucocytes and endothelial cells and, like integrins, they are important in many host-defence mechanisms involving those cells. In contrast to other cell adhesion molecules, selectins bind to carbohydrate residues located on the cell surface and the resulting binding forces are relatively weak.

Figure 5.6 illustrates how cell adhesion molecules allow the endothelium and circulating cells in the bloodstream to signal to each other. Shown is the fate of a circulating neutrophil that has been attracted by interleukin-8 released from a site of inflammation. Selectin-mediated interactions result in the formation of weak (transitory) bonds between the neutrophil and endothelial cells, promoting the rolling of the white blood cell along the endothelium towards the site of inflammation. Integrins expressed at the site of inflammation bind more tightly to the neutrophil and stop it in place, while ICAM-1 helps secure the adhesion to the endothelium. As a result, the cell leaves the bloodstream via the endothelium and moves into the inflamed tissue, where it can release leucotrienes (to cause

FIGURE 5.6 **Leucocyte diapedesis**

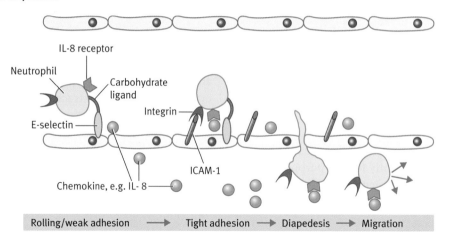

ICAM-1 = intercellular cell adhesion molecule 1 | IL-8 = interleukin-8

vasoconstriction and increase vascular permeability), free radicals and proteases as part of the inflammatory response.

Cell junctions

Cells are also able to interact with each other and communicate locally via specialised cell junctions. There are four major classes of junctions:

- tight junctions
- adherens junctions and desmosomes
- hemidesmosomes
- gap junctions.

The former three are adhering junctions, whereas gap junctions are communicating junctions.

Tight junctions essentially form an impermeable seal between two cells. In the gastrointestinal tract, tight junctions prevent the escape of digestive enzymes from the lumen into the intracellular space.

Adherens junctions and desmosomes bind the plasma membrane of adjacent cells at various spots, which gives strength and rigidity to the entire tissue.

Hemidesmosomes are junctions that connect a cell's intermediate filaments to the underlying extracellular matrix. These junctions firmly anchor epithelial cells, thereby increasing the rigidity of epithelial tissues.

Gap junctions are specialised cell–cell junctions that are formed from a mirror image of protein units (connexons) located in the plasma membranes of two cells. As a result, the cytoplasms of these cells are connected by narrow water-filled channels. These channels allow passage of small signalling molecules, such as Ca^{2+} and cAMP, but not of large molecules such as proteins.

In the myometrium, gap junctions provide low-resistance pathways between smooth muscle cells, thereby increasing their electrical coupling to allow increased coordination of myometrial contractility. During pregnancy, gap junctions are present at very low numbers in the myometrium; however, labour is associated with an increase in the number and size of gap junctions. This has led to the idea that gap junctions are essential, but not sufficient, for effective labour and delivery.

Cell cycle, cell growth and division and cancer

CELL DIVISION

To know when to divide, cells use their own internal clock known as the cell cycle (Figure 5.7). During each cycle, a series of events occurs in an orderly sequence. DNA is duplicated during the synthesis phase (S phase).

64

FIGURE 5.7 **Cell cycle and cell cycle checkpoints**

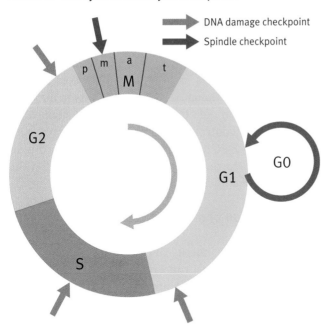

a = anaphase | G0 = quiescent phase | G1 = gap 1 | G2 = gap 2 |
m = metaphase | M = mitosis | p = prophase | S = synthesis phase |
t = telophase

The two DNA copies are then moved to opposite ends of the cell. Halving of the genome is called mitosis (M phase).

Mitosis is divided into several stages:

- During prophase the chromosomes condense.
- During metaphase sister chromatids produced by DNA replication during the S phase become aligned in the centre of the cell.
- During anaphase the sister chromatids separate and move to opposite poles of the mitotic apparatus/ spindle.
- During telophase the nuclear envelope breaks down and reforms around the segregated chromosomes. The final physical division of the cytoplasm to yield two daughter cells is called cytokinesis.

The period between M and S is called gap 1 (G1). The period between S and M is called gap 2 (G2). Both gap phases allow time for cell growth. The gaps also enable the cells to monitor the internal and external environment before committing to the S phase and then to mitosis. Nondividing cells exit the cell cycle and enter the quiescent state (G0).

CELL CYCLE CONTROL

Progress through the cell cycle involves important checkpoints (Figure 5.7):

- DNA damage checkpoints detect DNA damage before and during the S phase. If damage is detected, the activity of a protein called cyclin-dependent kinase 2 (CDK2) is inhibited and progression through the cell cycle is stopped. If the damage to the DNA is not repairable (for example using the DNA repair proteins BRCA1 and BRCA2), the cell undergoes apoptosis.
- Spindle checkpoints check that spindle fibres attach to kinetochores. If any fibres fail to attach, apoptosis occurs.

Several proteins have a key role in the regulation of the cell cycle. For example, a protein called adenomatous polyposis coli (APC) activates a transcription factor known as Myc, which induces the transcription of a number of genes for movement from G1 to the S phase of the cell cycle.

The protein p53 can detect DNA damage and inhibit the cell cycle by blocking CDK2. In addition, p53 has a key role in apoptosis.

Finally, the protein ataxia telangiectasia mutated (ATM) also detects DNA damage and stops the cell cycle (with help from p53) if required. In addition, ATM maintains normal telomere length, thereby counteracting the tendency of the chromosome to shorten with each round of replication.

DEVELOPMENT OF CANCER

Multiplication of cells is tightly regulated. It exceeds cell death in children so that they can increase in size to become adults. In adulthood, the half-life of cells varies a lot depending on the function of the cell. For example, intestinal cells have a half-life of a few days before being renewed, red blood cells have a half-life of about 100 days, liver cells rarely die and brain cells are slowly lost over a lifetime with no or very little renewal.

If the regulatory mechanisms that control cell growth and apoptosis break down, a clone of cells (tumour) can begin to appear in an area where this is not wanted. There are over 200 types of human cancer:

- Carcinomas are derived from endoderm or ectoderm.
- Sarcomas are derived from mesoderm.
- Leukaemias are a class of sarcomas that grow as individual cells in the blood.

Oncogenes and tumour suppressors

The types of protein involved in normal cell growth that can lead to cancer when mutated are as follows (Figure 5.8 provides an overview of these proteins):

- Growth factors or their receptors, signal transduction proteins and transcription factors can acquire gain-of-function mutations that turn the affected gene (the proto-oncogene) into an oncogene. Mutated oncogene alleles are usually dominant.
- Cell cycle control proteins usually act as tumour repressors and loss-of-function mutations in these proteins can make it more likely that a cell becomes a tumour cell. Mutated tumour repressor alleles tend to be recessive.

Virus-encoded proteins can also cause cancer by acting on growth factor receptors.

FIGURE 5.8 **Proteins involved in cell growth and cancer development**

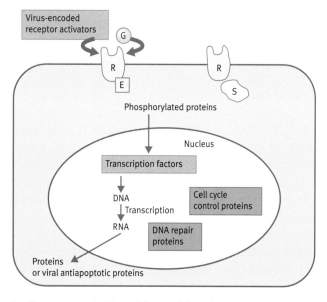

E = effector, e.g. tyrosine kinase | G = growth factor |
R = growth-factor receptor | S = signal transduction protein

Over 50% of cancers have mutations in the tumour suppressor protein p53, rendering p53 unable to function. This allows faulty mutant cells to continue through the cell cycle and to escape apoptosis. Both *p53* alleles must be mutated for the function of the protein to fail.

APC also acts as a tumour suppressor protein. Absence of a functional APC protein results in inappropriate activation of the transcription factor Myc, resulting in uncontrolled cell proliferation. Again, both alleles of the *APC* gene must be mutated for this to occur, as one normal copy of the gene can result in the production of sufficient APC protein.

Transformation of a normal cell into a cancer cell

Some individuals inherit cancer-causing mutations in the germline, but most cancers are caused by mutations in somatic cells (any cell other than a germ cell) and such mutations usually accumulate over years. The accumulation of a few right up to perhaps 20 mutations may be required to start off a cancer; hence, cancer is often a disease of the aged.

The example of colorectal cancer illustrates this point. Individuals with an inherited *APC* mutation are at increased risk of developing colorectal cancer. However, APC only has a role in the first stage of the development of cancer, namely the development of colorectal polyps. If the tumour is removed at the polyp stage, the prognosis is good. If not, polyp cells can accumulate further mutations starting with mutation of *Ras* into an oncogene and followed by other changes including loss of function of a tumour suppressor protein called defective in sister chromatid cohesion (DCC) and loss of function of p53. Another common genetic lesion in colorectal cancer involves mutations in the so-called mismatch repair proteins, which have a role in DNA repair.

This example shows that lesions in a single gene are generally not transforming. Instead, transformation usually involves the suppression of apoptosis followed by a series of other events that eventually lead to malignancy.

Oncogenic viruses

Some viruses can cause cancer by subverting normal cell control mechanisms. At some point in evolution, these viruses have incorporated normal cellular proto-oncogenes into their genome, and these proto-oncogenes have subsequently been mutated to become oncogenes. For example, the Harvey sarcoma virus contains the *Ha-ras* gene, which differs from the human *Ras* gene by the presence of a single point mutation. Over-expression of *Ha-ras* has been identified in human bladder tumours.

Another example is the viral Src (v-Src) protein produced by Rous sarcoma virus (Src is short for sarcoma). This protein is a constitutively active mutant of the cellular Src (c-Src) protein, a protein tyrosine kinase that, like Ras, is involved in signal transduction. The v-Src protein is produced at much higher levels than c-Src and continuously and inappropriately phosphorylates a number of target proteins.

Retroviruses such as Harvey sarcoma virus and Rous sarcoma virus contain an RNA genome. In a host cell, they first hijack the cell's replication process to make a DNA copy of their own viral RNA. The DNA is then inserted into the cell's chromosomal DNA, giving rise to the replication of the viral genome and the production of viral proteins, including oncogenes.

Many DNA viruses also contain oncogenes and, unlike retroviruses, they need the oncogenes for their own survival. Examples include the family of human papillomaviruses, which cause genital warts and other benign tumours of epithelial cells.

TUMOUR GROWTH AND SPREAD

Growth properties of cancer cells

Cancer cells are usually less well differentiated than normal cells and may start to lose their specific functions and instead exhibit features of rapidly growing cells. They can exist in one of three states:

- They go constantly through the cell cycle.
- They are in a quiescent state (G0), able to re-enter the cell cycle at any time.
- They are no longer able to divide but continue to contribute to the size of the tumour.

Drugs such as cisplatin, which belongs to the family of platinum compounds, only affect dividing cells. However, in some tumours, such cells may constitute as little

as 5% of the total tumour mass. Cisplatin does not affect the ability of tumour cells to spread and is indiscriminate in affecting all rapidly dividing cells; hence its associated adverse effects such as hair loss, nausea and suppression of bone marrow function. The drug has to be given at a dose that still allows enough normal cells to survive so the treated person can recover.

Metastasis

Tumours that do not spread are benign; an example would be a wart. An important feature of malignancy is the ability to spread. The process of spreading and establishment in secondary sites is called metastasis.

Metastatic cells break their adhesive contacts with other cells and are also able to overcome the movement restraint provided by the basal lamina (basement membrane). The basal lamina is a fibrous network of collagens and proteoglycans that support epithelial and other cells. Many tumour cells secrete plasminogen activator, which in turn converts plasminogen to the active protease plasmin.

Plasmin then digests the basal lamina allowing some of the tumour cells to enter and travel in the bloodstream.

To colonise another site, the tumour cell must attach to the endothelium at the site of metastasis and migrate across it to the tissue below. Fewer than 1 in 10 000 cancer cells that escape into the bloodstream survive. Those that do have acquired many new characteristics that allow them to grow in a tissue from which they did not originate.

Paradoxically, a number of primary tumours can secrete substances that inhibit metastasis of secondary tumours. In these cases, removal of the primary tumour can actually promote the metastatic process.

Angiogenesis

To grow beyond a mass of about 2 mm in diameter (about 10^6 cells), a tumour requires a blood supply or it will not be able to sustain further growth. Many tumours therefore release growth factors such as vascular endothelial growth factor (VEGF), basic fibroblast growth factor or transforming growth factor alpha. These growth factors can stimulate a process known as angiogenesis.

Angiogenesis involves degradation of the basement membrane of an adjacent capillary, migration of the endothelial cells towards the tumour and ultimately the formation of a new capillary that can supply nutrients to the tumour.

Current cancer research includes the search for treatments that can stop angiogenesis. Approaches include:

- blocking signals from the tumour; for example, the drug bevacizumab is approved to treat colon cancer by intercepting VEGF signals
- blocking VEGF receptors on endothelial cells
- using small-molecule drugs that can get inside endothelial cells and interfere with tyrosine kinase
- targeting the enzymes that clear the pathway for blood vessels to extend
- targeting oncogenes to prevent angiogenesis from starting.

DNA, RNA, the genetic code and protein synthesis

DNA contains all the information required to build the entire body. During transcription, DNA is copied into RNA, which has three roles in protein synthesis. Messenger RNA (mRNA) carries the message from DNA and specifies the correct order of amino acids during protein synthesis. Next, during translation, the amino acids are assembled into proteins. This requires the help of transfer RNA (tRNA), which interprets the message on the mRNA, and of ribosomal RNA (rRNA).

STRUCTURE OF DNA AND RNA

DNA and RNA are very similar in structure. Both are made up of nucleotides, which have three components:

- a nitrogen-containing base, which is either a purine or a pyrimidine; in DNA, the four bases are adenine, guanine, thymine and cytosine; in RNA, uracil replaces thymine; adenine and guanine are purines and consist of a pair of fused nitrogen-containing rings, whereas cytosine, thymine and uracil are pyrimidines and consists of a single nitrogen-containing ring.

- a five-carbon sugar (pentose); in RNA the sugar is a ribose, whereas in DNA the sugar is a deoxyribose
- a phosphate group linked to the pentose by a phosphodiester bond.

Each nucleotide has two distinctive ends: a 5-prime end, where a phosphate group is attached to carbon atom number 5 of the sugar ring, and a 3-prime end, where a hydroxyl group is attached to carbon atom number 3 of the sugar.

DNA molecules can contain up to several hundred million nucleotides. Figure 5.9 shows how the nucleotides link together to form nucleic acids.

DNA consists of two polynucleotide strands wound together to form a double helix. The two strands in the DNA backbone run antiparallel to each other: one of the DNA strands is built in the 5-prime to 3-prime direction, while the other runs in the opposite direction. The two sugar–phosphate backbones are on the outside of the double helix and the base pairs are on the inside.

The strands are held together through base pairing between the two strands. Adenine always pairs with thymine through two weak hydrogen bonds and cytosine always pairs with guanine through three weak hydrogen bonds. When two strands are paired as shown in Figure 5.9 they are said to be complementary.

By contrast, RNA can be fewer than 100 to thousands of nucleotides long and is usually single-stranded.

DNA SYNTHESIS

DNA replication begins with the unwinding of the DNA double helix by proteins called helicases, which break the hydrogen bonds. The junction between the unwound part and the open part is called a replication fork (Figure 5.10).

One of the template strands is the leading strand. DNA polymerase adds the complementary nucleotides and binds the sugars and phosphates. It follows the helicase as it unwinds and continuously forms new DNA. The leading strand is oriented in the 3-prime to 5-prime direction and DNA polymerase travels from the 5-prime to the 3-prime end of the new strand. It cannot add nucleotides in the opposite direction.

The other side of the ladder is the lagging strand, oriented in the 5-prime to 3-prime direction. DNA

FIGURE 5.9 **Structure of DNA**

A Building blocks of DNA

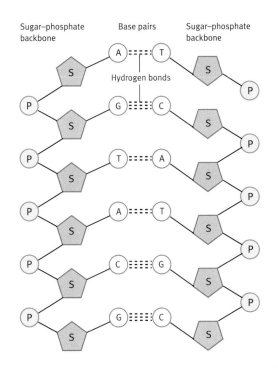

B DNA double helix

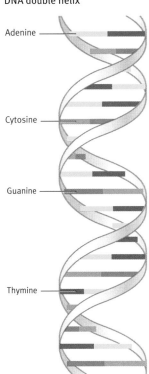

A = adenine | C = cytosine | G = guanine | P = phosphate group | S = sugar molecule | T = thymine

FIGURE 5.10 **DNA replication at a replication fork**

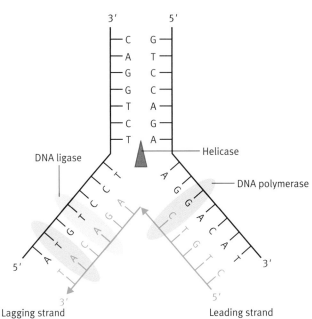

A = adenine | C = cytosine | G = guanine | T = thymine

polymerase also adds complementary nucleotides on this side but it is now travelling in the opposite direction (moving away from the helicase). As a result, the lagging strand is made in many discontinuous segments rather than continuously as for the leading strand. This process results in the creation of several fragments, called Okazaki fragments, which are then joined together by DNA ligase.

During replication, DNA synthesis occurs simultaneously at many points along the original strand (multiple replication forks). It would take a long time to go from one end of the parent DNA to the other; thus it is more efficient to open up several points at the same time.

RNA SYNTHESIS

To allow the DNA template to be copied into mRNA, the two DNA strands must first unwind (denature). Transcription begins with RNA polymerase binding to

69

the promoter region (upstream of the coding region) in the DNA (Figure 5.11). As in DNA replication, transcription proceeds in the 5-prime to 3-prime direction, but during RNA synthesis uracil replaces thymine. The single DNA strand that is copied to form the new strand is called the template strand and the strand that is not used is called the coding strand. Once the mRNA is released, the DNA strands reanneal.

Transcription can involve many RNA polymerases on a single DNA template, so that many RNA molecules can be produced during copying.

FIGURE 5.11 **Transcription**

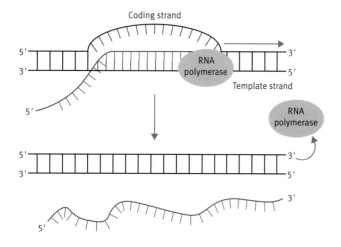

GENE SPLICING

The DNA sequence in genes contains exons (the DNA regions that are being transcribed to the final functional mRNA molecule) and introns (noncoding sequences). Following the production of an identical RNA transcript of the original DNA sequence, the introns are removed by a process known as splicing (Figure 5.12) and the exons are joined together. Although exons can include the sequences that code for amino acids, some exons are also noncoding.

The process of alternative splicing (Figure 5.12) allows a single gene to be translated into multiple proteins that are similar but have their own distinct function, such as targeting a particular cell. For example, alternative splicing of the VEGF transcription product results in the production of a family of VEGF variants that take on various roles in vasculogenesis and angiogenesis.

PROTEIN SYNTHESIS

Proteins are chains of polypeptides, which in turn are chains of amino acids. Amino acids are held together by strong peptide bonds. mRNA contains the code for the amino acid sequence.

To understand translation, it is important to first understand the genetic code (the rules by which mRNA is made,

FIGURE 5.12 **Gene splicing**

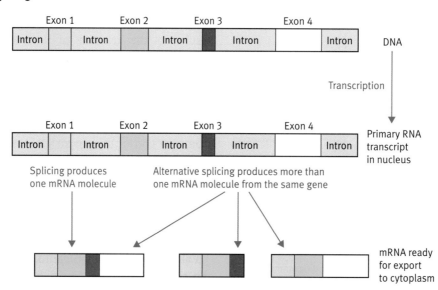

mRNA = messenger RNA

FIGURE 5.13 **Protein synthesis**

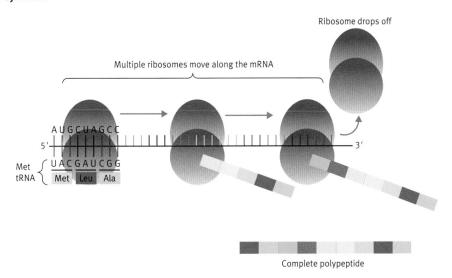

Ribosome drops off

Multiple ribosomes move along the mRNA

AUGCUAGCC

5'   3'

Met
tRNA   UACGAUCGG
       Met | Leu | Ala

Complete polypeptide

A = adenine | Ala = alanine | C = cytosine | G = guanine | Leu = leucine |
Met = methionine | mRNA = messenger RNA; tRNA = transferRNA | U = uracil

or translated, into proteins). Within an mRNA molecule, each triplet of nucleotides is called a codon. Each codon specifies an amino acid. The code is degenerate, meaning that more than one codon can specify the same amino acid but no codon specifies more than one amino acid.

Protein synthesis (translation) also requires tRNA and rRNA. The tRNA deciphers the code, with each amino acid having its own tRNA. One end of the tRNA molecule has a binding site for a particular amino acid and the other side contains the anticodon that can base-pair with the codon. As protein synthesis proceeds, the correct tRNA with its attached amino acid is added to the growing polypeptide chain (Figure 5.13). However, this also requires the help of the ribosome. The ribosome is a multiunit structure containing rRNA and proteins. As the ribosome moves along, the free tRNA that has donated an amino acid leaves the ribosome and is free to receive another amino acid. The next tRNA molecule then adds an amino acid and the polypeptide chain grows. At the end, the complete polypeptide is released and the ribosome drops off. Multiple ribosomes move along the mRNA, so that multiple copies of the polypeptide can be made more quickly.

The sequence of amino acids in a polypeptide chain is called the primary structure of a given protein. The term secondary structure refers to the folding of the polypeptide chain into one of two geometric arrangements, an alpha helix or a beta sheet stabilised by hydrogen bonds. The term tertiary structure refers to the folding of the polypeptide chain into an overall arrangement and this is achieved through hydrophobic interactions and disulphide bonds. The term quaternary structure refers to the arrangement of multiple polypeptide chains (subunits) in multimeric proteins.

POST-TRANSLATIONAL MODIFICATION

After translation, proteins can undergo chemical modification such as the addition of an acetyl group (acetylation), which affects the lifespan of the protein, addition of a phosphate group (phosphorylation), which is used to regulate the activity of a protein, and addition of carbohydrate chains (glycosylation). Many secreted proteins and membrane proteins are glycosylated.

Laboratory techniques

SOUTHERN BLOTTING

Southern blotting (Figure 5.14) is used to detect the presence and amount of a particular sequence of DNA

71

FIGURE 5.14 **Southern blotting**

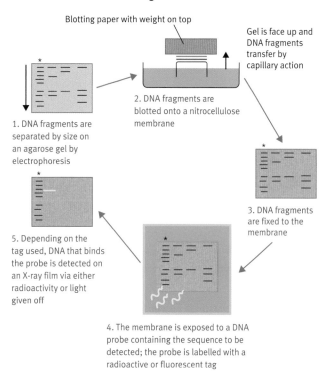

Blotting paper with weight on top

Gel is face up and DNA fragments transfer by capillary action

1. DNA fragments are separated by size on an agarose gel by electrophoresis

2. DNA fragments are blotted onto a nitrocellulose membrane

3. DNA fragments are fixed to the membrane

4. The membrane is exposed to a DNA probe containing the sequence to be detected; the probe is labelled with a radioactive or fluorescent tag

5. Depending on the tag used, DNA that binds the probe is detected on an X-ray film via either radioactivity or light given off

* DNA molecular weight markers

proteins through a gel matrix exposed to an electric current, with smaller proteins travelling faster leading to separation of the proteins) and immunoblotting with a specific antibody raised against the protein of interest.

Tissues are homogenised first to solubilise the proteins. The proteins are then denatured with reducing agents to break disulphide bonds and allow separation by molecular weight. They are also coated in sodium dodecyl sulphate (SDS), which gives them a negative charge.

Once the proteins have been separated and transferred to a membrane, the antibody is added. For example, a typical primary antibody for the detection of COX-1 in myometrial tissue homogenates would be antihuman COX-1 from goat (in other words, human COX-1 protein had been injected into goats to raise antibodies against the human protein). Thereafter, a secondary antibody is added. This could be an antigoat antibody from mouse, rabbit or another species (except goat or human).

The secondary antibody is linked to a radioactive, chromogenic, fluorescent or chemiluminescent tag. For example, if the tag is horseradish peroxidase, addition of a chemiluminescent substrate will result in the emission of light, which can be detected by a photographic film. The stronger the detection signal, the more protein is present.

POLYMERASE CHAIN REACTION

Polymerase chain reaction (PCR) is used to amplify a specific sequence of DNA or RNA, which can be present in a mixture with other DNA or RNA fragments. If RNA rather than DNA is being amplified, it must first be transcribed into complementary DNA (cDNA) by the enzyme reverse transcriptase.

The key ingredients in a PCR reaction are the four nucleotides (adenine, thymine, cytosine and guanine), a heat-stable DNA polymerase called *Taq* polymerase and primers. Primers are short nucleic-acid sequences that are complementary to the template-strand DNA. When the primer sequence is attached to the template strand, the *Taq* polymerase can then continue to add on further nucleotides. With this method, the number of DNA strands grows exponentially.

in a sample that contains many other DNA sequences, such as total cellular DNA. This technique was named after its inventor, Edwin Southern. The names of other blotting methods were chosen in reference to Edwin Southern's surname.

NORTHERN BLOTTING

Northern blotting is a very similar technique. It is used to detect the presence and amount of a particular RNA sequence in a sample containing a mixture of RNA molecules.

WESTERN BLOTTING

Western blotting is used to detect the presence and amount of a specific protein in a tissue sample. This technique employs gel electrophoresis (the movement of

PCR can be used to amplify very small amounts of DNA and has many applications in genetic testing, forensics and scientific research.

DNA MICRORARRAYS

DNA microarrays enable the simultaneous analysis of the expression of thousands of genes. Essentially, a DNA microarray is a collection of thousands of DNA spots (short oligonucleotides) that are bound to a solid surface. These microarrays can be purchased commercially and can be custom-made to include genes belonging to particular gene families that the researcher is interested in looking at.

Expression of the genes of interest can be assayed by synthesising fluorescently labelled cDNA from mRNA that has been isolated from cells exposed to different conditions. For example, a researcher might isolate mRNA from cultured myometrial cells that have been exposed to mechanical stretch and from cultured control cells that have been left untreated. The mRNA from each culture would then be converted into cDNA by reverse transcription. Subsequently, the DNA from each experiment would be labelled with a dye and added to separate microarray plates. That way, the researcher could see which genes in the cells were affected by the mechanical stretch.

BIOINFORMATICS

Bioinformatics is the term used to describe the computer methods for storing, distributing and analysing the huge number of DNA sequences that have been reported.

Several databanks around the world, one of the main ones being GenBank at the National Institutes of Health, USA, store all newly reported DNA sequences and allow scientists from all over the world access via the Internet. Researchers who have sequenced a DNA fragment can enter their sequence into such a databank and determine if their sequence is similar to any other sequences that have already been submitted. If so, and if the function of the encoded protein is already known, this will give them a hint on the function of the DNA they have sequenced. For example, mutations in the

BRCA1 gene convey a high risk of developing breast cancer. When this gene was sequenced and entered into a DNA databank, it was discovered that it was very similar to a yeast gene that produces a cell cycle checkpoint protein.

PROTEOMICS

Proteomics is the large-scale study of proteins and, in particular, their structures and function. The term proteomics was chosen to make an analogy with genomics, the study of genes. After genomics, proteomics is the next step in the study of a biological system.

However, proteomics is far more complex than genomics and provides a more accurate understanding of how the body works. This is primarily because an organism's genome is constant, whereas its proteome (the entire complement of proteins) varies from cell to cell and changes continuously. Protein expression is different in different parts of the body, at different stages of development and under different environmental conditions. On top of this, about 25 000 genes have been identified so far in humans, but there are probably more than 500 000 proteins derived from these genes. This is the result of events such as alternative splicing and post-translational modification (for example glycosylation, phosphorylation). It is also important to note that the level of transcription of a gene does not necessarily reflect the level of expression of the respective protein; mRNA can be degraded rapidly or not translated efficiently, so that large amounts of mRNA can result in only small amounts of protein. Finally, many proteins are only functional if they form complexes with other proteins or RNA molecules. Proteomics therefore also involves the study of protein interactions.

A number of methods are available in the field of proteomics. The traditional method for the study of protein interactions is yeast two-hybrid analysis, which detects physical interactions (such as binding) between two proteins or between a single protein and a DNA molecule. Other methods employed in proteomics include protein microarrays (similar to DNA microarrays).

Proteomics has a crucial role in the development of new drugs. If a protein is thought to be involved in a disease, information on its three-dimensional structure can be used to design drugs that interfere with, or block, the action of the protein. For example, in Alzheimer's disease, elevations in beta-secretase levels result in the creation of beta-amyloid, which is the principal constituent of the brain plaques that are associated with the development of dementia. Drugs targeting the enzyme beta-secretase decrease the production of beta-amyloid and so slow the progression of the disease.

Proteomics is also important in the discovery of disease biomarkers that can be used for diagnostic purposes.

CHAPTER 6

Steroids and prostaglandins

Anthony E Michael

Introduction

Steroids and prostaglandins are both classes of lipid hormones. However, they differ fundamentally in their molecular substrates, synthetic pathways, cellular receptors, mechanisms and speed of action, and physiological responses. The cellular actions of placental steroid hormones and prostaglandins on the myometrium need to be coordinated carefully to ensure timely delivery of the infant at term. This chapter covers these topics and ends with a discussion of the cellular mechanisms underlying the control of myometrial contractions.

Steroid hormones

STEROID SYNTHESIS AND METABOLISM

Origins, transport and metabolism of cholesterol

As shown in Table 6.1, steroid hormones can be broadly classified as:

- corticosteroids (synthesised in the adrenal cortex)
- gonadal steroids (synthesised in the ovary or testis).

All steroid hormones are derived from cholesterol by the sequential removal of carbon groups and addition of oxygen-containing groups (Figure 6.1).

Four major sources of cholesterol are used for steroid hormone biosynthesis:

- *de novo* cholesterol biosynthesis (from acetate)
- plasma membrane

- intracellular lipid droplets (containing cholesteryl esters, such as cholesteryl oleate)
- plasma lipoproteins (primarily low-density lipoprotein cholesterol).

The rate-determining step in the synthesis of steroid hormones is the removal of the 6-carbon side chain from the 27-carbon substrate cholesterol to generate the first 21-carbon steroid, pregnenolone (Figure 6.2). This reaction is catalysed by the cytochrome P450 (CYP)-based cholesterol side chain cleavage enzyme (CYP11A1, previously named $P450_{SCC}$), which is located in the inner mitochondrial membrane facing the matrix. The relevance of this fact is that the lipid substrate cholesterol has to be transported across the

TABLE 6.1 **Classification of steroid hormones**

Class of steroid	Number of carbon atoms	Major physiological example
CORTICOSTEROIDS[a]		
Mineralocorticoids	21	Aldosterone
Glucocorticoids	21	Cortisol
Androgens	19	DHEA
GONADAL STEROIDS[b]		
Progestogens	21	Progesterone
Androgens	19	Testosterone
Estrogens	18	Estradiol

[a] Made in zones of the adrenal cortex | [b] made in the ovary or testis | DHEA = dehydroepiandrosterone

FIGURE 6.1 **Overview of steroid hormone biosynthesis**

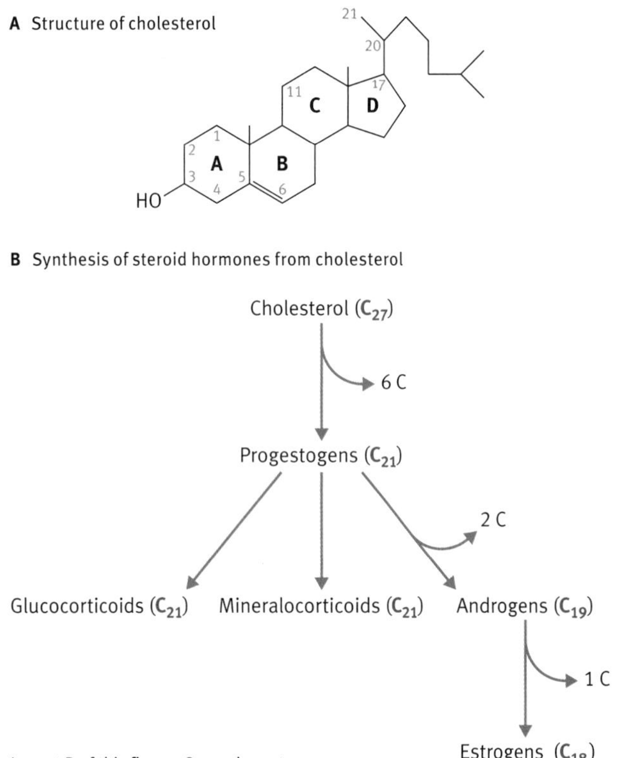

A Structure of cholesterol

B Synthesis of steroid hormones from cholesterol

Cholesterol (C_{27})

6 C

Progestogens (C_{21})

2 C

Glucocorticoids (C_{21})   Mineralocorticoids (C_{21})   Androgens (C_{19})

1 C

Estrogens (C_{18})

In part B of this figure, C = carbon atom

FIGURE 6.2 **Metabolism of cholesterol to pregnenolone**

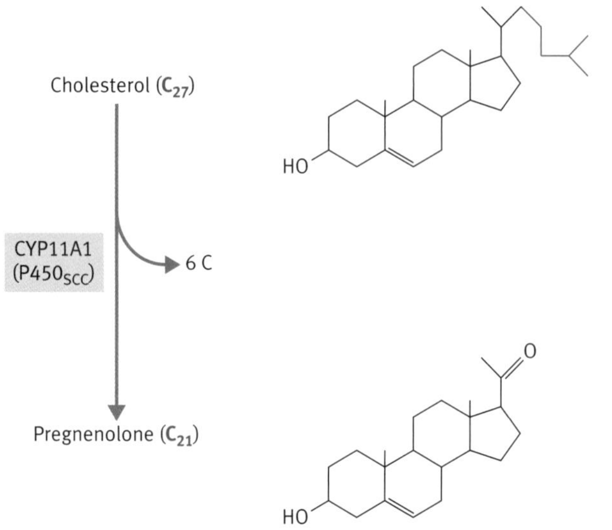

Cholesterol (C_{27})

CYP11A1 (P450$_{scc}$)   6 C

Pregnenolone (C_{21})

C = carbon atom | CYP11A1 (P450$_{scc}$) = cholesterol side chain cleavage enzyme

aqueous space that lies between the outer and the inner mitochondrial membranes. The intracellular trafficking of cholesterol to the CYP11A1 enzyme relies on the actions of:

- steroidogenic acute regulator (StAR) protein
- mitochondrial peripheral benzodiazepine receptors.

Cellular levels of StAR increase following stimulation of steroidogenic cells by luteinising hormone, follicle-stimulating hormone, human chorionic gonadotrophin or adrenocorticotrophic hormone. The StAR protein then acts as a ligand for the mitochondrial peripheral benzodiazepine receptors, which bring the mitochondrial membranes into apposition by activating voltage-dependent anion channels to mediate Cl⁻ efflux from the aqueous intermembrane space.

The significance of StAR in steroidogenesis is underscored in pregnancies complicated by lipoid congenital adrenal hyperplasia. In this condition, failure of StAR in the fetal adrenal glands prevents transport of cholesterol

into the mitochondria of the adrenocortical cells, leading to the accumulation of cholesteryl esters within engorged lipid droplets in the adrenal cortex. As a consequence, the fetal adrenal glands fail to make any of the cortico-steroid hormones. This rare condition is usually lethal *in utero*. If affected infants are delivered, they have problems inflating their lungs (because of the absence of fetal glucocorticoids *in utero*) and enter a salt-wasting crisis (because of the absence of aldosterone).

Steroidogenic enzymes

Although the pathways for steroid biosynthesis seem to be complex, they revolve around just two classes of enzyme:

- CYP enzymes
- hydroxysteroid dehydrogenase (HSD) enzymes.

The function of the CYP enzymes is to catalyse the hydroxylation reactions required to increase the solubility of the steroid hormones in aqueous media (blood, extracellular fluid and urine). In addition, some of the CYP enzymes – specifically CYP11A1 and steroid 17α-hydroxylase (CYP17A or P450$_{c17}$) – also act as lyase enzymes to cleave single carbon bonds.[1] The hydroxylase

FIGURE 6.3 **Operation of steroidogenic enzymes: cytochrome P450 enzymes**

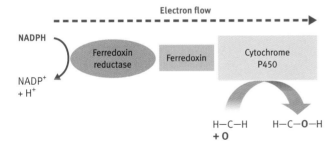

NADP⁺ = oxidised form of nicotinamide adenine dinucleotide phosphate | NADPH = reduced form of NADP

function of CYP enzymes relies on the transport of electrons from the reduced form of the nucleotide co-factor nicotinamide adenine dinucleotide phosphate (NADPH) to the haem centre of the CYP enzyme via ferredoxin reductase and ferredoxin (Figure 6.3).

The HSD enzymes (3β-HSD and 17β-HSD) are oxidoreductase enzymes that belong to the superfamily of short-chain alcohol dehydrogenases. As such, the HSD enzymes catalyse the oxidation of secondary alcohol groups and/or the reduction of ketone groups on steroid hormones at designated carbon positions (Figure 6.4). In addition, 3β-HSD acts as a Δ^5,Δ^4 isomerase to convert the weak steroids pregnenolone and dehydroepiandrosterone to the more potent steroid metabolites progesterone and androstenedione, respectively. During this reaction, the double bond between carbon positions 5 and 6 (signified by the symbol Δ^5) of the steroid B ring is relocated to carbon positions 4 and 5 (signified by the symbol Δ^4) of the A ring (Figure 6.5A). By contrast, the 17β-HSD enzymes act primarily as reductase enzymes,

FIGURE 6.4 **Operation of steroidogenic enzymes: hydroxysteroid dehydrogenase enzymes**

NAD(P)⁺ = oxidised form of nicotinamide adenine dinucleotide (phosphate) | NAD(P)H = reduced form of NAD(P)

FIGURE 6.5 **Steroid metabolism by hydroxysteroid dehydrogenase enzymes**

A 3β-Hydroxysteroiddehydrogenase

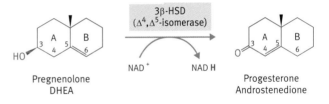

B 17β-Hydroxysteroiddehydrogenase

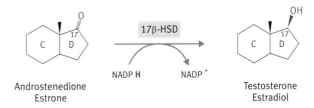

DHEA = dehydroepiandrosterone | HSD = hydroxysteroid dehydrogenase | NAD⁺ = oxidised form of nicotinamide adenine dinucleotide | NADH = reduced form of NAD | NADP⁺ = reduced form of NAD phosphate | NADPH = reduced form of NADP

reducing the ketone at carbon position 17 on androstenedione and estrone to the more potent beta-alcohol group at carbon position 17, characteristic of testosterone and estradiol (Figure 6.5B).

Tissue-specific patterns of steroidogenesis

The pathway of steroid biosynthesis within a given steroidogenic tissue depends on the precise pattern of CYP and HSD expression in that tissue:

- In testis Leydig cells, CYP11A1, CYP17A, 3β-HSD and 17β-HSD act in sequence to synthesise testosterone (Figure 6.6A).
- In the theca cells of ovarian follicles, CYP11A1, CYP17A and 3β-HSD act in sequence to synthesise androstenedione (Figure 6.6B).
- In the follicular granulosa cells, follicle-stimulating hormone upregulates the enzyme aromatase (CYP19 or P450$_{AROM}$), which converts androstenedione from the theca cells into estrone. Estrone can subsequently be reduced by 17β-HSD to the more potent estrogen, estradiol (Figure 6.6C).

FIGURE 6.6 **Tissue-specific steroidogenic pathways**

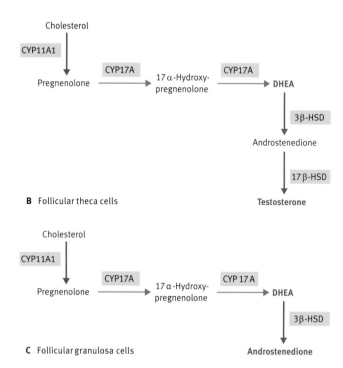

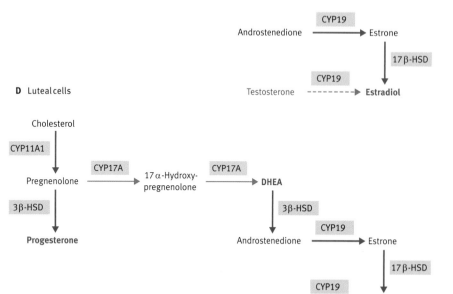

CYP11A1 = cholesterol side chain cleavage enzyme | CYP17A = steroid
17α-hydroxylase | CYP19 = aromatase | DHEA = dehydroepiandrosterone |
HSD = hydroxysteroid dehydrogenase

■ In the steroidogenic cells of the corpus luteum, CYP11A1, 3β-HSD, CYP17A, CYP19 and 17β-HSD are all expressed, enabling the luteal cells to synthesise both progesterone and estradiol (Figure 6.6D).

The pattern of steroid synthesis in the placenta is complicated by the fact that the placenta is an 'incomplete endocrine gland': it lacks the key enzymes required to synthesise the full range of steroid hormones. Most notably, the placenta does not express the CYP17A enzyme necessary to convert progestogens to androgens. As a consequence, for the placenta to synthesise estrogens, it has to work in concert with the fetal adrenal gland and maternal liver, with steroids passing back and forth between the placenta, fetal and maternal circulations. Importantly, 16α-hydroxyandrostenedione secreted from the fetal zone of the fetal adrenal cortex can, in the placenta, be aromatised to estriol, a unique steroid that is synthesised only by the placenta and that can be used as a surrogate marker to assess the functional status of the fetal adrenal gland.

Steroid metabolism and clearance

After their secretion, steroid hormones can undergo extensive metabolism at peripheral sites, including skin, bone and adipose tissue. For example, to induce virilisation of the external genitalia, testosterone must be converted within the genital skin fibroblasts to the androgen metabolite 5α-dihydrotestosterone by the steroid 5α-reductase 2 enzyme. By contrast, to cause closure of the epiphyses of the long bones, testosterone must be metabolised within the bone by CYP19 to generate estradiol, which acts on the epiphyses via the estrogen receptor, rather than the androgen receptor.

To be cleared from the body, steroid hormones have to be rendered more hydrophilic (water-soluble) so that they can pass out into the urine or faeces. This two-step process, catalysed primarily in the liver, typically involves the sequential actions of:

- CYP or HSD enzymes, which create polar hydroxyl (alcohol) groups
- conjugating enzymes (typically glucuronyltransferases or sulphotransferases), which catalyse condensation reactions to add polar or charged chemical groups (such as glucuronides and sulphates, respectively) to the polar hydroxyl/alcohol groups.

STEROID HORMONE ACTIONS

Steroid hormone receptors

Owing to their hydrophobicity, steroid hormones can pass easily through the plasma membrane of target cells and so exert their actions via intracellular receptors that serve as ligand-dependent transcription factors.[2] There are five different steroid hormone receptors, each of which binds a distinct class of steroid hormone with relatively high affinity (Table 6.2).

All steroid hormone receptors are composed of the same four functional domains:

- ligand-binding domain, which binds the steroid hormone in a hydrophobic binding pocket
- DNA-binding domain, which typically comprises a pair of zinc fingers to bind DNA

TABLE 6.2 **Classification of the steroid hormone receptors**

Receptor name	Conventional abbreviation	Physiological ligand
Progesterone receptor	PR	Progesterone
Mineralocorticoid receptor[a]	MR	Aldosterone (and deoxycorticosterone)
Glucocorticoid receptor[b]	GR	Cortisol
Androgen receptor	AR	5α-DHT (and testosterone)
Estrogen receptor	ER	Estradiol (and estrone)

[a] Also referred to as type 1 corticosteroid receptor | [b] also referred to as type 2 corticosteroid receptor | 5α-DHT = 5α-dihydrotestosterone

- dimerisation domain (located within the ligand-binding domain), which facilitates interactions between pairs of activated steroid receptors
- transactivating factor domains, which interact with proteins in the preinitiation transcription complex.

In the vacant state, steroid receptors may reside in either the cytoplasm or the nucleus. Following the binding of a steroid ligand, the activated receptors translocate into the nucleus, where they bind DNA to modulate the transcription of target genes.[2] Steroid receptors always act as molecular dimers, which can either be homodimers (for example glucocorticoid–glucocorticoid receptors) or heterodimers (for example glucocorticoid–progesterone receptors). The dimeric receptors either possess or recruit (via their transactivating domains) enzymes that remodel chromatin in such a way as to either increase or decrease the rate of transcription of the target genes.

Steroid hormone actions

Dimeric receptors bind to DNA at specific nucleotide sequences (termed steroid response elements) that are typically found in the promoter region of the target gene. The dimeric receptors are then able to interact with receptor-interacting proteins, which can act either as co-repressor or as coactivator proteins:

- Co-repressor proteins recruit histone deacetylase enzymes, which remove the acetyl groups from the neighbouring histone proteins. This has the effect of allowing the DNA to remain in the annealed, condensed state, thereby repressing the transcription of the target genes.
- Coactivator proteins recruit histone acetyltransferase enzymes, which exert the opposite action of acetylating the histones to decondense and open the DNA, thereby increasing the rate of gene transcription.

Owing to the complexity of their genomic mode of action, the speed of action of steroid hormones is relatively slow. Typically, it takes steroid hormones anything between 6 hours and several days to effect a change in cellular function by changing the repertoire of genes expressed in the target cell.

Prostaglandins

PROSTAGLANDIN SYNTHESIS AND METABOLISM

Arachidonic acid

All prostaglandins are synthesised from arachidonic acid, a polyunsaturated fatty acid (Figure 6.7).[3] In the cell, this polyunsaturate is typically found esterified to membrane phospholipids. Hence, the simplest way for arachidonic acid to be liberated for prostaglandin synthesis is by the action of phospholipase A_2 on membrane phospholipids to generate free arachidonate and the residual lysophospholipid molecules. The rate-determining cleavage of arachidonate by phospholipase A_2 is inhibited by lipocortin, which is in turn upregulated by the anti-inflammatory glucocorticoid steroids (for example cortisol and dexamethasone).

Cyclooxygenase enzymes

Once liberated, arachidonate is acted upon by the enzyme cyclooxygenase (COX, also called prostaglandin H_2 synthase) to synthesise prostaglandin G_2, an intermediate that is rapidly converted to prostaglandin H_2 (Figure 6.7). There are two forms of COX enzyme:

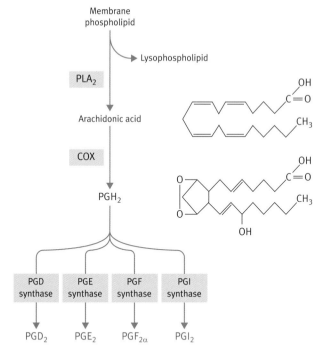

FIGURE 6.7 **Prostaglandin synthesis from membrane phospholipids**

COX = cyclooxygenase | PGD synthase = prostaglandin D synthase | PGD_2 = prostaglandin D_2 | PGE synthase = prostaglandin E synthase | PGE_2 = prostaglandin E_2 | PGF synthase = prostaglandin F synthase | $PGF_{2\alpha}$ = prostaglandin $F_{2\alpha}$ | PGH_2 = prostaglandin H_2 | PGI synthase = prostaglandin I synthase | PGI_2 = prostaglandin I_2 | PLA_2 = phospholipase A_2

- COX-1, a constitutively active isoenzyme
- COX-2, a hormone-responsive/inducible isoenzyme.

Both COX enzymes are inhibited by indometacin and other nonsteroidal anti-inflammatory drugs, such as aspirin.

Prostaglandin synthase enzymes

Once generated by the COX enzymes, prostaglandin H_2 can be metabolised by a range of prostaglandin synthase enzymes to generate various prostaglandins, each with a distinct array of actions. Specifically, prostaglandin H_2 can be acted upon by the prostaglandin D, prostaglandin E, prostaglandin F and prostaglandin I synthases to generate prostaglandin D_2, prostaglandin E_2, prostaglandin-$F_{2\alpha}$ and prostaglandin I_2 (prostacyclin), respectively (Figure 6.7).

TABLE 6.3 **Classification of the major prostaglandin receptors and the predominant signalling pathways activated by each class of receptor**

Prostaglandin	Receptor	Conventional abbreviation	Second messenger
D_2	D-prostanoid receptor	DP receptor	↑ cAMP
E_2	E-prostanoid receptor subtype 1	EP_1 receptor	↑ Ca^{2+}
E_2	E-prostanoid receptor subtype 2	EP_2 receptor	↑ cAMP
E_2	E-prostanoid receptor subtype 3	EP_3 receptor	↓ cAMP
E_2	E-prostanoid receptor subtype 4	EP_4 receptor	↑ cAMP
$F_{2\alpha}$	F-prostanoid receptor	FP receptor	↑ IP_3 /↑ Ca^{2+}
I_2	I-prostanoid receptor	IP receptor	↑ cAMP

↑ = increased | ↓ = decreased | cAMP = cyclic adenosine monophosphate | IP_3 = inositol trisphosphate

Prostaglandin metabolism

The biological activity of each prostaglandin relies on the presence of an alcohol group at carbon position 15. Hence, oxidation of this alcohol to a 15-carbon ketone by 15-hydroxyprostaglandin dehydrogenase results in the rapid inactivation of prostaglandins. The 15-hydroxyprostaglandin dehydrogenase enzyme is highly expressed in the lungs, such that around 65% of prostaglandins are inactivated with each pass through the pulmonary circulation. The susceptibility of prostaglandins to oxidative inactivation catalysed by 15-hydroxyprostaglandin dehydrogenase limits the actions of these lipid hormones to autocrine and paracrine effects on neighbouring cells.

PROSTAGLANDIN ACTIONS

Given that prostaglandins are lipid hormones synthesised from a fatty-acid substrate, they would intuitively be expected to have free access to the interior of target cells and hence to exert their actions via intracellular (probably nuclear) receptors, as is the case for steroid hormones. However, despite their lipid structure, prostaglandins exert their effects on target cells via G-protein-coupled receptors on the cell surface.

Specific information on the prostaglandin $F_{2\alpha}$ and prostaglandin E_2 receptors can be found in Table 6.3.

By way of overview:

- Prostaglandin $F_{2\alpha}$ generally acts via the F-prostanoid receptor to exert its cellular effects via the phospholipase C–inositol trisphosphate–Ca^{2+} signalling pathway.
- Prostaglandin E_2 can activate a series of four distinct E-prostanoid receptors, which generally transduce their signals via changes in the intracellular concentration of cyclic adenosine monophosphate (cAMP) and the activity of the cAMP-dependent protein kinase.

The ability of prostaglandin $F_{2\alpha}$ and prostaglandin E_2 to activate different signal transduction pathways probably accounts for the fact that their cellular actions are generally opposite and antagonistic. Through activation of protein kinases via second-messenger molecules/ions, prostaglandins are able to alter the function of pre-existing proteins and elicit cellular responses within seconds or minutes (rather than hours or days).

Regulation of myometrial contractility

The regulation of myometrial contractions involves a yin–yang balance between contractant molecules, which serve to increase myometrial contractions, and relaxant molecules, which antagonise the contractants so as to decrease the frequency and/or force of myometrial contractions (Figure 6.8).

FIGURE 6.8 **Balanced control of myometrial contractions**

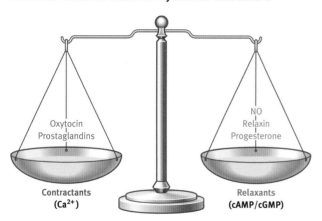

cAMP = cyclic adenosine monophosphate | cGMP = cyclic guanosine monophosphate | NO = nitric oxide

FIGURE 6.9 **Uterine oxytocin–prostaglandin $F_{2\alpha}$ spiral**

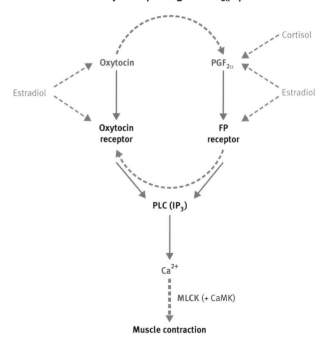

cAMK = Ca^{2+}/calmodulin-dependent kinase | IP_3 = inositol trisphosphate | MLCK = myosin light chain kinase | $PGF_{2\alpha}$ = prostaglandin $F_{2\alpha}$ | PLC = phospholipase C

The contractant molecules include:

- oxytocin, a peptide molecule that originates from the uterus, rather than the posterior lobe of the pituitary gland
- prostaglandins, specifically prostaglandin $F_{2\alpha}$.

Both of these hormones activate phospholipase C (via the oxytocin receptor and F-prostanoid receptor, respectively), leading to an increase in the intracellular Ca^{2+} concentration and activation of both myosin light chain kinase and Ca^{2+}/calmodulin-dependent protein kinase to increase the force of myometrial muscle contractions (Figure 6.9). The stimulation of myometrial contractions is augmented by the fact that oxytocin can stimulate uterine prostaglandin synthesis, while prostaglandin $F_{2\alpha}$ can, in turn, upregulate the expression of oxytocin receptors, culminating in a positive feedback loop that drives myometrial contractions (Figure 6.9). In addition, this loop is subject to modulation by steroid hormones, specifically by estradiol and cortisol. These steroids increase the expression of the genes that encode oxytocin, the oxytocin and F-prostanoid receptors and the enzymes required to synthesise prostaglandins.

The relaxant molecules act in opposition to oxytocin and prostaglandins and are therefore often referred to as anticontractant hormones. The relaxant/anticontractant pathways operate primarily via the cyclic-nucleotide second messengers cAMP and cyclic guanosine monophosphate (cGMP), which activate the cAMP-dependent

and cGMP-dependent protein kinases to dephosphorylate the myosin light chain and limit the force of contractions.

The major myometrial relaxant is progesterone, which impairs the synthesis and action of both oxytocin and prostaglandin $F_{2\alpha}$ via a combination of classic genomic and nonclassic (hence rapid) nongenomic pathways. In addition, progesterone increases the intracellular cAMP concentration and decreases the operation of gap junctions (impairing the ability of the myometrial myocytes to act as a functional syncytium).[4] The actions of progesterone are supplemented by the relaxant actions of:

- nitric oxide, which seems to relax the myometrium independently of its ability to stimulate soluble guanylyl cyclase and elevate cGMP levels
- relaxin, which increases cAMP levels
- prostacyclin, which also increases cAMP levels.

At term, the decline in placental output of progesterone, and hence in the ratio of progesterone to estradiol, causes a switch in the steroidal control of the myometrium from predominantly relaxant actions to the contractant actions that are required for the onset of labour.

Summary and revision

In conclusion, although steroids and prostaglandins are related in being classes of lipid hormone, they differ fundamentally in several respects. These include the precise nature of the molecular substrates, the enzymes required for hormone biosynthesis, the cellular receptors through which steroids and prostaglandins act, their mechanisms and speed of action and, most importantly, the physiological responses that steroid hormones and prostaglandins elicit.

REFERENCES

1. MILLER W L. Molecular biology of steroid hormone synthesis. *Endocr Rev* 1988;9:295–318.

2. CARSON-JURICA M A, SCHRADER W T, O'MALLEY B W. Steroid receptor family: structure and functions. *Endocr Rev* 1990;11:201–20.

3. SMITH W L. Prostanoid biosynthesis and mechanisms of action. *Am J Physiol* 1992;263:F 181–91.

4. MESIANO S. Myometrial progesterone responsiveness. *Semin Reprod Med* 2007;25:5–13.

CHAPTER 7

Fluid and acid–base balance

Mark Heining

Fluid and electrolyte balance in pregnancy

During the course of a normal pregnancy, extracellular fluid accumulates:

- plasma volume rises typically from 3 to 4.5 litres
- interstitial-fluid volume rises typically from 11 to 15 litres.

The intracellular fluid volume also rises minimally.

These changes account for about 6–8 kg of the weight gain experienced during pregnancy. There is an accompanying accumulation of Na^+ and K^+, so that there is no overall significant change in the concentrations of these ions.

Because of the accumulation of H_2O in the plasma compartment during a normal pregnancy, there is a fall in the concentration of plasma albumin and therefore a fall in the colloid osmotic pressure of plasma. This results in an imbalance in the so-called Starling forces, which control the movement of fluid across the capillary membrane:

- intravascular pressure pushes fluid out of the vessel
- colloid osmotic pressure tends to keep it in.

As a result of the drop in colloid osmotic pressure during pregnancy, accumulation of interstitial fluid and development of oedema become more likely, especially during the third trimester when arterial pressure rises.

It should be noted that in certain disease states, most importantly pre-eclampsia, there may be a fall in plasma volume.

Acid–base balance

SOME DEFINITIONS

Understanding of the acid–base balance is helped greatly by a clear understanding of the relevant terminology.

Acids and bases

An acid is a proton donor, meaning that it tends to give up H^+ ions. A base is a proton acceptor, meaning that it tends to take up H^+ ions. It follows that acids and bases may be anions, cations or electrically neutral.

For example, ammonium (NH_4^+) is an anionic acid in equilibrium with ammonia (NH_3):

$$NH_4^+ \rightleftharpoons NH_3 + H^+$$

Dihydrogen phosphate ($H_2PO_4^-$) is a cationic acid in equilibrium with hydrogen phosphate (HPO_4^{2-}):

$$H_2PO_4^- \rightleftharpoons HPO_4^{2-} + H^+$$

Hydrochloric acid (HCl) is a neutral acid in equilibrium with H^+ and Cl^-:

$$HCl \rightleftharpoons H^+ + Cl^-$$

These are all acids because they tend to give up H^+ ions.

pH value

The pH value of a solution is the negative logarithm to the base 10 of the H^+ concentration and is a dimensionless quantity (it has no units). This means that the higher the H^+ concentration (the more acidic the solution), the lower the pH value.

Acidaemia and acidosis

These terms are often used interchangeably in everyday clinical practice and this can be a source of confusion. Strictly speaking, acidaemia means that the blood is more acidic than normal, while acidosis refers to the underlying process (for example ketoacidosis, lactic acidosis) that may cause acidaemia. Alkalaemia and alkalosis have comparable meanings.

ACID LOAD

The normal pH value of the blood and extracellular fluid is about 7.4, with a range of about 7.35–7.45. Because of the logarithmic derivation of the pH value, this represents an H^+ concentration in the order of nmol/l. Table 7.1 shows how physiological pH values in the normal range correspond to the concentration of H^+.

Clearly, the pH value is normally controlled within a narrow range. The importance of this must be appreciated in the context of the amount of H^+ production that takes place in the body:

- 15 000 mmol/day from CO_2 production
- 50–150 mmol/day from the production of phosphoric acid and sulphuric acid
- 1000 mmol/day from lactic acid production.

The impact of this on the overall pH value of the extracellular fluid is minimised by three mechanisms:

TABLE 7.1 **Physiological pH values and corresponding concentrations of hydrogen ions**

pH	H^+ concentration (nmol/l)
7.0	100
7.2	63
7.4	40
7.6	25
7.8	16

- very quick response (within seconds) – buffer systems in the blood, proceeding with the speed of a chemical reaction
- quick response (within minutes) – changes in ventilation
- slow response (within days) – renal mechanisms for the adjustment of H^+ excretion.

BUFFERS

A buffer system is a system that tends to minimise changes in the pH value of a solution. It normally consists of a weak acid with its conjugate base (this is what remains when H^+ has left the acid molecule). An example would be:

$$R-COOH \rightleftarrows R-COO^- + H^+$$
$$\text{(acid)} \quad \text{(conjugate base)}$$

Addition of further H^+ ions will cause the reaction to shift towards the left, resulting in the formation of more undissociated acid because the conjugate base tends to combine with the extra H^+ ions, while the reverse happens if H^+ ions are removed from the system. The buffering power of a system is greatest when half the buffering groups are undissociated and half are dissociated; that is, when $[R-COOH]$ equals $[R-COO^-]$. The pH value at this point equals the pK value of the system, with the pK value being the negative logarithm to the base 10 of the dissociation constant, K.

The most important buffers in extracellular fluid are the bicarbonate (HCO_3^-) system and haemoglobin. Other proteins also contribute some buffering power.

Bicarbonate as a buffer

Carbonic acid (H_2CO_3) is a relatively strong acid, so the HCO_3^- system is a relatively weak buffer. Its importance lies in the link between H_2CO_3, HCO_3^- and dissolved CO_2:

$$CO_2 + H_2O \rightleftarrows H_2CO_3 \rightleftarrows H^+ + HCO_3^-$$

Hence the contribution of ventilation and CO_2 excretion to the acid–base balance.

The relationship between the components of the HCO_3^- buffer system can be described by the following equation, where K is the dissociation constant of H_2CO_3, α is the solubility coefficient for CO_2 in plasma and pCO_2 is the partial pressure of CO_2:

$$[H^+] = K \times \alpha PCO_2 / [HCO_3^-]$$

Taking negative logarithms yields the following equation:

$$pH = pK + \log[HCO_3^-]/\alpha PCO_2$$

This is the Henderson–Hasselbach equation, sometimes more familiar in the following form:

$$pH = pK + \log[base]/[acid]$$

It follows that by knowing any two of the three variables $[H^+]$, $[HCO_3^-]$ and PCO_2, the third may be calculated. This is important when interpreting results given by bench blood gas machines, as some machines calculate HCO_3^- concentration while others measure it.

Haemoglobin as a buffer

The importance of the haemoglobin buffer system lies in the fact that haemoglobin is present in high concentration and has multiple acidic and basic groups such as carboxyl (–COOH) and amino (–NH$_2$) groups, respectively. The former will release H^+ ions if the solution becomes more basic, while the latter will take up H^+ ions (forming –NH$_3^+$) if the solution becomes more acidic.

Reduced haemoglobin is a weaker acid than oxygenated haemoglobin and hence it is a more effective buffer. Therefore, as haemoglobin releases O_2 in the tissues, more H^+ ions are buffered. As more H^+ ions are buffered, more CO_2 will dissolve in the plasma to maintain H_2CO_3 concentration. This aids CO_2 transport and is known as the Haldane effect.

CARBON DIOXIDE CARRIAGE

CO_2 is carried in blood in three ways.

A small amount is carried in simple solution, with the dissolved CO_2 being in equilibrium with H_2CO_3 and hence with HCO_3^-:

$$CO_2 + H_2O \rightleftharpoons H_2CO_3 \rightleftharpoons H^+ + HCO_3^-$$

A slightly larger amount forms carbamino compounds with plasma proteins:

$$R\text{-}NH_2 + CO_2 \rightleftharpoons R\text{-}NHCOO^- + H^+$$

The H^+ ion may in turn be buffered.

Finally, the majority enters red blood cells, where three things happen:

- CO_2 stays in simple solution, as in plasma
- CO_2 forms carbaminohaemoglobin, facilitated by the reduction in haemoglobin, the Haldane effect and the extra buffering of H^+ ions by the high concentration of haemoglobin
- significant amounts of H_2CO_3 are formed in a reaction catalysed by the enzyme carbonic anhydrase (present in large amounts in red blood cells); H_2CO_3 in turn splits into H^+ and HCO_3^-; the H^+ ions are buffered by haemoglobin and the HCO_3^- ions diffuse out of the red blood cell into the plasma, in exchange for Cl^- ions.

Note that, just as the reduction of haemoglobin aids CO_2 carriage in the Haldane effect, an increase in the CO_2 content of the red blood cell aids O_2 release from haemoglobin in the Bohr effect. In the case of O_2 transfer in the placenta, there is a 'double Bohr effect' because CO_2 leaves the fetal side of the membrane and accumulates on the maternal side; maternal haemoglobin is more likely to release O_2, fetal haemoglobin more likely to bind O_2.

CLINICAL STATES OF ACID–BASE DISTURBANCE

Clinical states of acid–base disturbance are important since many physiological processes (such as enzyme activity and membrane stability) may be affected by changes in the pH value. In the following discussion, the suffixes -aemia and -osis will be used in their correct meanings as outlined at the beginning of this chapter.

Acidaemia and alkalaemia may both be caused by primarily respiratory or primarily metabolic processes, although the term metabolic needs to be interpreted flexibly. There are therefore four situations to describe:

- Acidaemia arising from respiratory acidosis. This is caused by underventilation with consequent build-up of CO_2.
- Alkalaemia arising from respiratory alkalosis. This is caused by overventilation with a consequent fall in CO_2 concentration. Such a situation may occur by

voluntary hyperventilation or by overvigorous artificial ventilation during anaesthesia or intensive care.

- Acidaemia arising from metabolic acidosis. The term metabolic refers to more than just metabolic processes (such as lactic acidosis or diabetic ketoacidosis) that cause increased production of acid. It may also refer to increased ingestion of acid (as in salicylate overdose) or failure to excrete acid (as in renal failure).

- Alkalaemia arising from metabolic alkalosis. 'Metabolic' is an even less appropriate term here because no metabolic process leads to a build-up of alkali. Metabolic alkalosis therefore refers to loss of acid (as in severe vomiting) or injudicious intake of alkali (as in overuse of alkali in the symptomatic management of peptic ulcers or overzealous use of intravenous HCO_3^- in the management of metabolic acidosis).

Clearly, the management of these situations depends on an understanding of the underlying processes and this in turn depends on accurate understanding of the information given by commercial blood gas machines.

INTERPRETATION OF BLOOD GASES

Normal ranges of blood gas values vary slightly from one machine to another and from one population to another. Approximate values are provided in Table 7.2.

In all the acid–base disturbances described earlier, physiological processes will tend to compensate for the acid–base imbalance, so that the change in pH value will

be smaller than predicted by the extent of the primary process. For example, a metabolic acidosis will normally be partially compensated by increased ventilation, which produces a respiratory alkalosis.

The success of treatment depends mainly on the correct identification of the primary disturbance (see also Box 7.1 and Table 7.3). An obvious starting point is to remember that compensation is rarely complete; the measured pH value will have changed in the direction of the primary disturbance. For example, a pH value that is more acidic than normal is usually caused by an acidosis as the primary event, whereas a pH value that is more alkaline than normal is usually caused by an alkalosis as the primary event.

BOX 7.1 Interpretation of blood gases

1. Remember this equation:

$$CO_2 + H_2O \rightleftharpoons H^+ + HCO_3^-$$

It satisfactorily explains acid–base disorders and their physiological compensation. If H^+ is generated, the reaction shifts to the left; if CO_2 is generated, the reaction shifts to the right.

2. Remember normal blood gas values:

- pH = 7.35–7.45
- PCO_2 = 4.5–5.8 kPa
- $[HCO_3^-]$ = 23–28 mmol/l

3. Then follow this algorithm:

- Start with the pH value: is it acidosis or alkalosis?
- Then CO_2: if the partial pressure is high, it is respiratory acidosis or at least has a respiratory component. If it is not high, then it is not respiratory acidosis.
- Lastly HCO_3^-: if the concentration is low, this confirms the presence of metabolic acidosis and vice versa.
- If CO_2 and HCO_3^- values are going in opposite directions (that is, one is higher and the other is lower than normal), it is a mixed disorder.

TABLE 7.2 **Normal blood gas values**

Parameter	Normal range
pH	7.35–7.45
PO_2	12.5–14.3 kPa
PCO_2	4.5–5.8 kPa
$[HCO_3-]$	23–28 mmol/l
Standard $[HCO_3-]$	24–30 mmol/l

$[HCO_3^-]$ = bicarbonate concentration | PO_2 = partial pressure of O_2 | PCO_2 = partial pressure of CO_2 | standard $[HCO_3^-]$ = bicarbonate concentration under standard conditions (PCO_2 = 40 mmHg, 37 degrees C, saturated with O^2)

TABLE 7.3 **Interpretation of blood gases**

Parameter measured	Acidosis	Alkalosis
pH	Low	High
PCO_2 (respiratory component)	High	Low
$[HCO_3^-]$ (metabolic component)	Low	High

$[HCO_3^-]$ = bicarbonate concentration | PCO_2 = partial pressure of CO_2

Next, the PCO_2 should be inspected. If low, this indicates a respiratory alkalosis; if high, there is a respiratory acidosis. Either may be the primary event or a compensatory response.

The presence of a metabolic disturbance may be indicated by a change in the HCO_3^- concentration: it falls in metabolic acidosis and rises in metabolic alkalosis. Again, either may be a primary or compensatory event.

When looking at the clinical context, it is worth remembering that respiratory compensation (for a primary metabolic event) occurs within a few seconds or minutes, whereas metabolic compensation depends on changes in the excretion of renal HCO_3^- and therefore takes hours to days.

However, over-reliance on the HCO_3^- concentration as an indicator of metabolic disturbance can be misleading, particularly if there is a mixed respiratory and metabolic acidosis or if a quantitative measurement of metabolic disturbance is required. Hence, over the years, a variety of other measurements has been introduced, including standard HCO_3^-, anion gap, buffer base and base excess.

Nowadays, base excess is regarded as the most useful quantitative index of metabolic acid–base derangement. The normal range is from –2 (slightly acidic) to +2 (slightly alkaline); there are no units. Severe metabolic acidosis is considered to be present when the base excess is more negative than –10. A negative base excess is sometimes called a base deficit.

CLINICAL CORRECTION OF AN ACID–BASE DISTURBANCE

Changes in the pH value affect many physiological processes, mainly enzyme activity and stability of excitable membranes (including those of nerves, striated muscle and cardiac muscle). Management of any acid–base disturbance therefore depends on the clinical context and the severity of the resulting physiological abnormality.

Respiratory acidosis, as already mentioned, is caused by hypoventilation. If treatment is clinically indicated, this is by taking over ventilation (by positive-pressure or negative-pressure ventilation) or by treatment of the cause (for example, the use of naloxone hydrochloride in an overdose of opioid).

Metabolic acidosis is treated by treatment of the underlying cause. For example, there is the standard management of diabetic ketoacidosis (involving rehydration and administration of insulin), or restoration of cardiac output in lactic acidosis arising from shock. If very severe and there are convincing clinical indications, treatment with intravenous sodium bicarbonate ($NaHCO_3$) may be needed. Great care is necessary with dose as it is easy to give too much and there is always a risk of causing intracellular alkalosis.

Both metabolic alkalosis and respiratory alkalosis are rare and difficult to treat.

ACID–BASE BALANCE IN PREGNANCY

Pregnancy is associated with a slight respiratory alkalosis. A compensatory fall in HCO_3^- concentration occurs, which reduces the change in pH value, but the low PCO_2 is necessary to maintain a diffusion gradient for CO_2 across the placenta.

During labour, maternal hyperventilation and respiratory alkalosis become more extreme. Because of the relatively short timescale, compensation by renal mechanisms does not occur and so the consequences of alkalosis are more marked.

Alkalosis causes a leftward shift of the oxyhaemoglobin dissociation curve and therefore an increased affinity of maternal haemoglobin for O_2. This may lead to a fall in the partial pressure of O_2 in the umbilical vein and even metabolic acidosis (owing to anaerobic metabolism) in the fetus. Additionally, the increased proportion of deoxygenated haemoglobin in the fetus allows more CO_2 to remain in solution and thus contributes to respiratory acidosis. Extreme maternal hyperventilation during labour may therefore contribute to both metabolic acidosis and respiratory acidosis in the fetus.

Fetal acid–base abnormalities

As suggested, acidaemia in the fetus is nearly always a mixed respiratory and metabolic disturbance, with blood gas measurements showing a low pH value, a raised PCO_2, a low HCO_3^- concentration and a raised base deficit (negative base excess). Treatment consists of correction of any underlying cause or aggravating factor, such as maternal shock.

Maternal acid–base abnormalities

Pregnant women do not only have a 'physiological' alkalosis but they may also be subject to the usual abnormalities that occur in nonpregnant individuals. If acidaemia is present, the cause may be (among other things) diabetic ketoacidosis, dehydration or shock.

Again, the management is correction of the cause by administration of fluids, administration of insulin if indicated or arrest of haemorrhage.

Treatment with $NaHCO_3$ is rarely necessary, especially since the associated hazards are well documented and the affected women are mostly fit and able to correct acidosis once organ perfusion is restored.

Calcium homeostasis and bones

Rosemary Bland

Calcium homeostasis

Ca^{2+} is essential for a number of physiological mechanisms such as muscle contraction, intra- and extracellular signalling (as a second messenger; see Chapter 5), activation of enzymes (as a co-factor), stabilisation of membrane potentials and nerve excitability and, of course, normal bone and tooth formation (Table 8.1). Consequently, circulating levels of Ca^{2+} are tightly regulated.

The adult body contains around 1.2 kg of Ca^{2+}. Approximately 99% of this is stored in the skeleton as hydroxyapatite, the mineral component of bone. About 1% is present intracellularly, although it is important to remember that Ca^{2+} does not occur free in the cytoplasm but is sequestered in intracellular organelles such as the endoplasmic reticulum, mitochondria and, in skeletal muscle, the sarcoplasmic reticulum and is available for rapid release if required.

The intracellular Ca^{2+} concentration is approximately 100 nmol/l. The concentration gradient across the cells is maintained by the plasma membrane Ca^{2+}-ATPase (PMCA) and, in some cells, the Na^+,Ca^{2+}-exchanger (also known as NCX). Extracellular Ca^{2+} accounts for only 0.1% of total body Ca^{2+}. This equates to a normal serum concentration of approximately 2.5 mmol/l (normal range 2.2–2.6 mmol/l).

TABLE 8.1 **Physiological functions of calcium**

Function	Notes
Bone mineralisation	Ca^{2+} is a component of hydroxyapatite, the mineral component of bones
Tooth formation	Ca^{2+} is a constituent of the mineral component of teeth
Muscle contraction	Binding of Ca^{2+} to troponin allows myosin to bind actin
Enzyme co-factor	Ca^{2+} is required by blood clotting enzymes [a]
First extracellular messenger	Ca^{2+} binds to a membrane-bound receptor
Second intracellular messenger	Ca^{2+} regulates a number of intracellular signalling proteins
Secretion and exocytosis	Ca^{2+} is used for neurotransmitter release from synapses and is required for exocytosis
Stabilisation of membrane potentials	Ca^{2+} is essential for the maintenance of membrane potentials and for depolarisation
Regulation of cellular division, proliferation and apoptosis	Ca^{2+} modifies many intracellular signalling pathways

[a] For example, the chelating agent EDTA is added to blood collection tubes to bind to Ca^{2+} and thereby inhibit these enzymes, so as to stop the blood clotting

Approximately 45% of serum Ca^{2+} circulates in the free ionised form, which is biologically active. The remaining 55% circulates in a bound form, with about 10% bound to anions, including lactate, phosphate (PO_4^{3-}) and bicarbonate, and about 45% bound to plasma proteins (mainly albumin). Consequently, a change in albumin levels will alter the ratio of free to bound Ca^{2+}. Values are therefore quoted as 'total adjusted' Ca^{2+} (the value for total Ca^{2+} has been corrected for albumin levels).

IMPORTANT POINT

Ca^{2+}

Clinicians usually order a total Ca^{2+} value to evaluate Ca^{2+} status, but it is the free, ionised Ca^{2+} that is biologically active. Conditions that alter the balance between free and bound Ca^{2+} will not alter the total Ca^{2+} concentration but will change the physiological responses. For example, in acidosis the H^+ ions compete with the Ca^{2+} ions for the binding of plasma proteins, so acidosis increases the concentration of free serum Ca^{2+} without altering the levels of total Ca^{2+}. The biochemistry of people with acidosis therefore seems to be normal even though they are hypercalcaemic.

Ca^{2+} is obtained from the diet. Ideally, adults should have an intake of approximately 1000 mg/day, although the current UK reference nutrient intake for adults (detailed in Table 8.2) is set slightly lower at 700 mg/day. This figure should be higher in adolescents and in pregnant and lactating women because of the increased requirements for Ca^{2+} for bone growth and milk formation.

TABLE 8.2 **Current UK reference nutrient intake for calcium**

Age	Reference nutrient intake (mg/day)
Infant	525
1–3 years	350
4–6 years	450
7–10 years	550
11–18 years	800 (women), 1000 (men)
Adults	700
Lactating women	1250

Absorption of Ca^{2+} from the diet is relatively inefficient, with only 20–30% of dietary intake being taken up by the body. Absorption varies with age (increased in children and decreased with advanced age), intestine function, diet (lactose increases absorption, oxalates and phytates decrease absorption by binding to the ingested Ca^{2+}) and vitamin D availability. Ca^{2+} absorption can occur throughout the gastrointestinal tract but the majority (60–70%) of all ingested Ca^{2+} is absorbed in the small intestine.

The control of Ca^{2+} homeostasis (Box 8.1) and the maintenance of serum Ca^{2+} levels require a complex interaction between Ca^{2+}, hormones (vitamin D, parathyroid hormone and calcitonin) and four main organs (the intestine, parathyroid glands, the kidneys and bone; see Table 8.3). This is described in more detail in the following sections.

MECHANISM OF CALCIUM ABSORPTION AND EXCRETION

Ca^{2+} is absorbed from the intestine via transcellular or paracellular routes (Figure 8.1). Transcellular absorption involves entry of Ca^{2+} into the cell via the epithelial Ca^{2+} channel 2 (TRPV6) in the microvilli of the brush border. Bound to Ca^{2+}-binding proteins (calmodulin and calbindin), Ca^{2+} then moves through the cell to the baso-lateral membrane. Export into the extracellular fluid of the lamina propria occurs by exocytosis or by the PMCA. Paracellular transport also requires the presence of Ca^{2+}-binding proteins.

All of the free (ionised) Ca^{2+} and the Ca^{2+} bound to anions is filtered by the glomerulus and most (99%) of the filtered Ca^{2+} is reabsorbed (Figure 8.2). Ca^{2+} is reabsorbed by passive paracellular (80%) and active transcellular (20%) processes. Transcellular transport requires the presence of epithelial Ca^{2+} channel 1 (TRPV5) in the apical membrane.

CALCIUM BALANCE

The Ca^{2+} balance depends on the amount of Ca^{2+} absorbed minus the amount of Ca^{2+} excreted, as well as the balance between the amount buffered in the bone and the concentration in the extracellular fluid.

BOX 8.1 Quick guide to the control of calcium homeostasis

The concentration of serum Ca^{2+} is detected by the Ca^{2+}-sensing receptor on the parathyroid glands. In response to low serum Ca^{2+} concentrations, parathyroid hormone (PTH) is released. It acts on the bone to stimulate bone resorption. In the kidney, PTH promotes resorption of Ca^{2+} and excretion of phosphate (PO_4^{3-}). It also increases the activity of the enzyme 25-hydroxyvitamin D_3 1α-hydroxylase, which catalyses the conversion of calcidiol to its active metabolite calcitriol.

Calcitriol increases bone turnover, increases absorption of Ca^{2+} from the intestine and enhances Ca^{2+} and PO_4^{3-} reabsorption in the kidney, resulting in an increase in serum Ca^{2+} concentration. Ca^{2+} and calcitriol provide negative feedback to the parathyroid gland to inhibit further secretion of PTH.

Calcitonin, produced in the thyroid gland, acts to decrease the serum Ca^{2+} concentration and is secreted in response to hypercalcaemia. It inhibits renal Ca^{2+} and PO_4^{3-} reabsorption and osteoclastic bone resorption.

Fibroblast growth factor 23, a phosphaturic hormone, is released from bone cells (mostly osteocytes) in response to stimulation by calcitriol and seeks to limit calcitriol-induced increases in serum PO_4^{3-} concentration.

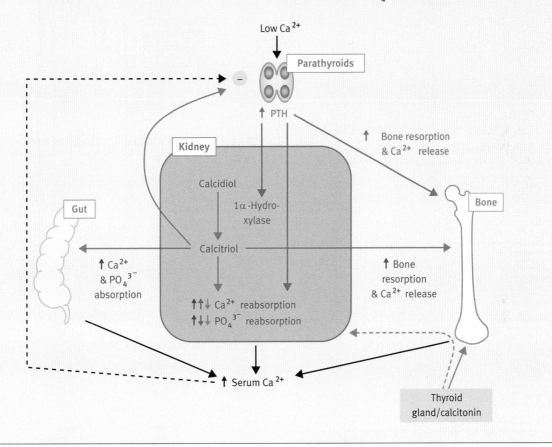

Generally, children have a positive Ca^{2+} balance, in adults the balance should be neutral (input equals output) and postmenopausal women and the elderly usually have a negative Ca^{2+} balance.

A disruption in Ca^{2+} homeostasis can result in hypocalcaemia or hypercalcaemia and it is important to remember that changes in Ca^{2+} homeostasis will usually alter PO_4^{3-} status.

Hormones that regulate serum Ca^{2+} levels

The three main hormones that regulate serum Ca^{2+} levels are parathyroid hormone (PTH) and vitamin D, which increase serum Ca^{2+} concentrations, and calcitonin, which reduces serum Ca^{2+} concentrations. Table 8.4 contains a summary of the characteristics and functions of these hormones.

TABLE 8.3 **Organs that regulate calcium homeostasis**

Organ	Function
Kidney	Response to Ca²⁺, PTH, vitamin D and calcitonin
	Activation of vitamin D
	Regulation of Ca^{2+} and PO_4^{3-} reabsorption and excretion
Bone [a]	Storage (buffer) of Ca^{2+}, PO_4^{3-} and Mg^{2+}
Parathyroid glands	Response to changes in serum Ca^{2+} (express the CaSR)
	Synthesis and secretion of PTH
Gastrointestinal tract	Absorption of Ca^{2+} and PO_4^{3-}
Thyroid glands	Response to changes in serum Ca^{2+} (express the CaSR)
	Synthesis and secretion of calcitonin

[a] Bone remodelling is regulated by PTH, calcitonin and vitamin D | CaSR = Ca^{2+}-sensing receptor | PTH = parathyroid hormone | PO_4^{3-} = phosphate

FIGURE 8.1 **Calcium absorption from the intestine**

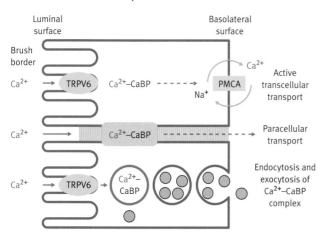

CaBP = Ca_2^+-binding protein | PMCA = plasma membrane Ca^{2+}-ATPase | TRPV6 = epithelial Ca^{2+} channel

Adapted with permission from Nussey S, Whitehead SA. *Endocrinology: An Integrated Approach*. Oxford: BIOS Scientific Publishers; 2001.

PARATHYROID HORMONE

PTH is a peptide hormone that is synthesised in the parathyroid glands. These glands (normally four) are located on the posterior of the thyroid gland. They

FIGURE 8.2 **Reabsorption of calcium along the nephron**

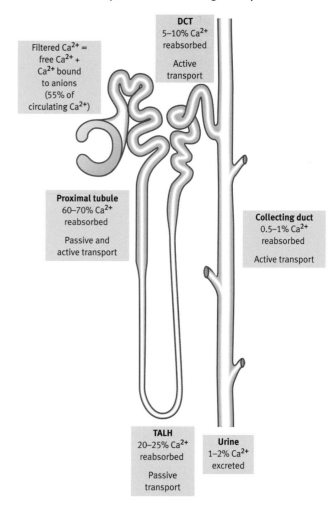

DCT = distal convoluted tubule | TALH = thick ascending loop of Henle

originate from the pharyngeal pouches, are small (3–8 mm long, 2–5 mm wide, 1.5 mm deep with a weight of less than 40 mg each) and are supplied by branches of the inferior thyroid arteries. The parathyroid glands contain two cell types: oxyphil cells, and chief cells, which synthesise and secrete PTH.

Synthesis and release of parathyroid hormone

PTH is synthesised as a 115-amino-acid compound called prepro-PTH. Cleavage reactions produce PTH, an 84-amino-acid molecule that is stored in vesicles until required. The release of PTH is initiated by the

TABLE 8.4 **Summary of the characteristics and physiological functions of the main hormones that regulate calcium homeostasis**

Hormone	Hormone type	Receptor	Site of synthesis	Signal for synthesis and/or secretion	Physiological actions	Net effect on Ca²⁺ homeostasis
PTH	Peptide	G-protein-coupled receptor (PTHR1)	Chief cells in the parathyroid glands	Low Ca^{2+}	Bone: ↑ bone resorption Kidney: ↑ PO_4^{3-} excretion Kidney: ↓ Ca^{2+} excretion Kidney: ↑ vitamin D activation	↑ Serum Ca^{2+} ↓ Serum PO_4^{3-}
Vitamin D (calcitriol)	Secosteroid	Nuclear receptor (VDR) A member of the steroid/thyroid receptor superfamily	Hydroxylated (activated) in the proximal convoluted tubules of the kidney Extra-renal activation of vitamin D can also occur	Low Ca^{2+} Low PO_4^{3-} PTH	Bone: ↑ bone formation and mineralisation Bone: ↑ bone remodelling GI tract: ↑ Ca2+ absorption Kidney: ↑ Ca^{2+} and PO_4^{3-} reabsorption	↑ Serum Ca^{2+} ↑ Serum PO_4^{3-}
Calcitonin	Peptide	G-protein-coupled receptor	C cells in the parathyroid glands	High Ca^{2+}	Kidney: ↑ PO_4^{3-} excretion Kidney: ↓ Ca^{2+} reabsorption Bone: inhibits osteoclast function	↓ Serum Ca^{2+}

↑ = increase I ↓ = decrease I GI = gastrointestinal I PO_4^{3-} = phosphate I PTH = parathyroid hormone I PTHR1 = PTH receptor type 1 I VDR = vitamin D receptor

Ca^{2+}-sensing receptor (CaSR) in response to hypocalcaemia. PTH secretion occurs within seconds and the parathyroids contain sufficient PTH to maintain secretion for approximately 60 minutes. If prolonged PTH secretion (secretion for hours to days) is required, PTH synthesis is increased.

If the hypocalcaemia is not corrected and PTH secretion needs to be sustained for days or even months, proliferation of the parathyroid gland cells increases and this results in hyperplasia and unregulated synthesis and release of PTH (secondary hyperparathyroidism).

Parathyroid-hormone receptors

PTH binds to the PTH receptor (PTHR), which is a G-protein-coupled receptor. Ligand binding activates cyclic adenosine monophosphate (cAMP) as a second messenger and results in the phosphorylation of intracellular proteins. There are at least two PTHR subtypes, PTHR1 and PTHR2. The first 34 amino acids of PTH bind to PTHR1 and it has classically been assumed that the biological activity of PTH is only attributable to these 34 amino acids. The function of other fragments of the PTH peptide is currently under investigation.

> **IMPORTANT POINT**
>
> **Parathyroid hormone receptors**
>
> If the receptor subtype is not specified, reference is probably made to PTHR1.

Physiological actions of parathyroid hormone

PTH acts on the bone and kidney. In bone, it causes bone resorption and, thereby, Ca^{2+} and PO_4^{3-} release. PTH binds to PTHRs on the osteoblasts, resulting in osteoblast-mediated activation of osteoclast differentiation. *In vitro* studies have also shown inhibition of collagen synthesis by PTH-activated osteoblasts.

In the kidney, PTH has three main actions. In the distal convoluted tubule, it increases Ca^{2+} reabsorption possibly by increasing the transport of Ca^{2+} that is mediated by TRPV5. In the proximal and distal convoluted tubules, PTH inhibits the reabsorption of PO_4^{3-} and so increases PO_4^{3-} excretion. In the proximal tubule, it blocks PO_4^{3-} resorption by reducing expression of the Na^+-dependent inorganic phosphate co-transporter type II (NPT2). PTH also increases the renal activation of vitamin D by increasing expression and activity of the enzyme 25-hydroxyvitamin D_3 1α-hydroxylase (CYP27B1; 1α-hydroxylase).

Hyperparathyroidism

Hyperparathyroidism results from excess synthesis and release of PTH and is associated with increased bone resorption. There are two main forms: primary and secondary hyperparathyroidism.

Primary hyperparathyroidism is caused by a defect of the parathyroid glands, normally a benign tumour. Malignant tumours are rare and may be associated with multiple endocrine neoplasia syndrome. Primary hyperparathyroidism is characterised by increased levels of PTH and calcitriol and decreased levels of PO_4^{3-} and hypercalcaemia. The increase in calcitriol levels and the decrease in PO_4^{3-} levels indicate that the kidneys are functioning. Individual cells respond normally to feedback signals but the increase in cell numbers means that, on balance, PTH is synthesised and released in excess.

Primary hyperparathyroidism is one of the most frequent causes of hypercalcaemia and is the third most common endocrine disorder after diabetes and hyperthyroidism (prevalence 1 in 500–1000).

Secondary hyperparathyroidism occurs as a result of defective feedback control. Most commonly, the primary defect is in the kidneys and the development of secondary hyperparathyroidism is usually associated with chronic kidney disease.

In renal disease, the kidney is unable to respond normally to PTH, so renal reabsorption of Ca^{2+} is not stimulated and vitamin D activation is not promoted. As a result, Ca^{2+} absorption from the intestine cannot be increased on demand. One consequence of this is that the bone is the only place where PTH can act to increase serum Ca^{2+} levels. The resulting loss of Ca^{2+} from the bone causes high bone turnover, bone demineralisation (osteomalacia) and chronic kidney disease – mineral and bone disorder. As a consequence of the failure to increase serum Ca^{2+} levels and the lack of vitamin D signalling, the normal negative feedback on the parathyroid glands is absent and they continue to produce and secrete PTH. This results in hyperplasia and eventually the parathyroid glands lose their sensitivity to Ca^{2+} and vitamin D.

Ultimately, secondary hyperparathyroidism will progress to tertiary hyperparathyroidism, which is almost exclusively associated with end-stage renal disease and should be treated in the same way as primary hyperparathyroidism.

Calcium-sensing receptor

The CaSR is a G-protein-coupled receptor that is sensitive to serum Ca^{2+} concentrations in the physiological range. The receptor was originally cloned from bovine parathyroid glands but is known to be expressed in a number of tissues including the kidneys, the intestine, vascular smooth muscle cells and bone. Synthetic allosteric activators of the CaSR (calcimimetics) for the treatment of hyperparathyroidism have been developed. The development of CaSR antagonists (calcilytics) is being explored.

Several disorders related to mutations in the CaSR exist. Familial hypocalciuric hypercalcaemia and neonatal severe hyperparathyroidism are associated with loss-of-function mutations and autosomal dominant hypoparathyroidism is associated with an activating mutation.

Parathyroid-hormone-related peptide

PTH-related peptide (PTHrP, also known as PTH-like peptide) is able to bind to PTHR1 (the first 34 amino acids of PTHrP are similar to those of PTH and the first 13 amino acids of the two peptides are almost identical) and therefore mimics PTH actions. It is produced by many cells including cancer cells and is often responsible for hypercalcaemia associated with malignancy. Its physiological functions are not completely understood. It regulates chondrocyte development and therefore endochondral bone formation, placental Ca^{2+} transport and fetal development.

VITAMIN D

The classification of vitamin D as a vitamin is incorrect because we make most of the vitamin D that we require and vitamin D is a pleiotrophic secosteroid. Dietary intake of vitamin D_2 may account for 10–20% of our vitamin D levels but the majority (80–90%) is synthesised in the skin as vitamin D_3. The final activation step occurs predominantly in the proximal convoluted tubule of the kidney, although extrarenal synthesis also occurs.

Vitamin D is required for normal bone remodelling and it increases serum levels of Ca^{2+} and PO_4^{3-} mainly by increasing their intestinal absorption. A number of different vitamin D metabolites exist. The metabolite that is considered to be the biologically active molecule is $1\alpha,25$-dihydroxyvitamin D_3 (calcitriol). All vitamin D metabolites are transported in blood bound to vitamin-D-binding protein. The major circulating form of vitamin D is 25-hydroxyvitamin D_3 (calcidiol), which is considered to be a good surrogate marker of vitamin D status. It is the metabolite of vitamin D that is usually measured clinically.

Vitamin D synthesis

The first step in vitamin D synthesis requires modification of 7-dehydrocholesterol in the keratinocytes to vitamin D_3 (cholecalciferol), a reaction that is mediated by ultraviolet light (sunlight). Vitamin D activation then occurs via a number of hydroxylation reactions. Vitamin D_2 (dietary vitamin D) and vitamin D_3 are hydroxylated in the liver by 25-hydroxylase into calcidiol, which is further hydroxylated into calcitriol in the proximal convoluted tubule of the kidney by the enzyme 1α-hydroxylase, a mitochondrial cytochrome P450 enzyme (Figure 8.3). In

FIGURE 8.3 **Synthesis of vitamin D**

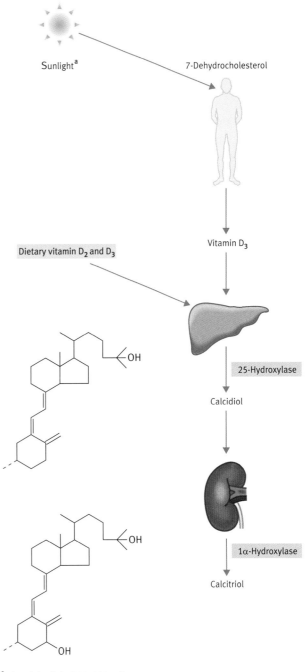

Sunlight[a]

7-Dehydrocholesterol

Dietary vitamin D_2 and D_3

Vitamin D_3

25-Hydroxylase

Calcidiol

1α-Hydroxylase

Calcitriol

[a] Ultraviolet light (290–320 nm)

contrast to 25-hydroxylase activity, which depends on substrate availability, the activity of 1α-hydroxylase is very tightly regulated and is increased by PTH, low Ca^{2+} levels, low PO_4^{3-} levels and calcitonin and is inhibited by calcitriol. Calcitriol is further metabolised (and inactivated) by 24-hydroxylase, an enzyme that is present in all vitamin D target tissues and induced by calcitriol.

The ability to activate vitamin D varies with sunlight exposure, age, ethnic status and mineral status and requires a functional liver and kidneys. Vitamin D insufficiency (less than 50 nmol/l) and deficiency (less than 30 nmol/l) are common throughout the world. Populations living at northern and southern latitudes have lower levels of vitamin D than people living nearer the equator. Elderly people often have insufficient vitamin D as they have lower 1α-hydroxylase activity and reduced mobility may result in decreased exposure to sunlight. Asian and black populations are also vitamin-D-deficient. To some extent, this can be attributed to a combination of dietary factors, reduced sunlight exposure (among those living in regions of low ultraviolet radiation intensity and among those who are required to wear clothing covering most of their skin or use of products containing an SPF) and reduced 1α-hydroxylase activity.

Vitamin D is also activated at nonrenal sites. This is associated with local paracrine/autocrine actions and does not contribute to circulating levels of calcitriol and appears to be unrelated to calcium homeostasis. Extrarenal activation is important for activation of the immune system. It contributes to the normal response to infection and helps to regulate inflammatory responses. It also has a role in cellular proliferation and development.

IMPORTANT POINT

Vitamin D availability and storage

The inactive metabolites of vitamin D (vitamin D_2, vitamin D_3 and calcidiol) are stored in body fat and can be released when required. This allows for storage of excess vitamin D produced during the summer, when sunlight is available, for release and activation during winter months.

Vitamin D receptor and vitamin D signalling

Vitamin D acts via a nuclear receptor. Vitamin D is lipophilic and it had been thought that vitamin D and

FIGURE 8.4 **Vitamin D signalling**

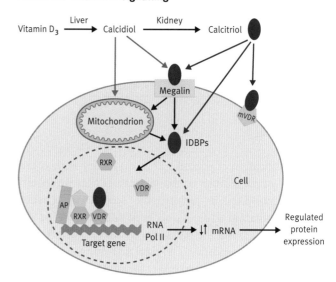

AP = accessory proteins | IDBP = intracellular vitamin-D-binding protein | mRNA = messenger RNA | mVDR = membrane-bound VDR | Pol II = polymerase II | RXR = retinoid X receptor | VDR = vitamin D receptor

other steroid hormones crossed cell membranes by diffusion. Although this may occur, it is now apparent that there are specific transport proteins in the cell membrane (Figure 8.4). Megalin, a large glycoprotein, has been identified as the membrane transporter for calcidiol and calcitriol. If required, calcidiol is hydroxylated to calcitriol in the mitochondria. Calcitriol translocates to the nucleus (bound to intracellular vitamin-D-binding proteins), where it binds to the vitamin D receptor (VDR). The ligand-bound VDR and its heterodimer partner, retinoid X receptor, bind to specific DNA sequences known as vitamin D response elements and, under the regulation of a number of accessory proteins, function as a transcription factor (Figure 8.4).

There is evidence that vitamin D is also able to act via a nongenomic pathway and a membrane receptor.

Physiological actions of vitamin D

Vitamin D is classically known to mediate Ca^{2+} homeostasis but a role has now also emerged as a potent regulator of a number of other cellular functions. Vitamin D regulates the development of cells within the immune system and plays a role in the modulation of inflammation. It has antiproliferative and prodifferentiation properties and has been shown to induce apoptosis and impair progression through the cell cycle in a number of cancer cell types.

Vitamin D affects Ca^{2+} homeostasis by acting on the bone, the intestine and the kidney. In bone, calcitriol regulates osteoblast activity to increase bone mass and calcification. Vitamin D is also required for chondrocyte development. Consequently, vitamin D deficiency results in defective bone mineralisation and growth plate abnormalities (rickets in children and osteomalacia in adults). Vitamin D also promotes osteoclast differentiation and so promotes bone resorption. By increasing the development and function of both osteoblasts and osteoclasts, vitamin D increases the rate of bone remodelling.

Ca^{2+} absorption in the intestine, as outlined in Figure 8.1, also requires adequate calcitriol levels. Vitamin D signalling increases the expression of TRPV6, calbindins, calmodulin and PMCA and can increase intestinal Ca^{2+} absorption three-fold.

In the kidney, vitamin D has three main actions. It increases Ca^{2+} reabsorption in the proximal and distal convoluted tubules. It increases PO_4^{3-} reabsorption in the proximal convoluted tubule and inhibits activation of vitamin D by inhibition of 1α-hydroxylase. In chronic kidney disease, mineral homeostasis is disrupted. The reduced activity of renal 1α-hydroxylase leads to reduced levels of calcitriol and eventually triggers secondary hyperpara-thyroidism and chronic kidney disease – mineral and bone disorder. Vascular calcification (arteriosclerosis) is also common in people with chronic kidney disease and is responsible for increased morbidity and mortality.

Vitamin D deficiency and rickets

Vitamin D deficiency can be of nutritional origin (poor diet or malabsorption), although this is rare, or caused by failure to synthesise vitamin D. Vitamin D activation may be limited in liver or kidney disease and insufficient vitamin D production is also associated with ultraviolet light deficiency (lack of sunlight).

Vitamin D deficiency causes rickets in children and osteomalacia in adults. These are conditions of decreased mineralisation of the bones, attributable to a lack of both Ca^{2+} and vitamin D and sometimes PO_4^{3-}.

In rickets, there is a failure to mineralise endochondral bone in the growth plate, which results in elongation of the growth plate and delayed calcification. Weight bearing produces deformity of the limbs. Other likely bone defects include soft skull bones (craniotabes), delayed closure of the anterior fontanel, Harrison sulcus (indentation of the chest wall; pigeon chest) and thickening of the ankles, knees and wrists. Affected children also suffer from bone pain, increased fractures, defects in tooth formation and muscle weakness.

In osteomalacia, there is a failure to mineralise newly formed osteoid. This leads to increased osteoid width and decreased bone mineralisation. Bones appear thin on X-ray and the most common feature is osteopenia/osteoporosis. Occasionally, looser zones may be apparent, which suggests osteomalacia. A bone biopsy may be needed to confirm the diagnosis.

Vitamin D resistance also presents as vitamin D deficiency. Two rare genetic conditions exist: vitamin D resistance type 1 or pseudovitamin D resistance, which is caused by a defect in the 1α-hydroxylase gene, and vitamin D resistance type 2 or hereditary vitamin-D-resistant rickets, where there is a defect in the gene encoding VDR.

CALCITONIN

Calcitonin is a peptide hormone that is produced by the C cells (parafollicular cells) in the thyroid gland in response to increased circulating Ca^{2+} levels. Calcitonin acts on the kidneys and bone but, in contrast to PTH and vitamin D, it decreases serum Ca^{2+} levels.

Calcitonin synthesis, receptors and release

Post-transcriptional processing of the calcitonin gene leads to the production of calcitonin and calcitonin-gene-related peptide. However, the physiological actions of calcitonin and calcitonin-gene-related peptide are distinct. This contrasts with the situation regarding PTH and PTHrP, which are the products of different genes but have some similar actions.

Calcitonin-gene-related peptide is a potent vasodilator but it also functions as a neurotransmitter. By contrast, calcitonin is released in response to hypercalcaemia, binds to a G-protein-coupled receptor and activates cAMP signalling.

Physiological actions of calcitonin

Calcitonin acts on the bone and kidney. In the kidney, calcitonin inhibits reabsorption of PO_4^{3-} and Ca^{2+} in the proximal tubule, promoting their excretion. In bone, it acts on the osteoclasts, causing them to shrink and reduce bone resorption and so preventing the release of Ca^{2+} and PO_4^{3-}. Interestingly, calcitonin seems to have a relatively minor role in Ca^{2+} homeostasis in humans.

IMPORTANT POINT

Hormone action

For each hormone you should know:

- the type of receptor through which it works
- where and how it is synthesised
- the signal for synthesis/release
- the target organ
- the biological action and physiological consequence.

Phosphate

As we have already seen, Ca^{2+} homeostasis is closely related to that of PO_4^{3-} but this chapter is not going to discuss the regulation of PO_4^{3-} homeostasis in detail. PO_4^{3-} ions are stored in bone and bone reabsorption and remodelling release PO_4^{3-} in addition to Ca^{2+}. Likewise, Ca^{2+}-containing foods generally also contain PO_4^{3-}, so an increase of dietary Ca^{2+} will often increase dietary PO_4^{3-}. Absorption of PO_4^{3-} from the diet is efficient, with about 80% of ingested PO_4^{3-} being absorbed.

PO_4^{3-} is required for the formation of high-energy compounds (for example ATP and creatinine phosphate) and second messengers (for example cAMP, inositol phosphates) and for the phosphorylation of enzymes. It is also a component of DNA, RNA, bone and membrane phospholipids.

Approximately 86% of PO_4^{3-} is stored in the bone and 14% is present intracellularly; the extracellular concentration of PO_4^{3-} is very low (0.03–0.1%). The normal serum concentration of PO_4^{3-} is 0.8–1.4 mmol/l and, in contrast to Ca^{2+}, only 10% of serum PO_4^{3-} is bound.

It is important to remember that the kidney is the only organ capable of excreting PO_4^{3-}. Hence, people with chronic kidney disease are at risk of hyperphosphataemia.

FIBROBLAST GROWTH FACTOR 23

Both bone reabsorption and an increase in vitamin D will lead to increases in the serum levels of PO_4^{3-} as well as Ca^{2+}. It is therefore important that there is a mechanism to prevent vitamin-D-mediated hyperphosphataemia. Fibroblast growth factor 23 is a PO_4^{3-}-regulating hormone (a phosphatonin). The phosphaturic molecule is produced by mineralised tissues, in particular osteocytes and possibly osteoblasts, in response to stimulation with vitamin D. It acts by reducing the expression of NPT2 in the apical membrane of the proximal tubule, which in turn increases PO_4^{3-} excretion in urine.

Pregnancy and calcium balance

Pregnancy and lactation are periods of increased Ca^{2+} requirement to enable the growth of fetal tissues and the production of milk, and are a huge drain on the mother's mineral resources. The fetus contains approximately 20–30 g of Ca^{2+} and is relatively hypercalcaemic compared with the mother (the ratio of the fetal to maternal Ca^{2+} concentration is 1.4 to 1.0). Most (80%) of the Ca^{2+} accumulation in the fetus occurs in the third trimester, when ossification occurs.

Ca^{2+} and PO_4^{3-} are transferred to the fetal circulation against a concentration gradient by use of various Ca^{2+} transporters. Many fetal tissues produce PTHrP, which plays a role in the regulation of placental Ca^{2+} transport by modifying placental calbindin or the PMCA.

The fetus can also synthesise PTH by week 12 of gestation (PTH does not cross the placenta) but serum levels of this hormone remain low for the first 2–3 days postpartum. At birth, the newborn baby has low PTH and high calcitonin levels.

To cope with the requirements of the fetus, the mother has decreased/normal levels of PTH, increased levels of calcitonin and increased levels of vitamin D. Ca^{2+} absorption from the intestine is also increased. These changes occur early in the pregnancy before the fetus requires significant amounts of Ca^{2+}. It is thought that this increases the mother's Ca^{2+} stores in preparation for the fetal requirement. Maternal bone mineral density (BMD) varies throughout pregnancy with changes in both cortical BMD (generally increased) and trabecular BMD (generally decreased). Bone turnover also increases in the third trimester.

FETAL DEVELOPMENT AND VITAMIN D

Studies have linked the vitamin D status of the mother to the development of the fetus. For example, studies of knockout mice that are deficient of the genes encoding VDR or 1α-hydroxylase have suggested that vitamin D is vital for fertility and fetal development. There is also a clear link between the development of diabetes (type 1 and type 2) and vitamin D levels in both the mother and the baby. All pregnant women, particularly Asian women, should receive vitamin D supplementation during pregnancy and breast feeding. A number of European countries also supplement children for the first few years of life.

Bone

Bone is a metabolically active tissue that has a number of functions:

- support
- protection (e.g. skull and ribs)
- production of blood cells from the bone marrow
- attachment of muscle, tendons and ligaments
- storage (buffer) of minerals (Ca^{2+}, PO_4^{3-} and Mg^{2+}).

BONE STRUCTURE

Normal bone comprises a protein matrix (osteoid) and a mineral component. Osteoid makes up about 25% of bone content and is secreted by osteoblasts. It consists of type 1 collagen (90%) and noncollagenous proteins (glyco-proteins and proteoglycans; approximately 10%). The mineral component (hydroxyapatite) makes up approximately 65% of bone content. Mineralisation requires high concentrations of Ca^{2+} and PO_4^{3-} for crystallisation to occur. The strength of bone is dependent on bone mineral content, but the structure is also extremely important. It is highly organised and can be considered analogous to reinforced concrete in that it requires strength and rigidity but also flexibility to complement the brittleness of the hydroxyapatite. Collagen provides resilience and the mineral component rigidity.

There are two types of bone tissue: trabecular (also referred to as cancellous) and cortical (or compact). Trabecular bone is strong, lightweight and has a spongy appearance. By contrast, cortical bone is extremely strong but heavy and forms the outer (cortical) layer of the bone. In the axial skeleton, there is only a thin layer of cortical bone. Trabecular bone has a very large surface area that is significantly greater than that of cortical bone. As a result, it provides a large area for interaction with the extracellular fluid, which makes it more important than cortical bone in Ca^{2+} and PO_4^{3-} homeostasis.

Histologically, bone can be classified as woven bone (new bone) or lamellar bone (mature bone). Woven bone results from rapid osteoid production, such as occurs in fracture healing. The collagen structure is haphazard and the resulting bone is weak. Lamellar bone is remodelled woven bone; it is highly organised with collagen fibres that are arranged in parallel lamellae (sheets).

BONE CELLS

There are three types of bone cells: osteoblasts, osteoclasts and osteocytes. Osteoblasts are the cell type responsible for bone production and arise from mesenchymal stem cells. They produce matrix components and mineralise osteoid. When inactive, they form flat bone-lining cells.

Osteoclasts reabsorb bone. They are multinucleated cells from the bone marrow lineage that act alone or in pairs. Attachment of the osteoclasts to the bone surface is essential for bone reabsorption.

Osteocytes are terminally differentiated osteoblasts trapped in the bone. They are located in lacunae (small cavities) and maintain contact with the surface by cellular extensions that pass through fluid-filled canaliculi (Figure 8.5). They respond to mechanical strain and release calcium via the canaliculi.

BONE REMODELLING

Bone remodelling occurs continuously on the surface of the bone to maintain good-quality bone and structural integrity. Remodelling can be periosteal (occurring at the periosteum–bone interface) and endosteal (occurring at the bone–bone marrow interface).

Remodelling occurs in small areas called osteons, as illustrated in Figure 8.5. The quiescent bone surface is

FIGURE 8.5 **Bone remodelling**

A Quiescent phase

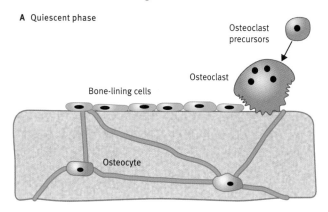

B Osteoclastic bone resorption

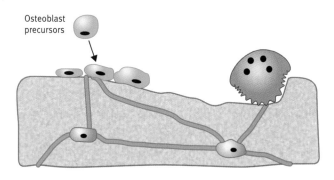

C Deposition of osteoid by osteoblasts and mineralisation of the new bone

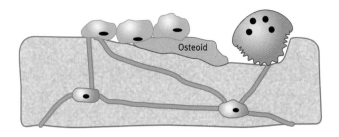

which is eventually mineralised. A complete cycle takes between 90 and 130 days.

Osteoclastic bone reabsorption and osteoblastic bone formation are normally tightly coupled. A disruption in this balance leads to altered bone mineral content and structure. For example, too much or too little bone may be produced (as in osteopetrosis or osteoporosis) or the structure may be modified (as in rickets and osteomalacia, where there is loss of mineral component).

A number of factors regulate bone remodelling and bone cell development and function, including hormones, cytokines and growth factors. Estrogen is vital for normal bone development in both men and women. It inhibits osteoclast function and osteoclastogenesis and may promote osteoblast survival. Its loss at the menopause is fundamental in the development of postmenopausal osteoporosis. Similarly, testosterone is required for bone strength in both men and women and hypogonadism accounts for approximately 20% of osteoporosis in men. Glucocorticoids (cortisol) are also required for bone development. However, excess levels of glucocorticoids are associated with decreased bone formation and increased bone loss as well as with decreased intestinal Ca^{2+} absorption and increased renal Ca^{2+} excretion. Key to osteoblast:osteoclast regulation is RANKL (RANK ligand). Produced by osteoblasts RANKL binds to RANK receptors on mature osteoclasts and osteoclast precursor cells increasing osteoclast formation, function and survival. Osteoprotegerin (OPG), which is also produced by osteoblasts, acts as a decoy receptor that binds excess RANKL and prevents it binding to the osteoclasts. Denosumab, a new anti-osteoporotic treatment, is a monoclonal antibody that mimics OPG. Sclerostin, which is primarily produced by osteocytes, inhibits bone formation. Mechanical stimulation of osteocytes (such as weight bearing exercise), reduces sclerostin and so promotes bone formation.

ASSESSMENT OF BONE REMODELLING AND BONE MINERAL DENSITY

BMD can be assessed by imaging and biochemical measurements. X-rays will often show defects in bone structure but dual energy X-ray absorptiometry (DEXA) is the diagnostic measure of BMD and bone mineral content (see Chapter 10 for further information on this technique). Areas of osteoblastic activity can be

lined with bone-lining cells (Figure 8.5A). Osteocytes embedded in the bone are connected to each other and the bone surface via a series of canaliculi. Following a 'bone resorption' signal, mature osteoclasts develop. These break down the bone structure, destroying both the hydroxyapatite and osteoid and leaving small pits (Howship lacunae) in the bone surface (Figure 8.5B). Osteoblast differentiation is triggered and osteoblasts then fill the resorption pits with osteoid (Figure 8.5C),

TABLE 8.5 **Biochemical measures of bone turnover**

Type of bone-cell activity measured	Serum markers	Urinary markers
Bone formation and/or remodelling	Bone-specific alkaline phosphatase [a]	
	Osteocalcin [a]	
	Propeptides of type 1 collagen [a]	
Bone resorption	TRAP [b]	Hydroxyproline
	Type 1 collagen	Pyridinolines
	Collagen cross-links	Collagen cross-links

[a] Produced by osteoblasts; raised levels indicate increased bone turnover, which usually reflects increased bone reabsorption produced by osteoclasts;
[b] raised levels indicate increased osteoclastic activity | TRAP = tartrate-resistant alkaline phosphatase produced by osteoclasts

identified following injection of a radionucleotide (often technetium) that targets areas of bone remodelling.

Biochemical markers of bone turnover can measure either bone formation or bone resorption; they are listed in Table 8.5.

If it is important to identify at a cellular level the pathological changes that have occurred, then a bone biopsy can be taken. Bone biopsies are not performed unless necessary because the procedure is invasive and painful.

OSTEOPOROSIS AND OSTEOPENIA

Osteoporosis, which means porous bones, is a common bone disease. One in two women and one in five men over the age of fifty years are at risk of an osteoporotic fracture. It is a combination of decreased BMD and a change in microarchitecture that can result in fractures following minimal trauma. Osteoporotic fractures are associated with increased morbidity and mortality.

Osteoporosis occurs when osteoclast resorption exceeds osteoblast bone formation. Consequently, in a normal bone-remodelling cycle, the resorption pits are not fully restored by the osteoblasts and microfractures are not effectively repaired. In osteoporosis, both collagen and mineral is lost, so in contrast to most other bone conditions, the remaining bone is normal but there is less of it.

Although osteoporosis is associated with bone pain, often the first sign of osteoporosis is a fracture. Compression fractures of the spine, which cause kyphosis, are a common feature of osteoporosis. Osteoporosis is frequently considered to be a female disease but it has been recognised recently that it is also common in men. The

increased numbers of men being diagnosed with osteoporosis is in part attributable to increased life expectancy.

Osteopenia is identical to osteoporosis but there is less loss of bone mineral. Management involves the prevention of progression to osteoporosis. Often nothing is done, except to offer dietary and lifestyle advice (increase Ca^{2+} intake, increase weight-bearing exercise, ensure the person is vitamin D-replete, reduce smoking and consumption of alcohol).

The possibility of identifying osteopenia, a forerunner to osteoporosis, raises the question of screening. Currently, DEXA scans are not performed unless there is a predisposition to osteoporosis, such as long-term steroid use, premature menopause, prolonged secondary amenorrhoea, a history of fragility fractures, radiological osteopenia, vertebral deformity or a family history of early and severe osteoporosis. If a screening programme were introduced, this would raise the question of what treatment to offer to those identified with osteopenia.

Diagnosis of osteoporosis and osteopenia

The World Health Organization diagnostic criteria for osteoporosis are outlined in Table 8.6. The diagnosis is made on the basis of the BMD value as determined by a DEXA scan.

What determines whether a person develops osteoporosis?

It is important to realise that it is perfectly normal to lose bone mineral, and so BMD, as we age. Bone loss

TABLE 8.6 **World Health Organization diagnostic criteria for osteoporosis**

Category	T-score [a]
Normal	Above −1.0
Osteopenia	−1.0 to −2.5
Osteoporosis	Below −2.5

[a] Defined as the number of standard deviations above or below the average bone mineral density value for a young healthy adult

occurs at almost every skeletal site with age. It becomes a problem when the BMD falls so low that it increases the fracture risk. It is very important to prevent fractures as osteoporotic fractures are associated with increased morbidity and mortality. So what determines how much bone an individual loses?

During childhood and early adult life, bone formation is greater than bone resorption and over 90% of adult bone mass is acquired, with the rate of bone mass acquisition being greatest during the pubertal growth spurt (Figure 8.6). The bone mass accrued by the time full skeletal maturation is achieved is known as the peak bone mass, which is higher in men than in women. Bone mass then remains fairly constant until around 40 years of age, at which point bone formation becomes less efficient and bone loss begins to occur. The rate of bone loss in men and women is similar, with the exception of the period around the menopause, when the loss of estrogen accelerates the rate of loss in women (Figure 8.6). Both the rate of bone loss and the peak

bone mass obtained are important factors that determine a person's chance of developing osteoporosis.

In women, the loss of estrogen at menopause is often the main cause of osteoporosis development. In men, hypogonadism and prescribed corticosteroids account for around 40% of osteoporosis; however, osteoporosis in men is often idiopathic.

Risk factors associated with an osteoporotic fracture include low BMD, low body weight, rheumatoid arthritis, cigarette smoking, alcohol consumption, poor nutrition, vitamin D and/or Ca^{2+} deficiency, physical inactivity, sex hormone deficiency and some drugs (corticosteroids, heparin). Endocrine disorders including hypogonadism, hyperparathyroidism, hyperthyroidism and Cushing syndrome and some malignancies are also associated with bone loss. It is thought that genetic factors account for 50–80% of the variance in BMD.

Why is the loss of BMD so damaging? The loss of bone strength seen in osteoporotic bone is greater than that attributable to the loss of bone mineral content alone. This is because in osteoporosis there is also a change in the structure of trabecular bone. The complex cross-linking of the trabeculae gives bone added strength and a loss of this cross-linking results in an additional loss of structural integrity.

INTERESTING FACTS

Osteoporosis

- Hip fractures in the UK cause as many deaths as breast cancer.
- Men experience more osteoporotic fractures than prostate cancer.
- Every 3 minutes someone in the UK has an osteoporotic fracture.

Management of osteoporosis

Minimising any further loss of bone and prevention of fractures are the main management strategies in osteoporosis. Peak bone mass cannot be altered once it has been obtained; therefore, management should focus on:

- maintenance of current BMD and reduction in the rate of bone loss
  - lifestyle and dietary advice

FIGURE 8.6 **Change in bone mass with age**

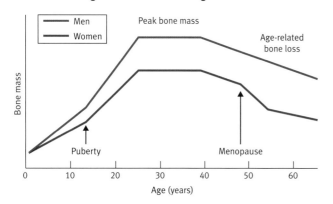

- drug treatment (most current osteoporosis drugs prevent further bone loss; anabolic drugs are likely to be important in the future)
- early detection (DEXA scan)
- prevention of fractures
  - minimising falls (good footwear, glasses, walking aids, muscle strength and balance)
  - lessening the impact of falls (hip protectors).

The National Institute for Health and Care Excellence (NICE) has produced guidelines for the prevention of primary and secondary osteoporotic fractures. At present, the drugs of choice are bisphosphonates. Selective estrogen receptor modulators, PTH and Denosumab are also covered by current NICE guidelines. Hormone replacement therapy, while effective, should not be prescribed for osteoporosis treatment unless other drugs are ineffective or not tolerated.

Pregnancy, lactation and osteoporosis

Pregnancy and breastfeeding are a significant drain on the mother's Ca^{2+} stores. For example, lactation requires 280–400 mg/day of Ca^{2+} and clinical osteoporosis, while rare, can occur. However, pregnancy-induced osteoporosis is difficult to assess (imaging techniques include exposure to radiation). It is usually identified in the third trimester (41%) or postpartum (56%). The presenting signs and symptoms are similar to those of age-related osteoporosis: pain, loss of height and vertebral fractures.

It is important to try and assess whether the osteoporosis is attributable to the pregnancy or whether the pregnancy has exacerbated a pre-existing condition. However, pregnancy-induced osteoporosis and lactation-induced osteoporosis usually resolve approximately 6 months after birth or weaning and neither presents an increased lifetime risk of osteoporosis.

Juvenile osteoporosis

Osteoporosis is rare in children. However, if it does occur, it can have a significant impact on the peak bone mass, as most bone accretion occurs during childhood. The rate of bone mass increase is most rapid during the first 3 years of life and most Ca^{2+} is deposited during puberty. In addition, as described earlier, the peak bone mass can determine the risk of developing osteoporosis and clinicians are concerned that current lifestyles of young and adolescent children will not promote the development of a good peak bone mass.

Although juvenile osteoporosis is often idiopathic, it can also be caused by an underlying condition (rheumatoid arthritis or an endocrine disorder), drugs (steroids are a particular risk factor) or lifestyle.

Calcium homeostasis and teeth

When considering Ca^{2+} homeostasis and abnormalities of bone, the teeth should not be forgotten. Teeth are embedded in bone and contain three types of mineralised tissues: enamel, dentine and cementum. The mineral component of teeth resembles hydroxyapatite and they contain cells similar to osteoblasts. Odontoblasts make dentine, cementoblasts produce cementum and ameloblasts synthesise enamel.

People with conditions that alter Ca^{2+} homeostasis, such as pregnancy and chronic kidney disease, often have problems with teeth. Defects of the teeth are also seen in genetic skeletal disorders, such as osteogenesis imperfecta and osteopetrosis. Likewise, metabolic bone disorders (vitamin D deficiency, rickets, hypophosphataemia, Paget's disease and osteoporosis) are associated with defective tooth development and mineralisation.

FURTHER READING

International Osteoporosis Foundation: www.iofbonehealth.org.

National Osteoporosis Society: www.nos.org.uk.

NUSSEY S S, WHITEHEAD S A. The parathyroid glands and vitamin D. In: NUSSEY S S, WHITE S A. Endocrinology: An Integrated Approach. Oxford: BIOS Scientific Publishers Ltd; 2001. p171–212.

SHOBACK D, SELLMEYER D, BIKLE D D. Metabolic bone disease. In: GARDNER DG, SHOBACK D, editors. Greenspan's Basic and Clinical Endocrinology. 8th ed. San Francisco: McGraw-Hill; 2007. p281–345.

Human metabolism: carbohydrates, fats and proteins

Mary Board

Introduction

In accordance with the principle of energy conservation, energy extracted from food is harnessed for energy-consuming processes such as mechanical work, biosynthesis, active transport and protein phosphorylation. The link between the metabolism of fuels and the consumption of energy is provided by the high-energy compound ATP (Figure 9.1) and metabolic pathways are strictly regulated to ensure maintenance of appropriate levels

FIGURE 9.1 **Maintenance of ATP levels**

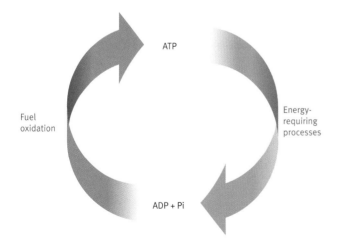

ATP

Fuel oxidation

Energy-requiring processes

ADP + Pi

ADP = adenosine diphosphate | ATP = adenosine trisphosphate |
Pi = inorganic phosphate

of ATP. The differing requirements of individual cells and tissues mean that the ways in which ATP supplies are maintained are quite diverse.

Carbohydrate metabolism

Carbohydrates are the only fuels that can be respired anaerobically and, moreover, glucose represents the most accessible energy source for many cells and tissues, most notably the brain and the erythrocyte.

FORMS OF CARBOHYDRATE

Dietary carbohydrate can be ingested in a wide variety of forms, ranging from simple mono- or disaccharides to huge polymers (polysaccharides) that contain hundreds or thousands of monosaccharide residues (Table 9.1). The mono- and disaccharides provide the body with readily available glucose and their ingestion produces a rapid increase in blood glucose level. By contrast, glucose polymers, which are most abundant in the form of storage compounds such as plant starches or animal glycogen (Table 9.1), take much longer to be digested.

One way or another, all dietary carbohydrate can be converted to glucose. When glucose is removed from the blood because of its consumption by tissues, it is quickly replenished by breakdown of hepatic glycogen or by synthesis via hepatic gluconeogenesis.

TABLE 9.1 **Examples of dietary carbohydrate**

Carbohydrate	Monosaccharide components	Source
MONOSACCHARIDES		
Glucose	Glucose	Fruit, honey
Fructose	Fructose	Fruit, honey
DISACCHARIDES		
Lactose (milk sugar)	Glucose, galactose	Milk
Sucrose (table sugar)	Glucose, fructose	Cane sugar, prepared foods
TRISACCHARIDES		
Trehalose	Glucose	Mushrooms
POLYSACCHARIDES		
Amylose	Glucose (linear)	Plant starch
Amylopectin	Glucose (branched)	Plant starch
Glycogen	Glucose (branched)	Meat

FIGURE 9.2 **Glycolysis**

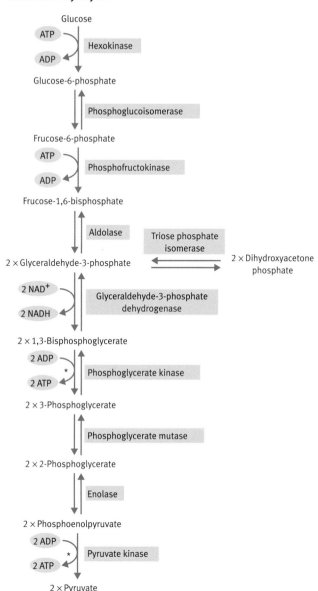

* Reactions responsible for the production of ATP by substrate-level phosphorylation | ADP = adenosine diphosphate | ATP = adenosine triphosphate | NAD$^+$ = oxidised form of nicotinamide adenine dinucleotide | NADH = reduced form of NAD

OVERVIEW OF GLUCOSE METABOLISM

Glucose is a versatile fuel: not only can it be consumed by all tissues, but it can also be respired anaerobically, unlike fats or proteins. Aerobic and anaerobic respiration of glucose share the initial pathway of glycolysis in the cytosol. In the absence of O_2, glycolysis leads to the conversion of 1 mole of glucose to 2 moles of lactate. This conversion brings about the formation of ATP via substrate-level phosphorylation and the production of the reduced co-factor nicotinamide adenine dinucleotide (NADH).

Aerobic respiration continues in the mitochondrion with the tricarboxylic acid (TCA) cycle and the electron transport chain and results in the complete oxidation of the glucose molecule to its combustion products, CO_2 and H_2O:

$$C_6H_{12}O_6 + 6\,O_2 \rightarrow 6\,CO_2 + 6\,H_2O$$

ANAEROBIC METABOLISM

All glucose metabolism begins with the anaerobic cytosolic pathway of glycolysis (Figure 9.2). The pathway converts the six-carbon glucose molecule into two molecules of the three-carbon compound pyruvate, with the net production of 2 moles of ATP per mole of glucose by substrate-level phosphorylation.

Under anaerobic conditions, pyruvate is reduced to lactate (Figure 9.3). Indeed, the appearance of lactate in

FIGURE 9.3 **Reduction of pyruvate to lactate**

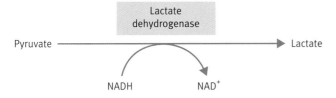

NAD^+ = oxidised form of nicotinamide adenine dinucleotide |
NADH = reduced form of NAD

the bloodstream is often used as an indicator of the occurrence of anaerobic respiration. The molecule represents a metabolic dead end: the body has no use for lactate other than to reconvert it to pyruvate. However, production of lactate from pyruvate by lactate dehydrogenase results in the regeneration of oxidised nicotinamide adenine dinucleotide (NAD^+) from NADH. This step is vital for the continued operation of glycolysis under anaerobic conditions because NAD^+ is a co-factor for the oxidation of glyceraldehyde-3-phosphate (Figure 9.2) and cytosolic supplies of NAD^+ are limited.

The glycolytic pathway can be reversed to bring about synthesis of glucose from noncarbohydrate sources (gluconeogenesis) in the liver. When this occurs, the irreversible reactions in Figure 9.2 (unidirectional arrows) must be bypassed by separate reactions catalysed in the reverse direction, whereas the reactions denoted by double arrows may be freely reversed.

AEROBIC METABOLISM: PYRUVATE DEHYDROGENASE REACTION AND TRICARBOXYLIC ACID CYCLE

Under aerobic conditions, the product of the glycolytic pathway is pyruvate, which becomes the substrate for the remaining steps of the oxidative metabolism that take place within the mitochondrion. The three-carbon pyruvate molecule is converted to the two-carbon acetyl coenzyme A (CoA) molecule by the enzyme pyruvate dehydrogenase (PDH), in a reaction that produces NADH. Acetyl CoA is then consumed by the TCA cycle (Figure 9.4) and converted to two molecules of CO_2. The cycle also produces three molecules of NADH, one molecule of the reduced form of flavin adenine dinucleotide ($FADH_2$) and one molecule of guanosine

triphosphate (GTP) per turn (Table 9.2). The reduced co-factors NADH and $FADH_2$ pass their electrons along the electron transport chain to elicit ATP synthesis and GTP may be converted to ATP.

The PDH reaction, which links the anaerobic and aerobic pathways, is irreversible and cannot be bypassed in the reverse direction. Thus, no pathway exists for the conversion of acetyl CoA into pyruvate. Moreover, while two carbon atoms enter the TCA cycle in the form of acetyl CoA, two carbon atoms are lost as CO_2, meaning that there is no net gain of carbon by any TCA cycle intermediate. Thus, there is no pathway for the synthesis of glucose from acetyl CoA. These observations achieve significance during starvation.

ATP YIELD FROM GLUCOSE

Aerobic respiration produces 30–32 moles of ATP per mole of glucose, compared with 2 moles of ATP obtained during anaerobic respiration. This means that aerobic respiration of glucose is 15–16 times more efficient than anaerobic respiration. Table 9.2 illustrates how the ATP yield is derived.

Quoted yields of ATP vary considerably from text to text. Some sources put ATP yields at 30–32 moles for aerobic respiration, others at 36–38 moles. This discrepancy represents more than just the usual inability of biochemists to agree among themselves. The higher figure is derived from theoretical considerations, where the amount of energy liberated when electrons travel along the electron transport chain is divided by the amount of energy required to synthesise an ATP molecule. Theoretical yields are 3 moles of ATP per mole of NADH and 2 moles of ATP per mole of $FADH_2$. The lower figure is based on empirical values, that is, those derived from experiment. Empirical yields for NADH and $FADH_2$ are 2.5 moles of ATP and 1.5 moles of ATP, respectively. These values are lower because some of the energy obtained from electron transport is used for the export of ATP from the mitochondrion as well as for the synthesis of ATP.

ANAEROBIC TISSUES

Several cells and tissues rely wholly or partly on anaerobic respiration, either in a constitutive manner or as

FIGURE 9.4 **Tricarboxylic acid cycle**

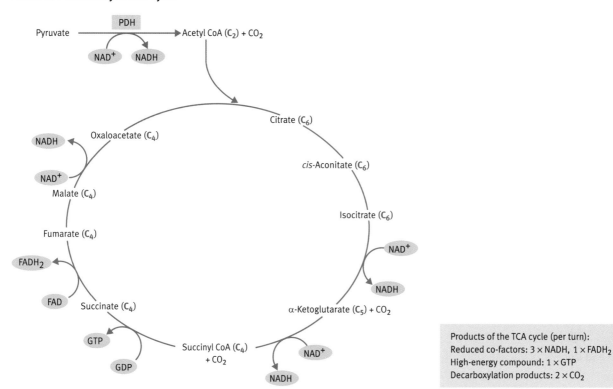

Note that 2 moles of acetyl CoA are produced per mole of glucose and that oxidation of this acetyl CoA requires two turns of the cycle.
CoA = coenzyme A | GDP = guanosine diphosphate | GTP = guanosine triphosphate | FAD = oxidised form of flavin adenine dinucleotide |
FADH$_2$ = reduced form of FAD | NAD$^+$ = oxidised form of nicotinamide adenine dinucleotide | NADH = reduced form of NAD |
PDH = pyruvate dehydrogenase | TCA = tricarboxylic acid

circumstances dictate. Partially anaerobic tissues include the kidney medulla, which is poorly perfused by blood and therefore receives little O$_2$, and the cells of the retina, where O$_2$ metabolism is not favoured lest it damage the light-sensitive pigments necessary for photoreception. More extreme examples are represented by the red blood cell and by vigorously exercising white (type 2) muscle fibres.

Red blood cells show great economy of volume to maintain a property of deformability, which allows them to travel unimpeded through narrow capillaries. One of the means by which this is achieved is the complete absence of intracellular organelles, including mitochondria. Thus, the red blood cell has zero capacity for oxidative metabolism and relies entirely on anaerobic conversion of glucose to lactate to meet its energy requirements.

By contrast, white muscle fibres do have mitochondria. These fibres compose fast-twitch muscles, which

are the 'fight or flight' muscles responsible for escape from danger (or, more mundanely, for sports such as sprinting). The rapid response of such muscles, and the ATP requirement involved, precludes use of the aerobic route for ATP generation. This is not because the aerobic route is longer and more time-consuming, but rather because the rate of O$_2$ diffusion into the muscle fibre is so slow by comparison with the rate of ATP consumption by the contracting muscle. However, the very rapid rates of the enzyme-catalysed reactions in the glycolytic pathway can be increased 1000-fold in an almost instantaneous manner and this is sufficient to cater for the muscle's energy requirements.

As with all anaerobic episodes, the only fuel that can be respired by white muscle fibres is glucose. The white muscle fibre has large stores of intracellular glycogen to produce glucose units for anaerobic respiration (Figure 9.5) and the breakdown of glycogen in

TABLE 9.2 **Steps contributing to ATP yield during anaerobic and aerobic respiration of glucose**

Reduced co-factors produced (moles per mole glucose)	Route of ATP synthesis	Resulting ATP yield[a] (moles per mole glucose)
GLYCOLYSIS		
	Substrate-level phosphorylation	2 ATP
2 NADH [b]	Oxidative phosphorylation	5 ATP
PDH REACTION		
2 NADH	Oxidative phosphorylation	5 ATP
TCA CYCLE		
	Substrate-level phosphorylation [c]	2 ATP
6 NADH	Oxidative phosphorylation	15 ATP
2 FADH$_2$	Oxidative phosphorylation	3 ATP

The blue bracket shows the scope of anaerobic respiration, the red bracket that of aerobic respiration; [a] estimated from empirical data; [b] NADH generated in the cytosol must be shuttled into the mitochondrion; [c] substrate-level phosphorylation during the succinyl coenzyme A synthetase reaction produces guanosine triphosphate, which can be used to synthesise ATP. | FADH$_2$ = reduced form of flavin adenine dinucleotide | NADH = reduced form of nicotinamide adenine dinucleotide | PDH = pyruvate dehydrogenase | TCA = tricarboxylic acid

FIGURE 9.5 **Fuels for anaerobically respiring muscle**

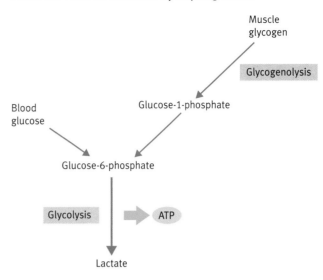

contracting muscle is stimulated by adrenaline, among other factors. The muscle cannot produce free glucose from glycogen because it lacks the enzyme glucose-6-phosphatase; therefore, glycogen is broken down to the glycolytic intermediate glucose-6-phosphate. The muscle may also take up glucose from the blood to fuel anaerobic ATP production. Ultimately, the source of blood glucose is likely to be liver glycogen.

CARBOHYDRATE METABOLISM DURING STARVATION

During starvation, the body has access to huge fat reserves (which are metabolised to acetyl CoA) but to very little carbohydrate. Glycogen reserves are substantially depleted by the overnight fast and are undetectable after about 24 hours of fasting. This brings the body to something of a crisis because the brain has an absolute

requirement for glucose. In the fed state, the brain consumes about 100 g/day of glucose and while this requirement can be reduced to about 25 g/day during starvation, it cannot be diminished any further. During such episodes, hepatic gluconeogenesis must maintain supplies of glucose.

However, the irreversibility of the PDH reaction now presents something of a stumbling block: although the abundant fat stores allow the production of large amounts of acetyl CoA, this cannot be converted to pyruvate, which would be a gluconeogenic substrate. There is also no way of synthesising another gluconeogenic intermediate from acetyl CoA because two carbon atoms are lost during TCA cycle activity. The net result of these observations is that fat can never be converted to glucose under any circumstances.

It is interesting to note that plants, perhaps as a result of occupying an evolutionary pinnacle, do have means of converting fat into glucose (the glyoxylate shuttle).

Given that the brain's glucose requirement must be satisfied for its continued function, glucose must be synthesised from non-carbohydrate, non-fat precursors.

This role is fulfilled by muscle protein and amino acids are released from wasting muscle relatively early on in starvation (Figure 9.6). Such wasting is not without its penalty, however, since loss of muscle protein leads to loss of function. Death from starvation (which occurs after around 60 days in a normal-sized adult) is most commonly caused by weakening of essential muscles.

FIGURE 9.6 **Release of glucogenic amino acids by muscle tissue during prolonged starvation**

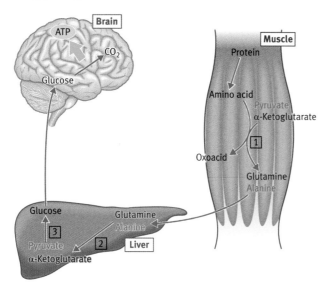

Transamination reactions (1) convert the constituent amino acids of muscle protein into the transportable glucogenic amino acids alanine and glutamine; the liver transdeaminates (2) alanine and glutamine and their carbon skeletons can be used to synthesise glucose through the pathway of gluconeogenesis (3).

MAINTENANCE OF BLOOD GLUCOSE CONCENTRATIONS IN THE NORMAL AND DIABETIC STATE

The body expends a great deal of effort and energy in maintaining blood glucose levels within very narrow limits (Figure 9.7). For a healthy individual without diabetes, for whom glucose homeostasis is strictly controlled, fasting blood glucose might be as low as 4 mmol/l and postprandial levels might rise as high as 8 mmol/l but values do not vary outside these limits. Blood glucose is maintained during the first 24 hours of starvation by mobilisation of liver glycogen and thereafter by muscle protein breakdown, followed by gluconeogenesis. Blood glucose concentrations are maintained at around 4 mmol/l for the duration of starvation, until death occurs.

By contrast, uncontrolled diabetes can result in vast fluctuations in blood glucose concentration with severe consequences (Figure 9.7). The brain is perfectly able to function when the blood glucose concentration is 4 millimoles/l but loses this ability at 2 mmol/l, when a hypoglycaemic coma is very likely to result (Figure 9.7).

When the blood glucose concentration is 2 mmol/l, there is still a total of 1.8 g of glucose present in the circulation (compared with 3.6 g at 4 mmol/l) but this glucose becomes much less accessible to the brain. These values are derived by assuming that an average-sized person has 5 l of blood (the molecular weight of glucose is 180 g). Here we can appreciate the importance of considering the concentration rather than the quantity of glucose. The brain takes up glucose by facilitated diffusion using the proteinaceous glucose transporter type 3 (GLUT3). GLUT3 has a K_M for glucose of 1.6 mmol/l, meaning that the transporter will be saturated with glucose and working at maximal capacity at all normal concentrations of blood glucose. If the blood glucose concentration drops below 3 millimoles/l, however, the brain's glucose transporter is no longer saturated and is not able to satisfy the brain's glucose requirement. Such a situation is characteristic of hypoglycaemic coma caused, for example, by the presence of diabetes or by overconsumption of alcohol.

The Michaelis constant K_M, represents the substrate concentration at which an enzyme-catalysed reaction or a transport process reaches half-maximum velocity. If the K_M is low, only a low substrate concentration is required for a process to occur at maximum velocity and vice versa. It is noteworthy that the glucose transporter in the brain has a lower K_M than those present in any other cell or tissue. To a certain extent, this allows the brain preferential access to the glucose present in the bloodstream. (The K_M is often quoted as an inverse index of the affinity of a transporter or enzyme for its substrate. This is not an equation that bears close scrutiny but it does provide a useful conceptual perspective: if the K_M is low, the affinity is high and vice versa.)

Fat metabolism

Fat molecules show great versatility in the uses to which they are put by the body. Table 9.3 outlines some of the diverse roles of fats. During the present chapter we will concern ourselves with their role in energy storage and oxidation.

In terms of both mass and caloric content, fat represents by far the largest energy depot in the body. Fat is stored as triacylglycerol (TAG or triglyceride) (Figure 9.8),

.

FIGURE 9.7 **Blood glucose levels**

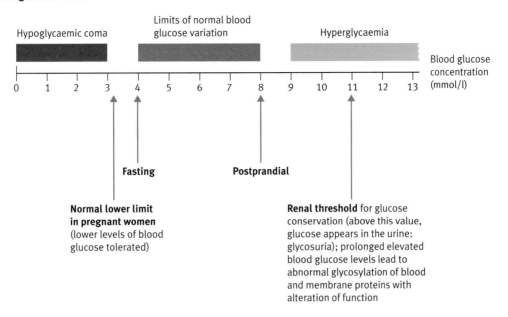

TABLE 9.3 **Major roles of fats in the body**

Role	Form
Energy storage	Triacylglycerol
Membrane formation	Phospholipids
Hormone synthesis	Eicosanoids (prostaglandins, thromboxanes, leucotrienes formed from essential fatty acids)
Intracellular signalling	Membrane phospholipids broken down to second messengers when hormone binds to its receptor
Regulation of gene transcription	Fatty acids (plus fat-soluble vitamins)

FIGURE 9.8 **Structure of triacylglycerol**

The presence of a double bond causes the fatty acid side chain to bend and adopt an angle of 135 degrees; such bends disrupt the packing of the side chains and thus the inclusion of unsaturated fatty acids is important in maintaining the fluidity of the TAG depot. [a] monounsaturated fatty acid | [b] saturated fatty acid | [c] polyunsaturated fatty acid | TAG = triacylglycerol

which forms liquid droplets in the cytosol of the adipocyte. This represents a particularly efficient form of energy storage for many reasons. The fatty acid side chains of the TAG molecule are long and contain many hydrogen atoms, which behave as a reservoir of reducing potential for the production of the reduced co-factors NADH and $FADH_2$. These co-factors pass their electrons along the electron transport chain and elicit ATP production. This translates into an energy yield per unit weight for fat that is more than twice that for either carbohydrate or protein (Table 9.4).

The storage of TAGs in an anhydrous form (much different from the highly hydrated glycogen deposits in liver and muscle tissue) also contributes to the density and efficiency of energy storage. Moreover, fat can be stored in limitless quantities around the human physique.

TABLE 9.4 **Energy content of the main dietary components**

Component	Energy yield (kJ/g)
Fat	37
Carbohydrate	17
Protein	17

The adipocyte is a remarkably flexible cell that can shrink or expand to adopt a spherical shape to accommodate changing requirements for fat storage.

MOBILISATION OF TRIACYLGLYCEROL

The TAG molecule (Figure 9.8) consists of a three-carbon glycerol backbone that is esterified to three fatty acid side chains and the free fatty acid molecule constitutes the accessible energy source for cells and tissues. The liberation of fatty acids from the TAG molecule is catalysed by the enzyme hormone-sensitive lipase (HSL) (Figure 9.9), in a reaction that is strictly controlled. Appropriate signals from adrenaline or glucagon ensure that fats are mobilised in response to a need for physical activity or during fasting, and the

opposing signal from insulin conserves fat depots during the fed state.

It follows that the level of HSL activity has a strong impact on the level of plasma fatty acids and we can see the results of this association in Table 9.5. Many conditions, such as fasting or exercising, produce an increase in the plasma concentration of fatty acids. A salutary note is sounded by the example of the racing driver (see the 'stress' entry in Table 9.5), who leads a stressful but sedentary lifestyle, which results in high levels of the stress hormone adrenaline. Adrenaline promotes the elevation of plasma fatty acid levels and prolonged elevation of blood fats is known to increase the risk of coronary heart disease (CHD). The propensity for atherosclerotic plaques to develop in the presence of high circulating levels of fats and cholesterol provides one of the links between CHD and the pursuit of a stressful lifestyle.

People with diabetes also have elevated plasma levels of fatty acids (Table 9.5). The absence or reduction of the antilipolytic insulin signal in diabetes causes HSL to continue producing fatty acids even in the fed state (Figure 9.9). Again, this situation has its consequence in an increased risk of CHD among individuals with long-term diabetes. The term metabolic syndrome (or syndrome X) describes the frequent co-occurrence of type 2 diabetes, hypertension and CHD.

FIGURE 9.9 **Lipolysis and its control**

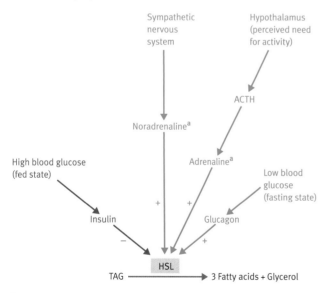

[a] Mediated by beta-3-adrenergic receptors | + indicates an increase in HSL activity | − indicates a decrease in HSL activity | ACTH = adrenocorticotrophic hormone | HSL = hormone-sensitive lipase | TAG = triacylglycerol

TABLE 9.5 **Level of fatty acids in the blood under various conditions**

Condition	Hormonal agent that influences HSL activity	Plasma fatty acids (mmol/l)
Normal (fed)	Balance between insulin and glucagon	0.1–0.3
Starvation[4]	Glucagon	2.2 [a]
Stress[5]	Adrenaline	1.7 [b]
Exercise[6]	Adrenaline	1.0 [c]
Diabetic coma[7]	Absence of insulin signal	3.0
Gestational diabetes mellitus[8]	Reduction of insulin signal	0.7

[a] Value refers to a prolonged period of starvation (8 days) | [b] value refers to the example of the racing driver | [c] value refers to 15 minutes of exercise followed by 15 minutes of rest | HSL = hormone-sensitive lipase

TRANSPORT OF FATS

Fats of all kinds, being hydrophobic and insoluble, are transported in the blood in complexes with proteins (Table 9.6). Different lipoprotein complexes have different fat components and fulfil different functions. Thus, the lipid profile of the blood (that is, the relative concentrations of the different lipoprotein complexes) can provide an index of health. High levels of low-density lipoprotein (LDL), often resulting from a high-fat diet but occasionally from a genetic disorder such as familial hypercholesterolaemia, are associated with an increased risk of CHD. By contrast, high levels of high-density lipoprotein (HDL), which imply active excretion of cholesterol, are associated with a lowered risk of CHD (Table 9.6).

Some dietary practices are considered to have a favourable impact on the lipid profile and to cause lowering of LDL and raising of HDL levels. Among these practices is the consumption of a diet rich in monounsaturated fats, such as olive oil (the Mediterranean diet) or certain nut oils including almond and walnut oils.

TABLE 9.6 **Lipoproteins in the circulation**

Lipoprotein	Main fat constituent	Function
Chylomicron	Dietary TAG	Transports TAG from the intestine to other tissues for oxidation or storage (fed state)
VLDL	Endogenous TAG, cholesterol	Transports TAG produced in the liver to other tissues where it can be oxidised (fasting state)
LDL	Cholesterol and cholesteryl ester	Transports cholesterol from the liver to other tissues
HDL	Cholesteryl ester	Scavenges cholesterol from many tissues and takes it to the liver for excretion
Fatty acid–albumin	Fatty acid	Transports fatty acids from adipose tissue to other tissues where they can be oxidised (fasting state)

HDL = high-density lipoprotein | LDL = low-density lipoprotein | TAG = triacylglycerol | VLDL = very-low-density lipoprotein

Another is the pursuit of the Atkins diet,[1,2] a weight-reducing diet that involves the consumption of very little carbohydrate but unlimited quantities of fat and protein. This last observation is difficult to explain. It has been suggested that the high protein content of the Atkins diet has a satiating effect on the appetite. Thus, caloric intake by a person on the Atkins diet tends to be lower than that by control subjects. If the reduced caloric intake includes a reduced intake of fat, then there will be a corresponding reduction in lipoprotein particles carrying dietary fat and cholesterol (chylomicrons and LDLs).

OXIDATION OF FATTY ACIDS

Many highly aerobic tissues, such as heart tissue and the red fibres of skeletal muscle, consume and oxidise fatty acids at a high rate. Once inside the cell, the fatty acid is activated by attachment of CoA. The fatty acyl CoA then constitutes the substrate for the beta-oxidation pathway.

Oxidation takes place inside the mitochondrion and repeated cycles of the beta-oxidation pathway (Figure 9.10) nibble away the hydrocarbon chain of the fatty acid. Each cycle produces one molecule of the two-carbon compound acetyl CoA as well as one molecule of $FADH_2$ and one molecule of NADH.

The shortened fatty acyl CoA rejoins the pathway for a repeat cycle. The acetyl CoA product is consumed by the TCA cycle in exactly the same way as that produced from pyruvate (Figure 9.4) and the reduced co-factors elicit ATP production. Table 9.7 shows the tally of ATP-production from the 16C fatty acid palmitate.

INTEGRATION OF FAT AND CARBOHYDRATE METABOLISM

We have already observed the disparity between carbohydrate and fat stores in the body. Fat can be stored in seemingly limitless quantities, whereas glycogen reserves are very limited, lasting for only about 24 hours of starvation in the adult. This means that, after the first day of starvation, fat becomes the predominant fuel for the body, and it is a very energy-dense and efficient form of fuel.

However, fat has some limitations as a fuel source for the whole body with its diverse tissue-specific requirements. We have already seen that fat cannot be

FIGURE 9.10 **Beta-oxidation pathway**

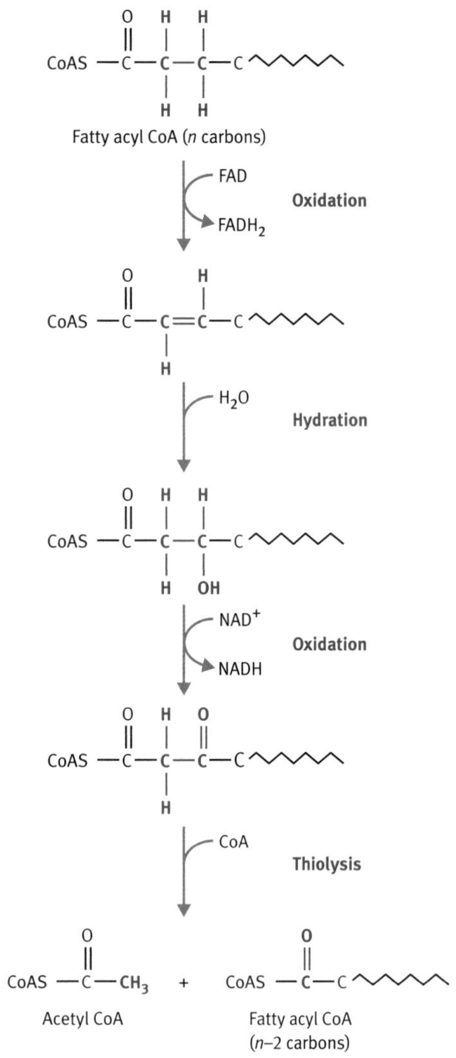

Fatty acyl CoA (n carbons)

— FAD

Oxidation

— FADH$_2$

— H$_2$O

Hydration

— NAD$^+$

Oxidation

— NADH

— CoA

Thiolysis

Acetyl CoA + Fatty acyl CoA (n–2 carbons)

Repeated cycles of these four reactions convert the fatty acid with n carbons into $n/2$ moles of acetyl CoA. CoA = coenzyme A | FAD = oxidised form of flavin adenine dinucleotide | FADH$_2$ = reduced form of FAD | NAD$^+$ = oxidised form of nicotinamide adenine dinucleotide | NADH = reduced form of NAD

TABLE 9.7 **ATP production from oxidation of palmitate**

Reduced co-factors/GTP produced (moles per mole palmitate)	ATP produced (moles per mole palmitate)
7 × BETA-OXIDATION	
7 NADH	17.5
7 FADH$_2$	10.5
8 × TCA CYCLE	
24 NADH	60
8 FADH$_2$	12
8 GTP	8
FATTY ACID ACTIVATION	
None	−2
TOTAL	
	106

oxaloacetate molecule (Figure 9.4). To accommodate any extra acetyl CoA produced from increased rates of fat oxidation, levels of oxaloacetate must rise, too. Since glycogen has been depleted and oxaloacetate cannot be produced from acetyl CoA (owing to the loss of two CO_2 molecules earlier in the cycle), the carbon needed for oxaloacetate synthesis must derive from muscle protein (Figure 9.11).

OXIDATION OF FATS DURING STARVATION: KETOGENESIS

An unusual situation exists inside liver cells because the liver is the only tissue performing significant rates of gluconeogenesis. During starvation, oxaloacetate is withdrawn from the TCA cycle in the liver to fuel gluconeogenesis (Figure 9.12). Since the liver also takes up fatty acids and rates of beta-oxidation remain high in this tissue, the imbalance between levels of acetyl CoA and oxaloacetate in the liver mitochondria is exaggerated (Figure 9.12). This imbalance stimulates the liver to channel excess acetyl CoA into ketogenesis.

The resulting ketone bodies are released into the blood for use by many tissues, most notably the brain. Ketone bodies supply about 75% of the brain's energy requirements during prolonged starvation. Ketone body

converted into glucose and is, therefore, useless in satisfying the brain's glucose requirement. Moreover, the brain itself cannot consume fatty acids as a fuel because lipoproteins do not cross the blood–brain barrier. Thus, oxidation of fatty acids cannot supply the 75% shortfall generated in the brain's energy requirements by its reduced glucose consumption during the starved state.

There is another factor to consider. When acetyl CoA is consumed by the TCA cycle, it must condense with an

FIGURE 9.11 **Metabolism during starvation: oxidation of fats by peripheral tissues**

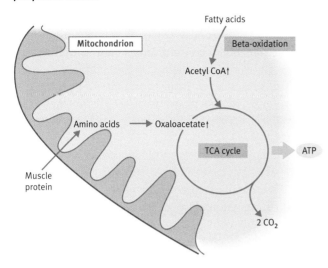

↑ = increased | CoA = coenzyme A | TCA = tricarboxylic acid

FIGURE 9.12 **Metabolism during starvation: gluconeogenesis and ketogenesis in the liver**

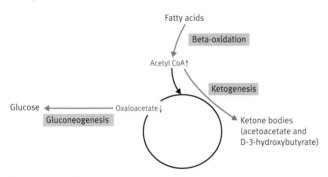

↑ = increased | ↓ = decreased | CoA = coenzyme A

production increases sharply after the first 24 hours of starvation and levels are sustained (at around 8 mmol/l) until death occurs.

DIABETIC KETOACIDOSIS

An interesting complication arises for individuals with diabetes, in whom impaired control of HSL means that the plasma concentration and rates of oxidation of fatty acids persist at high levels even in the fed state. Since the rates of beta-oxidation and ketogenesis are little regulated other than by supply of their substrates (fatty acids and acetyl CoA, respectively), the loss of control of HSL

leads to the uncontrolled production of ketone bodies. These compounds can achieve concentrations in the blood of people with diabetes that are several times higher than the normal maximum of 8 mmol/l.

Ketone bodies are acidic molecules, as are fatty acids. The acidic burden presented by the co-presence of ketone bodies and fatty acids in high concentrations can have an overwhelming effect on the buffering capacity of the blood, leading to a drop in pH (acidosis).

Diabetic ketoacidosis can be a severe condition, leading to a hypoxic coma. It is characteristic of type 1 diabetes, particularly when insulin therapy is interrupted or when a concurrent illness is present. The sequence of events is outlined in Figure 9.13. The drop in pH, although superficially small, disturbs many important interactions, perhaps most notably that of haemoglobin and O_2, which is pH-dependent. The erythrocyte attempts to rectify this situation by adjusting levels of 2,3-bisphosphoglycerate, a small molecule that mediates the affinity of haemoglobin for O_2.

Treatment for diabetic ketoacidosis, which centres on a slow infusion of insulin (given in the presence of glucose to avoid abrupt change in the blood glucose level), was in the past accompanied by administration of isotonic sodium bicarbonate if the blood pH was below 7. However, any clinical adjustment of the pH value must be made gradually to allow the erythrocyte time to readjust levels of 2,3-bisphosphoglycerate and this is a difficult balance to achieve. Hence, treatment with sodium bicarbonate is not a current practice. The dose of insulin administered is relatively low: sufficient to suppress hepatic glucose output but not high enough to stimulate glucose uptake by tissues.

GESTATIONAL DIABETES MELLITUS

The consequences, outlined previously, of a loss or reduction of insulin control apply to any type of diabetes, but a word could profitably be said about the special case of gestational diabetes mellitus (GDM). Mild insulin resistance seems to affect all pregnant women and may be necessary to ensure that maternal uptake of glucose and other nutrients does not compromise fetal requirements. GDM represents a more severe situation but it is difficult to tell whether this disorder occurs at the extreme end of the normal insulin

FIGURE 9.13 **Metabolic disturbances in diabetic ketoacidosis**

Loss of antilipolytic insulin signal

↓

High plasma concentration of fatty acids, high plasma concentration of ketone bodies

↓

Drop in blood pH (from 7.4 to 6.9)

↓

Kidney excretes H^+, electrolytes and water; osmotic diuresis develops as a result of hyperglycaemia and glycosuria

↓

Dehydration

↓

Reduced blood flow

↓

Inefficient delivery of O_2 to peripheral tissues (which begin to respire anaerobically, producing lactate, which contributes to the acidic burden)

↓

Hypoxia

↓

Subject takes huge gulping breaths ('air hunger') in an attempt to rectify the hypoxia and exhales CO_2

↓

Lowering of PCO_2 in blood

Clinical symptoms:
- hyperglycaemia and glycosuria
- ketonaemia and ketonuria
- low blood pH, K^+ and PO_4^{3-}
- low blood PO_2 and PCO_2

PCO_2 = partial pressure of CO_2 | PO_2 = partial pressure of O_2 | PO_4^{3-} = phosphate ion

resistance spectrum in pregnancy or whether it represents an incipient form of type 2 diabetes.

There is some evidence to suggest that women who suffer from GDM, which normally persists only for the duration of pregnancy, may be at higher risk of developing type 2 diabetes later in life.[3] Some characteristics of GDM strongly resemble those of type 2 diabetes. Insulin levels are normal or raised but accompanied by high levels of plasma fatty acids and ketone bodies (high blood ketone body concentrations and ketonuria are often considered to be diagnostic for GDM). This indicates the presence of insulin resistance. Postprandial glucose levels in the blood are also greatly increased, presumably because of impaired uptake by maternal tissues.

The high glucose levels stimulate uptake by the fetus, which has a high metabolic requirement for this substrate. The rate of glucose uptake by the fetus is predictive of birth weight, and the raised blood glucose levels in GDM probably contribute to the fetal macrosomia that is associated with this condition.

Protein metabolism

Rates of protein degradation are accelerated in two situations. The first concerns the consumption of a high-protein diet, when intake exceeds requirements, since excess protein cannot be stored. The second involves the increased breakdown of muscle protein during starvation, which is designed to release amino acids for glucose synthesis. In either event, proteins are degraded to their constituent amino acids.

Amino acids, the building blocks of proteins, contain the elements nitrogen, carbon, hydrogen and oxygen. The nitrogenous amino group is disposed of separately from the carbon skeleton. This separation is necessary to maintain nitrogen balance in the body and prevent accumulation of toxic nitrogenous compounds such as the ammonium ion (NH_4^+).

The removal of the amino group is the first stage in amino acid metabolism. The amino group is incorporated into urea by the hepatic urea cycle and the remaining carbon skeleton contributes to one of the branches of metabolism already encountered in this chapter.

REMOVAL OF THE ALPHA-AMINO GROUP

Amino acids undergo a combination of transamination reactions, where the amino group is transferred to a

118

FIGURE 9.14 **Removal of the alpha-amino group in amino acid metabolism**

A Transamination

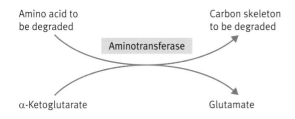

B Deamination

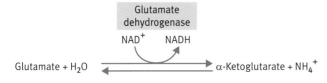

NH_4^+ = oxidised form of nicotinamide adenine dinucleotide | NADH = reduced form of NAD | NH_4^+ = ammonium ion

different carbon skeleton (Figure 9.14 A), and deamination, where the amino group is released as NH_4^+ (Figure 9.14 B). The transamination step is necessary to transfer the amino group from the target amino acid to α-ketoglutarate, thereby forming the amino acid glutamate. Glutamate is the substrate for the glutamate dehydrogenase reaction, which is able to accomplish the removal of the amino group in the form of NH_4^+.

One of the consequences of this sequence of reactions is that the pathway of amino acid degradation includes many aminotransferase enzymes with specificity for individual amino acids but only one enzyme (glutamate dehydrogenase) with deaminating activity.

UREA CYCLE

The urea cycle in the liver serves to detoxify NH_4^+. It incorporates 2 moles of nitrogen (1 mole derived from NH_4^+ and 1 mole from aspartate) into 1 mole of urea. Figure 9.15 shows the conversion achieved by the five reactions that constitute the urea cycle. The cycle consumes energy and spans both the cytosolic and the mitochondrial compartments. The product, urea, is a soluble, nontoxic vehicle for the transport of nitrogen atoms and is transported to the kidney for excretion.

Inborn errors of metabolism that result in deficiencies have been reported for all five enzymes that participate in the urea cycle. Such deficiencies result in hyperammonaemia and symptoms become manifest shortly after birth. The severity of the symptoms, which include swelling of the brain, lethargy and, ultimately, mental restriction, indicate the toxicity of NH_4^+ at high concentrations and justify the effort that the body expends in maintaining low concentrations.

The concentration of NH_4^+ does not normally exceed about 20 micromoles/l in the arterial and venous circulation (excluding the hepatic portal vein, where concentrations can be ten-fold higher). If concentrations are allowed to achieve values of 200 micromoles/l, then toxic symptoms appear. Even toxic concentrations are relatively low compared with those of most other blood-borne compounds and are insufficient to disturb the pH balance of the blood. Instead, high concentrations of NH_4^+ disturb some of the metabolic equilibria we have already met.

The two deamination reactions that convert glutamine to α-ketoglutarate produce NH_4^+, plus a reduced co-factor and a TCA cycle intermediate (Figure 9.16). Both reactions are reversible and can be displaced in the reverse direction if NH_4^+ concentrations exceed normal

FIGURE 9.15 **Synthesis of urea**

$$NH_4^+ + \text{Bicarbonate} + \underset{\text{(amino acid)}}{\text{Aspartate}} \xrightarrow[\text{3 ATP}]{\text{2 ADP} + \text{AMP}} \text{Urea} + \underset{\substack{\text{(TCA cycle} \\ \text{intermediate)}}}{\text{Fumarate}}$$

ADP = adenosine diphosphate | AMP = adenosine monophosphate | TCA = tricarboxylic acid

FIGURE 9.16 **Equilibria displaced by high concentrations of NH4+**

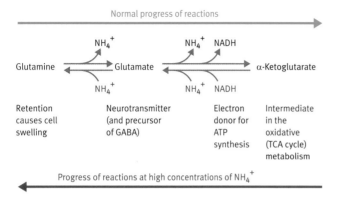

GABA = γ-aminobutyric acid | NADH = reduced form of nicotinamide adenine dinucleotide | NH$_4^+$ = ammonium ion | TCA = tricarboxylic acid

metabolism on which the brain depends for energy generation. Levels of the neurotransmitter glutamate are also depleted, leading to functional impairment. Moreover, the ultimate product of the displacement, glutamine, accumulates and, by an unknown mechanism, leads to cell swelling.

DEGRADATION OF AMINO-ACID CARBON SKELETONS

Each carbon skeleton has its individual pathway of de-gradation; but there are seven eventual degradation products for all 20 amino acids. These products are shown in Figure 9.17 and all represent intermediates on pathways previously encountered in this chapter.

Given that one of the situations identified when amino acid degradation occurs at high rates is that of starvation, an important property of amino acids concerns whether or not they may contribute to glucose synthesis.

levels. The consequences of this displacement, however, are deleterious for the brain for a number of reasons. If the reactions shown in Figure 9.16 are displaced to the left-hand side, α-ketoglutarate and NADH are depleted and both of them are vital components of the oxidative

FIGURE 9.17 **Degradation of carbon skeletons derived from amino acid metabolism**

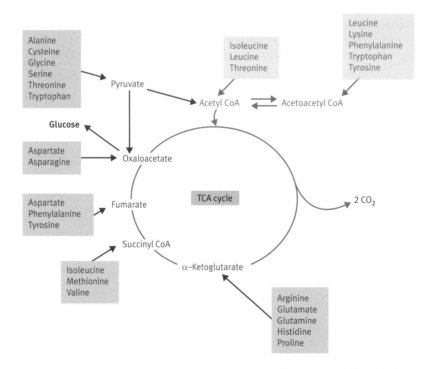

Glucogenic amino acids and intermediates are shown in red; ketogenic amino acids and intermediates are shown in blue. | CoA = coenzyme A | TCA = tricarboxylic acid

GLUCOGENIC AND KETOGENIC AMINO ACIDS

Amino acids can be classified according to whether their carbon skeleton can contribute to the synthesis of glucose (glucogenic amino acids) or ketone bodies (ketogenic amino acids). Inspection of Figure 9.17 will show that any carbon skeleton converted to α-ketoglutarate or a later TCA cycle intermediate or to pyruvate can eventually become an intermediate of the gluconeogenic pathway and produce glucose. By contrast, amino acids that are converted to acetyl CoA or to acetoacetyl CoA cannot contribute to glucose synthesis (because of the loss of CO_2 from the cycle). Instead, this second group of carbon skeletons can produce ketone bodies.

Both glucose and ketone bodies are important fuels during intermediate and prolonged starvation: both can be oxidised by many tissues (including the brain) to produce ATP. However, an especial significance attaches to the provision of glucose during starvation, because blood glucose levels must be maintained above

3 mmol/l to retain the accessibility of this substrate for the brain's glucose transporter.

Thus, when muscle protein breakdown accelerates during starvation, alanine and glutamine represent 60–70% of all amino acids released by muscle tissue. This does not reflect the composition of muscle protein, which is made up of a wide variety of the 20 amino acids available. Rather, it reflects the occurrence of transamination reactions within the muscle tissue that convert the constituent amino acids of muscle protein into alanine and glutamine. These two amino acids represent a stable means of transporting carbon to the liver, where the pathway of gluconeogenesis occurs (Figure 9.6).

Once in the liver, further rounds of transamination and deamination convert alanine and glutamine into pyruvate and α-ketoglutarate, respectively, which join the gluconeogenic pathway by the routes shown in Figure 9.18. Pyruvate is an intermediate on the cytosolic gluconeogenic pathway and is directly converted to glucose. α-Ketoglutarate is converted to oxaloacetate by reactions of the TCA cycle and then must be

FIGURE 9.18 **Conversion of glucogenic amino acids to glucose**

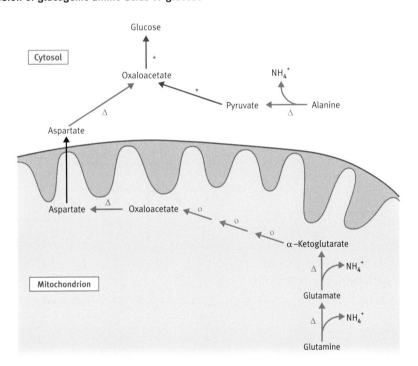

* = gluconeogenic pathway | ○ = tricarboxylic acid cycle | Δ = transamination reactions | NH_4^+ = ammonium ion

transaminated to aspartate to leave the mitochondrion because the membrane is impermeable to oxaloacetate. Once in the cytosol, aspartate is transaminated to oxaloacetate, an intermediate on the gluconeogenic pathway.

Protein metabolism makes a vital contribution to the provision of glucose for the brain during starvation. This is an expensive process, however, since loss of muscle protein is accompanied by loss of function. To maximise the utility of glucogenic substrates, such as amino acids, starvation conditions are characterised by the adoption of a glucose-sparing strategy: tissues that are able to use substrates other than glucose do so during starvation and, thus, spare the precious glucose resources for the brain.

Quantitatively, the most significant among the tissues that adopt such a strategy is skeletal muscle, largely because of the huge mass it represents. During starvation, when plasma fatty acids are abundant but levels of glucose and insulin are low, muscle relies heavily on uptake and oxidation of fatty acids and high rates of these processes serve to inhibit its uptake of glucose.

INTEGRATION OF METABOLIC PATHWAYS IN THE LIVER DURING STARVATION

Owing to its role in glucose homeostasis, the liver bears the brunt of adaptation to starvation conditions. It is the only tissue that performs appreciable rates of gluconeogenesis and is the sole site of ketogenesis. We have seen that these two pathways are integrated (Figure 9.12) and that the balance between the gluconeogenic intermediate, oxaloacetate, and the ketogenic substrate, acetyl CoA, is crucial in determining rates of ketone body synthesis.

Now we can see that protein metabolism has an impact on this scheme, too. The supply of glucogenic amino acids, along with activation of gluconeogenesis by the hormones glucagon and cortisol, maintains appropriate rates of glucose synthesis (Figure 9.6).

Inborn errors of metabolism

A short word could profitably be said about inborn errors of metabolism, a disproportionate number of which seem to affect the metabolism of amino acids. We have already noted the effects of such disorders with respect to the urea cycle. Such conditions are characterised by genetic mutations that affect pathway enzymes. When the mutation produces an enzyme of greatly diminished activity, the result is that a substrate commonly present in the diet cannot be metabolised. A relatively common inborn error with potentially disastrous consequences is phenylketonuria.

PHENYLKETONURIA

Phenylketonuria occurs in approximately 1 in 10 000 babies born in the UK and around 300 polymorphisms are thought to result in the same phenotype. The disorder is characterised by the absence or greatly diminished activity of the enzyme phenylalanine hydroxylase, with the result that the common amino acid, phenylalanine cannot be metabolised (Figure 9.19).

The consequences are various. Phenylalanine levels rise so that the amino acid takes part in unusual side reactions that produce phenylpyruvate, phenyllactate and phenylacetate (Figure 9.19). These compounds would normally be undetectable but appear in the urine when phenylketonuria is present.

The accumulation of phenylalanine itself interferes with uptake of many other amino acids by competition

FIGURE 9.19 **Molecular basis of phenylketonuria**

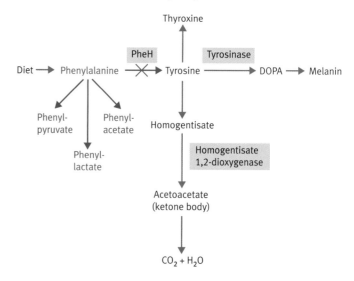

pheH = phenylalanine hydroxylase | DOPA = 3,4-dihydroxyphenylalanine

with the saturable amino acid transporter. This has a severe impact on the developing brain, which has a large requirement for amino acids for the synthesis of neuro-transmitters and myelin and to promote growth. In addition, phenylpyruvate probably interferes with the oxidative metabolism by competing with pyruvate for mitochondrial uptake. Again, this has a severe impact on the brain, a highly oxidative tissue that relies heavily on the oxidation of pyruvate generated from glucose to fuel its energy requirements.

It is, unfortunately, rather predictable that the most severe symptoms suffered by those with untreated phenylketonuria concern gross mental restriction (IQ below 50). However, screening programmes mean that phenylketonuria is readily detected by means of the Guthrie test, which is carried out 6–14 days after birth. A spot of the baby's blood is used to supplement the medium of a bacterial strain that requires phenylalanine for growth. If the blood levels are above 240 micro-moles/l, the bacteria flourish and phenylketonuria can be diagnosed.

Treatment involves the pursuit of a dietary regimen that excludes all but the minimal amounts of phenyl-alanine necessary for protein synthesis but includes sufficient amounts of tyrosine and other amino acids. Since accumulation of phenylalanine mainly affects the developing brain, the diet must be followed strictly until the age of around 11 years, but can then be relaxed. It must be resumed during pregnancy to protect the fetal brain. Many commercial protein substitutes are available to control phenylalanine intake but noncompliance (possibly owing to the unpalatability of the protein substitutes) is common. As a consequence, many phenylketonuria sufferers, although diagnosed and treated, endure some degree of cognitive deficit.

Inspection of Figure 9.19 reveals that the metabolism of phenylalanine is closely linked to that of the amino acid tyrosine, a precursor for the pigment melanin. As a consequence of disruption of the melanin synthetic pathway, partial albinism accompanies the other symptoms of phenylketonuria. Other inborn errors of metabolism can also affect the pathways shown in Figure 9.19; lack of tyrosinase causes occulocutaneous albinism and lack of homogentisate 1,2-dioxygenase causes alkaptonuria.

Metabolic adaptation

Fuels used and metabolic pathways available vary hugely over the lifespan and a good example of this is the difference between fetal and neonatal metabolism.

METABOLISM IN THE MATERNAL–FETAL UNIT

After an initial increase in insulin sensitivity in early pregnancy, mild insulin resistance develops in maternal tissues. Sensitivity can be reduced by 50–70% by the third trimester. This means that anabolic activities, such as lipogenesis and deposition of fat and glycogen by maternal tissues, are favoured in the first trimester but, by late pregnancy, nutrient uptake by the fetus is favoured at the expense of that by the mother.

During the late phase of pregnancy, maternal tissues take up little glucose but oxidise the abundant circulating fatty acids and ketone bodies at high rates (Figure 9.20). By contrast, the fetus consumes and oxidises glucose at high rates, aided by the maternal insulin resistance. Maternal blood glucose levels (which can rise steeply if GDM is present) are predictive of birth weight.

The fetus has little, if any, oxidative capacity for ketone bodies and fatty acids, although placental lipo-protein lipase activity increases in late gestation to allow storage of fat in preparation for birth. Overall, fetal

FIGURE 9.20 **Fuel in the maternal–fetal unit**

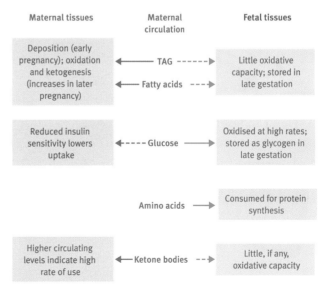

nutrition is oriented very much towards the consumption of glucose.

METABOLISM IN THE NEWBORN BABY

The baby's metabolism matures enormously around the time of birth, with many metabolic pathways becoming active that cannot be detected in the fetus. The newborn liver is replete with glycogen and this, together with the emergent pathway of gluconeogenesis (inactive in the fetus), serves to regulate blood glucose levels (Figure 9.21).

The capacity of the liver for fatty acid oxidation also increases dramatically to meet energy requirements and supply the newly active ketogenic pathway with substrate. Hepatic lipogenic capacity, however, remains low during suckling, when fats are supplied through milk, and only increases markedly on weaning. The metabolic pathways available to newborn babies equip them for consumption of a relatively high-fat diet

(human milk has a fat content of approximately 42g/l). Lipoprotein lipase activity in tissues such as heart, skeletal muscle and brown adipose tissue increases dramatically during suckling to increase the availability of dietary fats to those tissues. This high enzymatic activity is maintained until weaning.

Dietary fats are vital for several purposes, other than energy generation. Human milk is rich in polyunsaturated fats, such as the omega-3 fatty acid α-linoleic acid. Long-chain derivatives of α-linoleic acid, such as docosahexaenoic acid (DHA), are crucial for development of the specialised membranes of the central nervous system. About two-thirds of the central nervous system content of DHA is laid down during the last trimester of gestation with the remaining third being incorporated during the first 3 months of life. Even a small interruption of DHA supply during these crucial periods can lead to impairment of cognitive development and compromise visual acuity.

Moreover, fatty acids are the fuel consumed by a specialised thermogenic organ, brown adipose tissue (Figure 9.21). Human newborns lack the appropriate muscular development to enable heat generation by shivering. Instead, they have large deposits of brown adipose tissue, especially in the interscapular region. Owing to the partial uncoupling of electron transport from ATP synthesis in brown adipose mitochondria, this tissue is able to harness the chemical energy contained in fatty acids for heat production (instead of for ATP generation) in a process of nonshivering thermogenesis (Figure 9.21).

FIGURE 9.21 **Summary of energy-yielding pathways in the newborn**

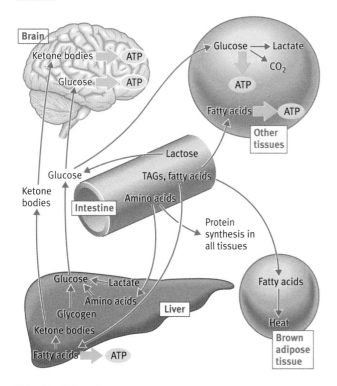

TAG = triacylglycerol

REFERENCES

1. STERN L, IQBAL N, SESHADRI P, CHICANO K L, DAILY D A, MCGRORY J, *et al.* The effects of a low-carbohydrate versus conventional weight loss diet in severely obese patients: one-year follow-up of a randomized trial. *Ann Intern Med* 2004;140:778–85.

2. YANCY W S JR, OLSEN M K, GUYTON J R, BAKST R P, WESTMAN E C. A low carbohydrate, ketogenic diet versus a low fat diet to treat obesity and hyperlipidaemia. *Ann Intern Med* 2004;140:769–77.

3. OATS J N, BEISCHNER N A, GRAND P T. The emergence of diabetes and impaired glucose tolerance in women who had gestational diabetes. In: WEISS P A M, COUSTAN D R, editors.

Gestational Diabetes. New York: Springer-Verlag; 1988. p.199–207.

4. ALBRINK M J, NEWIRTH R S. Effect of previous starvation on the response of plasma lipids and free fatty acids to a fat meal. *J Clin Invest* 1960;39:441–6.

5. TAGGART P, CARRUTHERS M. Endogenous hyperlipidaemia induced by emotional stress of racing driving. *Lancet* 1971; i:363–6.

6. FRIEDBERG S J, HARLAN W R, TROUT D L, ESTES E H. The effect of exercise on the concentration and turnover of plasma non-esterified fatty acids. *J Clin Invest* 1960;39:215–20.

7. WATKINS P J, HILL D M, FITZGERALD M G, MALINS J M. Ketonaemia in uncontrolled diabetes. *Br Med J* 1970;4:522–5.

8. MEYER B, CALVERT D, MOSES R. Free fatty acids and gestational diabetes mellitus. *Aust N Z J Obstet Gynaecol* 1996;36:255–7.

Biophysics

CHAPTER 10

Biophysics

Nazar N Amso and Neil Pugh

Introduction

Most obstetricians and gynaecologists use a wide range of equipment and instruments in their clinical practice, including ultrasound, X-rays and electronic instruments for monitoring the heart. However, not all practitioners fully appreciate the background principles on which these techniques are based. It is not so much the complex knowledge of physics and formulae that is required but rather a knowledge of how the principles of physics are applied in clinical practice. This is fundamental to a better understanding of the techniques as well as their safe, optimal and efficient use. In this chapter, each of the principal sections outlines the scientific foundations and uses of a procedure frequently used in our obstetric and gynaecological practice.

Principles and use of electrocardiography

Electrocardiography is a commonly used noninvasive procedure for the recording of electrical changes in the heart. The printed record, called electrocardiogram (ECG or EKG), traces the electrical impulses that are generated during each cardiac cycle. The waves in a normal record are labelled P, Q, R, S and T. The test evaluates cardiac function and identifies any problems that might exist in the frequency and rhythm of the heart rate or in the size and position of the heart's chambers; the test also assesses whether there is any myocardial damage.

RELATIONSHIP BETWEEN THE CARDIAC CYCLE AND ELECTROCARDIOGRAM

Electrical stimulation of the myocardium (depolarisation) is followed by restoration of the electrical potential of the myocardial cell (repolarisation). The electrical stimulation starts at the sinoatrial node, which acts as the natural cardiac pacemaker. The electrical signal then propagates through the internodal tracts of the atria to the atrioventricular node and subsequently activates the ventricles via the His–Purkinje system. This system consists of a bundle of fibres that divides into right and left branches. The left branch further divides into left anterior and posterior hemifascicles (Figure 10.1).

In an ECG, the P wave represents atrial depolarisation, while atrial repolarisation occurs during ventricular

FIGURE 10.1 **His–Purkinje system**

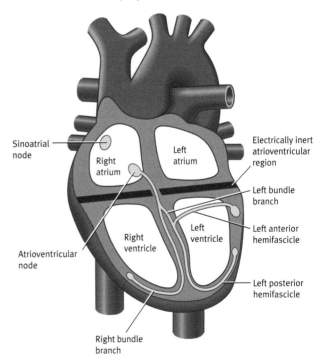

Adapted by permission from: BMJ Publishing Group Ltd. Meek S, Morris F. ABC of clinical electrocardiography. Introduction. I – Leads, rate, rhythm, and cardiac axis. *Br Med J* 324:415–8.

depolarisation and hence is not visualised. The QRS wave represents ventricular depolarisation, while the T wave represents ventricular repolarisation.

The ECG is recorded onto standard paper travelling at a rate of 25 mm/second. The paper is divided into large squares, each measuring 5 mm in width and representing 0.2 seconds. Each large square is divided into 25 small squares; a small square is 1 mm wide and represents 0.04 seconds.

ELECTRODE PLACEMENT AND SKIN PREPARATION

ECG lead electrodes are placed either in a bipolar or in a unipolar arrangement. In the bipolar lead arrangement, the electrical activity at a single positive electrode is compared with that at a single negative electrode. In the unipolar lead arrangement, the electrical potential at a single positive electrode, the so-called exploring electrode, is compared with the average electrical activity at several other electrodes, which serve as the negative pole.

The limb leads (I, II, III) are bipolar leads, while the augmented voltage leads (aVR, aVL, aVF) are unipolar leads. These six leads explore the electrical activity of the heart in the frontal plane (the orientation of the heart seen when looking directly at the anterior chest; see Figure 10.2).

The chest leads (V1, V2, V3, V4, V5, V6) explore the electrical activity of the heart in the horizontal plane (Figure 10.2). The reference point for the chest leads is obtained by connecting the left-arm, right-arm and left-leg electrodes together. The position of the six chest electrodes for standard 12-lead electrocardiography is depicted in Figure 10.3.

In a standard 12-lead ECG:

- leads II, III and aVF 'view' the inferior surface of the heart
- leads V1 to V4 view the anterior surface of the heart
- leads I, aVL, V5 and V6 view the lateral surface of the heart
- leads V1 and aVR view the right atrium and the cavity of the left ventricle.

The shape of the QRS complex in any lead depends on the orientation of that lead to the vector of depolarisation.

To obtain good electrical contact, the skin is cleaned and gel is applied before placing the electrodes. After removal of the electrodes at the end of the procedure,

FIGURE 10.2 **Vertical and horizontal perspectives of the electrode leads**

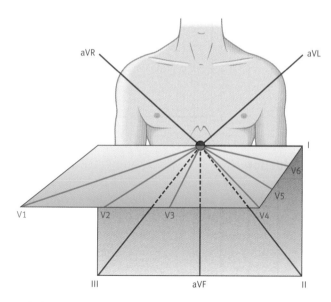

Red = frontal plane of the heart; green = horizontal plane of the heart.

Adapted by permission from: BMJ Publishing Group Ltd. Meek S, Morris F. ABC of clinical electrocardiography. Introduction. I – Leads, rate, rhythm, and cardiac axis. *Br Med J* 324:415–8.

FIGURE 10.3 **Position of the six chest electrodes for standard 12-lead electrocardiography**

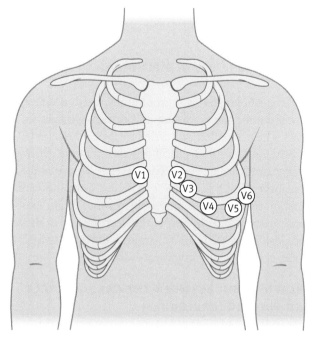

Adapted by permission from: BMJ Publishing Group Ltd. Meek S, Morris F. ABC of clinical electrocardiography. Introduction. I – Leads, rate, rhythm, and cardiac axis. *Br Med J* 324:415–8.

the skin should be thoroughly cleaned again to avoid skin irritation from the salty gel. No special precautions are required and no complications from this procedure have been observed.

FEATURES OF A NORMAL ELECTROCARDIOGRAM

Normal sinus rhythm on an ECG has the following cardinal features:

- The heart rate is 60–99 beats/minute.
- The cardiac rhythm is regular except for minor variations with respiration.
- The P wave is upright in leads I and II.
- The normal duration of the PR interval is 0.12–20 seconds. This is the time required for the completion of atrial depolarisation, conduction through the atrioventricular node and His–Purkinje system and arrival at the ventricular myocardial cells.
- Each P wave is usually followed by a QRS complex.
- The normal duration of the QRS interval is 0.06–0.10 seconds. This represents the time required for ventricular cells to depolarise.
- Normal values for the QT interval are between 0.30 and 0.43 seconds (0.30–0.45 seconds for women). This is the time required for depolarisation and repolarisation of the ventricles.

Young healthy individuals, especially athletes, may also display various other rhythms, especially during sleep. For example, respiration may cause sinus arrhythmia, characterised by beat-to-beat variation in the RR interval, with the heart rate increasing during inspiration. This is a vagally mediated effect in response to the increased volume of blood that returns to the heart during inspiration. Other normal findings noted in healthy individuals include tall R waves, prominent U waves (reflecting repolarisation of the papillary muscles or His–Purkinje fibres), ST segment elevation, exaggerated sinus arrhythmia, sinus bradycardia and first-degree heart block.

Principles and use of ultrasound

Diagnostic ultrasound uses the transmission of mechanical vibrations through matter to obtain some information about that matter. Ultrasound allows us to:

- determine the nature of a tissue (for example cystic or solid)
- assess the movement of tissues (such as fetal heart, bowel)
- measure blood flow (for example in the ovarian/follicular circulation, fetal circulation)
- measure structures (such as follicular diameter, femur length).

Ultrasound has an advantage over other imaging modalities because it is noninvasive and does not use ionising radiation. For these reasons, ultrasound can be used as a screening test and repeated examinations can be made with relative safety. Therefore, ultrasound is ideally suited for use in obstetrics and gynaecology.

THE SOUND WAVE AND ITS GENERATION

Sound is a pulsating pressure wave (that is, a mechanical disturbance of a medium) that passes through the medium at a fixed speed. Any sound wave can be defined by two main parameters, namely its amplitude, which is related to its acoustic power, and its frequency. Sound waves with frequencies above 20 kHz are termed ultrasound, with medical ultrasound operating in the low MHz range. Figure 10.4 shows the range of ultrasound frequencies used in the medical environment.

To produce ultrasound, there is the need to generate a pressure wave. This is achieved by incorporating a piezoelectric crystal within a transducer that is placed in contact with the tissue under investigation. The piezoelectric crystal converts electrical energy into mechanical energy and vice versa. When excited by a high-voltage current, the crystal oscillates at a given frequency, which is determined by the thickness of the crystal.

Two types of ultrasound can be produced, namely continuous-wave ultrasound and pulsed-wave ultrasound. For imaging purposes, pulsed-wave ultrasound

FIGURE 10.4 **Typical range of ultrasound frequencies used in clinical practice**

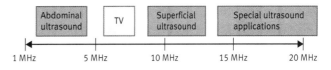

TU = transvaginal ultrasound

FIGURE 10.5 **Temporal profile of pulsed-wave ultrasound**

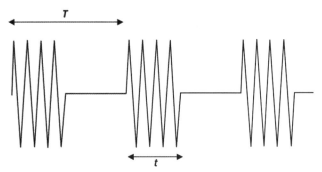

T = pulse repetition period | *t* = pulse length

is used. It consists of bursts or 'packets' of ultrasound that are sent out at a given frequency. The rate at which these bursts of ultrasound are sent out is known as the pulse repetition frequency. Figure 10.5 shows the temporal profile of pulsed-wave ultrasound. The advantage of this type of ultrasound is that it is possible to obtain spatial information and therefore imaging is possible.

INTERACTIONS OF ULTRASOUND WITH TISSUE

To build up an ultrasound image, the ultrasound pressure wave needs to interact with the tissue under investigation. The pressure wave then needs to return to the piezoelectric crystal to be converted from mechanical into electrical energy. There are three principal interactions with tissue:

- reflection
- scatter
- absorption.

Reflection occurs at interfaces between tissues with different characteristics. The tissue property that determines the degree of reflection is called the acoustic impedance (*Z*), which is related to the density (ρ) of the tissue and the velocity (*c*) of ultrasound in that particular tissue:

$$Z = \rho \times c$$

The greater the difference in acoustic impedance between two tissues, the greater the degree of reflection.

Scatter occurs when ultrasound interacts with a structure whose dimensions are similar to, or smaller than, the wavelength of the ultrasound wave. This is known as

Rayleigh scattering and the resulting wave is scattered in all directions (360 degrees scattering). This type of interaction typically occurs when ultrasound interacts with very small structures such as blood cells or parenchyma. The intensity of the scattered wave depends primarily on the dimensions of the target tissue and the wavelength of the ultrasound wave. Generally, the intensity of the scatter increases very rapidly with the frequency of the ultrasound pressure wave, which puts an upper limit on the frequency of ultrasound that can be used in clinical practice.

Absorption is the conversion of mechanical (ultrasound) energy into heat or internal molecular energy. This can obviously have detrimental results in that the heating effect can produce unwanted bioeffects. In addition, energy is lost from the ultrasound beam, reducing the penetration of the beam. Absorption increases with frequency, which effectively puts an upper limit of 20 MHz on the frequency of ultrasound that can be used.

The echoes generated from the reflection at tissue boundaries and the scattering within tissues and organs give rise to the complex echo trains from which the diagnostic information is derived.

REAL-TIME B-MODE (BRIGHTNESS MODE) ULTRASOUND SCANNING

Ultrasound scanning is a highly operator-dependent technique. To produce a B-mode ultrasound image, the ultrasound beam needs to be swept across the field of view (Figure 10.6A). Typically, 200 effective ultrasound beams will be used to produce an image (Figure 10.6B).

Figure 10.7 illustrates the main components of a typical B-mode ultrasound scanner. We will now discuss the role of these components in image formation.

The transducer houses the piezoelectric crystal and generates the ultrasound beam. Modern transducers tend to be broadband transducers with selectable frequencies. Transducers come in different shapes and sizes, depending on the frequencies used and the specific applications.

The power control allows adjustment of the amount of electric voltage that is applied to generate the ultrasound pulses.

FIGURE 10.6 **Image acquisition with ultrasound**

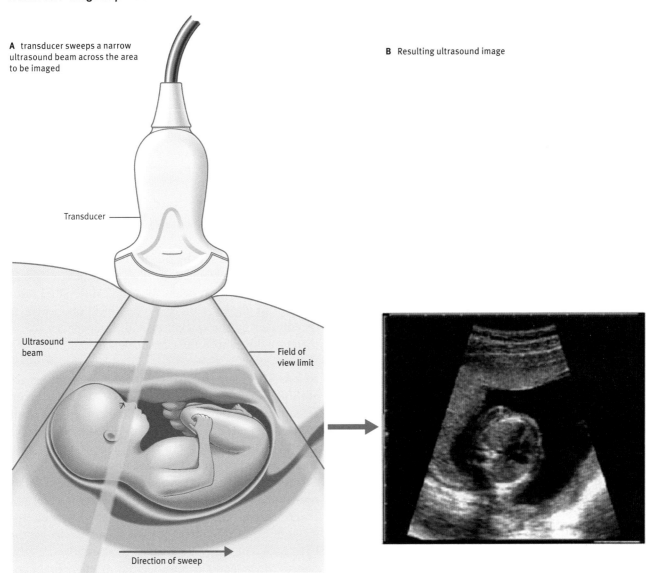

A transducer sweeps a narrow ultrasound beam across the area to be imaged

B Resulting ultrasound image

Transducer

Ultrasound beam

Field of view limit

Direction of sweep

The echoes received from the tissues are converted into electrical signals by the transducer. However, the received signal is much weaker than the transmitted signal and therefore a receiver amplifier boosts the returning signals to useful levels. As an analogy, the gain control acts like the volume control on a radio.

Owing to the attenuation of ultrasound pulses with depth, echoes from similar reflectors reduce in amplitude as the tissue depth increases. To ensure that echoes from similar reflectors at different depths are displayed at the same amplitude, it is necessary to compensate for attenuation. This is achieved using a technique called time-gain compensation, which essentially employs a series of amplifiers that can be adjusted to increase the image amplification at specific depths.

The scan converter controls the way in which the image is presented. It basically consists of computer memory elements that store grey-scale information and produces a digital image that is comprised of tiny picture elements (pixels). Each pixel has a unique address where the value of the echo amplitude is stored. This allows the appropriate shade of grey for each pixel

FIGURE 10.7 **Main operator-dependent components of a typical B-mode ultrasound scanner**

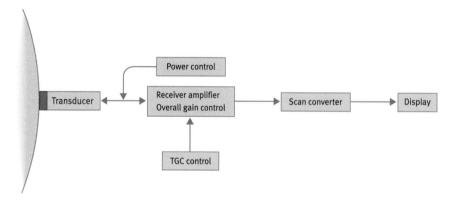

TGC = time-gain compensation

to be displayed on the screen. In the scan converter, various parameters such as preprocessing and postprocessing curves can be altered, which can improve image quality.

Flat screens or conventional monitors are used to display the images.

Limitations of real-time B-mode scanning

B-mode ultrasound scanning has several practical limitations including:

- inadequate spatial resolution
- inadequate penetration
- poor image quality (grey scale)
- low frame rate
- compromised field of view
- low line density.

Spatial resolution is the minimum distance between two reflectors or scattering surfaces that is necessary to be able to distinguish two separate echo signals. There are two main components to spatial resolution. Firstly, axial resolution, which is the minimum distance between two points that are located along the beam axis. The axial resolution is determined by the pulse length, which is shorter at higher frequencies. In fact, the axial resolution is equal to half the pulse length and this is why higher frequencies are used to give better axial resolution. The second component of spatial resolution is lateral resolution, which is the minimum distance between two points that are located at the same range or depth within

the tissue (objects side by side in the image). The lateral resolution is determined by the beam width and is highly dependent on beam focusing. The spatial resolution also depends on the slice thickness, which is determined by the thickness of the transducer and is therefore inherent in the transducer's design.

Penetration is reduced by the attenuation of ultrasound. The main factors influencing penetration are absorption and scatter. As alluded to earlier, both absorption and scatter increase with increasing frequencies. Hence, lower frequencies have to be used to achieve greater penetration. As a result, better penetration comes at the price of poorer resolution.

Image quality depends on several factors: the contrast resolution, which is influenced by the preprocessing and postprocessing carried out in the scan converter; the dynamic range (the range of echo strengths that can be handled by the amplifiers), which dictates how the echo train is converted to a grey scale; and the temporal resolution, which depends on the number of frames displayed per second (frame rate). All of these factors need to be optimised to obtain the best possible image quality.

Frame rate, line density (the number of scan lines in the image) and field of view (the size of the image displayed) are all interrelated. Ideally, one would like to have a fast frame rate, a high line density and a large field of view to obtain the best possible image. Unfortunately, the interrelation of these factors means that something has to be compromised and, depending on the scan being performed, one has to decide which of the factors are the most important to optimise.

134

DOPPLER ULTRASOUND

The wavelength recorded by an observer depends on the movement of the source and the observer relative to one another. This phenomenon can be used in medical ultrasound to give two pieces of useful information:

- the speed at which the target is moving
- the direction of the motion.

The difference in frequency between the returning echo and the transmitted ultrasound wave is known as the Doppler frequency shift; in medical ultrasound, it is particularly used to assess blood flow.

Doppler equation

If the red blood cells are moving through a blood vessel at velocity v and the angle of insonation between the red blood cells and the ultrasound beam is θ degrees (Figure 10.8), then the Doppler frequency shift (f_d) is given by the following equation:

$$f_d = \frac{2 f_t v \cos \theta}{c}$$

where c is the velocity of ultrasound in soft tissue and f_t is the frequency of the ultrasound wave transmitted by the ultrasound transducer.

Doppler instrumentation

The simplest way to detect blood flow is by use of continuous-wave ultrasound. Instruments of this kind will give us no imaging capability and the devices therefore tend to be fairly basic, designed to assess the pulse or the fetal heart beat.

To get more information about the nature of blood flow, the Doppler information needs to be coupled with an imaging device. To this end, the main instrument now available is a colour flow scanner, which combines a B-mode real-time grey-scale imaging system with pulsed-wave Doppler and colour flow imaging. Colour flow images display direction and velocity information pictorially (Figure 10.9). Information on the direction of blood flow is colour-coded; generally, flow towards the transducer is red and flow away from the transducer is blue. Information on the velocity of red blood cells is

FIGURE 10.8 **Doppler frequency shift**

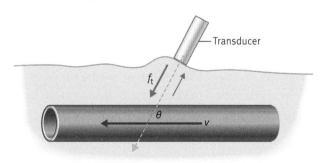

An ultrasound wave is transmitted towards a blood vessel; the ultrasound echo reflected by the red blood cells moving through the vessel incurs a Doppler frequency shift that is proportional to the velocity of the blood flow. | f_t = frequency of the transmitted ultrasound wave | v = velocity of the red blood cells | θ = angle between the transmitted ultrasound wave and the direction of the blood flow

FIGURE 10.9 **Colour flow Doppler scan of a carotid artery**

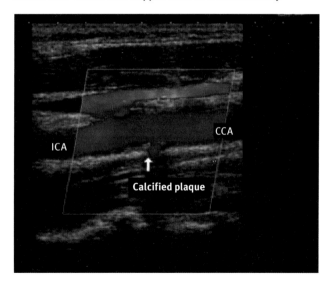

Red signifies flow towards the direction of the colour box; blue signifies flow away from the box; the hue of each colour represents the mean velocity. | CCA = common carotid artery | ICA = internal carotid artery

also colour-coded, with dark hues representing low velocities and bright hues representing high velocities.

SAFETY OF DIAGNOSTIC ULTRASOUND

Diagnostic ultrasound has been used for many years with no proven adverse effects, so why should we worry? Modern ultrasound equipment uses a broader range of ultrasound intensities than were ever used before; there is an increased use of Doppler imaging, which requires higher intensities than B-mode and M-mode ultrasound (M-mode stands for movement mode and is used exclusively in cardiac application); and in some circumstances there is the use of microbubble contrast agents. All of these factors in combination produce the potential for bioeffects. The following bioeffects have been variably reported in epidemiological studies:

- effects on isolated cells *in vitro*
- functional changes in multicellular organisms
- reduction in birth weight
- increase in childhood malignancies
- changes in neurological development
  - dyslexia
  - handedness
  - speech development.

The interactions of ultrasound with tissue can give rise to potentially harmful bioeffects, the most important of these being heating and mechanical effects.

Heating

As stated earlier, absorption of ultrasound energy can lead to the heating of tissue. Heating is more likely to occur at sites in the body where the absorption is higher than in the surrounding tissue. For example, bone absorbs energy more strongly than soft tissue does and therefore the surrounding soft tissue can experience secondary heating as a result of conduction from the bone. This is particularly important as fetal bone matures, when large increases in absorption have been documented. Consequently, heating effects during routine fetal assessment need to be considered. Diagnostic ultrasound can produce temperature rises that are hazardous to sensitive organs and the developing embryo.

To this end, the thermal index has been developed in an attempt to account for the possibility of bioeffects resulting from heating. This index is an estimate of the rise in tissue temperature that might be possible under 'reasonable worst-case conditions' and is defined as the ratio of the acoustic power emitted to the power required to heat a particular target tissue by 1 degree C. As heating is tissue-specific, there are in fact three thermal indices: the thermal index in soft tissues (TIS),

the thermal index in bone (TIB) and the thermal index in the cranium (TIC).

The responsibility for safety issues is with the operator. The operator should therefore continually monitor the thermal index and keep it as low as is consistent with achieving a diagnostic result. Regarding the safe use of ultrasound in obstetric investigations, the British Medical Ultrasound Society (BMUS) recommends monitoring of the TIS during scans carried out in the first 8 weeks following conception and monitoring of the TIB during subsequent scans.

Cavitation

Since the early days of ultrasound, it has been known that ultrasound can lyse or otherwise damage cells in suspension. This effect is not a result of the thermal properties of ultrasound; instead, it is attributable to the presence of gas-filled cavities in tissue exposed to ultrasound waves. These cavities can either oscillate or collapse under the pressure of the ultrasound beam, producing either considerable shear forces or high pressures and temperatures that can damage cell membranes or produce highly reactive free radicals. This phenomenon is known as cavitation. Gas in the lung, in the intestine and in contrast agents increases the likelihood of cavitation and mechanical damage.

Once again, an index has been developed in an attempt to account for the possibility of bioeffects resulting from mechanical effects. This is known as the mechanical index and is related to the maximum negative pressure and frequency in an ultrasound field.

The importance of cavitation has been summed up by the European Federation of Societies for Ultrasound in Medicine and Biology (EFSUMB) as follows: 'biological effects of nonthermal origin have been reported in animals but, to date, no such effects have been demonstrated in humans, except when a microbubble contrast agent is present.'

Guidelines and recommendations for the safe use of diagnostic ultrasound

There are a number of guidelines and recommendations for the safe use of diagnostic ultrasound and these change or are updated at regular intervals. A good review of the current guidelines and recommendations can always be found on the website of the BMUS [www.bmus.org]. The BMUS also provides recommended thermal and mechanical index values. The EFSUMB [www.efsumb.org] and the American Institute of Ultrasound in Medicine [www.aium.org] also publish their latest documents on their websites.

Principles and use of X-rays, computed tomography and magnetic resonance imaging

X-RAYS

X-radiation is a form of electromagnetic radiation. X-rays have a wavelength in the range of 10–0.01 nm, corresponding to frequencies in the range of $0.03–30 \times 10^{18}$ Hz and energies in the range of 120 eV to 120 keV. They are longer than gamma rays but shorter than ultraviolet rays. X-rays with energies below 12 keV are classified as soft X-rays and those above as hard X-rays, owing to their penetration abilities.

Radiography is considered to be a noninvasive medical test method that is primarily used for diagnostic purposes. It is the oldest and most frequently used form of medical imaging. As a result, the term X-ray is used to refer to a radiographic image produced using this method as well as to the method itself. X-rays are a form of ionising radiation and as such can be dangerous. X-rays were listed as a carcinogen by the US government in 2005.

The sievert (Sv) is the SI unit of measure of radiation and denotes the amount of energy delivered to a human body by gamma radiation or X-radiation (ionising radiation). The old-fashioned counterpart is the rem; 1 Sv is equivalent to 100 rem. Commonly, the radiation exposure from an X-ray is in the microsievert range, whereby 1 mrem equals 10 microsievert. The average person living in the USA receives approximately 3 mSv annually from background sources alone.

Beam formation and detection

X-rays are produced by accelerating electrons, which are then made to collide with a metal target; the precise nature of the metal target depends on the type of application. In the X-ray tube, the electrons suddenly decelerate upon collision with the metal target and can knock out an electron from the inner shell of the metal atom. Electrons from higher energy levels then fill up the vacancy and X-ray photons are emitted as a result. The process is extremely inefficient and a considerable amount of energy and heat has to be wasted to produce a reasonable flux of X-rays.

X-rays were originally detected by use of a photographic plate and later by use of an X-ray film in a cassette. These devices are generally referred to as image receptors. Plates and films have been largely replaced in hospitals by computed and digital radiography, although film technology is still used in some countries and for industrial applications. Computed and digital technologies have several advantages: they do not require wet processing facilities on site; they do not require the use of silver, which is a nonrenewable resource; and the archiving and retrieval of digital images is considerably easier, with additional space-saving benefits.

Use of X-rays in clinical practice

The body region to be imaged is positioned between the X-ray source and the image receptor, which captures a shadow image of internal body structures. X-rays may be blocked (attenuated) by dense tissues such as bone but pass more easily through soft tissues. On the X-ray, the areas where the image receptor is exposed to high X-ray energy will appear black. Soft tissue and bone will appear as shades of grey or white because some of the radiation energy is lost on its way from the source to the receptor.

X-rays are useful for identifying skeletal disease as well as chest, lung and abdominal pathologies. Their use in some cases, such as in the imaging of muscle or brain structures, is debatable and alternative imaging methods such as computed tomography (CT), magnetic resonance imaging (MRI) or ultrasound might be more appropriate.

Radiopaque contrast agents are used to highlight organs or vessels depending on the mode of their administration. They are often used in real-time procedures carried out with a so-called X-ray image intensifier resulting in a sequence of images that are projected on to a fluorescent screen or a television-like monitor. Such procedures

FIGURE 10.10 **Hysterosalpingogram showing an anterior view of the uterine fundus and patent tubes**

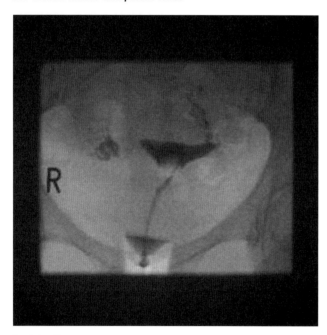

R = right side

include barium meal or enema, hysterosalpingography and uterine artery embolisation for the treatment of uterine fibroids.

In gynaecology, hysterosalpingography is frequently used to assess tubal patency in subfertile women (Figure 10.10). The procedure is usually performed in the first 10 days of the menstrual cycle to avoid inadvertent exposure of early pregnancy to radiation. There is no need for anaesthesia, although pain relief medications and antispasmodics are often given orally.

Hysterosalpingography has the following advantages:

- radiation does not persist after the procedure
- the procedure is minimally invasive
- complications are rare
- the procedure is relatively quick
- the procedure can provide valuable information on the appearance of the uterine cavity and the patency of the fallopian tube
- X-rays usually have no immediate adverse effects in the diagnostic range.

The effective radiation dose from hysterosalpingography is about 1 mSv, which is about the same as the amount received by the average person from background radiation in 4 months. The procedure carries the following risks:

- a very small risk of cancer from excessive exposure to radiation
- risk of flare-up of undiagnosed chronic pelvic infection or untreated sexually transmitted disease
- risk of inadvertent exposure of an unsuspected early pregnancy to X-ray
- small teratogenic risk associated with ovarian irradiation.

DUAL ENERGY X-RAY ABSORPTIOMETRY

Bone density scanning is also called dual energy X-ray absorptiometry (DEXA) or bone densitometry. In this test, the machine sends two beams of low-dose X-rays (approximately one-tenth that of a standard chest X-ray) with distinct and differing energy levels through the bones being examined. One beam is absorbed mainly by soft tissue and is subtracted from the total beam. The bone mineral density (BMD) can be calculated from the absorption of each beam by bone, although small and usually insignificant changes may be observed between scans owing to differences in positioning. The machine's special software calculates and displays the BMD measurements on the monitor. A DEXA image of the lumbar spine is shown in Figure 10.11.

DEXA is the most widely used BMD measurement technology. The test results are plotted as a graph and are also presented in the form of two scores: T score and Z score.

The T score is used to estimate an individual's risk of developing a fracture and compares the amount of bone in this individual with that in a young adult of the same gender with peak bone mass. A score above −1 is considered to be normal. A score between −1 and −2.5 is classified as osteopenia, the first stage of bone loss. A score below −2.5 is indicative of osteoporosis.

The Z score reflects the amount of bone in an individual compared with other individuals in the same age group and of the same size and gender. This is particularly relevant in children, where BMD is lower than in adults; hence, comparison with the reference data of adults would result in overdiagnosis of osteopenia in children.

FIGURE 10.11 **Dual energy X-ray absorptiometry scan of the lumbar spine**

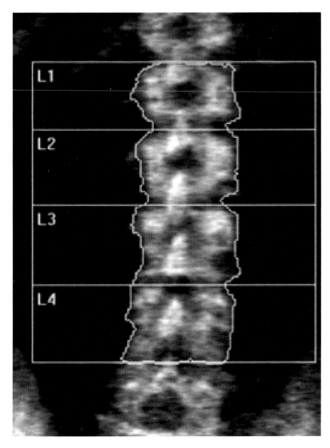

L1–4 = lumbar vertebrae

FIGURE 10.12 **Bone densitometry machine**

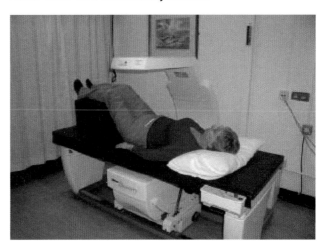

When interpreting the results, the bone size should also be considered. DEXA tends to overestimate the BMD of taller subjects and underestimate the BMD of smaller subjects. This error is attributable to the way in which the BMD is calculated: the DEXA scanner divides the bone mineral content by the area scanned by the machine (a two-dimensional figure), whereas density is actually defined as mass divided by volume (a three-dimensional figure).

Two types of DEXA equipment are available. In central devices, the X-ray generator is positioned below a large, flat table and a detector, or imaging device, is suspended overhead (Figure 10.12). Central devices measure BMD in the hip and spine. Peripheral devices are much smaller; they measure BMD in the wrist, heel or fingers.

COMPUTED TOMOGRAPHY

Ultrasound is usually the modality of first choice to assess female pelvic disease but CT is also used as part of the assessment of pelvic tumours and other abdominal disease. CT scanning uses X-rays and the principles of X-ray formation, detection and contrast outlined previously apply here as well. CT, however, produces transverse cross-sectional images of the body by reconstructing the attenuation of fine X-ray beams passed through the body. This gives images of higher contrast resolution than plain radiography does.

Recent software developments enable the reconstruction and display of three-dimensional images. These images are generated by stacking a series of two-dimensional planes on top of each other to generate a volumetric display of the area under examination. Advanced three-dimensional rendering techniques such as surface and volume rendering allow the construction of different three-dimensional models, with each anatomical structure being represented by a different colour. It is also possible to remove certain unwanted structures from the image through a process known as segmentation.

MAGNETIC RESONANCE IMAGING

MRI is another imaging technique used to visualise the structure and function of the body. Unlike CT, MRI does not use ionising radiation. Instead, a powerful

FIGURE 10.13 **MRI scan of a fibroid uterus**

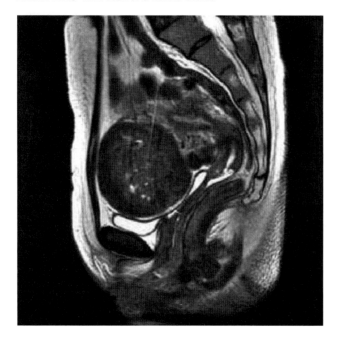

magnetic field is created to align the H$^+$ ions (protons) present in tissue H$_2$O molecules. A radiofrequency pulse is then used to disrupt the alignment of these protons with the main magnetic field. Following the pulse, the protons drift back into alignment with the magnetic field, emitting a detectable radiofrequency signal as they do so. Contrast agents may be injected directly into the area being examined or intravenously to enhance the appearance of vessels, tumours or inflammatory tissue.

In clinical practice, MRI is used to differentiate pathological tissue such as brain or ovarian tumours from normal tissue (Figure 10.13). The spatial resolution (the ability to distinguish two structures that are very close to each other as separate) provided by MRI is comparable with that of CT, but its contrast resolution (the ability to distinguish between two similar but not identical tissues) is far better because modern MRI scanners include a complex library of pulse sequences that can be employed to characterise different tissues on the basis of their interaction with the pulse signal.

Magnetic resonance imaging and pregnancy

No harmful effects of MRI have been demonstrated on the fetus, especially as no ionising radiation is used.

However, as a precaution, MRI in pregnant women should be undertaken only where necessary, especially in the first trimester. Contrast agents, for example gadolinium-based compounds, are known to cross the placenta and their use during pregnancy is controversial. Nevertheless, on the basis of the available evidence, European Society of Radiology guidelines conclude that gadolinium-based contrast agents seem to be safe in pregnancy and that any gadolinium that reaches the fetus would rapidly be eliminated into urine. Gadolinium use should therefore be considered if the diagnostic study is important for the health of the mother and MRI also plays a role in the diagnosis and monitoring of congenital defects of the fetus.

Interventional magnetic resonance imaging

In view of its safety record, MRI is well suited for interventional radiology, where the images produced by an MRI scanner are used to guide minimally invasive procedures. Such procedures, naturally, must be done in the absence of any ferromagnetic instruments. A sub-specialty of interventional MRI is that of intraoperative MRI, where systems have been developed to allow imaging concurrent with the surgical procedure. More typical, however, is the temporary interruption of the surgical procedure so that MRI scans can be acquired to verify the success of the procedure or guide subsequent surgical work.

Radiation therapy simulation

MRI is used to locate tumours within the body before the initiation of radiation therapy. The person to be treated is placed in a specific, reproducible, body position and scanned. The MRI system then computes the precise location, shape and orientation of the tumour mass, correcting for any spatial distortion inherent in the system. The person is then marked with triangulation points that will permit the delivery of precise, targeted radiation therapy.

Magnetic-resonance-guided focused ultrasound

MRI is also used to guide ultrasound surgery, in which a high-energy ultrasound beam is focused on a small spot in a target tissue such as a uterine fibroid. The ultra-sound beam heats the tissue to a temperature of more than 65 degrees C, destroying it completely. The three-dimensional view of the target tissue offered by MRI allows accurate focusing of the ultrasound energy as well as monitoring of the treatment cycle, resulting in precise ablation of the diseased tissue.

Drawbacks of magnetic resonance imaging

Claustrophobia is one of the most common reasons for people to refuse to undergo an MRI examination. Traditionally, owing to the construction of the original machines, the person under investigation had to be placed in the centre of the magnet and, coupled with a somewhat lengthy examination time, the experience was often unpleasant. Modern scanners have short bores and faster scan times, so the procedure is better tolerated. Certain groups of people, such as children, obese individuals and pregnant women, are difficult to accommodate within the machine without special provisions. Acoustic noise associated with the operation of an MRI scanner can also exacerbate the discomfort associated with the procedure. Metal fragments in the eyes (welders), neurosurgical clips, pacing wires and other ferrous prostheses are contraindicated.

Guidance and safety notes on the use of MRI were first published by the American College of Radiology in 2002,[1] with an update published in 2007.[2] In the UK, the Medicines and Healthcare products Regulatory Agency published its *Safety Guidelines for Magnetic Resonance Imaging Equipment in Clinical Use* in December 2007.[3]

Principles and use of electrosurgery

The use of thermal energy for therapy dates back many centuries. Hippocrates (460–370 BC) already recorded the use of heat for incising suprapubic abscesses. With the advent of electricity in the early 1800s, electrically heated surgical instruments became available. Surgical diathermy machines were first introduced in the late 1920s.

A diathermy machine converts the mains low-frequency current (230V, 50Hz) into a high-frequency current in the radiofrequency range (between 200kHz and 3.3MHz) to obtain a desired surgical effect, such as cutting, coagulation (clotting of blood), vaporisation and/or destruction.

INTERACTIONS OF ELECTRIC CURRENT WITH TISSUE

Low-frequency versus high-frequency currents

The effect of an electric current on tissues depends on the frequency of the current. A low-frequency current causes cyclic polarisation and depolarisation of cells owing to the transmembrane exchange of ions, resulting in neuromuscular stimulation. Depending on the actual frequency, this manifests as clonic or tetanic contraction.

By contrast, a high-frequency current changes direction so rapidly that ionic exchange at the cellular level does not happen because of the fixed time that such ions require to move through nerve tissue. Hence, no neuromuscular stimulation takes place. Nevertheless, the high energy delivered to tissue produces collision of intracellular ions and other materials, which manifests as heat.

Grounded versus isolated electrosurgery systems

Earthed (grounded) diathermy systems allow the current to return back to the unit via earth. If the return electrode is faulty or poorly applied, an alternative return pathway such as the treated person's skin is used, resulting in severe burns. By contrast, in an isolated system, minimal or no current flows to earth and the circuit through the human body is isolated. Hence, should there be a faulty connection or appliance, the current does not return to the machine and there is no risk of burns.

The return electrode, or patient plate, in grounded diathermy systems provides a safe return pathway for the passage of the current from the active electrode through the human body. As the current that passes through the tissues produces a greater current density and heat intensity under the smaller electrode (Figure 10.14), the surface area of the return electrode should be much larger than that of the active electrode. Generally, a minimum surface area of $69cm^2$ or $10inch^2$ is recommended to keep the temperature increase at very low levels.

FIGURE 10.14 **Impact of electrode size on current density**

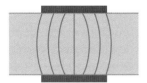

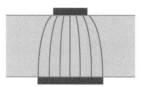

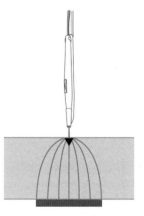

A Two electrodes of equal size: the heating effect is the same beneath each electrode

B Unequal electrodes: the heating effect is greater under the smaller electrode

C Current density and thermal effects are highest when the electrode is pointed

Monopolar versus bipolar electrosurgery

Surgical diathermy can be either monopolar or bipolar. During monopolar surgical diathermy, the electric current is transported through the human body and back to the generator. An electrode used in monopolar diathermy may be a blade, a ball, a needle tip or an open or closed loop. It is important to remember that the smaller the tip, the greater the heating effect will be because the current density will be concentrated at the smaller area (Figure 10.14). The monopolar electrode is connected to the diathermy machine (Figure 10.16),

which in turn is connected to a return plate that is attached to another body part of the person undergoing the operation.

In bipolar diathermy, the current flows between the tips of a forceps' blades (Figure 10.15), which are separated by an insulating material. One blade acts as an active electrode and the other as a return. The tissue in between the blades acts as the conducting medium for the current. Many bipolar diathermy generators incorporate a facility for autocoagulation (Figure 10.17), where the degree of coagulation is sensed by the generator and the current is discontinued when the optimum effect has been achieved. Unlike monopolar diathermy, where

FIGURE 10.15 **Electrosurgery electrodes**

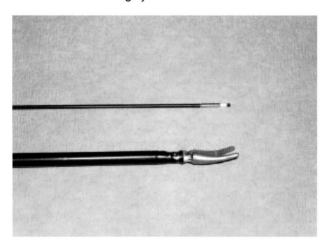

Bipolar electrode used in hysteroscopic surgery (top); a grasping bipolar electrode used in laparoscopic surgery (bottom).

FIGURE 10.16 **Generator for monopolar and bipolar electrosurgery applications**

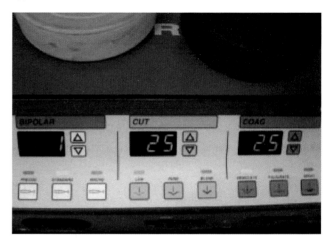

FIGURE 10.17 **Bipolar diathermy generator with autocoagulation capability**

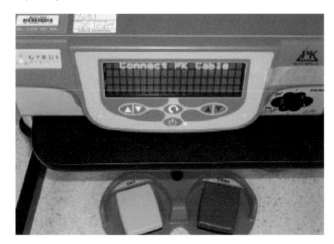

FIGURE 10.19 **Cutting effect**

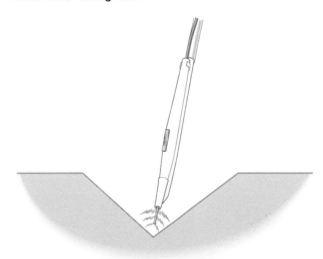

cutting and coagulation modes are possible, bipolar diathermy only permits coagulation with no cutting. Several new bipolar electrodes are now available on the market.

Tissue effects of various waveforms

Electrosurgical generators can produce current in several modes (Figure 10.18), with distinct tissue effects for each modality.

A cutting current is produced with a continuous unmodulated sinusoidal waveform, with a relatively low voltage needed to produce the desired tissue vaporisation effect (Figure 10.18A). The tip of the electrode is held just above the target tissue. Electric arcs are formed

FIGURE 10.18 **Modes of electrosurgical currents**

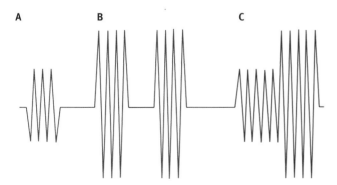

A Cutting mode | B Coagulation mode | C Blended mode

between the cutting electrode and the tissue, generating points of extremely high temperatures that vaporise cells in such a way that a clean tissue cut is achieved (Figure 10.19). There is insufficient time for the heat to dissipate to adjacent tissue; hence there is less tissue trauma and cutting occurs without significant haemostasis.

A coagulation effect is produced with a higher voltage current than that used for cutting, but the current is applied intermittently (Figure 10.18B) and modulated with a duty cycle that is on for about 6% of the time, although this may vary depending on the desired effect. This modulation, or dampening, allows the tissue to cool between heating bursts. Thus, no vaporisation occurs but the current causes coagulation, a complex process that is an important part of haemostasis. Higher voltage with longer modulation intervals results in greater coagulation or haemostatic effect.

Desiccation is the process of extreme drying, whereby tissues are coagulated while being heated to 70–100 degrees C. Soft coagulation uses a peak voltage of about 200 volts or less and the power output is precisely limited or minimal leading to minimal carbonisation, quick coagulation and as little sticking to the electrode as possible. Desiccation and soft coagulation both require contact by the active electrode with the tissue.

Monopolar or bipolar instruments can be used to desiccate tissues and the effect can be produced with either the cutting mode or the coagulation mode of the

FIGURE 10.20 **Desiccation effect**

FIGURE 10.21 **Fulguration effect**

A Desiccation accomplished by use of a low-voltage 'cutting' waveform with 100% duty cycle

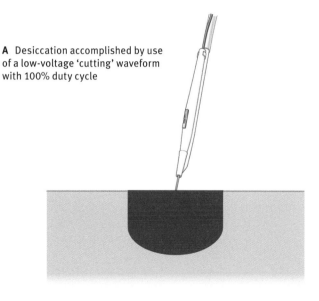

B Desiccation accomplished by use of an intermittent high-voltage 'coagulation' waveform

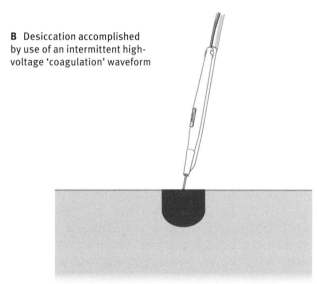

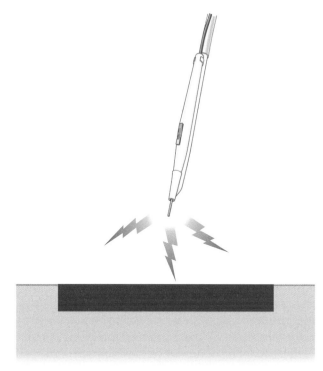

generator (Figure 10.20), although the cutting mode is the preferred option. A blended waveform combines bursts of low-voltage (cutting) and high-voltage (coagulation) currents (Figure 10.18C) and produces cutting with coagulation effects.

Other variables can impact the tissue effect, namely the duration of application, the power setting and the precise type of active electrode. Too long an activation should be avoided as it may lead to adherence of the coagulum to the electrode and subsequent tearing of the

coagulum from the vessels, resulting in inadequate haemostasis. Modern generators may monitor the flow of current through the tissue to optimise the coagulation effect.

Fulguration (electrofulguration) or forced coagulation results when a high-powered current is used to produce a sparking effect to coagulate a large bleeding area or to char tissue without touching the tissue with the electrode (Figure 10.21). This effect produces deeper coagulation than can be achieved with soft coagulation and is used in specific circumstances only.

Argon-enhanced electrosurgery was introduced in the late 1980s. The inert, nonreactive argon gas wraps the electrosurgical current and concentrates and delivers the spark to the tissue in a beam-like fashion, creating a smoother, more malleable dry scab.

SAFETY OF ELECTROSURGERY

In the past 15 years, considerable improvements in electrosurgical safety have been achieved. Modern generators produce efficient and effective cutting and coagulation currents, automatically measure tissue impedance and adjust the output, monitor and warn of any potentially dangerous low-frequency leaks of current from the human body to earth and warn of incomplete application of the return electrode. These features reduce the risk of adverse effects to people undergoing electrosurgery. Additionally, modern generators have two separate return plates and the resistance is constantly measured in each. If for any reason there is a difference in the resistance of the return plates, the system will automatically be turned off. It is also important that the diathermy machine displays the power output and that the surgeon uses the lowest effective power setting, for example 30 W. Higher outputs are required when using diathermy with glycine, such as in transcervical resection or rollerball ablation of the endometrium.

Hazards associated with the use of active monopolar electrodes also include direct coupling, insulation failure and capacitive coupling, each of which may cause severe injury.

Direct coupling occurs when the electrode is activated in close proximity or direct contact with another conductive instrument within the body. This risk is avoidable or greatly minimised through the adoption of strict safety rules during surgery.

Insulation failure occurs when the coating that covers the active electrode is compromised. This may result from repeated use or incorrect handling of instruments and may not be detected by the surgeon or theatre staff.

Capacitive coupling may occur between two conductors that are separated by an insulator. For example, if an insulated active electrode is inserted down a metal cannula, the electric current can be transferred from the active electrode through its insulation and into the conductive metal cannula, which can discharge electrical energy if it comes into contact with body structures.

The following practices are recommended to ensure the safe use of electrical surgical instruments:

- Check the instrument's isolation before surgery.
- Use the lowest possible power and voltage settings to achieve the desired effect.
- Activate the electrode only when necessary.
- Never activate the electrode when in close proximity or direct contact with a metal or conductive object.

Consideration should also be given to the following points:

- Bipolar instruments are safer than monopolar devices.
- An all-metal or all-plastic cannula system is the safest option.
- Active-electrode monitoring systems reduce the risk of capacitive coupling.

Principles and use of lasers in endoscopic surgery

The term laser is an acronym for light amplification by stimulated emission of radiation. The laser device emits light photons (electromagnetic radiation) through a process called stimulated emission to vaporise, dissect and coagulate tissue. Laser beams additionally have a natural sterilisation effect as they evaporate bacteria, viruses and fungi and seal nerve endings, thus decreasing postoperative pain. Laser devices used in endoscopic surgery are either gas (CO_2 or argon ions) or solid-state lasers and are described as class 4 lasers with a capacity to cause fires, burns and retinal damage. Lasers can interact with tissues in four ways, namely photothermally (commonly employed in gynaecology), photochemically, photomechanically and photoablatively.

CARBON DIOXIDE GAS LASERS

CO_2 gas lasers have a wavelength of 10 600 nm and are absorbed to a high degree by soft tissues that contain water. This enables precise tissue cutting and dissection with minimal lateral damage. The vaporisation capability of CO_2 lasers is useful for the removal of endometriotic implants, especially near the ureters. However, the beam has to be transmitted from the generator to the endoscope by a system of articulated arms and mirrors, which are expensive and difficult to clean, and is then sent through a semiflexible fibre that runs down the endoscopic operating channel. As CO_2 lasers are invisible to the human eye, an additional visible aiming laser is needed to assist with treatment. Overall, the depth of the CO_2 laser is very limited, making it unsuitable for laparoscopic surgery.

SOLID-STATE LASERS

Solid-state lasers are commonly made by 'doping' a crystalline solid host with ions that provide the required energy states. Examples include the neodymium-doped yttrium aluminium garnet (Nd:YAG) laser, which can produce high-energy beams in the infrared spectrum at 1064 nm and can be transmitted down a fibreoptic cable to the operating site. The Nd:YAG laser provides good cutting and haemostatic effects as well as being able to vaporise tissue. When the beam is transmitted down a bare quartz fibre, it penetrates deeply into tissues, a property that may be useful for hysteroscopic surgery but may be unsafe in laparoscopic procedures. In laparoscopic procedures, the beam should be focused at the tip (the focal spot size varies from approximately 0.1 mm to 0.4 mm) to limit the amount of unintended tissue damage to 0.2–1.0 mm.

Passage of the Nd:YAG beam through a crystal of potassium titanyl phosphate (KTP) results in doubling of the original frequency and a wavelength that is half the original, with beam characteristics that are somewhere between those of the CO_2 laser and the Nd:YAG laser. The KTP laser produces a visible beam at a wavelength of 532 nm, is easily transmitted down flexible fibreoptic cables and penetrates tissue for about 1–2 mm. The beam can vaporise, cut and coagulate tissue with a single, bare and reusable quartz fibre.

During the use of Nd:YAG and KTP lasers, staff must wear protective goggles and the person undergoing laser surgery must be provided with suitable protection to prevent inadvertent exposure and injury to the retina by the beam.

Principles and use of radiotherapy

Radiation therapy or radiotherapy is the use of ionising radiation as a medical intervention, primarily for the treatment of cancer. The amount of radiation used is measured in gray (Gy). Use of radiotherapy for nonmalignant conditions is very limited because of concerns about the risk of radiation-induced cancers.

Radiotherapy acts by damaging cellular DNA. This damage may be caused by photons, electrons, protons, neutrons or ion beams and may occur either directly or indirectly. The indirect effect is the most common

mechanism of action and results from the ionisation of H_2O molecules, which generates H^+ and hydroxyl (OH^-) ions and free radicals ($H^{\bullet}$ and $OH^{\bullet}$) that damage the DNA. This can lead to the irreversible loss of the cells' reproductive integrity and their eventual death.

Radiotherapy also affects intracellular processes that are necessary for cellular growth, senescence and apoptosis and the intrinsic ability to repair damage. Cell survival curves depend on the dose of radiation, the position of the cell in the mitotic cycle, the O_2 tension, the intrinsic cellular radiosensitivity and the cellular environment. Tissue hypoxia increases resistance to the effects of radiation as O_2 makes the radiation damage to DNA permanent. Several strategies have been developed to increase tissue oxygenation and enhance the effectiveness of radiotherapy, including the practice of total dose fractionation (spreading the dose out over time). Details of logarithmic survival curves and information on how manipulation of the cellular environment alters these curves are provided in the literature.

When protons (positively charged particles) are used, their biological effects are the same as those of other particles. However, unlike photons (soft X-rays), protons release their energy at the point of impact within the tumour, with a rapid fall-off in dose in the healthy tissue beyond. Adverse effects are minimised and a higher dose can be used for treatment.

Radiotherapy may be used as primary therapy, in conjunction with either surgery, chemotherapy or endocrine therapy or in combination with one or more of these modalities.

When used as a primary therapeutic modality where there is survival benefit, it can be curative (resulting in the radical removal of disease) or palliative (where the aim of treatment is symptom control or the local control of disease).

When used as an adjuvant therapy, radiotherapy is usually given after the surgical removal of all detectable disease and its aim is to improve disease-specific and overall survival. Thus, adjuvant radiotherapy is essentially administered to minimise the risk of recurrence, rather than for the treatment of a proven disease, and a proportion of people who receive adjuvant therapy will already have been cured by their primary surgery.

When radiotherapy is given before the main treatment, it is described as neoadjuvant therapy and its aim is to reduce the size of the tumour so as to facilitate more-effective surgery.

If administered at the same time as other therapies, it is described as concomitant or concurrent therapy.

DELIVERY OF RADIOTHERAPY

External-beam radiotherapy

Linear accelerator (linac) machines deliver two-dimensional beams from several (one to four) directions to the area being treated. In conventional techniques, the treatment is first simulated on a specially calibrated diagnostic X-ray machine known as the simulator, which has the same geometry as the linear accelerator employed during treatment. Treatment simulation is used for tumour localisation, treatment plan verification and treatment monitoring.

An enhancement of virtual simulation is three-dimensional conformal radiotherapy (CRT), which uses a variable number of beams with the profile of each radiation beam being shaped to fit the profile of the target. As the shape of the treatment volume matches the shape of the tumour, the relative toxicity of radiation to the surrounding normal tissues is reduced, allowing a higher dose of radiation to be delivered to the tumour than possible with conventional techniques.

Intensity-modulated radiation therapy (IMRT) is the next generation of three-dimensional CRT. In this form of high-precision radiation therapy, the intensity of each radiation beam can be modulated so that a given treatment field may be targeted by beams of variable intensity. This allows for greater control of the distribution of the dose within the target, thereby creating limitless possibilities to sculpt the radiation dose to the tumour itself.

Despite such advances, the limitations of radiotherapy include the inability to identify microscopic disease with accuracy, the difficulty of immobilising the treated person/tumour for the duration of a treatment session (with IMRT this is typically 15–30 minutes) and problems arising from tumour shrinkage with treatment.

The next challenge in radiation oncology is therefore to accommodate changes in the position of the treated person and/or movement or shrinkage of the tumour during treatment. Incorporating real-time imaging with real-time adjustment of the therapeutic beams, an approach commonly called four-dimensional CRT, allows 'online' imaging of the individual during treatment and real-time reconstruction of the actual daily delivered dose on the basis of the individual's and the tumour's changing anatomies. This approach results in adaptive radiotherapy – the modulation of prescription and delivery on the basis of the actual daily delivered dose as opposed to the planned dose.

Internal-beam radiotherapy

Internally delivered radiotherapy may be in the form of:

- sealed-source radiotherapy
- unsealed-source radiotherapy.

Brachytherapy involves the use of sealed sources, which are placed directly into, or adjacent to, the volume of tissue to be irradiated. The advantage is that it allows the tumour to be treated at very short distances and the radiation passes through less healthy tissue. In addition, brachytherapy sources generally emit lower-energy radiation compared with external-beam radiotherapy. The proximity of the radiation source in brachytherapy allows the dose to be better localised to the tumour volume. The clinician can therefore treat the tumour with very high doses while the dose to the surrounding healthy tissue is minimised.

Brachytherapy is used to treat many gynaecological cancers including vaginal, cervical, ovarian and uterine cancer. The radioactive material, such as caesium-137 (^{137}Cs) or iridium-192 (^{192}Ir), is placed temporarily inside or near a tumour for a specific amount of time and then withdrawn. It may be administered at a low or high dose. Occasionally, radioactive seeds or pellets, such as iodine-125 (^{125}I) seeds, are placed in or near the tumour and are left there permanently. After several weeks or months, the radioactivity level of the implants eventually diminishes to nothing. The seeds then remain in the body with no lasting effect.

Radioisotope therapy is an unsealed form of radiotherapy. It is delivered by injection, for example intravenous infusion of a radioisotope substance to treat neuroblastoma, or by ingestion, for example ingestion of iodine-131 (^{131}I) to treat thyroid cancer or thyrotoxicosis.

Other examples of radioisotope therapy are the intravenous administration of hormone-bound lutetium-177

(^{177}Lu) and yttrium-90 (^{90}Y) to treat neuroendocrine tumours in what is called peptide receptor radionuclide therapy, and the injection of radioactive glass or resin microspheres into the hepatic artery to radioembolise liver tumours or liver metastases.

Further developments include the introduction of a monoclonal antibody against CD20 conjugated to a radioisotope molecule such as ^{131}I or ^{90}Y for the treatment of refractory non-Hodgkin lymphoma. This is referred to as radioimmunotherapy.

SAFETY OF RADIOTHERAPY

Acute adverse effects of radiotherapy include:

- damage to epithelial surfaces (such as skin, oral and bowel mucosa)
- oedema and swelling of soft tissues as part of the inflammatory reaction, which may be ameliorated with steroids

- infertility caused by damage to the radiation-sensitive gonads
- generalised fatigue.

Medium-term and long-term adverse effects depend on the particular area being treated and may be minimal. These include:

- fibrosis and diffuse scarring of the irradiated tissue
- hair loss
- dryness as a result of damage to the salivary and tear glands or vaginal dryness as a result of damage to the cervical glands
- fatigue and lethargy
- cancer secondary to irradiation
- death.

Reirradiation may cause additional acute or intermediate adverse effects or exacerbation of already existing adverse effects and people undergoing reirradiation must be monitored closely.

REFERENCES

1. KANAL E, BORGSTEDE JP, BARKOVICH AJ, BELL C, BRADLEY WG, FELMLEE JP, et al. American College of Radiology White Paper on MR Safety. Am J Roentgenol 2002;178:1335–47.

2. KANAL E, BARKOVICH AJ, BELL C, BORGSTEDE JP, BRADLEY WG JR, FROELICH JW, et al. ACR Guidance Document for Safe MR Practices. Am J Roentgenol 2007;188:1–27. [www.acr.org/SecondaryMainMenuCategories/quality_safety/MRSafety/safe_mr07.aspx].

3. Medicines and Healthcare Products Regulatory Agency. Safety Guidelines for Magnetic Resonance Imaging Equipment in Clinical Use. Device Bulletin DB2007(03). London: MHRA; 2007. [www.mhra.gov.uk/home/idcplg?LdcService=GET_FILE&dDocName=CON2033065&RevisionSelectionMethod=LatestReleased].

FURTHER READING

Electrocardiography

MORRIS F, BRADY W, CAMM J, editors. ABC of Clinical Electrocardiography. 2nd ed. London: BMJ Books; 2008.

Ultrasound

CLAUDON M, COSGROVE D, ALBRECHT T, BOLONDI L, BOSIO M, CALLIADA F, et al. Guidelines and good clinical practice recommendations for contrast enhanced ultrasound

(C E U S) – update 2008. Ultraschall Med 2008;29:28–44 [www.efsumb.org/mediafiles01/ceus-guidelines2008.pdf].

KREMKAU F W. Diagnostic Ultrasound: Principles and Instruments. 7th ed. Philadelphia: Saunders/Elsevier; 2005.

X-ray, CT and MRI

DE WILDE J P, RIVERS A W, PRICE D L. A review of the current use of magnetic resonance imaging in pregnancy and safety implications for the fetus. Prog Biophys Mol Biol 2005;87:335–53.

Electrosurgery

MANE S, PENKETH R. Hysteroscopy. In: SHAW R W, SOUTTER W P, STANTON S L, editors. Gynaecology. 3rd ed. London: Churchill Livingstone; 2003. p.37–53.

SMITH A R B, PARSONS J. Diathermy and lasers. In: SHAW R W, SOUTTER W P, STANTON S L, editors. Gynaecology. 3rd ed. London: Churchill Livingstone; 2003. p.67–77.

Radiotherapy

BUCCI M, BEVAN A, ROACH M. Advances in radiation therapy: conventional to 3D, to IMRT, to 4D, and beyond. CA Cancer J Clin 2005;55:117–34 [http://caonline.amcancersoc.org/cgi/content/full/55/2/117].

POULIOT J, XIA P, AUBIN M, VERHEY L, BANI-HASHEMI A, GHELMANSARAI F, et al. Low-dose megavoltage cone-beam C T for dose-guided radiation therapy. Int J Radiat Oncol Biol Phys 2003;57 Suppl 1:S183–4.

Embryology

CHAPTER 11

Early embryology

Ram Sharma

Overview

Human development begins when a sperm fertilises an ovum. By definition, an embryo consists of cells and tissues formed once mitosis of a zygote begins, thus even at the two-cell stage it is an embryo. These few cells multiply in number over an 8-week period into a fetus, by which time it will consist of many millions of cells. Table 11.1 summarises the major events of the prenatal stages of development. The critical phase during which there is potential for malformation is in the embryonic period, when the embryo is most vulnerable to environmental agents such as viruses and other teratogens.

Gametogenesis

Gametogenesis is a process in which female and male germ cells (called oogenesis and spermatogenesis respectively) undergo cytoplasmic and chromosomal changes to form the definitive oocyte and the spermatozoon. There are, however, a number of differences between the two processes. Oogenesis is a cyclical event, while spermatogenesis begins at puberty and continues throughout

adult life. The monthly female cycle consists of maturation of a single (usually) oocyte and is accompanied by changes in the hormone secretion. There are concurrent changes in the endometrium to prepare the uterus for pregnancy.

The primordial germ cells arise from the wall of the yolk sac during the second week of development. In the sixth week they migrate into the body of the embryo to occupy the gonadal ridges. The primordial germ cells undergo rapid mitotic divisions. However, the pattern of proliferation of these cells differs in the two sexes. In the female, the germ cells differentiate into oogonia and multiply rapidly in the embryonic ovary until the fifth month to reach up to 7 million in number. After this period, large numbers of oogonia undergo degeneration (atresia). In the male, primordial germ cells form spermatogonia, in contrast to female germ cells, which continue to proliferate from puberty throughout life.

Both oogenesis and spermatogenesis require two meiotic cell divisions, which reduce the number of chromosomes from diploid to haploid (covered in Chapters 29 and 30 on female and male reproductive physiology). Meiosis also allows random assortment of maternal and paternal chromosomes and redistribution of genetic information through the process of crossing over. Thus,

TABLE 11.1 **Stages of development before birth**

Time period	Stage	Main events
Conception to week 2	Pre-embryonic	Fertilised ovum undergoes mitosis, formation of morula; appearance of blastocyst; blastocyst implanted; germ layers develop
Week 2 to week 8	Embryonic period	Germ layers and placenta develop; main body systems form
Week 9 to birth	Fetal period	Further growth and development of organs; locomotor system becomes functional

reshuffling of genes adds to the genetic variability among the offspring.

OOGENESIS

The process of oogenesis begins during the fetal period but is not completed until after puberty. During fetal life, the majority of oogonia proliferate by mitosis and differentiate into primary oocytes. At birth, most of the surviving primary oocytes enter the prophase of first meiotic division and remain suspended in the diplotene phase until puberty. This meiotic arrest is produced by secretion of oocyte maturation inhibitor (OMI), a small peptide produced by follicular cells surrounding the primary oocyte. A primary oocyte surrounded by a single layer of follicular cells is called a primary follicle.

As the primary oocyte grows during puberty, the follicular cells become stratified to produce a layer of granulosa cells. The primary oocyte becomes surrounded by a layer of glycoprotein secreted by the granulosa cells, and the ovarian connective tissue cells around the follicle condense to form theca folliculi; this layer then differentiates into an inner vascular and secretory layer, the theca interna, and an outer fibrous layer, the theca externa.

SPERMATOGENESIS

Spermatogenesis is the process by which the primitive germ cells or spermatogonia are transformed into spermatozoa. Spermatogonia, which have formed in the fetal period, remain dormant in the seminiferous tubules of the testes until puberty, when they increase in number after several mitotic divisions.

Fertilisation

The ovulated oocyte enters the abdominopelvic cavity and soon reaches the ampulla of the uterine tube, where it may be fertilised. Fertilisation takes place approximately 12–24 hours after ovulation. Fertilisation is a series of events that begins with penetration of a sperm into an oocyte and ends with a combination of maternal and paternal chromosomes at metaphase of the first mitotic division of the zygote. The several sequential events of fertilisation are:

- sperm activation and penetration of corona radiata
- attachment to zona and penetration of the zona pellucida
- fusion of the oocyte and sperm cell membranes
- completion of meiosis in the oocyte and formation of pronuclei
- formation of the zygote.

SPERM ACTIVATION AND PENETRATION OF CORONA RADIATA

Before the sperm reach the distal uterine tube, they must undergo a process of capacitation, which makes them capable of penetrating the ovum. During this phase, the glycoprotein and cholesterol of the acrosomal membrane are removed by the secretions from the cervix and the uterine tube. When viable sperm come in contact with the corona radiata surrounding a secondary oocyte, they surround it, undergo an acrosomal reaction and release the enzyme hyaluronidase, which is needed to penetrate the corona radiata. The active movements of sperm also play an important role in penetration.

ATTACHMENT TO AND PENETRATION OF THE ZONA PELLUCIDA

Once the path has been cleared through the cells of the corona radiata, a sperm binds to the zona pellucida and releases its acrosomal enzymes. The enzymes responsible for penetration include esterases, neuraminidase and acrosin. A spermatozoon binds to the zona pellucida and initiates a zona reaction, changing its physical properties to prevent attachment of any more sperm. The zona reaction is believed to result from a cortical reaction in which the cortical granules release their lysosomal enzymes into the space between the zona pellucida and oocyte cell membrane.

FUSION OF THE OOCYTE AND SPERM CELL MEMBRANES

Once the sperm makes its way through the zona pellucida into the privitelline space, it comes in contact with the cell membrane of the oocyte, resulting in the fusion of the membranes of the sperm head and oocyte. After this fusion, the cell membranes of sperm and egg break down at the area of their contact.

COMPLETION OF MEIOSIS IN THE OOCYTE AND FORMATION OF PRONUCLEI

Soon after entry of spermatozoa, the oocyte resumes second meiotic division, forming a mature oocyte and a second polar body. The chromosomes of the oocyte and sperm condense and enlarge to form pronuclei. As the pronuclei grow and approach each other, their haploid chromosomes become arranged on a spindle and split longitudinally to form chromatids.

FORMATION OF THE ZYGOTE

When the male and female pronuclei meet, their membranes break down and the chromosomes mix to produce a single cell called a zygote. At this stage, the process of fertilisation is completed and the zygote prepares for its first mitotic division.

The first week

A fertilised ovum has a diploid number of chromosomes and, once the second meiotic division has been completed, the stage of cleavage can begin. This consists of a series of rapid mitotic cell divisions in which the zygote divides over a period of about 3 days, resulting in the so-called 16-cell-stage embryo (Figures 11.1 and 11.2). Each cell is known as a blastomere. After each cleavage division, while the number of cells increases, the size of each cell diminishes. The solid sphere of cells that forms is known as a morula (Figure 11.2A). Each of these new daughter cells is, at this stage, pluripotential.

The morula soon shows signs of further differentiation. Cavities appear within the centre of the sphere of cells, forming a blastocyst, the cavity itself being the blastocoele (Figure 11.2B and C). Once this stage has been reached, the outer layer of the blastocyst soon thins to single-cell thickness to become the trophoblast, enclosing the enlarging fluid-filled blastocyst cavity. The central group of cells moves to one pole of the blastocyst

FIGURE 11.1 **Stages of pre-embryonic development during the first week**

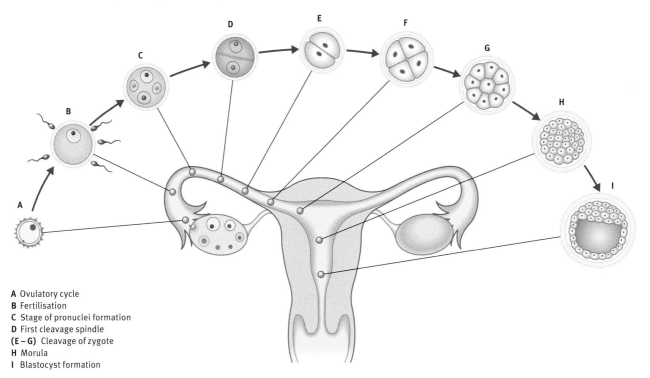

A Ovulatory cycle
B Fertilisation
C Stage of pronuclei formation
D First cleavage spindle
(E–G) Cleavage of zygote
H Morula
I Blastocyst formation

FIGURE 11.2 **Early stages of implantation**

A Morula at day 3

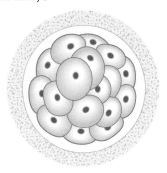

B Blastocyst at day 5

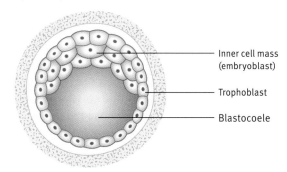

Inner cell mass (embryoblast)

Trophoblast

Blastocoele

C Blastocyst at day 6 making contact with uterine wall

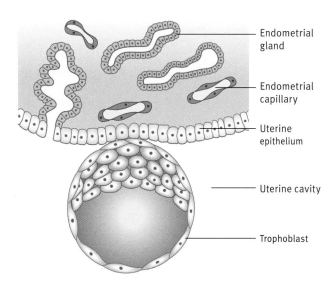

Endometrial gland

Endometrial capillary

Uterine epithelium

Uterine cavity

Trophoblast

Reproduced with permission from: Embryology:
An Illustrated Colour Text. Mitchell B, Sharma R. London: Churchill Livingstone; 2009.
Copyright Elsevier.

FIGURE 11.3 **Implantation of blastocyst**

A Blastocyst at day 7 beginning to implant

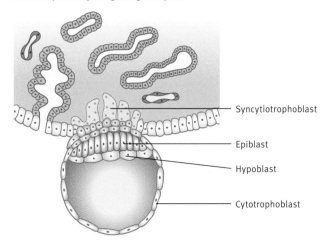

Syncytiotrophoblast

Epiblast

Hypoblast

Cytotrophoblast

B By day 8 the amniotic cavity appears

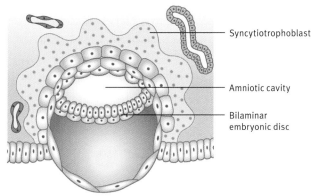

Syncytiotrophoblast

Amniotic cavity

Bilaminar embryonic disc

C By day 9 the syncytiotrophoblast invades the uterine glands and capillaries

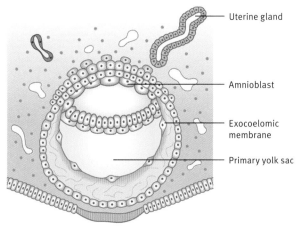

Uterine gland

Amnioblast

Exocoelomic membrane

Primary yolk sac

(the embryonic pole) to form the inner cell mass from which the whole embryo itself will form. The trophoblast contributes to the fetal component of the placenta.

The process of morula and blastocyst formation occurs while the sphere of dividing cells is in transit along the uterine tube (Figure 11.1). The first mitotic division of cleavage will be completed by the time the two-cell stage embryo reaches the middle of the tube, at about 30 hours post-fertilisation. By 3 days the morula of 12–16 cells will have reached the junction of the uterine tube and the uterus. By 4–5 days the fully formed blastocyst reaches the uterine lumen in preparation for implantation, which occurs a day later (Figure 11.2).

The second week – implantation and formation of bilaminar embryonic disc

At this stage the embryo is partly implanted in the endometrium. The implantation process initiates the decidual reaction or decidualisation in the uterine stroma, the cells of which contribute the maternal component of the placenta. The trophoblast begins to differentiate: its inner part becomes a single layer of cells, hence its name the cytotrophoblast (Figure 11.3A). The outer layer is more extensive and is the invasive layer. It is a syncytium and, at this stage, although it has invaded the endometrium, it has not invaded endometrial blood vessels. It is known as the syncytiotrophoblast. By this stage, the inner cell mass of the blastocyst has differentiated into two layers: the epiblast and the hypoblast (Figure 11.3A). These two layers are in contact and form a bilaminar embryonic disc (Figure 11.3B). Within the epiblast a cavity develops, the amniotic cavity, which fills with amniotic fluid. Some epiblast cells become specialised as amnioblasts and they secrete the amniotic fluid. The exocoelomic membrane is derived from the hypoblast and lines the cavity that appears beneath the endoderm, the primary yolk sac (Figure 11.3C). The fluid contained in this sac is the source of nutrition for the embryo before the placenta is fully formed and functional.

By 12 days there have been significant changes, particularly in the trophoblast. Small clefts, called lacunae, appear in the syncytiotrophoblast. These lacunae communicate with the maternal endometrial sinusoids, thereby deriving nutritional support for the developing embryo (Figure 11.4). Concurrent with this is the further development of the cytotrophoblast, which is thickest at the embryonic pole of the conceptus. Clefts appear between the exocoelomic membrane and the cytotrophoblast (Figure 11.4). These clefts merge to form the extra-embryonic coelom, which almost completely surrounds the embryo.

By day 13 the lacunae have enlarged substantially. The cytotrophoblast has begun to form primary chorionic villi, which are finger-like protrusions into the lacunae. The embryo proper consists of two layers, the epiblast and the hypoblast, still closely applied to each other. The two cavities continue to enlarge, with the amniotic cavity above the epiblast and the yolk sac below the hypoblast, now known as the secondary yolk sac because of the presence of the chorionic cavity. The embryo is connected to the cytotrophoblast by a connecting stalk of extra-embryonic mesoderm. This stalk is the forerunner of the umbilical cord. By this stage the uterine epithelium has reformed, thus completely engulfing the conceptus. The largest development of trophoblastic lacunae is on the deepest surface of the conceptus. By the end of the second week, the syncytiotrophoblast produces the hormone human chorionic gonadotrophin (hCG), which maintains the corpus luteum in the ovary, which in turn sustains the thickness of the endometrium. The hormone is secreted in the urine and thus its presence is an early indicator of pregnancy.

The third week – further development of the embryo and formation of trilaminar disc

The embryo develops further by forming three germ layers, the process known as gastrulation. Two layers have already formed: the epiblast and the hypoblast. These two closely apposed layers take up the form of two elliptical plates and together are termed the bilaminar embryonic disc. From this point the epiblast becomes known as the ectoderm and the hypoblast as the endoderm.

The ectoderm gives rise to the third layer that comes to lie between the two original germ layers, the intra-embryonic mesoderm. As a useful generalisation, the ectoderm (the outer skin) forms the covering of the body (the epidermis) as well as the nervous system; the endoderm (the inner skin) forms the lining of the

FIGURE 11.4 **Implanted blastocyst**

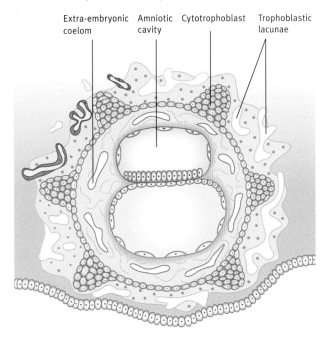

Extra-embryonic coelom   Amniotic cavity   Cytotrophoblast   Trophoblastic lacunae

At day 12 cavities develop that coalesce to form the extra-embryonic coelom.

Reproduced with permission from: Embryology: An Illustrated Colour Text. Mitchell B, Sharma R. London: Churchill Livingstone; 2009. Copyright Elsevier.

gastrointestinal and respiratory systems; and the mesoderm (the middle skin) forms the skeletal, connective and muscle tissues of the body. The main tissue derivatives of germ layers are shown in Figure 11.5.

Development of the ectoderm

PRIMITIVE STREAK FORMATION

By the end of the second week of development there is a groove-like midline depression in the caudal end of the bilaminar embryonic disc. This marks the appearance of the primitive streak. By the beginning of week 3 the streak deepens. At the cephalic end of the streak the primitive node develops. Cells of the ectoderm layer migrate towards the streak and then detach from it, spreading out laterally beneath it. This migration forms a new germ layer, the intra-embryonic mesoderm. The new germ layer spreads out in all directions to lie between the ectoderm and the endoderm, except in two locations where the original two germ layers remain in contact: the prochordal plate, at the cephalic end of

FIGURE 11.5 **Germ layer derivatives**

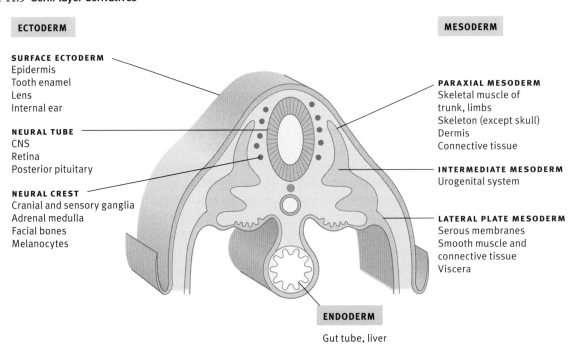

ECTODERM

SURFACE ECTODERM
Epidermis
Tooth enamel
Lens
Internal ear

NEURAL TUBE
CNS
Retina
Posterior pituitary

NEURAL CREST
Cranial and sensory ganglia
Adrenal medulla
Facial bones
Melanocytes

MESODERM

PARAXIAL MESODERM
Skeletal muscle of trunk, limbs
Skeleton (except skull)
Dermis
Connective tissue

INTERMEDIATE MESODERM
Urogenital system

LATERAL PLATE MESODERM
Serous membranes
Smooth muscle and connective tissue
Viscera

ENDODERM
Gut tube, liver

156

FIGURE 11.6 **Dorsal view of the embryonic disc showing the formation of the notochord**

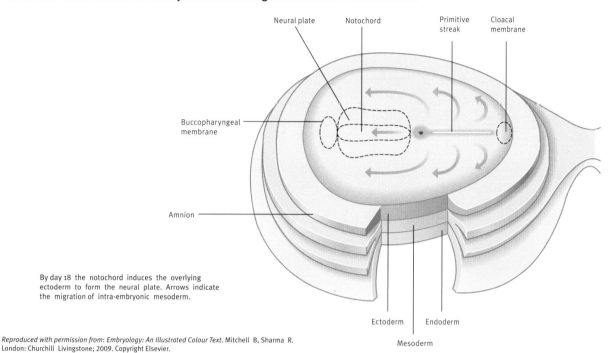

By day 18 the notochord induces the overlying ectoderm to form the neural plate. Arrows indicate the migration of intra-embryonic mesoderm.

the disc, and the cloacal plate at the caudal end of the disc (Figure 11.6). The prochordal plate is soon replaced by the buccopharyngeal membrane, which forms a temporary seal for the future oral cavity. In week 4 this membrane breaks down to establish communication between the gut tube and the amniotic cavity. The cloacal plate is replaced by the cloacal membrane.

NOTOCHORD FORMATION

Cells derived from the primitive node migrate cranially towards the buccopharyngeal membrane (Figure 11.6). This results in the appearance of the notochordal plate, which in turn folds in to form the solid cylinder of the notochord. The notochord thus comes to underlie the future neural tube (the future brain and spinal cord) and forms both a longitudinal axis for the embryo and the centres (nuclei pulposi) of the intervertebral discs of the vertebral column.

NEURULATION

The process of the formation of the brain and spinal cord is known as neurulation. The ectoderm germ layer gives rise to neuroectoderm, which gives rise to most of the major components of the nervous system. At about 19 days, at the cranial end of the primitive streak, the underlying mesoderm and notochord induce the ectoderm to form the neural plate (Figure 11.6), which rounds up to form the neural folds. The neural plate enlarges initially at the cranial end. At 20 days, the neural plate in the mid-region of the embryo remains narrowed, but it expands at the caudal end. The plate deepens to form the neural groove from which the neural tube forms. The cranial and caudal ends of the tube are open and are known as the anterior and posterior neuropores; these eventually close. At the edges of the neural tube, where the neuro-ectoderm is continuous with the surface ectoderm, the neural crests are formed. The neural crest cells detach themselves from the rest of the neural groove, before the tube forms, forming discrete aggregations of neural crest cells (Figure 11.7). They contribute to the formation of dorsal root, cranial, enteric and autonomic ganglia, connective tissues of the face and bones of the skull, the adrenal medulla, glial cells, Schwann cells, melanocytes, parts of the meninges and parts of the teeth.

FIGURE 11.7 **Transverse sections of the embryo showing the origin and migration of neural crest cells between days 19 and 21**

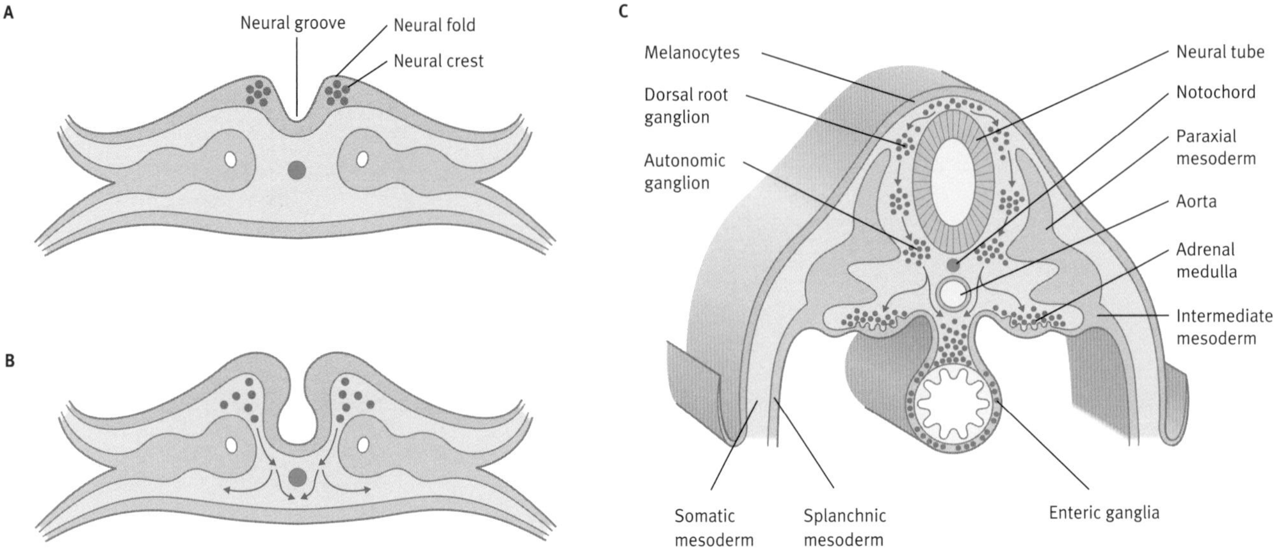

A

Neural groove · Neural fold · Neural crest

B

C

Melanocytes · Neural tube
Dorsal root ganglion · Notochord
Autonomic ganglion · Paraxial mesoderm
Aorta
Adrenal medulla
Intermediate mesoderm

Somatic mesoderm · Splanchnic mesoderm · Enteric ganglia

Further development of the mesoderm

As the number of mesodermal cells increases on either side of the notochord, by day 17 the layer becomes thickest closest to the midline, which is known as the paraxial mesoderm. The parts further out are known as the intermediate and lateral plate mesoderm (Figure 11.7C). At day 19, clefts begin to appear in the lateral plate. The mesoderm of the lateral plate is continuous with the extra-embryonic mesoderm covering the amniotic sac and the yolk sac (Figure 11.7A and B). The mesoderm covering the amniotic sac is termed the parietal or somatic layer and that covering the yolk sac the visceral or splanchnic layer (Figure 11.7B). The diverging limbs of the extra-embryonic mesoderm open into the extra-embryonic coelom. The clefts that appear within the lateral plate merge to form the intra-embryonic coelom, a cavity which is the forerunner of the serous cavities (the pericardial, pleural and peritoneal cavities). The intra-embryonic and extra-embryonic coeloms are therefore continuous.

Arising between the paraxial and lateral plate mesoderm is the intermediate mesoderm from which the urogenital system develops (Figure 11.7C).

Segmentation of the mesoderm

PARAXIAL MESODERM

The paraxial mesoderm undergoes further differentiation in paired blocks of tissue in a craniocaudal direction on each side of the notochord, called somites. The first pair of somites forms at about 20 days and thereafter at a rate of about three per day until 42–44 pairs are formed, though not all persist into adulthood. The age of an embryo is related to the number of somite pairs present. From the beginning of the fourth week, the somites undergo further differentiation to form dermomyotomes (which form connective tissue and skeletal muscle) and sclerotomes (which form bone and cartilage) (Figure 11.8). Cells from the sclerotomes surround the notochord and spinal cord and give rise to the vertebral column.

SOMITE DEVELOPMENT

In the fourth week, the medially placed mesenchymal cells of the somites migrate towards the notochord to form sclerotomes (mesenchyme is the loosely arranged embryonic connective tissue in the embryo). The ventro-lateral

FIGURE 11.8 **Transverse sections of the embryo showing development of the somite**

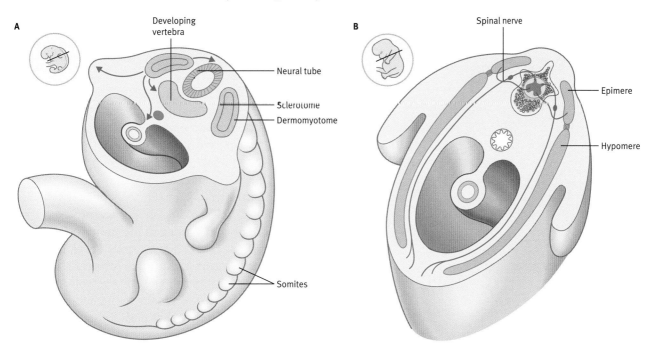

A

Developing
vertebra

Neural tube

Sclerotome

Dermomyotome

Somites

B

Spinal nerve

Epimere

Hypomere

cells of the somites become the myotomes, and those remaining become the dermatomes (Figure 11.8A). The myotomes split into dorsal epimeres and ventral hypomeres. The dorsal epimeres give rise to epaxial muscles, the erector spinae muscles. The ventral hypomeres give rise to hypaxial muscles, which include muscles of the body wall (Figure 11.8B). The ventrolateral parts of the somites in the regions of the future limb buds that remain after the sclerotomal portion has formed migrate to differentiate into limb musculature. The dermatomes form the dermis of the skin and, thus, these cells come to lie beneath the surface ectoderm, which forms the uppermost layer of the skin, the epidermis. It is important to appreciate that, as the myotomes and dermatomes migrate to their adult position, they bring with them their innervation, from the segment of origin of the developing spinal cord.

LATERAL PLATE MESODERM

The two layers of the lateral plate mesoderm enclose the intra-embryonic coelom. The mesodermal cells of the lateral plate arrange themselves as thin layers, which become the serous membranes of the body: the pleura, pericardium and peritoneum. These two continuous layers differentiate therefore to become a lining for the future body wall, a covering for the future endodermal gut tube and the smooth muscle and connective tissue of the gut wall. The serous layer in contact with the future body wall is the parietal layer; the serous layer in contact with the endodermal gut tube is the visceral layer. Other names for these two layers are somatopleure and splanchnopleure (Figure 11.7B and C).

ENDODERM

The epithelial lining of the gastrointestinal tract is derived from the endoderm germ layer. The formation of the endodermal gut tube depends on the transverse and longitudinal folding of the embryo. In addition to the lining of the gastrointestinal and respiratory systems, the endoderm also gives rise to the parenchymal cells of the liver and pancreas and of

159

FIGURE 11.9 **Formation of the lateral body folds between day 18 and day 21 in transverse sections of the embryo**

A Day 18

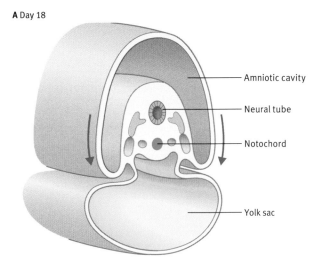

- Amniotic cavity
- Neural tube
- Notochord
- Yolk sac

B Day 21

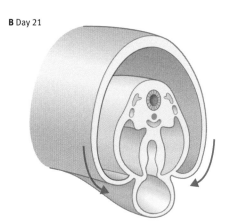

C Day 24

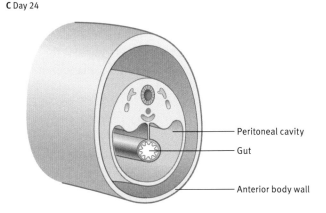

- Peritoneal cavity
- Gut
- Anterior body wall

Arrows indicate the lateral folds. By day 24 lateral folding is complete.

Reproduced with permission from: Embryology: An Illustrated Colour Text.
Mitchell B, Sharma R. London: Churchill Livingstone; 2009. Copyright Elsevier.

the thyroid and parathyroids, as well as the lining of the urinary bladder.

The fourth week – folding of the embryo

Folding takes place in two directions: longitudinal (also referred to as cephalocaudal) and lateral (or transverse). Longitudinal folding occurs mainly as a consequence of the rapid enlargement of the cranial end of the neural tube to form the brain. Lateral folding is a consequence of the enlargement of the somites. The process of lateral folding is illustrated in Figure 11.9.

Longitudinal folding, which occurs between days 21 and 24, results in bending of the embryo so that the head and tail are brought closer together (Figure 11.10). The endoderm forms a tube-like structure with an initially wide communication with the yolk sac: this communication narrows as the longitudinal folding increases. The amniotic cavity pushes in at the cranial and caudal ends of the embryonic disc, thus increasing the degree of longitudinal folding at the head and tail

FIGURE 11.10 **The process of longitudinal folding by day 25 in a saggital section of an embryo**

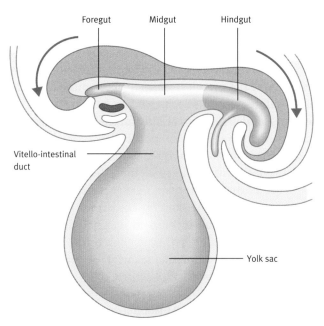

- Foregut
- Midgut
- Hindgut
- Vitello-intestinal duct
- Yolk sac

Arrows indicate the formation of head and tail folds.

Reproduced with permission from: Embryology: An Illustrated Colour Text.
Mitchell B, Sharma R. London: Churchill Livingstone; 2009. Copyright Elsevier.

folds. The amniotic cavity also pinches the connection of the yolk sac and gut to form the narrowed communication of the vitello-intestinal (or vitelline) duct (Figure 11.10). Later, this duct is lost.

The yolk sac plays a role in the early nutrition of the embryo, but this is lost after the first month or so and a vestigial yolk sac lies freely in the chorionic cavity.

Development of the urogenital tract

Vivek Nama

Development of the urogenital system

The urogenital system develops from the intermediate mesoderm. A longitudinal elevation of the intermediate mesoderm appears on either side of the aorta known as the urogenital ridge. The part that develops into the urinary system is known as the nephrogenic cord and the part that develops into the genital system is known as the gonadal ridge. The urinary system develops before the genital system (Box 12.1). The origins of the different parts of the fully formed urogenital system are listed in Table 12.1.

> BOX 12.1 **Useful time points in the development of the urinary system and the gonads**
>
> **URINARY SYSTEM**
> - Pronephros – week 4, never functional
> - Mesonephros – week 4, functions from weeks 6–10
> - Metanephros – week 4, functions from week 12
>
> **GONADS**
> - Primordial germ cells develop in the endodermal yolk sac – week 4
> - Germ cells migrate to mesodermal endothelium – week 5
> - Gonads remain as indifferent – week 6
> - Interstitial cells produce testosterone – week 8
> - Secondary sex cords (cortical cords) – weeks 10–12
> - Primordial follicles – week 16

Development of the kidney

Figure 12.1 shows the structures present early in embryonic development, at week 3. Three types of excretory organs are formed in a cranial to caudal sequence – the pronephros, mesonephros and metanephros – which are shown schematically in Figure 12.2.

The pronephros that appears at the beginning of week 4 of gestation is rudimentary and nonfunctional. It is seen as seven solid cell groups in the cervical region. All the elements of the pronephros disappear a week after their appearance. The pronephric ducts persist and are used by the mesonephros.

The mesonephros appears at week 4, becomes functional between weeks 6–10 and disappears by the end of week 10. The mesonephric ducts function as interim kidneys for 4 weeks (see Figure 12.4). They originate from the intermediate mesoderm between the upper thoracic and the upper lumbar segment (L3). They form

excretory tubules that lengthen and acquire a tuft of capillaries. The tubules immediately adjacent to the vascular tuft differentiate into the Bowman's capsule and, laterally, the tubules open into the wolffian duct. The tubules then degenerate but the wolffian ducts persist and participate in the formation of the genital system in the male but disappear in the female.

The metanephros forms the permanent kidney that appears in week 5 and urine production starts by week 12. The excretory units develop from the metanephric mesoderm (metanephric blastema). The collecting ducts develop from the ureteric bud, which is an outgrowth of the mesonephric duct close to its entrance to the cloaca. This bud penetrates the metanephric mesoderm, the stalk of the ureteric bud forms the ureter and the expanded part forms the renal calyx. Each newly formed collecting

TABLE 12.1 **Embryonic structures, adult derivatives and vestigial remnants in male and female**

Male	Embryonic structure	Female
Testis	Indifferent gonad	Ovary
Seminiferous tubules	Cortex	Ovarian follicles
Rete testis	Medulla	Rete ovarii
Gubernaculum testis	Gubernaculums	Ovarian ligament and round ligament
Efferent ductules	Mesonephric tubules	Epoophoron, paroophoron
Duct of epididymis, also appendix of epididymis	Mesonephric duct (wolffian)	Duct of epoophoron, appendix vesiculosa
Ductus deferens		Duct of Gartner
Ejaculatory duct and seminal vesicle		No homologue
Ureter, renal pelvis, calyces, collecting tubules		Ureter, renal pelvis, calyces, collecting tubules
Appendix of testes	Paramesonephric duct	Uterine tube, uterus, hydatid
Urinary bladder	Urogenital sinus	Urinary bladder
Urethra		Urethra
Prostate gland		Urethral and paraurethral glands
Prostatic utricle		Vagina
Penis	Genital tubercle	Clitoris
Glans penis		Glans clitoridis
Ventral aspect of penis	Urethral folds	Labia minora
Scrotum	Genital swellings	Labia majora

tubule is covered at its distal end by a metanephric tissue cap. The mesoderm adjacent to the collecting tubule develops into cells known as the metanephric vesicle. These vesicles differentiate later into the renal tubules and acquire a tuft of capillaries that later form glomeruli. Hence, the uriniferous tubule consists of the nephrons derived from the metanephric mass of intermediate mesoderm and a collecting tubule derived from the metanephric diverticulum. The glomerular integrity depends on signalling between the three major cell lineages: podocytes, and endothelial and mesangial cells. These tubules, together with their glomeruli, form nephrons. Hence, the kidney develops from two sources: metanephric mesoderm and the ureteric bud. In animal models, kidney formation is known to be controlled by

FIGURE 12.1 **The intermediate mesoderm and the development of the urogenital organs in the early embryo (week 3)**

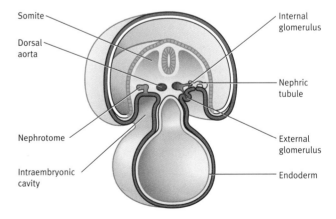

Somite
Dorsal aorta
Nephrotome
Intraembryonic cavity
Internal glomerulus
Nephric tubule
External glomerulus
Endoderm

FIGURE 12.2 **Schematic representation of the three types of excretory organs formed in the human embryo**

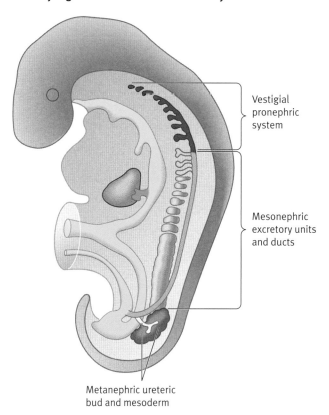

Vestigial pronephric system

Mesonephric excretory units and ducts

Metanephric ureteric bud and mesoderm

the proteins RET (rearranged during transfection protooncogene), GDNF (giant cell line-derived neutrophilic factor) and GFRA1 (GDNF family receptor alpha-1) (Table 12.2). Mutations in *RET* are found in both unilateral (20%) and bilateral (37%) renal agenesis.

POSITION OF THE KIDNEY

The kidney develops in the pelvic region and later ascends to a more cranial position. The change in position is due to the differential growth of the lumbar and sacral regions. As the kidney ascends, it rotates by 90 degrees and derives its blood supply from the aorta, and the lower vessels disappear.

Clinical correlates

- Wilms tumour occurs as a result of mutation in WT1, which regulates the mesoderm to respond to induction by the ureteric bud.
- Renal agenesis can occur if the ureteric bud fails to contact and/or induce the metanephric mesoderm. Unilateral renal agenesis occurs in 1 in 1000 infants. It is more common on the left side and in males. Unilateral renal agenesis is associated with a single umbilical artery. Bilateral renal agenesis is associated with oligohydramnios and characteristic facial appearance and occurs in 1 in 3000 births.
- Duplication of the ureter results from early splitting of the ureteric bud. Splitting may be partial or complete and metanephric tissue may be divided into two parts, each with its own renal pelvis and ureter. Partial division results in a divided kidney with a bifid ureter and complete division results in a double kidney with a bifid ureter.
- Accessory renal arteries occur from the persistence of embryonic vessels formed during the ascent of the kidney. About 25% of adult kidneys have two to four renal arteries. Accessory renal arteries usually arise from the aorta. Accessory arteries are about twice as common as accessory veins.
- Polycystic kidney disease is an autosomal that occurs because of the wide dilatation of the nephrons, particularly the loop of Henle. Gene mutations and faulty signalling have been implicated.

TABLE 12.2 **Development of the kidney and its regulators**

Embryo	Adult derivatives
Pronephros	Not functional and completely regresses, paramesonephric duct forms internal genitalia of the female
Mesonephros	Completely regresses but the mesonephric duct forms the internal male genital organs
Metanephros	
Ureteric bud	Collecting duct, minor calyx, major calyx, renal pelvis, ureter (regulated by WT1, GDNF9 glial cell line-derived neurotrophic factor, C-RET9 tyrosine kinase receptor)
Metanephric mesoderm	Renal glomerulus, renal capsule, proximal convoluted tubule, loop of Henle, distal convoluted tubule, connecting tubule (regulated by fibroblast growth factor 2, bone morphogenetic protein 7, GFRA1, WNT11)

Development of the bladder

During weeks 4 and 7 of development, the cloaca is divided into the urogenital sinus anteriorly and the anal canal posteriorly by the urogenital septum. The urogenital septum is a layer of mesoderm and its tip forms the perineal body. The urogenital sinus now develops into three parts. The cranial part forms the urinary bladder, which is continuous with the allantois. The narrower middle pelvic part forms the prostatic and membranous urethra in the male and the entire urethra in the female. The caudal, or phallic, part forms the genital organs (Figure 12.3). Later, the lumen of the allantois becomes obliterated to form the urachus (median umbilical ligament). During differentiation of the cloaca, caudal portions of the mesonephric ducts are absorbed into the wall of the urinary bladder. Consequently, the ureters outgrow the mesonephric ducts and enter the bladder separately. Since both mesonephric ducts and ureters originate in the mesoderm, the mucosa of the bladder (trigone) formed by the incorporation of the ureteric and ejaculatory ducts is mesodermal in origin.

Development of the urethra

The epithelium of the urethra in both sexes originates in the endoderm; the surrounding connective and smooth muscle tissue is derived from the mesoderm. In males, the cranial part of the prostatic urethral epithelium forms numerous outgrowths that form the prostate. In females, the cranial part gives rise to the urethral and paraurethral glands.

CLINICAL CORRELATES

- When the lumen of the intraembryonic portion of the allantois persists, a urachal fistula drains urine into the umbilicus. If only a small area persists, then a urachal cyst is formed.
- Congenital megacystis is a pathologically large bladder and results from maldevelopment of the ureteric bud. It is usually associated with renal failure and pulmonary hypoplasia unless intrauterine treatment is performed.
- Exstrophy of the bladder is caused by a lack of mesodermal migration and incomplete closure of the

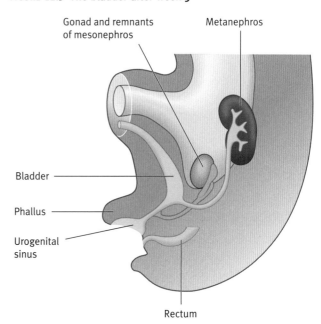

FIGURE 12.3 **The bladder after week 5**

Gonad and remnants of mesonephros

Metanephros

Bladder

Phallus

Urogenital sinus

Rectum

inferior abdominal wall between the umbilicus and genital tubercle followed by rupture of the thin layer of ectoderm. It occurs in 10 in 40 000 births. The anomaly is characterised by protrusion of the posterior wall of the bladder. Complete exstrophy is associated with epispadias and wide separation of the pubic bones.
- Exstrophy of the cloaca occurs because of the failure of migration of mesoderm to the midline. The defect includes exstrophy of the bladder, spinal defects, imperforate anus and usually omphalocele.

Development of the genital system

The genital system consists of gonads, gonadal ducts and external genitalia. All three components go through an indifferent stage, during which they may develop into either male or female.

GONADS

Gonadal development begins at week 4 and starts as an area of thickened mesothelium on the medial side of the mesonephros (Figure 12.4). The gonads appear initially as a pair of longitudinal ridges, the genital or gonadal

FIGURE 12.4 **Transverse section of the embryo at week 6 showing the genital ridge and the mesonephros**

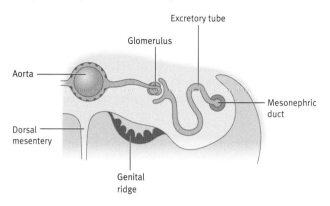

differentiation of the gonads. The SRY protein is the testis-determining factor; under its influence male development occurs and in its absence female development (Figure 12.5).

The testis

If the embryo is genetically male, the primordial germ cells carry an XY sex chromosome complex. Under influence of the *SRY* gene on the Y chromosome, which encodes the testis-determining factor, the primitive sex cords continue to proliferate and penetrate deep into the medulla to form the testis or medullary cords. A layer of dense connective tissue appears which separates the cords from the surface epithelium and later forms the tunica albuginea (white covering). The enlarging testis becomes separated from the mesoderm and develops its own mesentry, the mesochorium. The cords of cells, now called seminiferous cords, develop into seminiferous tubules: tubuli seminiferi recti (straight seminiferous tubules) and rete testis. The Sertoli cells are derived from the surface epithelium of the gland and interstitial cells of Leydig from the mesenchyme of the gonadal ridge. By week 8, Leydig cells begin production of testosterone and are able to influence sexual differentiation of the genital ducts and external genitalia. The seminiferous tubules canalise at puberty, which in turn enter the ductuli efferentes (excretory mesonephric tubules),

ridges, and remain indifferent until week 7. Finger-like epithelial cords, the gonadal cords, grow into the underlying mesenchyme, dividing the ridge into the external cortex and the internal medulla. Primordial germ cells from the yolk sac migrate by amoeboid movement along the dorsal mesentery, invading the genital ridges in week 6. If they fail to reach the ridges, the gonads do not develop and there is a lack of the inductive influence of these cells on the development of the gonad into ovary or testis.

The sex of the embryo is determined by its genotype. The sexual differentiation in the genital ducts and external genitalia is then determined by the type of gonad. The *SRY* (sex-determining region on Y) gene located on the short arm of chromosome Y (Yp11) determines the

FIGURE 12.5 **Events in the differentiation of the gonadal ridge based on the genotype and hormones produced**

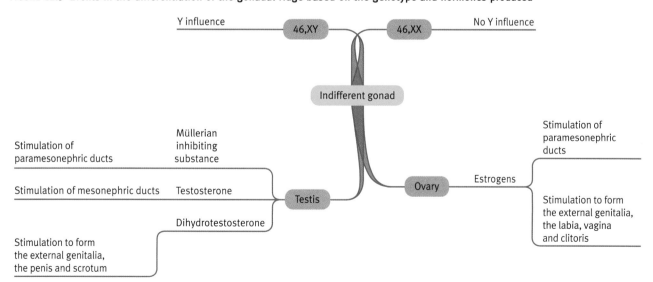

which link the rete testis and the mesonephric duct, which becomes the ductus deferens (mesonephric duct) (Figure 12.6).

The ovary

In embryos with XX chromosomes, the sex cords dissociate into irregular cell clusters. The germ cells in the medullary part of the ovary are replaced by vascular stroma but the surface epithelium continues to multiply, forming cords of cells. During multiplication, the primordial germ cells are incorporated into the cords. At month 4, these cords split into isolated cell clusters surrounding the primitive germ cells. Later, the germ cells develop into oogonia and the epithelial cells surrounding the oogonia form follicular cells (Figure 12.7).

FIGURE 12.6 **The embryonic testis**

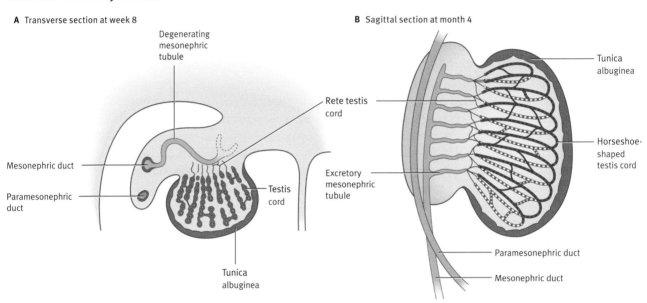

A Transverse section at week 8

B Sagittal section at month 4

FIGURE 12.7 **The embryonic ovary**

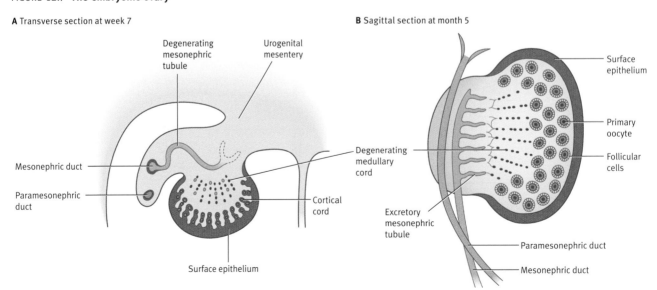

A Transverse section at week 7

B Sagittal section at month 5

GENITAL DUCTS

There are two pairs of genital ducts: wolffian (mesonephric) ducts and müllerian (paramesonephric) ducts.

In the male embryo

The mesonephric ducts under the influence of testosterone form the epididymis, ductus deferens and ejaculatory duct. As the mesonephros regresses, the tubules divide into epigenital and paragenital tubules. The epigenital tubules join the rete testis and form the efferent ductules, whereas the paragenital tubules do not join the rete testis and form the paradidymis. The mesonephric ducts below the paradidymis elongate and convolute to form the epididymis. The seminal vesicle grows as an outbudding from the tail of epididymis and the region beyond the seminal vesicle is called the ejaculatory duct. The paramesonephric ducts degenerate in the male to form the appendix testis (Figure 12.8).

In the female embryo

The paramesonephric ducts arise as a longitudinal invagination of the mesothelium on the lateral surface of the urogenital ridge. Cranially, the duct opens into the abdominal cavity and caudally it merges with the paramesonephric duct of the opposite side to form the uterovaginal primordium. The caudal tip then projects into the posterior wall of the urogenital sinus causing a small swelling known as the müllerian tubercle. As the ducts fuse in the midline, they take a sheet of peritoneum with them, which forms the broad ligament of the uterus. The fused paramesonephric ducts give rise to the corpus and cervix and the surrounding layer of mesenchyme forms the myometrium. The mesonephric ducts open into the urogenital hiatus on either side of the müllerian tubercle. The female may retain some parts of the excretory tubules known as epoophoron and paroophoron. Small cranial portions of the mesonephric duct persist in the epoophoron. If the caudal part persists, then it may

FIGURE 12.8 **The male genital ducts**

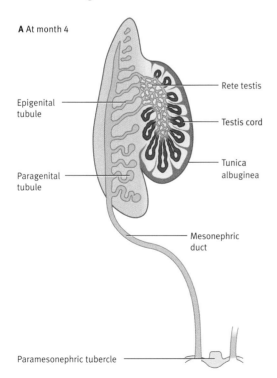

A At month 4

Epigenital tubule
Rete testis
Testis cord
Paragenital tubule
Tunica albuginea
Mesonephric duct
Paramesonephric tubercle

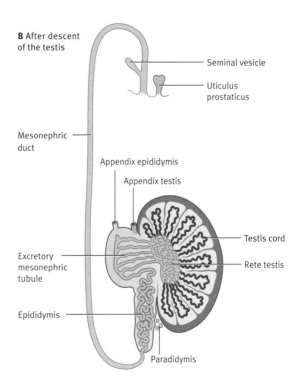

B After descent of the testis

Seminal vesicle
Uticulus prostaticus
Mesonephric duct
Appendix epididymis
Appendix testis
Testis cord
Excretory mesonephric tubule
Rete testis
Epididymis
Paradidymis

FIGURE 12.9 **The female genital ducts**

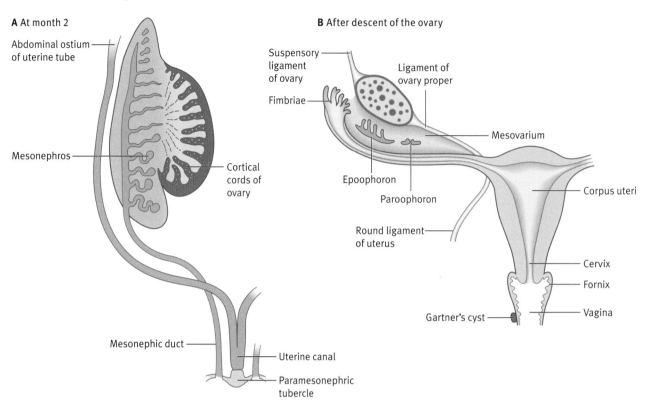

A At month 2

- Abdominal ostium of uterine tube
- Mesonephros
- Cortical cords of ovary
- Mesonephic duct
- Uterine canal
- Paramesonephric tubercle

B After descent of the ovary

- Suspensory ligament of ovary
- Ligament of ovary proper
- Fimbriae
- Mesovarium
- Epoophoron
- Paroophoron
- Round ligament of uterus
- Corpus uteri
- Cervix
- Fornix
- Gartner's cyst
- Vagina

develop into a cyst in the uterus or the vagina known as a Gartner's cyst (Figure 12.9).

EXTERNAL GENITALIA

Indifferent stage

At week 3, the mesenchyme around the cloacal membrane becomes slightly elevated to form the cloacal fold. The folds cranial to the cloacal membrane unite to form the genital tubercle and caudally they are divided into urethral folds anteriorly and anal folds posteriorly. As the urorectal septum fuses with the cloacal membrane, it divides the cloacal membrane into a dorsal anal membrane and a ventral urogenital membrane. On either side of the urethral fold, another pair of swellings becomes more apparent, known as genital swellings. The genital swellings will form the scrotal swellings in the male and the labia majora in the female (Figure 12.10).

In the male embryo

In the presence of androgens secreted by the testis, the genital tubercle elongates and is now called the phallus. As the phallus elongates it pulls the urethral folds forward so that they form the lateral walls of the urethral groove. The epithelial lining of the groove originates in

FIGURE 12.10 **Indifferent stages of external genitalia**

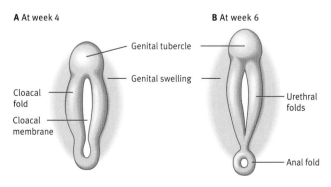

A At week 4

- Genital tubercle
- Genital swelling
- Cloacal fold
- Cloacal membrane

B At week 6

- Urethral folds
- Anal fold

FIGURE 12.11 **Male external genitalia**

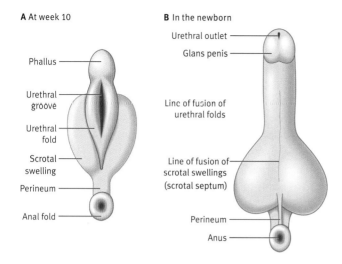

A At week 10

Phallus

Urethral groove

Urethral fold

Scrotal swelling

Perineum

Anal fold

B In the newborn

Urethral outlet

Glans penis

Line of fusion of urethral folds

Line of fusion of scrotal swellings (scrotal septum)

Perineum

Anus

FIGURE 12.12 **Female external genitalia**

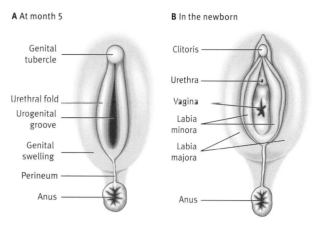

A At month 5

Genital tubercle

Urethral fold

Urogenital groove

Genital swelling

Perineum

Anus

B In the newborn

Clitoris

Urethra

Vagina

Labia minora

Labia majora

Anus

the endoderm and forms the urethral plate, which extends from the phallic portion of the urogenital sinus. The two urethral folds close over the urethral plate to form the penile urethra. Ectodermal cells penetrating inward and joining the urethra from the tip of the glans form the external urethral meatus. The corpora cavernosa and corpus spongiosum develop from mesenchyme in the phallus. The labioscrotal swellings fuse to form the scrotum (Figure 12.11).

Clinical correlates

- Androgen insensitivity syndrome occurs in 1 in 20 000 births and is phenotypically female but genotypically male. The external genitalia are female but end in a blind pouch. The uterus and uterine tubes are absent or rudimentary. It results from a defect in the androgen receptor mechanism.
- Hypospadias occurs as a result of failure of the fusion of the urethral folds near the glans or at the shaft or near the base of the penis. It is the most common anomaly of the penis and occurs in 1 in 300 male infants. Hypospadias is said to occur because of inadequate production of androgens by the fetal testes.
- Epispadias is the result of the genital tubercle developing in the region of the urorectal septum instead of the cranial end of the cloacal membrane.

This places the urethra on the dorsum of the penis. It occurs in 1 in 30 000 male infants and is often associated with exstrophy of the bladder.

In the female embryo

As the paramesonephric ducts reach the urogenital sinus, two solid evaginations grow out of the pelvic part of the urogenital sinus. These evaginations are known as the sinovaginal bulbs, which proliferate and form a solid vaginal plate. Proliferation of the cranial end of the plate continues until it reaches the cervix. The lower part of the paramesonephric ducts are absorbed into the sinovaginal bulbs. Hence, the vaginal fornices develop from the paramesonephric ducts. Later, the vaginal plate acquires a lumen by the breakdown of the central cells to form the vagina. In the presence of estrogens, the genital tubercle elongates only slightly to form the clitoris and the urethral folds develop into the labia minora. The genital swellings enlarge and form the labia majora and the urogenital groove forms the vestibule (Figure 12.12).

DESCENT OF GONADS

The urogenital mesentery attaches the testis and mesonephros to the posterior abdominal wall. With the degeneration of the mesonephros, the attachment serves as a mesentery for the gonad. Caudally it becomes ligamentous (caudal genital ligament). The gubernaculum is a band of mesenchyme extending from the tip of the testis and ending in the anterior abdominal wall. As the fetus grows and the testis passes through the inguinal canal, the lower part of the gubernaculum develops from the scrotal floor and joins the intra-abdominal part. The testis reaches the inguinal canal by week 12, migrates through the inguinal canal by week 28 and reaches the scrotum by week 33. As the testis descends, the peritoneum covering the testis is called a processus vaginalis (vaginal process), which later forms the tunica vaginalis. The communication between the abdominal cavity and the tunica vaginalis is obliterated at birth. The transversalis fascia (transverse fascia) forms the internal spermatic fascia, the internal abdominal oblique muscle forms the cremasteric fascia and muscle and the external oblique forms the external spermatic fascia.

The descent of the ovary is considerably less and settles below the rim of the true pelvis. The cranial genital ligament forms the suspensory ligament of the ovary, whereas the caudal genital ligament forms the ligament of the ovary proper and the round ligament of the uterus.

Clinical correlates

- Absence of vagina and uterus occurs in 1 in 4000–5000 female births. The failure of the sinovaginal bulbs to develop and form the vaginal plate leads to absent vagina. It is usually associated with an absent uterus as the sinovaginal plates are induced by the paramesonephric ducts fusion and migration to the urogenital sinus.
- Vaginal atresia is failure of canalisation of the vaginal plate, which results in vaginal atresia. This leads to formation of the transverse vaginal septum usually located at the junction of the middle and superior thirds of the vagina.
- Cryptorchidism or undescended testes occur in 30% of premature infants and 3–4% of infants born at term. In most cases, the testes descend into the scrotum by the end of the first year; if they remain within the abdominal wall, by the end of 1 year sterility is common. Deficient production of androgen by the fetal testes plays a role in its causation.

SUGGESTED FURTHER READING

KEITH L, MOORE T V N P, editors. *The Developing Embryo*, 7th ed. Philadelphia: Saunders; 2003.

QUAGGIN S E, KREIDBERG J A. Development of the renal glomerulus: good neighbors and good fences. *Development* 2008;135:609–20.

THOMAS W, SADLER J L, LELAND J, editors. *Langman's Medical Embryology*, 10th ed. Philadelphia: Lippincott Williams & Wilkins; 2006.

CHAPTER 13

Development and congenital anomalies of the gastrointestinal tract

Rohan D'Souza

Development of the digestive system

The primitive gut is formed during week 4 of development, when the embryo folds cephalocaudally and laterally, thereby incorporating a portion of the endoderm-lined yolk sac cavity (Figure 13.1). This gut system extends from the buccopharyngeal membrane to the cloacal membrane and is divided into the pharyngeal gut, foregut, midgut and hindgut, the derivatives of which are shown in Table 13.1. The relative contributions of the three germ layers of the primitive gut are outlined in Table 13.2 while the arterial supply is outlined in Table 13.3.

FOREGUT

Development of the oesophagus

In week 4, a respiratory diverticulum (lung bud) appears in the ventral wall of the foregut just beneath the pharyngeal gut. This diverticulum gradually gets partitioned from the dorsal part of the foregut by the tracheoesophageal septum. Thus, the foregut divides into a ventral respiratory primordium and a dorsal oesophagus. The oesophagus rapidly lengthens as the heart and lungs descend. The characteristics of the muscle coat of the oesophagus are outlined in Table 13.4.

FIGURE 13.1 **Sagittal sections showing the cephalocaudal folding of the embryo and the formation of the primitive gut**

A Presomite embryo

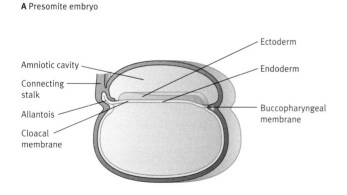

B Embryo at 22 days

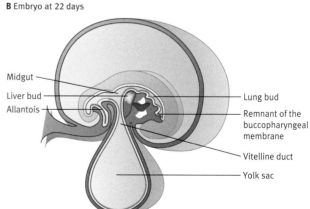

TABLE 13.1 **Derivatives of the primitive gut**

Pharyngeal gut	Pharynx and related glands
Foregut	Oesophagus
	Trachea and lung buds
	Stomach
	Duodenum proximal to the entrance of the bile duct
	Liver, biliary apparatus and pancreas
Midgut	Duodenum distal to the opening of the bile duct
	Small intestine
	Caecum and appendix
	Ascending colon and two-thirds of the transverse colon
Hindgut	Distal third of the transverse colon, descending colon and sigmoid colon
	Rectum and the superior part of the anal canal
	Epithelium of the urinary bladder and most of the urethra

TABLE 13.2 **Contributions of germ layers in development of the gut**

Germ layer	Derived components
Endoderm	Epithelium of the digestive system
	Parenchyma of the derivates of the gut
Splanchnic mesoderm	Connective tissue
	Muscular components
	Peritoneal components
Ectoderm	Distal part of the anal canal

TABLE 13.3 **Arterial supply of the primitive gut**

Portion of primitive gut	Arterial supply
Foregut	Branches of the coeliac trunk
Midgut	Branches of the superior mesenteric artery
Hindgut	Branches of the inferior mesenteric artery

TABLE 13.4 **Characteristics of the oesophageal muscle coat**

Portion of oesophagus	Muscle type	Nerve supply
Upper two-thirds	Striated	Vagus nerve
Lower third	Smooth	Splanchnic plexus

TABLE 13.5 **Rotational changes during development of the stomach**

Rotational change	Effects
90° clockwise rotation around its longitudinal axis	The original left side now faces anterior and the original right side faces posterior
	The left vagus nerve consequently innervates the anterior wall and the right innervates the posterior wall
Anteroposterior rotation	The cephalic and caudal ends of the stomach no longer lie in the midline
	The caudal or pyloric part moves to the right and upward and the cephalic or cardiac portion moves to the left and slightly downward

FIGURE 13.2 **Schematic representation of the rotation of the stomach on its anteroposterior axis**

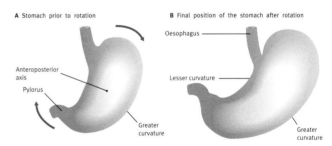

A Stomach prior to rotation

B Final position of the stomach after rotation

Anteroposterior axis

Pylorus

Greater curvature

Oesophagus

Lesser curvature

Greater curvature

Development of the stomach

The stomach appears as a fusiform dilation of the foregut during week 4. It subsequently rotates around a longitudinal and an anteroposterior axis (Figure 13.2). The effects of this rotation have been summarised in Table 13.5.

FIGURE 13.3 **The formation of the omental bursa and the greater omentum**

A Transverse section at 4 weeks, showing the formation of the omental bursa and lesser omentum

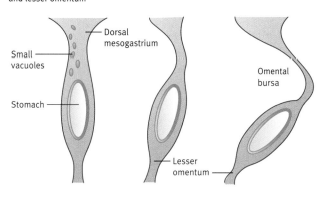

B Sagittal section at 4 months, showing the final position of the omental bursa and the greater omentum

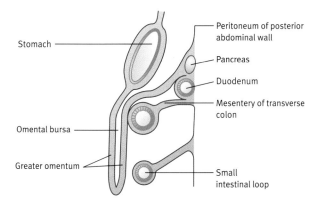

During rotation, the original posterior wall (now on the left) grows faster than the anterior portion (now on the right), forming the greater and lesser curvatures respectively. The stomach thus assumes its final position, its axis running from above left to below right.

Mesenteries of the stomach

The stomach is suspended from the dorsal wall and ventral body wall by mesenteries, known as the dorsal and ventral mesogastrium respectively. Its rotation and disproportionate growth alter the position of these mesenteries.

The dorsal mesogastrium is pulled to the left, creating a space behind the stomach called the omental bursa (lesser peritoneal sac). It continues to grow down, forming a double-layered sac – the greater omentum (Figure 13.3). The two leaves of the greater omentum later fuse with each other and with the mesentery of the transverse colon.

The ventral mesogastrium is pulled to the right, forming the lesser omentum (which passes from the liver to the lesser curvature of the stomach) and the falciform ligament (which extends from the liver to the ventral abdominal wall). On its way from the umbilical cord to the liver, the umbilical vein passes in the free border of the falciform ligament (Figure 13.4).

Development of the duodenum

The duodenum also develops early in week 4. Since it develops from both the terminal part of the foregut and

FIGURE 13.4 **The effect of rotation of the stomach on the position of the mesenteries**

A Embryo at week 5

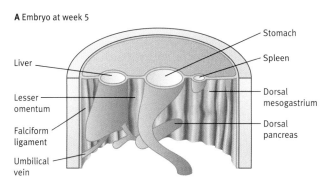

B Embryo at week 11

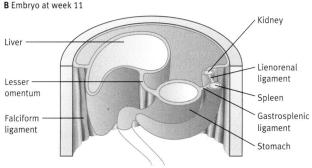

FIGURE 13.5 **Sagittal sections showing the penetration of the septum transversum by the rapidly proliferating cells of the hepatic diverticulum (liver bud) and the subsequent development of the liver and the biliary apparatus**

A Embryo at day 25

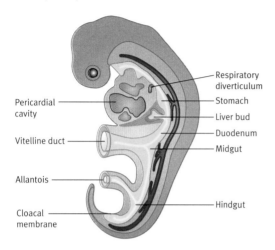

B Embryo at day 36

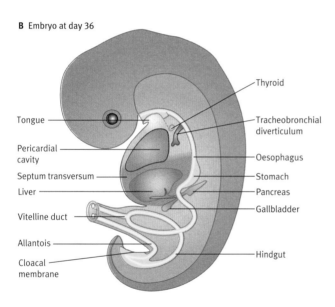

5–6, proliferation of epithelial cells results in temporary obliteration of the lumen of the duodenum, but this is recanalised by the end of the embryonic period.

Development of the liver and biliary apparatus

Rapidly proliferating cells at the distal end of the foregut result in the formation of a ventral outgrowth early in week 4. This is the hepatic diverticulum (liver bud), which then penetrates the septum transversum and goes on to form the liver and the biliary apparatus (Figure 13.5). The bile duct is formed when the connection between the hepatic diverticulum and the foregut (duodenum) subsequently narrows. The bile duct develops a small ventral outgrowth that then goes on to form the gallbladder and the cystic duct.

The surface mesoderm of the liver differentiates into visceral peritoneum, except on the cranial surface, where the liver remains in contact with the rest of the original septum transversum. This portion of the septum, which comprises densely packed mesoderm, forms the central tendon of the diaphragm, and the surface of the liver that is in contact with the future diaphragm forms the bare area of the liver. This area is never covered by peritoneum. The liver grows rapidly and, by week 9, accounts for approximately 10% of the body weight. Initially, the right and left lobes are approximately the same size, but the right lobe soon becomes larger.

Haematopoiesis begins during week 6, giving the liver a bright red appearance. Bile formation by hepatic cells begins during week 12. When the cystic duct joins the hepatic duct to form the bile duct, bile enters the gastrointestinal tract and its contents take on a dark green colour. This entrance of the bile duct is initially anterior but, because of positional changes of the duodenum, it moves posteriorly and finally comes to lie behind the duodenum. The origin of various hepatic cells is outlined in Table 13.6.

Development of the pancreas

Two separate buds, the ventral and dorsal pancreatic buds, originate from the endodermal lining of the duodenum and grow rapidly between the layers of

the proximal part of the midgut, it is supplied by branches of both the coeliac artery and the superior mesenteric artery. The junction of these two parts is just distal to the origin of the bile duct. As the stomach rotates, the duodenum takes on the form of a C-shaped loop, rotates to the right and becomes retroperitoneal. The region of the duodenal cap, however, retains its mesentery and remains intraperitoneal. During weeks

the dorsal mesentery. These go on to form the pancreas (Figure 13.6). The larger dorsal pancreatic bud appears first and develops cranial to the ventral pancreatic bud, which in turn develops near the entry of the bile duct into the duodenum. Rotation of the duodenum causes the ventral bud to move dorsally and finally to lie immediately below and behind the dorsal bud. Subsequently, the parenchyma and the duct systems of the two buds fuse and the main pancreatic duct enters the duodenum along with the bile duct at the major papilla. The accessory pancreatic duct (when present) enters the duodenum at the minor papilla. Figure 13.6 and Table 13.7 provide more details.

The main pancreatic duct, together with the bile duct, enters the duodenum at the site of the major papilla; while the accessory duct (when present) enters at the site of the minor papilla, which is located approximately 2 cm cranial to the major papilla. In 10% of cases, the duct system fails to fuse and the original double system persists.

The origin of various cell-types in the pancreas is outlined in Table 13.8. Insulin secretion begins at approximately month 5.

Development of the spleen

The spleen is derived from a mass of mesenchymal cells located between the layers of the dorsal mesogastrium. It begins to develop during week 5. In the fetus, the spleen is lobulated and functions as a haemopoietic centre. The splenic lobules normally disappear before

TABLE 13.6 **Origin of hepatic cells and sinusoids**

Origin	Cell type
Mesoderm of the septum transversum	Haematopoetic cells
	Kupffer cells
	Connective tissue cells
Liver cords	Parenchyma (liver cells) lining the biliary ducts
Intermingling of epithelial liver cords with vitelline and umbilical veins	Hepatic sinusoids

TABLE 13.7 **Origin of parenchyma and duct system of the pancreas**

Origin	Final structure
Ventral pancreatic bud	Uncinate process and inferior part of head of pancreas
Dorsal pancreatic bud	Entire pancreas except for the above
Ventral pancreatic duct and the distal part of dorsal pancreatic duct	Main pancreatic duct (of Wirsung)
Proximal part of dorsal pancreatic duct (if and when it persists)	Accessory pancreatic duct (of Santorini)

FIGURE 13.6 **Development of the pancreas**

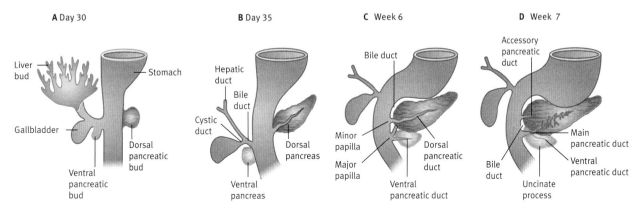

A Day 30

Liver bud
Stomach
Gallbladder
Dorsal pancreatic bud
Ventral pancreatic bud

B Day 35

Hepatic duct
Bile duct
Cystic duct
Dorsal pancreas
Ventral pancreas

C Week 6

Bile duct
Minor papilla
Major papilla
Dorsal pancreatic duct
Ventral pancreatic duct

D Week 7

Accessory pancreatic duct
Bile duct
Main pancreatic duct
Ventral pancreatic duct
Uncinate process

TABLE 13.8 **Origin of pancreatic cells and connective tissue**

Origin	Cell / tissue
Parenchymatous pancreatic tissue	Pancreatic islets (of Langerhans)
	Glucagon- and somatostatin-secreting cells
Splanchnic mesoderm surrounding the pancreatic buds	Connective tissue

TABLE 13.9 **Derivatives of the midgut**

Part of the midgut	Derivatives
Cephalic limb of the primary loop	Distal part of the duodenum
	Jejunum
	Part of the ileum
Caudal limb of the primary loop	Lower part of the ileum
	Caecum and appendix
	Ascending colon
	Proximal two-thirds of the transverse colon

birth, but the potential for blood cell formation is retained even in adult life. The splenic artery is the largest branch of the coeliac trunk.

MIDGUT

The portion of the gut that is supplied by the superior mesenteric artery undergoes rapid elongation and forms the primary loop. Its derivatives are outlined in Table 13.9. At its apex, it remains in open connection with the yolk sac by way of the vitelline duct.

Physiological umbilical herniation and subsequent retraction of herniated loops

The primary loop, and especially its cephalic limb, elongates rapidly. As a result of this, as well as the rapid growth and expansion of the liver, the abdominal cavity temporarily becomes too small to contain all the intestinal loops. During week 6 of development, the loops therefore enter the extraembryonic cavity in the umbilical cord. This is known as physiological umbilical herniation.

During week 10, regression of the mesonephric kidney, reduced growth of the liver and expansion of the abdominal cavity cause these herniated intestinal loops to return to the abdominal cavity. The first part to re-enter the cavity is the proximal part of the jejunum, which comes to lie on the left side. The loops that enter later settle more and more to the right.

Rotation of the midgut

The primary intestinal loop rotates around an axis formed by the superior mesenteric artery, by approximately 270 degrees in the anti-clockwise direction. This rotation occurs during herniation (about 90 degrees) as well as during return of the intestinal loops into the abdominal cavity (remaining 180 degrees).

Caecum and appendix

The caecal bud, which appears at about week 6 as a small conical dilation of the caudal limb of the primary intestinal loop, is the last part of the gut to re-enter the abdominal cavity. At first it lies in the right upper quadrant below the right lobe of the liver. Later it descends into the right iliac fossa and during this process its distal end forms a narrow diverticulum, the appendix. The appendix grows rapidly in length and at birth it is a relatively long tube arising from the distal end of the caecum. After birth, as a result of unequal growth of the caecal wall, it comes to lie medially, although it may sometimes lie posterior to the caecum and colon.

Fixation of the intestines

The enlarged colon presses the duodenum and pancreas against the posterior abdominal wall resulting in the absorption of most of the duodenal mesentery. Similarly, when the ascending and descending colon obtain their definitive positions, their mesenteries press against the peritoneum of the posterior abdominal wall and are eventually absorbed. The following structures therefore become retroperitoneal:

- duodenum (except for the first 2.5 cm)
- ascending colon
- descending colon.

The following structures, however, retain their free mesenteries:

- other derivatives of the midgut loop (the jejunum and ileum)
- lower end of the caecum and the appendix
- transverse colon (although its mesentery fuses with the posterior wall of the greater omentum)
- sigmoid colon.

The line of attachment of the fan-shaped mesentery of the small intestine passes from the duodenojejunal junction inferolaterally to the ileocaecal junction.

HINDGUT

Partitioning of the cloaca

The cloaca is the expanded terminal part of the hindgut. It is an endoderm-lined chamber that is in contact with the surface ectoderm at the cloacal membrane. This membrane is composed of endoderm of the cloaca on the inside and ectoderm of the proctodeum (anal pit) on the outside. As illustrated in Figure 13.7, at week 5, the allantois enters the anterior portion of the cloaca (the future urogenital sinus), while the hindgut enters the posterior portion (the future anorectal canal). A layer of mesoderm, the urorectal septum, separates the region between the allantois and hindgut. By week 6, the urorectal septum moves closer to the cloacal membrane, although the two

never make contact. At the end of week 7, breakdown of the cloacal membrane creates the anal opening for the hindgut and a ventral opening for the urogenital sinus. The tip of the urorectal septum forms the perineal body.

Proliferation of the ectoderm of the proctodeum closes the lowermost region of the anal canal but this region recanalises during week 9.

Anal canal

The superior two-thirds of the anal canal originate in the endoderm of the hindgut, while the inferior one-third originates in the ectoderm of the proctodeum. The junction between these regions is delineated by the pectinate line (also called the anocutaneous line or simply the 'white line'), just below the anal columns. The differences in blood supply, nerve supply and venous and lymphatic drainage of the superior and inferior parts of the anal canal are clinically important and are outlined in Table 13.10. The other layers of the wall of the anal canal are derived from the splanchnic mesoderm.

Congenital anomalies of the gut

ABNORMALITIES OF THE FOREGUT

Oesophageal atresia

Oesophageal atresia occurs in about 1 in 3000–4500 live births. When associated with a tracheo-oesophageal fistula (85–90%), it occurs as a result of posterior deviation of the tracheo-oesophageal septum. When it occurs as an isolated abnormality, the cause is failure of recanalisation of the oesophagus during week 8 of development.

FIGURE 13.7 **Partitioning of the cloaca**

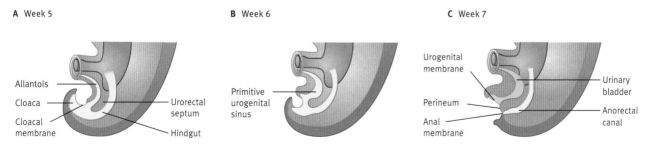

A Week 5

B Week 6

C Week 7

TABLE 13.10 **Distinctive features of the two parts of the anal canal**

Feature	Superior two-thirds	Inferior one-third
Origin	Endoderm (hindgut)	Ectoderm (proctodeum)
Length	25 mm	13 mm
Epithelium	Columnar	Stratified squamous
Arterial supply	Superior rectal artery (continuation of the artery of the hindgut, the inferior mesenteric artery)	Inferior rectal arteries, branches of the internal pudendal artery
Venous drainage	Superior rectal vein, a tributary of the inferior mesenteric vein	Inferior rectal vein, a tributary of the internal pudendal vein that drains into the internal iliac vein
Lymphatic drainage	Inferior mesenteric lymph nodes	Superficial inguinal lymph nodes
Nerve supply	Autonomic nervous system (hence 'painless carcinomas')	Inferior rectal nerve (hence 'painful carcinomas')

This may be associated with anorectal atresia and anomalies of the urogenital system.

Oesophageal atresia manifests as polyhydramnios in fetal life and excessive drooling and regurgitation after birth. Diagnosis is suspected when there is an inability to pass a catheter through the oesophagus and confirmed on radiography when the nasogastric tube is arrested in the proximal oesophageal pouch. This abnormality can be corrected surgically.

Congenital hiatal hernia

Congenital hiatal hernia results from the failure of the oesophagus to elongate sufficiently as the neck and thorax develop. The stomach therefore gets pulled into the oesophageal hiatus through the diaphragm. This condition generally manifests in middle age.

Congenital hypertrophic pyloric stenosis

Congenital hypertrophic pyloric stenosis occurs in 1 in 150 males and 1 in 750 females. There is a marked muscular thickening of the circular muscles and, to a lesser degree, the longitudinal muscles in the pylorus. Its cause is unknown, but genetic factors may be involved: there is a high rate of concordance in monozygotic twins.

Neonates present with projectile vomiting and marked distension of the stomach. Management is essentially surgical (pyloromyotomy).

TABLE 13.11 **Frequencies of atresias and stenoses of the gut**

Type of anomaly	Percentage
Loss of a region of the bowel	50
Fibrous cord remnant	20
Narrowing of lumen with a thin diaphragm separating the larger and smaller pieces of bowel	20
Stenoses	5
Multiple atresias	5

Duodenal stenosis and atresia

The frequencies of occurrence of atresias and stenoses of the gut are shown in Table 13.11.

Duodenal stenosis results when there is incomplete recanalisation of the duodenum. This generally involves the horizontal (third) and/or fourth parts of the duodenum.

Duodenal atresia results when the duodenal lumen fails to recanalise. This almost always occurs at the junction of the bile duct and pancreatic duct, but rarely in the third part of the duodenum. Duodenal atresia shows autosomal recessive inheritance and may be associated with other anorectal and cardiovascular abnormalities or annular pancreas. One-third of affected infants have Down syndrome.

Duodenal atresia presents as polyhydramnios in fetal life and bilious vomiting and distension of the epigastrium after birth. Diagnosis is made on X-ray (double bubble sign) or ultrasound.

ABNORMALITIES OF THE HEPATOBILIARY APPARATUS

Liver abnormalities

Major liver anomalies are rare, but minor variations of liver lobulation, accessory hepatic ducts and a duplicated gallbladder are common. These are of surgical importance.

Extrahepatic biliary atresia

Extrahepatic biliary atresia occurs in 1 in 10 000–15 000 live births. It results from infections, immunological reactions or the failure of the remodelling process at the hepatic hilum. It commonly occurs at or just above the porta hepatis, a deep transverse fissure on the visceral surface of the liver.

The main signs are pathological jaundice after birth and clay-coloured stools. Surgical correction is by Kasai hepatoportoenterostomy or liver transplant.

Intrahepatic biliary atresia or hypoplasia

Intrahepatic biliary atresia occurs in 1 in 100 000 live births. It may be caused by fetal infections. It can be lethal or may run an extended benign course.

Annular pancreas

Migration of the left portion of the ventral bud of the pancreas in the opposite direction results in the formation of a ring (annulus) around the pancreas. Annular pancreas may be associated with Down syndrome, intestinal atresia, imperforate anus, pancreatitis and malrotation of the gut. Males are affected more frequently. Although uncommon, an annular pancreas can result in serious duodenal obstruction, especially when inflamed.

Accessory pancreatic tissue

Accessory pancreatic tissue is extrapancreatic tissue that shows all the histological characteristics of the pancreas.

The tissue lies most frequently in the mucosa of the stomach or in a Meckel diverticulum.

Accessory spleens

Accessory spleens are seen in approximately 10% of people. They are usually isolated but may be attached to the spleen by thin bands.

ABNORMALITIES OF THE ANTERIOR ABDOMINAL WALL

Omphalocele (exomphalos)

Defects of the anterior abdominal wall include gastroschisis, omphalocele (exomphalos) and congenital umbilical hernia. The main differences between gastroschisis and omphalocele are outlined in Table 13.12.

Gastroschisis

Gastroschisis occurs in 1 in 10 000 live births, but the frequency is increasing, especially among young mothers and probably related to cocaine use. Its occurrence is more common in males.

Gastroschisis is herniation of abdominal contents, not covered by peritoneum/amnion, through the body wall. This herniation occurs lateral to the umbilicus, usually on the right, through a region weakened by regression of the right umbilical vein. Since it is not associated with chromosomal abnormalities or severe defects, the prognosis is generally excellent. However, a volvulus, resulting in a compromised blood supply, may damage large regions of the intestine and lead to fetal death.

Congenital umbilical hernia

Congenital umbilical hernia refers to the herniation of abdominal contents through an imperfectly closed umbilicus. There is a defect in the linea alba, the fibrous band between the rectus muscles. The protruding mass is generally omentum and/or small bowel and is covered by subcutaneous tissue and skin. The condition presents as an umbilical swelling that becomes prominent during crying or coughing.

TABLE 13.12 **Differences between gastroschisis and omphalocele (exomphalos)**

	Gastroschisis	Omphalocele
Definition	Herniation of abdominal contents, not covered by peritoneum/ amnion, through the body wall	Herniation of abdominal viscera (which may include liver, bowel, spleen and gallbladder) covered in amnion, through an enlarged umbilical ring
Defect	Para-umbilical (usually right sided) and diameter mostly <4cm	Central
Incidence	0.5–4.5/10 000 live births and increasing	2–3:10 000 live births
Aetiology	'Teratogenic effects on the lateral body folds' – Duhamel, 1963. (Formerly believed to be the result of vascular disruption involving the right omphalo-mesenteric artery. However, this artery supplies the intestine and not the abdominal wall)	Failure of the bowel to return to the body cavity from its physiological herniation during weeks 6–10
Genetics	Combination of genetic and environmental factors. Only 1.2% cases have associated chromosomal abnormalities and single gene disorders are even rarer 22 teratogens have been implicated	Probably caused by genetic insults with a smaller environmental component. 50% have associated chromosomal abnormalities 9 teratogens have been implicated
Associations	Young mothers (<20 years). Short time interval between menarche and first pregnancy Nicotine, alcohol, drug abuse Low educational and socio-economic status History of >1 abortions Male fetuses Intrauterine growth restriction (IUGR)	Cardiac defects: 50% Neural tube defects: 40% Mortality rates: 25%
Correction	Surgical repair after birth	Surgical repair. In infants with very large omphalocele, delayed closure is recommended to avoid complications from pulmonary and thoracic hypoplasia
Prognosis	Generally very good	Depends on associated anomalies

Surgery is not performed unless it persists beyond 3–5 years.

GUT ROTATION DEFECTS

Abnormal/incomplete rotation of the gut and its effects

Rotation by 90 degrees results in the colon and caecum returning first to the abdominal cavity and being situated to the left, while the small bowel returns to the right. The caecum lies just inferior to the pylorus of the stomach and is fixed to the posterolateral abdominal wall by peritoneal bands that pass over the duodenum. The peritoneal bands and the twisting of the intestines result in duodenal obstruction. Infants may present with bilious vomiting. The diagnosis is confirmed by a simple contrast study.

In cases where there is malrotation of the gut, the intestine remains improperly positioned and improperly fixed. This may lead to a catastrophic twisting of the gut (midgut volvulus), wherein the superior mesenteric vessels can be obstructed, resulting in infarction and gangrene of the intestine.

Rotation sometimes occurs by 90 degrees in the clockwise direction. This reversed rotation results in the duodenum lying anterior to the superior mesenteric artery and the transverse colon lying posterior to it. The transverse colon may be obstructed by pressure from the superior mesenteric artery.

OTHER ABNORMALITIES OF THE MIDGUT

Meckel diverticulum

A Meckel diverticulum occurs in 2–4% of the population. It is the most common anomaly of the digestive tract and is 3–5 times more prevalent in males. There is a persistence of a small portion of the vitelline duct, forming an outpocketing of the ileum. In the adult, it lies approximately 40–60 cm from the ileocaecal valve on the antimesenteric border of the ileum.

Inflammation (diverticulitis) mimics appendicitis. The wall may contain small patches of gastric and pancreatic tissues. The ectopic gastric mucosa often secretes acid, producing ulceration and bleeding. Variations, in the form of vitelline cysts and fistulae are also described, which could present with features of a volvulus or faecal discharge at the umbilicus, respectively.

Duplications of intestinal loops and cysts

Duplications may occur anywhere along the length of the gut but are most frequently found in the region of the ileum. The duplicated segment lies on the mesenteric side. Thirty-three percent are associated with other defects, such as intestinal atresias, imperforate anus, gastroschisis and omphalocele. Symptoms usually occur early in life. The duplicated intestine often contains ectopic gastric mucosa, which may result in local peptic ulceration and lower gastrointestinal bleeding.

Gut atresias and stenoses

Gut atresias and stenoses occur in 1 in 1500 live births. They may occur anywhere along the intestine, although most occur in the duodenum and fewest occur in the colon. Atresias in the upper duodenum are usually due to a lack of recanalisation, while those distal to this region are usually caused by deficient blood supply to the gut.

Apple-peel atresia accounts for 10% of atresias. Here, the intestine is short and the atresia is in the proximal jejunum, with the portion distal to the lesion coiled around a mesenteric remnant. Babies with this defect have low birth weight and other abnormalities.

Subhepatic caecum and appendix

Subhepatic caecum and appendix occurs in 6% of fetuses and is more common in males. The caecum adheres to the inferior surface of the liver where it returns to the abdomen and is drawn superiorly as the liver diminishes in size. This malposition can pose difficulty in the diagnosis of appendicitis and during appendicectomy.

ABNORMALITIES OF THE MESENTERIES

Mobile caecum

Mobile caecum occurs in 10% of the population. A failure of the ascending colon to fuse to the posterior abdominal wall results in the persistence of a portion of mesocolon. In the most extreme form, the long mesentery allows abnormal movements of the gut or even a volvulus of the caecum and colon. In unusual cases, it may herniate into the right inguinal canal.

Retrocolic hernia

A retrocolic hernia is an entrapment of portions of the small intestine behind the mesocolon. It is generally asymptomatic and often is only discovered at autopsy.

ABNORMALITIES OF THE HINDGUT

Low anomalies

Rectoanal atresias and fistulae occur in 1 in 5000 live births. They are caused by abnormalities in the formation of the cloaca, generally due to ectopic positioning of the anal opening and not due to defects in the urorectal septum.

Imperforate anus occurs in 1 in 5000 live births and is more common in males. There is no anal opening. This defect occurs because of a lack of recanalisation of the lower portion of the anal canal. It requires surgical correction.

Anal stenosis is seen when the anus is in the normal position but the anus and anal canal are narrow. It is probably caused by a slight dorsal deviation of the urorectal septum as it grows caudally to fuse with the cloacal membrane.

Membranous atresia of the anus is seen when the anus is in the normal position but a thin layer of tissue separates the anal canal from the exterior. It results from the failure of the anal membrane to perforate at the end of week 8.

Congenital megacolon (aganglionic megacolon or Hirschsprung disease) occurs in 1 in 5000 live births and males are four times more likely to be affected. Congenital megacolon accounts for 33% of all neonatal obstructions. It is a dominantly inherited, multigenic disorder with incomplete penetrance and variable expressivity. There is an absence of parasympathetic ganglia in the bowel wall. This occurs because neural crest cells fail to migrate into the wall of the colon during weeks 5–6. Of the genes so far identified, the *RET* proto-oncogene is the major susceptibility gene, accounting for most cases. In most cases the rectum is involved and in 3% the entire colon is affected.

High anomalies

Anorectal agenesis, with or without fistula, is the most common type of anorectal anomaly. The rectum ends blindly, superior to the puborectalis muscle, often with a fistula to the bladder, urethra or vestibule of the vagina. This is the result of incomplete separation of the cloaca by the urorectal septum. The main symptom is the passage of meconium or flatus in urine or in the vestibule of the vagina.

Rectal atresia is seen when the rectum and anus are separated; sometimes the two segments of bowel are connected by a fibrous cord. This may be caused by abnormal recanalisation or deficient blood supply.

FURTHER READING

BATES M D, BALISTRERI W F. Development and function of the liver and biliary system. In: BEHRMAN R E, KLIEGMAN R M, JENSON H B, editors. *Nelson Textbook of Paediatrics*, 17th ed. Philadelphia: WB Saunders; 2004. p.1304–8.

CHRISTISON-LAGAY E R, KELLEHER C M, LANGER J C. Neonatal abdominal wall defects. *Semin Fetal Neonatal Med* 2011,16:164–72.

GOSCHE J R, VICK L, BOULANGER S C, ISLAM S. Midgut abnormalities. *Surg Clin North Am* 2006;86:285–99.

LAU S T, CATY M G. Hindgut abnormalities. *Surg Clin North Am* 2006;86:301–16.

LEDBETTER D J. Gastroschisis and omphalocele. *Surg Clin North Am* 2006;86:249–60.

MAGNUSON D K, PARRY R L, CHWALS W J. Selected abdominal gastrointestinal anomalies. In: MARTIN R J, FANAROFF A A, WALSH M C, editors. *Fanaroff and Martin's Neonatal-perinatal Medicine. Diseases of the Fetus and Infant*, 8th ed. Philadelphia: Mosby; 2006. p.1381–402.

MOORE K L, PERSAUD T V N. The gastrointestinal system. In: *The Developing Human: Clinically Oriented Embryology*, 8th ed. Philadelphia: W B Saunders; 2008. p.211–42.

NAIK-MATHURIA B, OLUTOYE O O. Foregut abnormalities. *Surg Clin North Am* 2006;86:261–84.

NIEVELSTEIN R A J, VAN DER WERFF J F A, VERBEEK F J, VERMEIJ-KEERS C. Normal and abnormal development of the anorectum in human embryos. *Teratology* 1998;57:70–8.

ORENSTEIN S, PETERS J, KHAN S, YAUSSEF N, HUSSAIN S Z. Congenital anomalies. Esophageal atresia and tracheoesophageal fistula and function of the esophagus. In: BEHRMAN R E, KLIEGMAN R M, JENSON H B, editors. *Nelson Textbook of Paediatrics*, 18th ed. Philadelphia: W B Saunders; 2007. chap. 316.

SADLER T W. The gastrointestinal system. In: *Langman's Medical Embryology*, 10th ed. Baltimore: Lippincott Williams & Wilkins; 2006. p.203–27.

SADLER T W. The embryologic origin of ventral body wall defects. *Semin Pediatr Surg* 2010;19:209–14.

CHAPTER 14

Development of the heart and the fetal circulation

Rohan D'Souza

Development of the heart

The cardiovascular system is the first major system to function in the embryo. The primordial heart and vascular system appear in the middle of week 3, to satisfy the nutritional and oxygen requirements of the developing embryo.

The cardiogenic field

Cardiac progenitor cells lie in the epiblast, immediately lateral to the primitive streak (Figure 14.1). They migrate through the streak and then proceed towards the cranium, coming to lie in the splanchnic layer of the lateral plate mesoderm. They are then induced to form

FIGURE 14.1 **Embryo at day 18 showing the cardiogenic field and the formation of the pericardial cavity**

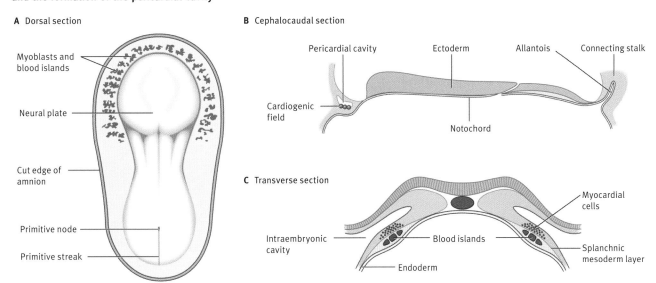

A Dorsal section

Myoblasts and blood islands

Neural plate

Cut edge of amnion

Primitive node

Primitive streak

B Cephalocaudal section

Pericardial cavity

Ectoderm

Allantois

Connecting stalk

Cardiogenic field

Notochord

C Transverse section

Myocardial cells

Intraembryonic cavity

Blood islands

Splanchnic mesoderm layer

Endoderm

Myoblasts and blood islands can be seen in the splanchnic mesoderm in front of the neural plate and on each side of the embryo. Note the position of the pericardial cavity and the cardiogenic field in **(B)**.

185

cardiac myoblasts. Blood islands also appear in this mesoderm, where they form blood cells and vessels by the process of vasculogenesis. With time, the islands unite and form a horseshoe-shaped endothelial-lined tube surrounded by myoblasts. This region is known as the cardiogenic field. The intra-embryonic cavity over it later develops into the pericardial cavity.

THE HEART TUBE

The embryo folds both cephalocaudally and laterally (Figures 14.2 and 14.3). As a result of cephalocaudal folding, as well as the rapid growth of the brain, the cardiogenic area moves caudally to the thorax. As a result of the lateral folding of the embryo, the caudal regions of the paired cardiac primordia merge, except at their caudal-most ends. The heart now becomes a continuous tube consisting of an inner endothelial lining (the future endocardium), which is separated from an outer muscular layer (the future myocardium) by a gelatinous connective tissue called cardiac jelly (Figures 14.3 and 14.4A). The pericardium is formed from mesothelial cells that arise from the external surface of the sinus venosus. This outer layer is responsible for formation of the coronary arteries, including their endothelial lining and smooth muscle.

FIGURE 14.2 **Cephalocaudal sections through an embryo**

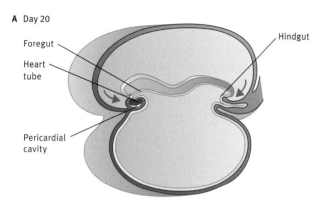

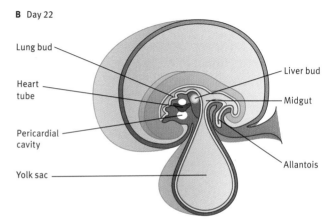

The effects of the rapid growth of the brain on the positioning of the heart can be seen. The cardiogenic field moves from in front of the buccopharyngeal membrane to the thorax.

FIGURE 14.3 **Transverse sections through an embryo**

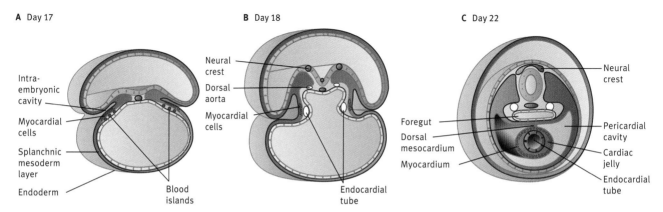

The effect of the lateral folding of the embryo and the merging of the paired cardiac primordial to form the endocardial tube can be seen.

FIGURE 14.4 **Ventral views of the developing heart**

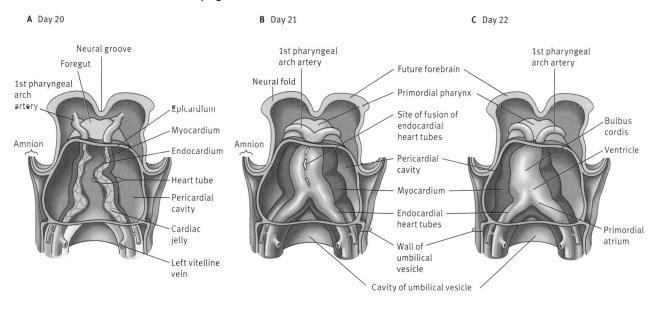

A Day 20

- Neural groove
- Foregut
- 1st pharyngeal arch artery
- Amnion
- Epicardium
- Myocardium
- Endocardium
- Heart tube
- Pericardial cavity
- Cardiac jelly
- Left vitelline vein

B Day 21

- 1st pharyngeal arch artery
- Neural fold
- Amnion
- Future forebrain
- Primordial pharynx
- Site of fusion of endocardial heart tubes
- Pericardial cavity
- Myocardium
- Endocardial heart tubes
- Wall of umbilical vesicle
- Cavity of umbilical vesicle

C Day 22

- 1st pharyngeal arch artery
- Bulbus cordis
- Ventricle
- Primordial atrium

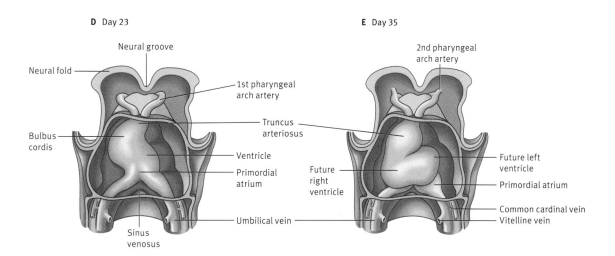

D Day 23

- Neural groove
- Neural fold
- 1st pharyngeal arch artery
- Bulbus cordis
- Truncus arteriosus
- Ventricle
- Primordial atrium
- Umbilical vein
- Sinus venosus

E Day 35

- 2nd pharyngeal arch artery
- Future right ventricle
- Future left ventricle
- Primordial atrium
- Common cardinal vein
- Vitelline vein

Fusion of the two heart tubes begins at the cranial ends of the heart tubes and extends caudally. A single tubular heart is formed as a result of the fusion of heart tubes. The heart elongates, forming regional segments and begins to fold on itself. This folding is completed by day 28 to form an S-shaped heart.

THE CARDIAC LOOP

The tubular heart elongates and develops alternate dilatations and constrictions (Figure 14.4). The primordial heart is composed of four chambers – the bulbus cordis (conotruncus), ventricle, atrium and sinus venosus. The cranial part of the bulbus cordis is the truncus arteriosus and is continuous cranially with the aortic sac. The sinus venosus receives the umbilical, vitelline and common cardinal veins from the chorion, umbilical vesicle and embryo, respectively. Because the bulbus cordis and ventricle grow faster than other regions, the heart bends upon itself, forming a S-shaped loop: the cardiac loop or the bulboventricular loop. This is completed by day 28. The developing heart bulges more and more into the pericardial cavity. Eventually, it is suspended in the cavity, remaining attached only at the cranial and caudal ends by blood vessels.

PARTITIONING OF THE PRIMORDIAL HEART

The partitioning of the various chambers of the primordial heart begins simultaneously around the middle of week 4 and is largely completed by the end of week 8.

Partitioning of the atrioventricular canal

In week 4 of development, endocardial cushions form on the dorsal and ventral walls of the atrioventricular canal. They approach each other and fuse, dividing the common atrioventricular canal in to right and left atrioventricular canals (Figure 14.5). These canals partially separate the primordial atrium from the primordial ventricle.

Partitioning of the atrium

The partitioning of the atrium occurs between day 27 and day 37 (week 4 to week 6) (Figure 14.6). A thin crescent-shaped membrane, the septum primum, grows from the roof of the primordial atrium towards the endocardial cushions, partially dividing the primordial atrium into right and left halves. This septum primum bears a large opening called the foramen primum

(ostium primum), which serves as a shunt, enabling oxygenated blood to pass from the right to left atrium. As the septum primum fuses with the endocardial cushions, the foramen primum becomes progressively smaller and then disappears. Before this can happen, however, perforations appear in the central part of the septum primum, which subsequently coalesce to form a new opening, the foramen secundum (ostium secundum). Thus, although the foramen primum closes, shunting of blood from the right to the left atrium continues via the foramen secundum. Now, a thick crescentic muscular fold grows from the ventrocranial wall of the right atrium, just adjacent to the septum primum. As this grows downwards, the upper part of the septum primum disappears, thus forming a flap-like valve between the two, called the foramen ovale (oval foramen). Owing to the flap-like mechanism, the foramen ovale allows only unidirectional flow of blood from the right atrium to the left during fetal life.

Partitioning of the sinus venosus

Partitioning of the sinus venosus occurs between week 4 and week 10 (Figure 14.7). Initially, the sinus venosus opens into the centre of the dorsal wall of the primordial atrium and its right and left horns are approximately of the same size. During weeks 4–5, left-to-right shunts in the venous system cause the right sinus horn to enlarge progressively. The left sinus horn rapidly loses its importance as the right umbilical vein and the left vitelline vein obliterates during week 5. At week 10,

FIGURE 14.5 **Partitioning of the atrioventricular canal**

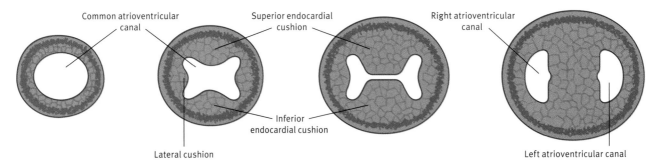

Endocardial cushions grow into the common atrioventricular canal (day 23) and result in the formation of the atrioventricular septum and the atrioventricular canals by day 35.

FIGURE 14.6 **Partitioning of the atrium**

A Coronal section through an embryo at day 30

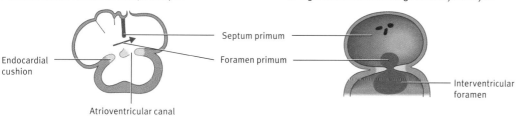

Endocardial cushion

Septum primum

Foramen primum

Atrioventricular canal

B Right lateral section through an embryo at day 30

Septum primum

Foramen primum

Interventricular foramen

C Coronal section through an embryo at day 33

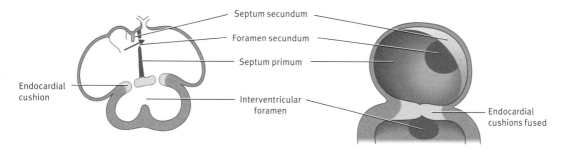

Septum secundum

Foramen secundum

Septum primum

Endocardial cushion

Interventricular foramen

D Right lateral section through an embryo at day 33

Endocardial cushions fused

E Coronal section through an embryo at day 37

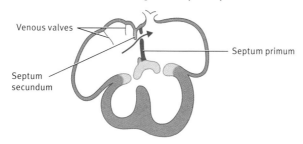

Venous valves

Septum secundum

Septum primum

F Coronal section through a newborn heart

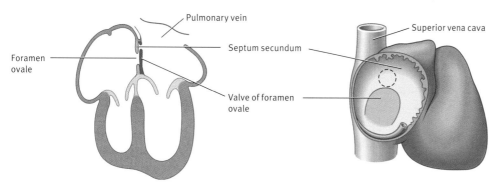

Pulmonary vein

Foramen ovale

Septum secundum

Valve of foramen ovale

G Right lateral section through a newborn heart

Superior vena cava

A and **B** show the formation of septum primum and foramen primum; note the development of perforations in the septum primum as the foramen primum begins to shrink. **C** and **D** show the formation of foramen secundum by the coalescence of perforations within the septum primum; note the formation of septum secundum as a growth from the ventrocranial wall of the right atrium. **E** shows the further growth of the septum secundum and the obliteration of the upper part of the septum primum, allowing unidirectional flow of blood from the right to left atrium. **F** and **G** show the foramen ovale and its flap-like valve formed by the lower part of the septum primum.

FIGURE 14.7 **Partitioning of the sinus venosus**

A Dorsal view at approximately day 26

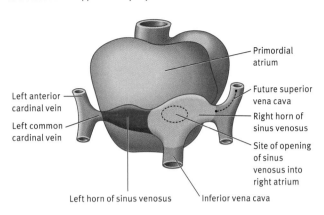

Primordial atrium

Left anterior cardinal vein

Left common cardinal vein

Future superior vena cava

Right horn of sinus venosus

Site of opening of sinus venosus into right atrium

Left horn of sinus venosus

Inferior vena cava

B Dorsal view in week 8

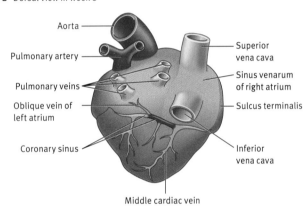

Aorta

Pulmonary artery

Pulmonary veins

Oblique vein of left atrium

Coronary sinus

Superior vena cava

Sinus venarum of right atrium

Sulcus terminalis

Inferior vena cava

Middle cardiac vein

Red = fully oxgenated blood | blue = deoxygenated blood | purple = mixed blood

FIGURE 14.8 **Development of the left atrium**

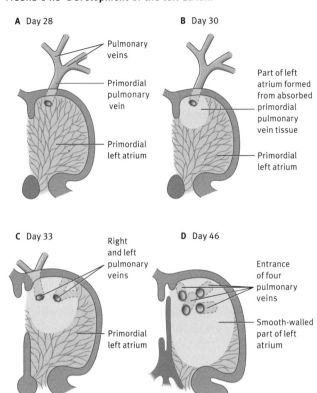

A Day 28

Pulmonary veins

Primordial pulmonary vein

Primordial left atrium

B Day 30

Part of left atrium formed from absorbed primordial pulmonary vein tissue

Primordial left atrium

C Day 33

Right and left pulmonary veins

Primordial left atrium

D Day 46

Entrance of four pulmonary veins

Smooth-walled part of left atrium

Partitioning of the ventricles

A muscular septum arises in the floor of the primordial ventricle, near its apex. This interventricular septum contains a crescent-shaped interventricular foramen, which permits communication between the two ventricles, until week 7. After the closure of this foramen, the pulmonary trunk communicates with the right ventricle and the aorta with the left ventricle (Figure 14.9).

Partitioning of the bulbus cordis and truncus arteriosus

During week 5, mesenchymal cells in the walls of the bulbus cordis proliferate actively and form bulbar ridges. Similar ridges that are continuous with the bulbar ridges form in the truncus arteriosus. The bulbar and truncal ridges (conotruncal ridges) then undergo 180-degrees spiralling, resulting in the formation of a spiral aorticopulmonary septum when the ridges fuse.

the left common cardinal vein also obliterates and now all that remains of the left sinus horn is the oblique vein of the left atrium and the coronary sinus. The enlarged right horn begins to receive all blood from the cranial and caudal regions of the body via the superior and inferior vena cava and gets incorporated into the wall of the right atrium forming the smooth-walled part of the right atrium, the sinus venarum. The remainder of the right atrial wall has a rough trabeculated appearance. The smooth and rough parts are demarcated internally by a vertical ridge, the crista terminalis, and externally by a shallow groove, the sulcus terminalis.

Most of the wall of the left atrium is formed by incorporation of the primordial pulmonary vein and is therefore smooth (Figure 14.8).

FIGURE 14.9 **Closure of the interventricular foramen**

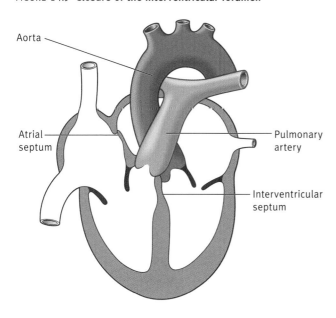

This septum divides the bulbus cordis and the truncus arteriosus into two distinct channels, the ascending aorta and pulmonary trunk. Because of the spiralling of the aorticopulmonary septum, the pulmonary trunk twists around the ascending aorta (Figure 14.10).

Formation of the cardiac valves

ATRIOVENTRICULAR VALVES

After the fusion of the atrioventricular endocardial cushions, each atrioventricular orifice is surrounded by proliferations of mesenchymal tissue. The bloodstream hollows out and thins these tissue proliferations on the ventricular surface, resulting in the formation of valves. These valves remain attached to the ventricular wall by muscular cords. Over time, the muscular tissue in the cords degenerates and is replaced by dense connective tissue. The valves then consist of connective tissue covered by endocardium. They are connected to thick trabeculae in the wall of the ventricle, the papillary muscles, by means of chordae tendineae (Figure 14.11). In this manner, two valve leaflets (mitral valve) form in the left atrioventricular canal, and three valve leaflets (tricuspid valve) form on the right side.

SEMILUNAR VALVES

At the time of partitioning of the truncus arteriosus, three swellings of subendocardial tissue develop around the orifices of the aorta and pulmonary trunk. These swellings are hollowed out and reshaped to form three thin-walled cusps, the future semilunar valves (Figure 14.12).

The conducting system of the heart

In the early stages of development, the function of pacemaker is assumed by the atrium and later by the sinus venosus. As the sinus venosus is incorporated into the right atrium, pacemaker tissue comes to lie near the opening of the superior vena cava, resulting in the formation of the sinoatrial node by week 5. The atrioventricular node and bundle (bundle of His) are derived from cells in the left wall of the sinus venosus and the atrioventricular canal. Fibres from the atrioventricular bundle pass from the atrium into the ventricle, split into right and left bundle branches and are distributed throughout the ventricular myocardium (Figure 14.13). Innervation of the sinoatrial node, atrioventricular node and atrioventricular bundle occurs later.

Congenital heart defects

Abnormalities of the cardiovascular system account for 1% of malformations among liveborn infants and almost 10% among stillborn babies, making up the largest category of human birth defects. Some defects cause very little disability and their impact may only become apparent at birth. Some others are incompatible with extrauterine life.

FACTORS LINKED WITH CONGENITAL HEART DEFECTS

The following factors are linked with congenital heart defects.

Genetic and chromosomal factors

It is estimated that 8% of cardiac malformations are due to genetic factors. Congenital heart defects are associated

FIGURE 14.10 **Partitioning of the bulbus cordis and truncus arteriosus**

A Ventral view through an embryo at week 5

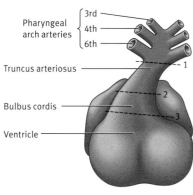

Pharyngeal arch arteries
- 3rd
- 4th
- 6th

Truncus arteriosus — 1

Bulbus cordis — 2
— 3

Ventricle

B Transverse section through an embryo at week 5   **C** Coronal section through an embryo at week 5

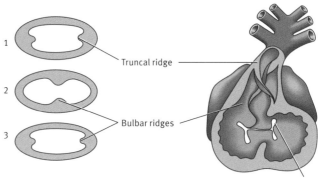

1

Truncal ridge

2

3

Bulbar ridges

Left atrioventricular canal

D Ventral views through an embryo at week 6

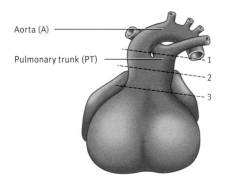

Aorta (A)

Pulmonary trunk (PT)

1
2
3

E Transverse section through an embryo at week 6   **F** Coronal section through an embryo at week 6

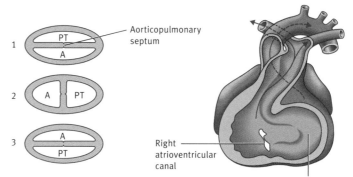

1   PT / A   Aorticopulmonary septum

2   A / PT

3   A / PT

Right atrioventricular canal

Interventricular septum

G Spiral form of the aorticopulmonary septum

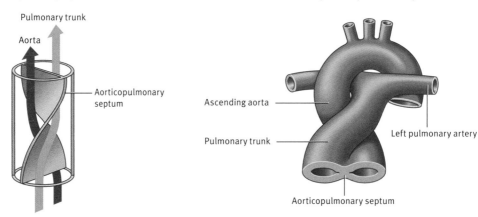

Pulmonary trunk

Aorta

Aorticopulmonary septum

H Aorta and pulmonary trunk twisting around each other

Ascending aorta

Pulmonary trunk

Left pulmonary artery

Aorticopulmonary septum

(A–C) show the truncal and bulbar ridges at 5 weeks. (D), (E) and (F) show the aorticopulmonary septum at 6 weeks. (G) and (H) show the final position of the ascending aorta and pulmonary trunk at the end of 8 weeks, twisting around each other as they leave the heart.

FIGURE 14.11 **Schematic coronal section through a ventricle, showing the formation of atrioventricular valves**

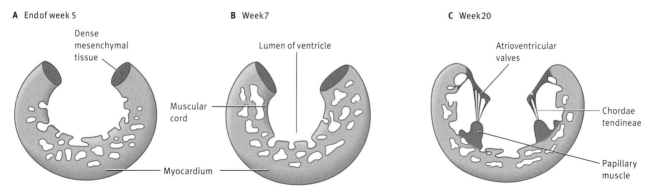

The atrioventricular orifice is surrounded by local proliferations of mesenchymal tissue. The tissue on the ventricular surface of these proliferations thins and forms valves, which remain attached to the ventricular wall by muscular cords. The muscular tissue in the cords degenerates by week 20 and is replaced by dense connective tissue forming chordae tendineae, which now connect valves with the papillary muscles.

FIGURE 14.12 **Formation of the semilunar valves**

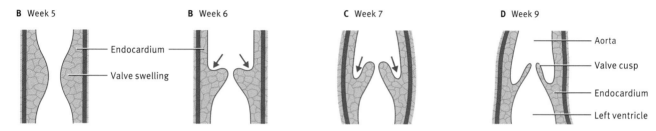

Longitudinal sections through the semilunar valves illustrate successive stages in the hollowing (shown by arrows) and thinning of the valve swellings to form valve cusps.

FIGURE 14.13 **The conducting system of the heart at week 20**

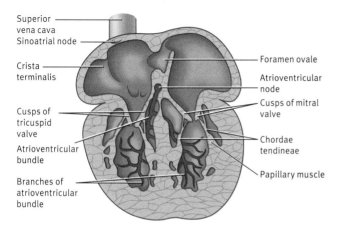

with a number of genetic syndromes such as DiGeorge, Goldenhar and Down syndromes. Of those children with chromosomal abnormalities, 33% have a congenital heart defect, with an incidence of nearly 100% in children with trisomy 18. Of newborns with congenital heart defect, 6–10% have an unbalanced chromosomal abnormality.

Environmental factors

A small proportion (2%) of congenital heart defects are due to environmental agents. Classic examples of cardiovascular teratogens include alcohol, the rubella virus and drugs such as thalidomide and isotretinoin (vitamin A). Raised first-trimester blood glucose and, more recently, hypertension have been linked to congenital heart defects.

Multifactorial inheritance

In most cases, the causes of congenital heart defects are unknown and are believed to occur as a result of a complex interplay between a number of factors, genetic and environmental.

POSITIONAL ANOMALIES

Dextrocardia

With dextrocardia, the heart lies on the right side of the thorax instead of the left. It is the most frequent positional anomaly of the heart and is caused when the heart loops to the left instead of the right. Dextrocardia may coincide with situs inversus, where there is a complete reversal of symmetry in all organs, or heterotaxy, where the position of some organs is randomly reversed. Generally these conditions are associated with normal physiology, although there is a slightly increased risk of heart defects.

Ectopia cordis

With ectopia cordis, the heart is in an abnormal location, most commonly partly or completely exposed on the surface of the thorax. It is also sometimes found to protrude through the diaphragm, into the abdomen. The thoracic form results from faulty development of the sternum and pericardium. Death from infection, cardiac failure or hypoxemia occurs in most cases during the first few days of life. Surgical correction is required and the clinical outcome has now improved, with a few patients surviving to adulthood.

ENDOCARDIAL CUSHIONS AND HEART DEFECTS

Abnormalities in endocardial cushion formation contribute towards many cardiac malformations because of their key location. Since neural crest cells, which contribute to the development of the head and neck, also populate the conotruncal cushions, abnormalities of these cells often produce both heart and craniofacial defects in the same individual.

Atrial septal defects

Atrial septal defects (ASDs) occur in 6.4 in 10 000 births with girls twice as likely to be affected than boys. There is a two in one prevalence in girl versus boy infants. The most common form of ASD is a **patent foramen ovale**, which may be present in up to 25% of the population. It is generally not clinically significant unless forced open because of other cardiac defects. There are four clinically significant types of ASD.

Foramen secundum ASD is characterised by a large opening between the atria. It is caused either by excessive cell death and resorption of the septum primum or by inadequate development of the septum secundum. It is generally tolerated well in childhood; symptoms of pulmonary hypertension usually appear after the third decade of life.

Endocardial cushion defects with foramen primum ASD include a group of abnormalities resulting from a common developmental defect: deficiency of the endocardial cushions and the atrioventricular septum. Here, the septum primum does not fuse with the endocardial cushions.

Sinus venosus ASD is the rarest type of ASD. It results from incomplete incorporation of the sinus venosus into the right atrium or abnormal development of the septum secundum. It is commonly associated with partial anomalous pulmonary venous connections.

Common atrium (cor triloculare biventriculare) refers to the complete absence of the atrial septum and represents the combination of all above ASDs. It is the most serious abnormality in this group.

Ventricular septal defect

Ventricular septal defect (VSD) is the most common type of congenital heart defect, accounting for approximately 25% of defects. It occurs more commonly in boys than in girls. It may be found as an isolated lesion or associated with abnormalities in partitioning of the conotruncal region. Dyspnoea, pulmonary hypertension and cardiac failure are known to occur depending on the size of the defect and associated conditions. The following subtypes have been identified.

Membranous VSD results from the failure of development of the membranous part of the interventricular septum and is the most common type of VSD with an incidence of 12 in 10 000 births. About 30–50% of these defects close within the first year of life.

Muscular VSD is less common and may appear anywhere in the muscular part of the interventricular septum. Sometimes there are multiple small defects, producing what is sometimes called the 'Swiss cheese VSD'.

Single ventricle (cor triloculare biatriatum) VSD is a complete absence of the interventricular septum. It is an extremely rare anomaly resulting in a three-chambered heart, where both aorta and pulmonary trunk arise from the common ventricle.

Atrioventricular septal defect (AVSD) is a failure of fusion of the endocardial cushions and results in a large defect in the centre of the heart. Although rare, it occurs in approximately 20% of people with Down syndrome.

ABNORMALITIES OF THE CONOTRUNCAL REGION

Four of the most common abnormalities of the conotruncal region are discussed below and illustrated in Figure 14.14.

Tetralogy of Fallot

Tetralogy of Fallot is the most frequently occurring abnormality of the conotruncal region. It occurs in 9.6

in 10 000 births and is not fatal. In this condition, an anterior displacement of the conotruncal septum results in an unequal division of the conus and produces four cardiovascular alterations: pulmonary stenosis (obstruction of right ventricular outflow), VSD, dextroposition of aorta (overriding or straddling aorta) and right ventricular hypertrophy. Cyanosis is an obvious sign of this condition, but may not be present at birth. Primary surgical repair in early infancy is the treatment of choice.

Persistent truncus arteriosus

Persistent truncus arteriosus occurs in 0.8 in 10 000 births. Here, the truncal ridges and aorticopulmonary septum fail to develop normally. This can result in the failure of division of the truncus arteriosus into aorta and pulmonary trunk, such that the undivided truncus overrides both ventricles and receives blood from both sides. It can also result in a VSD, because the ridges participate in the development of the interventricular septum.

Transposition of the great vessels

Transposition of the great vessels occurs in 4.8 in 10 000 births. It is the most common cause of cyanotic heart disease in newborn infants. Here, the conotruncal septum

FIGURE 14.14 **Abnormalities of the conotruncal region**

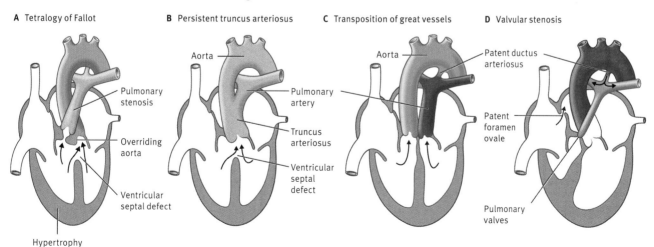

A Tetralogy of Fallot

Pulmonary stenosis
Overriding aorta
Ventricular septal defect
Hypertrophy

B Persistent truncus arteriosus

Aorta
Pulmonary artery
Truncus arteriosus
Ventricular septal defect

C Transposition of great vessels

Aorta

D Valvular stenosis

Patent ductus arteriosus
Patent foramen ovale
Pulmonary valves

Red = fully oxgenated blood | blue = deoxygenated blood | purple = mixed blood

runs straight down, instead of following a spiral course. This results in the aorta originating from the right ventricle and the pulmonary artery originating from the left ventricle. This condition may be associated with a membranous VSD or a patent ductus arteriosus. Death would ensue within a few months if not surgically corrected.

Valvular stenosis

Valvular stenosis of the pulmonary artery and aorta occurs in 3–4 in 10 000 births. It is caused by fusion of the semilunar valves. Stenosis could occur over a variable distance and could be either a mild narrowing or complete atresia. In valvular stenosis of the pulmonary artery, the trunk of the pulmonary artery is narrow or even atretic. Here, the patent oval foramen forms the only outlet for blood from the right side of the heart, while the patent ductus arteriosus is the only access route to the pulmonary circulation. In aortic valvular stenosis, the size of the aorta is usually normal. However, in aortic valvular atresia, the aorta, left ventricle and left atrium are markedly underdeveloped. Here the patent ductus arteriosus delivers blood into the aorta.

Tricuspid atresia

Tricuspid atresia is the absence or fusion of the tricuspid valves and results in obliteration of the right atrioventricular orifice. It is associated with a patent foramen ovale, a VSD, an underdeveloped right ventricle and a hypertrophied left ventricle.

ABNORMALITIES OF THE CONDUCTING SYSTEM

Abnormalities of the conducting system are the most common cause of sudden infant death syndrome in developed countries, accounting for 40–50% of infant deaths in the first year. No mechanism has been identified, although there is a suggestion that they have an abnormality in the autonomic nervous system.

Fetal circulation

The umbilical vein carries blood from the placenta to the fetus. Figure 14.15 illustrates the passage of blood

TABLE 14.1 **Mixing of oxygenated and deoxygenated blood, as shown in Figure 14.15**

Label	Site	Source of deoxygenated blood
I	Liver	Blood returning from the portal system
II	Inferior vena cava	Blood returning from lower extremities, pelvis and kidneys
III	Right atrium	Blood returning from the head and upper extremities
IV	Left atrium	Blood returning from lungs
V	Junction of ductus arteriosus and descending aorta	Blood from the proximal aorta

from the umbilical vein through the fetal heart to the umbilical arteries. The blood in the umbilical vein is nutrient-rich and 80% saturated with oxygen and it loses its high oxygen content as a result of mixing with deoxygenated blood at various places (Table 14.1) This is discussed in greater detail in Chapter 32.

Most of this blood bypasses the liver and flows directly through the ductus venosus into the right atrium at the junction with the inferior vena cava. A smaller amount enters the liver sinusoids and mixes with blood from the portal circulation. The flow of umbilical blood through the sinusoids is said to be regulated by a sphincter mechanism in the ductus venosus close to the entrance of the umbilical vein. This sphincter supposedly closes when a uterine contraction renders the venous return too high, thereby preventing sudden overloading of the heart.

In the inferior vena cava, placental blood mixes with deoxygenated blood returning from the lower limbs. It then enters the right atrium, from where most of the blood is guided through the foramen ovale to the left atrium. A small amount remains in the right atrium where it mixes with deoxygenated blood returning from the head and arms via the superior vena cava. Blood in the left atrium mixes with a small amount of deoxygenated blood returning from the lungs through the pulmonary veins.

Blood from the left atrium enters the left ventricle and ascending aorta. The coronary and carotid arteries are the first branches of the ascending aorta, ensuring that the heart and the brain are supplied with well-oxygenated blood.

Blood from the superior vena cava flows into the right ventricle and the pulmonary trunk. Since resistance in the pulmonary vessels is high during intrauterine life, most of this blood passes through the ductus arteriosus into the descending aorta, where it mixes with blood from the proximal aorta.

Blood from the descending aorta flows toward the placenta by way of the two umbilical arteries. The oxygen saturation in the umbilical arteries is about 58%.

Circulatory changes at birth

Cessation of placental blood flow and the beginning of respiration bring about profound changes in the vascular system: compare Figures 14.15 and 14.16.

CLOSURE OF THE UMBILICAL ARTERIES

Thermal and mechanical stimuli along with a change in oxygen tension bring about contraction of the smooth muscle in the walls of the umbilical arteries. Functional

FIGURE 14.15 **Fetal circulation *in utero***

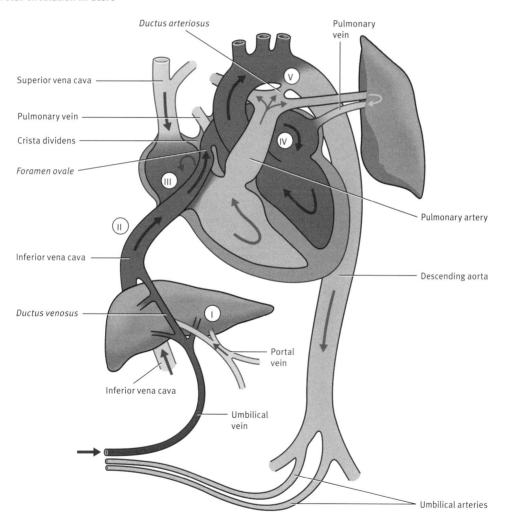

Red = fully oxygenated blood | blue = deoxygenated blood | red/blue = mixed blood | *Shunts in italics*

FIGURE 14.16 **Circulatory changes at birth**

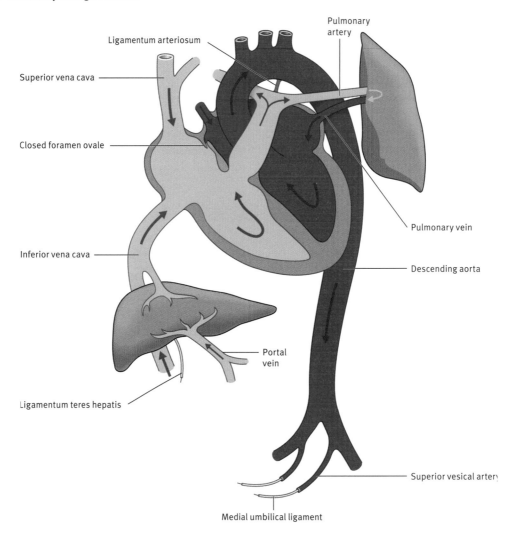

Pulmonary artery

Ligamentum arteriosum

Superior vena cava

Closed foramen ovale

Pulmonary vein

Inferior vena cava

Descending aorta

Portal vein

Ligamentum teres hepatis

Superior vesical artery

Medial umbilical ligament

closure of the arteries occurs a few minutes after birth, although actual obliteration of the lumen by fibrous proliferation could take 2–3 months. The proximal portions of the arteries remain open as the superior vesical arteries, while the distal portions form the medial umbilical ligaments.

CLOSURE OF THE UMBILICAL VEIN AND DUCTUS VENOSUS

The umbilical vein and ductus venosus close shortly after the umbilical arteries. After obliteration, the umbilical vein forms the ligamentum teres hepatis (round ligament of the liver) in the lower margin of the

falciform ligament, while the ductus venosus forms the ligamentum venosum, which courses from the ligamentum teres hepatis to the inferior vena cava.

CLOSURE OF THE DUCTUS ARTERIOSUS

Closure of the ductus arteriosus is mediated by bradykinin, a substance released from the lungs during initial inflation. Immediately after birth, its muscular wall contracts, but complete anatomical obliteration by proliferation of the intima is thought to take 1–3 months.

When the ductus arteriosus closes, there is a rapid increase in the amount of blood flowing through the lung vessels. This increases pressure in the left atrium. The obliterated ductus arteriosus forms the ligamentum arteriosum.

CLOSURE OF THE OVAL FORAMEN

There already is increased pressure in the left atrium as a result of closure of the ductus arteriosus and reduced pressure in the right atrium as a result of interruption of placental blood flow. Now, when the first breath is taken, the septum primum presses against the septum secundum, resulting in functional closure of the oval foramen.

This closure is reversible during the first days of life and when the baby cries a right-to-left shunt is created, accounting for cyanotic periods in the newborn. Constant apposition gradually leads to fusion of the two septa at about one year of age.

FURTHER READING

BRUYER H J, KARGAS S A, LEVY J M. The causes and underlying developmental mechanisms of congenital cardiovascular malformation: a critical review. *Am J Med Genet* 1987;3:411–31.

CLARK E B. Cardiac embryology: its relevance to congenital heart disease. *Am J Dis Child* 1986;140:41–4.

FISHMAN M C, CHIEN K R. Fashioning the vertebrate heart: earliest embryonic decisions. *Development* 1997;124:2099–117.

HIRAKOW R. Development of the cardiac blood vessels in staged human embryos. *Acta Anat* 1983;115:220–30.

MOORE, K L, PERSAUD, T V N. The cardiovascular system. In: *The Developing Human: Clinically Oriented Embryology*, 8th ed. Philadelphia: W B Saunders; 2008. p.285–337.

NODEN D M. Origins and assembly of avian embryonic blood vessels. *Ann N Y Acad Sci* 1990;588:236–49.

SADLER T W. Cardiovascular system. In: *Langman's Medical Embryology*, 11th edn. Baltimore: Lippincott Williams & Wilkins; 2010. p.165–200.

SCHERPTONG R W, JONGBLOED M R, WISSE L J, *et al.* Morphogenesis of outflow tract rotation during cardiac development: the pulmonary push concept. *Dev Dyn* 2012; 241(9):1413–22.

SKANDALAKIS J E, GRAY S W. *Embryology for Surgeons: The Embryological Basis for the Treatment of Congenital Anomalies*, 2nd edn. Baltimore: Williams & Wilkins; 1994.

WALDO K, MIYAGAWA-TOMITA S, KUMISKI D, KIRBY M L. Cardiac neural crest cells provide new insight into septation of the cardiac outflow tract: aortic sac to ventricular septal closure. *Dev Biol* 1998;196:129–44.

Endocrinology

Placental structure and function

Des Holden

Introduction

The placenta anchors the developing pregnancy within the uterus, is responsible for nutrient and waste exchange, is important in preventing the mother from recognising and rejecting paternally derived antigens, has important endocrine functions that equip the mother to survive childbirth and is involved in the signalling to initiate labour. This highly evolved organ has also been implicated in the aetiology of miscarriage, fetal growth restriction, pre-eclampsia and abruption. In this chapter, the mechanisms by which some of these functions are accomplished will be discussed. Definitions of terms are shown in Table 15.1.

The early conceptus

The fertilised egg is moved along the fallopian tube by cilial and muscular action. The first cleavage division takes place in the ampulla, within 30 hours of fertilisation, with subsequent divisions every 12 hours to the 16-cell stage. The daughter cells (blastomeres) remain totipotent until this stage is reached. This redundancy allows preimplantation diagnosis in the field of assisted conception by the removal of a single cell. These early divisions are directed by maternally derived proteins and RNA. The embryo enters the uterus at the eight-cell stage. Differences in the development of the early embryo in different species are shown in Table 15.2.

TABLE 15.1 **Terminology of pregnancy**

Term	Definition
Morula	The conceptus up until approximately 16-cell stage, prior to fluid collection and development of the inner cell mass
Blastocyst	The next stage of development from the morula, with fluid separating inner cell mass from outer cells, which become trophoblast
Blastomere	Individual cells of the blastocyst
Zona pellucida	Glycoprotein layer surrounding the oocyte, which persists to the morula/blastocyst stage, allowing growth in cell number without loss of cells prior to trophoblast invasion of the decidua
Trophoblast	Derived from the outer cell layer of the blastocyst, forms cytotrophoblast (retain single nucleus per cell) and syncytiotrophoblast, a true syncytium. The trophoblast is the key placental cell for synthesis, invasion and anchoring the pregnancy in the uterus
Decidua	Specialised modulation of the uterine endometrium, with species-specific alteration of blood vessels, connective tissue and leucocyte content
Haemochorial placenta	Maternal blood in direct contact with the chorionic (syncytio)trophoblast

TABLE 15.2 **Comparison of mouse, sheep and human early pregnancies**

Species	Cleavage to 4 cells	Transcriptionally active stage	Conceptus enters uterus	Formation of blastocyst	Time of attachment	Time to luteal regression if not pregnant	Pregnancy duration
INVASIVE							
Mouse	1.5–2	2 cell	3	3	4.5	10–12	19–20
Human	2	4–8 cell	3.5	4.5	7–9	12–14	270–290
NON-INVASIVE							
Sheep	4	8 cell	2–3	6–7	16	16–18	144–152

Values are time in days unless otherwise stated.

The development of the conceptus from the eight-cell stage to the time of implantation is shown in Figure 15.1. From the 16-cell morula stage, subcellular differentiation of organelles occurs with a greater concentration seen at the apex compared with the basal pole. The apical surface develops numerous microvilli. The outer cells of the morula (which are destined to become the trophoblast and placenta) develop tight intercellular junctions (gap junctions and desmosomes). Fluid collects in this outer layer, separating it from the cells that will become the inner cell mass (and ultimately the fetus). At this stage the morula becomes much more metabolically active, with increased protein synthesis and increased oxygen consumption. The energy fuelling these processes is derived from pyruvate rather than glucose metabolism.

In the preimplantation phase, new trophoblast develops from the base of the inner cell mass (polar trophoblast). This is the blastocyst stage of development. It is at this morula–blastocyst stage that one of the two X chromosomes of a female embryo becomes deactivated and condensed as a Barr body.

Implantation

Placental attachment to the maternal uterine wall is fundamental to successful human reproduction. Inadequate invasion of the decidua by the trophoblast is associated with various pregnancy complications, while excessive invasion compromises the health of the mother and, therefore, the infant.

The characteristics of trophoblast cells are:

- paternal X chromosome inactivation
- unmethylated DNA
- ability to form multinucleated cells
- variable expression of major histocompatibility complex (MHC) class 1 antigens; no MHC class 2 antigen expression.

The functions of the trophoblast cells are:

- attachment of the placenta to the uterine wall
- transport of nutrients, oxygen and maternal immunoglobulins to the fetus
- elimination of fetal waste products
- synthesis and secretion of proteins and hormones
- barrier between maternal and fetal circulations
- contact site between maternal immune system and conceptus.

Implantation can be thought of in three phases.

APPOSITION

Initially at the site of contact between the polar trophoblast and the endometrium, but subsequently more widely, the endometrium increases mitotic activity and undergoes localised changes in stromal cell morphology and intercellular matrix composition. There is also an influx of cells associated with host defence, including natural killer (NK) cells. This process is called decidualisation. The endometrium develops pinopodes, which remove fluid from the uterine cavity (by pinocytosis) and allow closer apposition between the blastocyst and the decidua.

FIGURE 15.1 Development of the conceptus from the eight-cell stage to the time of implantation

A Eight-cell stage

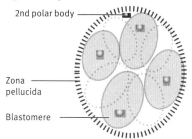

- 2nd polar body
- Zona pellucida
- Blastomere

B Sixteen-cell stage

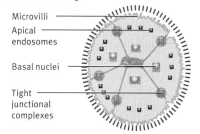

- Microvilli
- Apical endosomes
- Basal nuclei
- Tight junctional complexes

C Morula

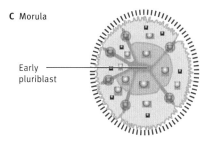

- Early pluriblast

D Blastocyst

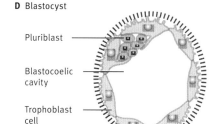

- Pluriblast
- Blastocoelic cavity
- Trophoblast cell

E Attached blastocyst

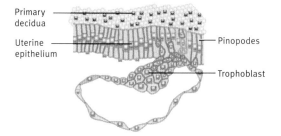

- Primary decidua
- Uterine epithelium
- Pinopodes
- Trophoblast

Adhesion

Adhesion is accompanied by destruction of the zona pellucida, allowing contact between maternal and trophoblast cells. Within a few hours of attachment, the surface epithelium adjacent to the trophoblast becomes eroded. This, and the destruction of the zona pellucida, is accomplished by a variety of metalloproteases and by the expression of adhesion molecules on the trophoblast cell membrane that are specific for ligands on the forming decidua.

PENETRATION

The production of metalloproteases by trophoblast allows the digestion of the extracellular matrix. This facilitates trophoblast invasion into the uterine decidua and makes a variety of lipids, proteins, nucleotides and sugars available as metabolic substrates and fuel. Trophoblast cells can actively transport small molecules across their cell membranes and are able to transport large molecules and cellular fragments by pinocytosis and phagocytosis. This early nutrition is independent of any placental circulation. Trophoblast cells contain microfilaments as part of their internal cytoskeleton. These allow the trophoblast cells to squeeze between endometrial cells and the blastocyst to thereby invade the underlying stroma so deeply that the surface epithelium becomes restored over it (interstitial implantation).

The biochemical signalling involved in these processes is incompletely understood. There may be considerable biochemical redundancy in this control as well, because transgenic mice with genes inactivated for each of the supposed key control cytokines (so-called 'knockout mice') are still able to reproduce successfully. The peptide hormone vascular endothelial growth factor

From the eight-cell stage, the conceptus becomes compacted with maximum contact between adjacent cell membranes. After cell division and differentiation, the cells become wedge-shaped and develop tight intercellular junctions that prevent intercellular diffusion. The nuclei become basally located and the polarised cells develop microvilli centrally and at their outer (zonal) ends. Further cell division to 16–32 cells leads to early division into an outer layer (destined to be trophoblast) and an inner, pluriblast layer. By the 64-cell stage (blastocyst), fluid has accumulated within the blastocoelic cavity, facilitated by tight intercellular junctions. The pluriblast is eccentric and will form the inner cell mass. After attachment, the zona pellucida is lost and the trophoblast is starting to penetrate the uterine epithelium.

FIGURE 15.2 **Formation of the intervillous space and primary stem villi**

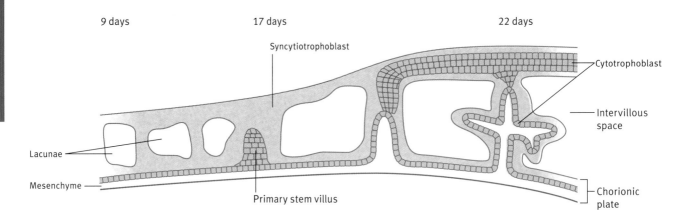

Anatomy of the developing placenta

The trophoblast differentiates into two layers: an inner layer of cytotrophoblast, where the cells remain recognisably individual, and an outer syncytiotrophoblast layer, where cellular walls are largely lost (Figure 15.2). Before implantation is complete (11–12 days), lacunae form in the polar syncytiotrophoblast. These trophoblast-lined lacunae will eventually be the intervillous space, allowing circulation of maternal blood in the placental bed. By 13 days after conception, some cells from the trophoblast shell will invade deeply through the decidua and into the myometrium, providing a supportive or attaching function. Also by the end of week 2, primary villous stems are formed. These comprise an outer layer of syncytiotrophoblast cells with a core of cytotrophoblast, which itself has a core of extraembryonic mesoderm (Figure 15.2).

Differentiation of the extraembryonic mesoderm allows vascularisation of the stem villus, which then becomes continuous with the vessels of the body stalk (which will become the umbilical vessels) during week 3 (Figure 15.3). The primary villous stems give rise to syncytiotrophoblast buds, again with a cytotrophoblast and mesodermal core, which become primary villi.

(VEGF) is made in the endometrium with a time course that suggests a key role in the changes in vascularity within the decidua.

Those primary villi adjacent to the uterine cavity regress to form the chorion laeve (nonplacental part of the chorion). The villi on the decidual side of the conceptus (chorion frondosum) undergo further growth and branching as secondary and tertiary villi, filling the intervillous space to form the definitive placenta. It is from the tertiary villi that the true placental villi arise. The elaboration of villi centred on a single primary stem villus is called a placental lobule, of which the placenta

FIGURE 15.3 **Formation of tertiary stem villi, which provide the architecture of the placenta**

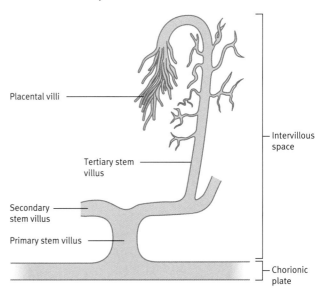

FIGURE 15.4 **Types of placentation and relationships between fetal trophoblast cells and maternal blood**

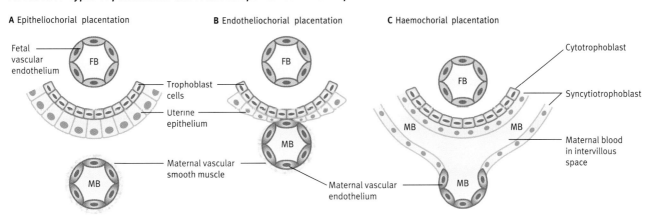

A Epitheliochorial placentation   **B** Endotheliochorial placentation   **C** Haemochorial placentation

Fetal vascular endothelium

Trophoblast cells

Uterine epithelium

Maternal vascular smooth muscle

Maternal vascular endothelium

Cytotrophoblast

Syncytiotrophoblast

Maternal blood in intervillous space

FB = fetal blood | MB = maternal blood

has approximately 200. This process is complete by 8–10 weeks of gestation. There is no relation between placental lobules, or groups of lobules, and the cotyledons (or lobes) seen when examining the maternal surface of the term placenta.

By 12 weeks, the placenta has reached its definitive form and subsequently enlarges laterally. The placenta exceeds the weight of the fetus until about 17 weeks and typically weighs about one-sixth of the fetus at term.

THE CHORIONIC VILLUS

Several different patterns of placental function (Figure 15.4) have developed in different mammalian species and these can be classified on the basis of the cell types intervening between maternal and fetal blood cells. In epitheliochorial placentation, the trophoblast cells attach to the surface epithelium of the uterus (no invasion). Endotheliochorial placentation sees trophoblast invasion of the uterine epithelium but no invasion of maternal blood vessels. Haemochorial placentation shows the greatest invasion, with maternal blood vessels invaded by trophoblast cells, which become bathed in maternal blood. Species with epitheliochorial placentation increase maternal blood flow to the placental bed through decidual angiogenesis (an increased number of similar-sized vessels). This contrasts with human (haemochorial) pregnancy where an increase in blood flow through the placental bed is achieved through trophoblast invasion of the spiral arteries of the decidua and outer myometrium.

In the nonpregnant state, the spiral artery is a muscular high-resistance vessel. In pregnancy, trophoblast invasion converts the spiral artery to a wider bore capacitance vessel, allowing blood flow through the uterus to increase 10–15-fold. The mechanism by which trophoblast cells invade decidual spiral arteries and replace the vascular endothelium is only just beginning to be understood. It seems likely that trophoblast cells recognise vascular smooth muscle and endothelial cells through specific adhesion molecule expression. This recognition can induce an intracellular sequence of events that alters trophoblast motility, induces apoptosis in the vascular myocytes and endothelial cells and causes the functional and histological changes in spiral arteries (reduced muscular wall and endothelial lining replaced by trophoblast cells) that are the characteristics of haemochorial placentation.

Two observations about placental architecture in pre-eclampsia have remained constant despite the growing understanding of placental development. Placental villi are less developed in placentas taken from pre-eclamptic pregnancies, with fewer branches and less complex vascular loops than placentas associated with normal pregnancy outcome. The second observation is that change in spiral artery architecture is less evident or patchy when the placental bed is examined histologically at placental bed biopsy (Figure 15.5).

FIGURE 15.5 **Differences in placental architecture for a normal pregnancy and a pre-eclamptic pregnancy**

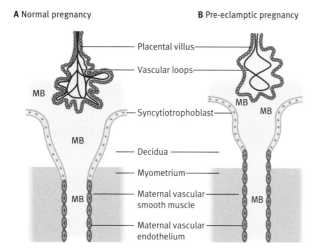

A Normal pregnancy   **B** Pre-eclamptic pregnancy

- Placental villus
- Vascular loops
- Syncytiotrophoblast
- Decidua
- Myometrium
- Maternal vascular smooth muscle
- Maternal vascular endothelium

MB

In **A** the placental villus contains an elaborate fetal vasculature and the spiral artery wall has been replaced by the endovascular syncytiotrophoblast; in **B** the fetal villous vessels are less branched and the spiral artery has remained as a narrow, high-resistance vessel with reduced replacement by the endovascular trophoblast. | MB = maternal blood

Immunology of pregnancy tolerance

While there are advantages of close contact between the trophoblast of placental villi and maternal blood (nutrition and waste elimination) as seen in the haemochorial placenta, the disadvantage is that the circulations are no longer separated by an epithelial barrier. Trophoblastic cells in human pregnancy are therefore exposed to potential allogenic immune responses by the mother.

Advances have been made in understanding the immune reactions of pregnancy by focusing on the relationship between trophoblast – the outermost layer of fetal cells – and the cells with which they are in contact. These are the cells of the uterus that undergo highly specialised differentiation during decidualisation. The most obvious features include enlargement of the uterine stromal cells and the presence of a distinct lymphocyte population of uterine NK cells. The presence of NK cells is seen widely in all species with a decidual response to invasive placentation. Similar cells are not seen in other tissues. The roles and characteristics of uterine NK cells are as follows:

- CD56hiCD16– uterine NK cells represent 70% of leukocytes at the implantation site and increase in number in the late luteal phase of the menstrual cycle and in early pregnancy.
- Uterine NK cells are similar to a minor (10%) fraction of blood NK cells, but have phenotypic differences, including unusual adhesion molecule expression and poor cytotoxicity.
- The origin of decidual NK cells, as discrete lineage, or differentiated from circulating NK cells, is unclear.
- Decidual NK cells produce a range of soluble products including angiogenic cytokines (angiopoietin-2 and vascular endothelial growth factor), immunoregulatory cytokines and chemokines and lytic enzymes.
- The reduced cytotoxicity of decidual NK cells may relate to a lack of intracellular cytoskeletal and lytic granule organisation.
- Diagnostic tests on NK cells in peripheral blood of women with reproductive failure give no information about decidual NK cell function.
- Possible roles for decidual NK cells include maintenance of mucosa and blood vessel stability, modification of spiral arteries in the decidua and regulation of trophoblast invasion of the decidua and its structures.

The relationship between the decidual response in the uterus and invasion has been argued both to permit and to control the degree of invasion. Both roles may occur, allowing the balance of sufficient placental invasion without excess. Uncontrolled trophoblast cell invasion is seen where the decidua is deficient or absent (for example, in tubal ectopic pregnancy or implantation on scar tissue within the uterus). Trophoblast cells implanted at distant ectopic sites (in animal experiments and in *in vitro* cell culture) show inherent invasive growth. Overinvasion of the fetal–maternal interface compromises the mother's health, resulting in haemorrhage in the absence of medical intervention.

At the opposite end of the spectrum, the decidua may prevent adequate invasion into the spiral arteries. This shift of fetal–maternal interface in favour of the mother is associated with reduced blood supply to the placental bed and a growth restricted, hypoxic fetus. Pre-eclampsia has a high maternal and fetal mortality and yet has an incidence of 5–10% in first-time mothers. That natural selection has not removed this complication may be a trade in human reproduction: balancing human trophoblasts' highly invasive tendencies against the consequent risk of maternal haemorrhage, death and subsequent compromise of neonatal survival. Exactly how the degree of trophoblast invasion is controlled is not yet understood, although there is evidence that apoptosis in invasive trophoblast may be a limiting and controlling factor.

PLACENTA–UTERUS IMMUNE INTERACTION

A mother does not biologically reject her pregnancy but would reject a tissue graft from a genotypically dissimilar donor. The rejection of an allograft (for example, renal or heart transplant) is through powerful antibody and T-cell-mediated responses to allogeneic MHC molecules expressed by the vascularised graft. However, the fetus is not in contact with the mother's immune system but is shielded by the trophoblast of the placental interface. Trophoblast cells never express MHC class 2 molecules and are thereby unable to present antigen to maternal CD4+ T cells. In humans, the placental trophoblast encounters the maternal immune system in two locations: (i) the villous syncytiotrophoblast is bathed by maternal blood; and (ii) the extravillous cytotrophoblast interacts with uterine tissue.

The syncytiotrophoblast expresses no MHC antigens, which is consistent with the concept that the placenta is immunologically neutral. This theory also fits with the observation that while fetal cells that enter the maternal circulation provoke an immune reaction (for example, rhesus isoimmunisation and haemolytic disease of the newborn), no such systemic T- or B-cell immune response to trophoblast cells has been described.

The second area of contact is between the decidua and the invasive, anchoring, extravillous cytotrophoblast. Unlike the syncytiotrophoblast, the extravillous trophoblast expresses unusual combinations of cell surface human leucocyte antigen (HLA) C, G and E molecules, but does not express polymorphic HLA-A and HLA-B, the molecules that are important in initiating allograft rejection. Polymorphic HLA-C is expressed but does not lead to allograft rejection. There are a number of hypotheses to explain this.[1] One difference from allograft rejection is that CD8+ regulatory T cell populations present in the uterus in pregnancy are specific for a carcinoembryonic antigen-like ligand, rather than

being MHC restricted. Another mechanism by which the placenta might alter the local immune environment is that trophoblast HLA-G binds with high avidity leukocyte immunoglobulin-like receptors on myelomonocytic cells. Increased expression of these receptors is associated with graft tolerance, possibly through reduced MHC class 2 pathways, and may be important in the decidua where macrophages and dendritic cells expressing MHC class 2 are found.

UTERINE NATURAL KILLER CELL RECOGNITION BY TROPHOBLAST CELLS

Uterine, but not peripheral, NK cells express an array of receptors for trophoblast MHC class 1 antigens. One of the C-type lectins (CD94-NKG2A) binds HLA-E and reduces NK cell cytotoxicity. All NK cells also express a killer cell immunoglobulin-like receptor family antigen, KIR2DL4, that can bind HLA-G, the effect of which is the upregulation of proinflammatory and proangiogenic cytokines. This may be a mechanism by which the placenta can enhance its blood supply, while soluble HLA-G entering the systemic circulation might interact with blood NK cells and contribute to the systemic vascular and inflammatory changes of pregnancy.

The polymorphic HLA-C expressed by trophoblast also interacts with NK cell KIR ligands, of which there are both activating (KIR2DS) and inhibitory (KIR2DL) receptor types. Hence, there are two polymorphic gene systems, maternal KIRs and fetal HLA-C antigens, at this site of the maternal–fetal interface. Decidual invasion by the trophoblast therefore has the potential to vary in different pregnancies, as some ligand–receptor interactions are likely to favour trophoblast invasion while others may prevent adequate placentation.

The placenta and maternal–fetal exchange

The placenta acts as a barrier between the maternal and fetal circulations. Simple diffusional exchange between the circulations is only significant for low-molecular-weight substances (such as gases, sodium, urea and water) and for nonpolar molecules (such as unconjugated steroids and fatty acids). This simple diffusion changes with gestation as the anatomy of the terminal villus changes. In early pregnancy, the terminal villi are large (diameter 150–200 micrometres) and the fetal vessels are located centrally, beneath 10 micrometres of syncytiotrophoblast, so metabolites need to diffuse relatively far to access the fetal circulation. As pregnancy progresses, the villi are smaller (40 micrometres diameter) and the vessels are more eccentric, giving a 90% reduction in diffusional distance. While the diffusion rate of most molecules is inversely proportional to this distance, oxygen is highly soluble and its diffusion is dependent more on blood flow than thickness of the intervening barrier.

OXYGEN AND CARBON DIOXIDE

Oxygen consumption in pregnancy is proportional to the growing conceptus. Cardiac output and blood flow through the uterus and placental bed increase and ventilation increases, reducing carbon dioxide and bicarbonate concentrations in maternal plasma. Concentration gradients promote oxygen and carbon dioxide diffusion into and out of the fetus, respectively. Fetal oxygen carriage, however, is approximately equal to that of maternal blood. This is due to the greater intrinsic affinity for oxygen and reduced binding for 2, 3-diphosphoglycerate with embryonic and fetal haemoglobin. Oxygen transfer to the fetus is also promoted by fetal blood in the placenta increasing in pH, which favours the uptake of oxygen by haemoglobin, while the reduction in maternal blood pH as it picks up carbon dioxide favours maternal haemoglobin giving up oxygen (double Bohr effect).

GLUCOSE AND CARBOHYDRATE

As gestation progresses, maternal tissues become relatively less sensitive to insulin. This can allow latent diabetes to appear, but also allows more of the plasma glucose to be taken up by the fetal–placental unit and relatively less to be taken up by maternal tissues. Placental uptake of glucose is by facilitated diffusion in which specific carriers use concentration gradients to drive the uptake of d-glucose. The maximum rate of transfer for this transport is 0.6 mmol/minute/g placenta. This transport only becomes saturated at 20 mmol/l glucose. The placenta metabolises considerable amounts of glucose to lactate and this is available to the fetus as fuel at about one-third the availability of glucose. The rate of fetal use of glucose is largely related to fetal insulin production.

Amino acids and urea

Deamination of amino acids by the maternal liver is reduced in pregnancy and the maternal excretion of resultant urea also falls. This makes more ingested and absorbed amino acids available to the placenta and fetus. Some amino acids are synthesised within the trophoblast cells (for example, acidic nonessential amino acids and neutral straight-chained amino acids). There are also a number of active transport systems for different groups of amino acids (neutral branched-chain and basic amino acids) in the placenta, which are used as building blocks for the placenta itself and for the dependent fetus. These concentrate amino acids within the trophoblast to five times the maternal plasma concentration. The urea generated by fetal amino acid metabolism diffuses passively back across the placenta into the maternal circulation, which has a reduced urea concentration.

Water and electrolytes

Exchange of water between mother and fetus occurs at two main sites: the placenta and the remainder of the nonplacental chorion. The amnion and chorion are freely permeable to water and either diffusion or hydrostatic forces must account for transfer. A large difference in hydrostatic pressure between maternal and fetal circulations within the placenta does not occur and it is likely that the necessary flux of water from fetus to mother is accomplished across small and intermittent hydrostatic gradients. Isotope studies have shown that sodium trafficking across the placenta occurs as co-transport for various active transport molecules and also by paracellular diffusion.

Fetal blood contains iron at between two and three times the concentration of maternal blood. This iron is delivered by active transport across the placenta and an intratrophoblast ferritin-binding stage has been described. Calcium and phosphate are transferred to the fetus against a concentration gradient by an active transport system that is sensitive to metabolic and competitive inhibitors.

AMNIOTIC FLUID

The volume of amniotic fluid increases during pregnancy from about 15 ml at 8 weeks to 450 ml at 20 weeks, after which net production declines to zero by 34 weeks (approximate volume 750 ml). The composition of amniotic fluid suggests that it is initially a transudate. Towards term, the total solute concentration in amniotic fluid falls but the concentrations of urea, creatinine and uric acid rise. Amniotic fluid is in a dynamic state, with complete exchange of its water occurring approximately every 3 hours.

PLACENTAL MEMBRANES

The amnion arises as an epithelial layer between the ectodermal disc of the inner cell mass and the trophoblast (chorion). The amnion has five layers: cuboidal epithelium (with prominent intracellular canals and vacuoles), basement membrane, compact layer, fibroblast layer and spongy layer of mucoid reticular tissue (remnant of extraembryonic coelom). The amniotic cavity lies between the amnion and the ectodermal disc.

The chorion has four layers: fibroblasts, reticular layer, basement membrane and trophoblast layer. The trophoblast layer is 2–10 cells thick, lies immediately adjacent to the deciduas and is continuous with placental trophoblast. Obliterated chorionic villi have been described.

Neither the amnion nor the chorion has blood vessels, lymphatics or nerves.

Hormonal control of placental synthesis

HUMAN CHORIONIC GONADOTROPHIN

For a pregnancy to survive, it is necessary that the corpus luteum does not involute during the first trimester. In humans, human chorionic gonadotrophin (hCG) is secreted by the syncytiotrophoblast from as early as 6–7 days post-fertilisation. It consists of two amino acid chains (alpha and beta) linked by noncovalent bonds and has a relative molecular weight of 38 400 kDa. Both

chains have attached carbohydrate residues. hCG is chemically and functionally similar to pituitary luteinising hormone (LH), with the alpha subunit being similar to all glycoprotein hormones: LH, follicle-stimulating hormone (FSH), thyroid-stimulating hormone. The beta subunit of hCG is similar to LH but with an additional 30 amino acids at the carboxy terminus. Immunoassays directed at this beta-subunit terminus are therefore specific for hCG and the basis for urinary pregnancy tests. The levels of hCG in maternal serum and urine rise rapidly in early pregnancy, peak at about 12 weeks of gestation and then decline. hCG binds to LH receptors in the corpus luteum. That hCG is the luteotrophic hormone of human pregnancy is suggested by observations that the corpus luteum does not involute in women who are not pregnant but are given parenteral hCG injections, and by the observation in animal studies that antibodies directed at hCG that prevent binding at the LH receptor site cause involution of the corpus luteum and abortion.

PROGESTERONE

hCG maintains the progestogenic activity of the corpus luteum, but within 2 weeks of fertilisation the conceptus is also synthesising all the steroid hormones required for pregnancy. Although the corpus luteum remains active throughout pregnancy, it is not essential after about 6 weeks and contributes only a small amount to the total pregnancy production of progesterone. In blighted ovum pregnancies, where no embryo forms, and in choriocarcinoma or hydatidiform moles, progesterone production by the conceptus is unaffected. This observation and immunocytochemical studies of the trophoblast *in vitro* have localised production of progesterone to the trophoblast itself. This synthesis uses maternal cholesterol and appears autonomous to the placenta (with no external control identified). The peak concentration of progesterone in human pregnancy is at term when it is ten-fold greater than the luteal phase of the ovarian cycle. The main maternal urinary excretion product is pregnanediol.

ESTROGEN

The main estrogen in pregnancy is not the ovarian-cycle steroid 17-estradiol but the less potent estriol. The synthesis of this steroid is severely reduced in molar and choriocarcinoma pregnancies and production requires the presence of a fetus (unlike the production of progesterone). Estriol synthesis occurs in the placenta but uses dehydroepiandrosterone (DHEA), derived from the fetal adrenal cortex, as a substrate. DHEA is hydroxylated to 16-hydroxy DHEA in the fetal liver and this product undergoes aromatisation of the A-ring in the trophoblast to form estriol. Deficiency of fetal adrenal activity (congenital adrenal hyperplasia and anencephaly) is associated with low estriol levels. In fetal blood, 16-hydroxy DHEA circulates as a sulphate conjugate and a placental sulphatase is essential for estriol synthesis. This sulphination of the steroid in the fetus and desulphination in the placenta is important as sulphination creates a steroid that is water soluble and inactive. This allows the fetus to be less exposed to the biological effects of a steroid that in the mother is bioactive and important in a range of pregnancy adaptations. Maternal estriol concentration rises to 100 times the nonpregnant estrogen concentration at term. Estrone and estradiol are also synthesised by the placenta, but in smaller amounts than estriol and from maternal precursors.

HUMAN PLACENTAL LACTOGEN

As the trophoblast makes less hCG towards the end of the first trimester of pregnancy, it synthesises human placental lactogen, a 21 600kDa single-peptide protein with 191 amino acids, two disulphide bridges and a plasma half-life of 15 minutes. It is chemically and functionally similar to prolactin and pituitary growth hormone but less biologically active. Its plasma concentration plateaus after 35 weeks and, while it may have a role in modifying carbohydrate metabolism, pregnancies lacking any human placental lactogen appear to progress normally.

Abnormal placentation

MULTIPLE PREGNANCY

One of the functions of the zona pellucida is to prevent the blastomeres of the early conceptus from falling apart during early cleavage. If the conceptus does become divided into two distinct groups of cells at this stage,

monozygotic twins result. If this division occurs early, then two completely separated pregnancies occur with implantations that may be separated within the uterus or may be coincidentally close to each other. In either case, the placentas are anatomically and functionally separate from each other. If division into two pregnancies occurs after 9 days from conception, then there will be either two distinct fetuses in a single amniotic sac with a single placenta (monoamniotic twins) or, if later still, then conjoined fetuses will result. If cleavage occurs between 4 and 8 days after conception, monochorionic diamniotic twins will result: two fetuses in two amniotic sacs but with a single chorion and a single placenta. In this placental arrangement, while most placental cotyledons will drain oxygenated blood to the umbilical vein of the same cord which has supplied it with deoxygenated blood, some cotyledons drain to the other cord and twin and one twin can become a net donor of blood to its sibling (the recipient). This is called twin-to-twin transfusion, with the recipient becoming hypervolaemic, with excessive amniotic fluid, a hyperdynamic circulation and a high haemoglobin concentration. Its donor becomes anaemic, oliguric and growth restricted (twin-to-twin transfusion syndrome).

MOLAR PREGNANCY

The chromosome complement within the developing trophoblast can have profound effects on the phenotype of the developing placenta. Clinically, this effect is seen most commonly with molar pregnancy. Molar, or hydatidiform molar, pregnancies are classified as partial or complete on the basis of their chromosome complement and the presence or absence of fetal tissue. A complete molar pregnancy occurs with fertilisation of an oocyte where the maternally derived chromosomes are lost and the paternally derived chromosomes are duplicated. There are 46 chromosomes in each cell, but they comprise 23 chromosomes from a single spermatozoon, duplicated to 46. As there are no maternally derived chromosomes, no fetal tissue forms. In a partial mole, there are 69 chromosomes in each cell, two sets paternally derived and one set from the oocyte. In this case, fetal tissue does form. In both situations, the trophoblast is more invasive than normal and secretes more pregnancy hormones per gestational stage than a normal conceptus.

UNIPARENTAL DISOMY

Uniparental disomy results in an imbalance between paternally and maternally derived chromosomes in the conceptus, with effects on placental structure and function. It occurs when conception produces a 46-chromosome complement, but one pair is formed by loss of the maternal or paternal chromosome and duplication of the remaining one; hence, 22 chromosomes are derived from one parent and 24 from the other. The best-characterised example of this relates to chromosome 15. Loss of maternal chromosome 15, with duplication of the paternal chromosome, is a rare cause of Angelman syndrome, while the reverse of this situation, with maternal disomy for chromosome 15, gives rise to Prader–Willi syndrome.

REFERENCE

1. MOFFAT A, LOKE C. Immunology of placentation in eutherian mammals. *Nature Rev Immunol* 2006;324:584–94.

FURTHER READING

CARTER A M. Evolution of placental function in mammals: the molecular basis of nutrient transfer, hormone secretion and immune responses. *Physiol Rev* 2012;92:1543–76.

HUPPERTZ B, PEETERS L L H. Vascular biology in implantation and placentation. *Angiogenesis* 2005;8:157–67.

JOHNSON M, EVERITT B. *Essential Reproduction*. Oxford: Blackwell Science; 2000.

REZENDE-FILHOE J, CASTRO P, PEREIRA LEITE S, BARBOSA MONTENEGRO CA, DE LOURDES DE ALMEIDA LIMA M. Pre-eclampsia: an overview in placentation, endothelial dysfunction and flow-mediated vasodilatation. *Ultrasound Rev Obstet Gynecol* 2005;5:242–53.

CHAPTER 16

Hypothalamus and pituitary gland

Gul Bano

Anatomy

The pituitary gland or hypophysis weighs approximately 0.5g in adult life and measures roughly 10–15mm in each dimension. It protrudes from the bottom of the hypothalamus at the base of the brain, rests in a small bony cavity (the sella turcica) in the sphenoid bone and is covered by a dural fold called the diaphragma sellae. The pituitary gland is in close proximity to the optic chiasm, the cavernous sinus and the floor of the third ventricle. It is heavier in women than in men and becomes larger during pregnancy.

The pituitary gland is composed of two main lobes: the anterior pituitary or adenohypophysis and the posterior pituitary or neurohypophysis. These two lobes are functionally distinct structures and also differ in their embryologic development and anatomy. The adenohypophysis can be subdivided into distinct lobes, the pars distalis (anterior lobe) and pars tuberalis. The neurohypophysis is composed of the pars nervosa, the pituitary stalk (also known as infundibular stalk or infundibulum) and the median eminence.

The pituitary stalk connects the pituitary gland and the hypothalamus. The hypothalamus is bounded anteriorly by the optic chiasm, laterally by the sulci formed with the temporal lobes and posteriorly by the mammillary bodies. Dorsally, it is delineated from the thalamus by the hypothalamic sulcus. The pituitary stalk descends from its central region, which is termed the median eminence. This stands out because of its dense vascularity, which is formed by the primary plexus of the hypophysial portal system. The long portal veins run along the ventral surface of the pituitary stalk. The hypothalamus has neuronal connections to the posterior pituitary and endocrine connections to the anterior pituitary.

The blood supply to the hypothalamo–pituitary axis is complex (Figure 16.1). The hypothalamus receives its blood supply from the circle of Willis, whereas the neurohypophysis and adenohypophysis receive blood from the inferior and superior hypophyseal arteries, respectively. The capillary plexus of the inferior hypophyseal artery drains into the dural sinus, although some of these capillaries in the neural stalk form short portal veins that drain into the anterior pituitary gland. This constitutes only a small fraction of the circulation of the anterior lobe, which is one of the best vascularized mammalian tissues. The major portion of the circulation arises from the long portal veins. These are formed from the capillary network of the superior hypophyseal arteries that invest the nerve endings of the neurosecretory cells in the median eminence. Here, the portal veins form a secondary capillary network into which the hormones of the anterior pituitary are secreted. The venous channels from the anterior pituitary gland drain into the cavernous sinuses and from there into the superior and inferior petrosal sinuses and into the jugular vein.

Histology of the hypothalamo-pituitary region

There are three types of hypothalamic neurosecretory cells. Magnocellular neurons secrete arginine vasopressin

FIGURE 16.1 **Blood supply to, and venous drainage from, the hypothalamo–pituitary axis**

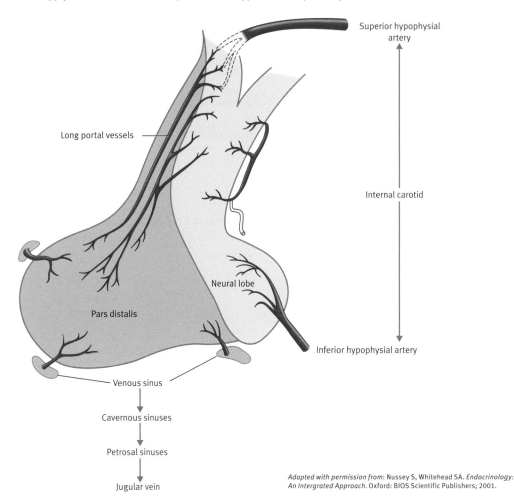

Adapted with permission from: Nussey S, Whitehead SA. *Endocrinology: An Intergrated Approach.* Oxford: BIOS Scientific Publishers; 2001.

(AVP) or oxytocin (OXY). The cell bodies, which are located in the supraoptic or paraventricular hypothalamic nucleus, project their neuronal processes via the pituitary stalk into the posteriorneural lobe and neurohormones are released from nerve endings into the blood. Hypophysiotrophic neurons are located in nuclear groups, including the paraventricular and arcuate and the arcuate nucleus in the medial basal hypothalamus. The hypophysiotrophic neuropeptides are released into the hypothalamo–hypophysial portal system and regulate the secretion of hormones from the pituitary. Hypophysiotrophic neuropeptides include thyrotrophin-releasing hormone (TRH), corticotrophin-releasing hormone

(CRH), somatostatin, growth-hormone-releasing hormone (GHRH), gonadotrophin-releasing hormone (GnRH) and dopamine.

Projection neurons are found in the paraventricular and arcuate nuclei and in the lateral hypothalamic area. These neurons project to autonomic preganglionic neurons in the brain stem and spinal cord.

Microscopic examination of the conventionally stained adenohypophysis reveals three distinctive cell types termed acidophils, basophils and chromophobes. This pattern of staining reflects the chemical character of intracellular hormone-laden granules within the pituitary cells.

The neurohypophysis is an extension of the hypothalamus and is composed of bundles of axons from hypothalamic neurosecretory neurons intermixed with glial cells.

Embryology of the hypothalamo–pituitary region

The anterior lobe of the pituitary gland or adenohypophysis develops from an evagination of ectodermal cells of the oropharynx in the primitive gut and is recognisable at weeks 4–5 of gestation. This evagination, known as the Rathke pouch, is eventually pinched off from the oral cavity and becomes separated by the sphenoid bone of the skull. The lumen of the pouch is reduced to a small cleft, while the upper portion of the pouch surrounds the neural stalk and forms the pars tuberalis. This, together with the anterior lobe, is called the adenohypophysis. When cells from the Rathke pouch are left behind and form tumours, these are called craniopharyngiomas.

The posterior lobe develops from neural crest cells as a downward evagination of the floor of the third ventricle of the brain. The lumen of this pouch closes as the sides fuse to form the neural stalk, while the upper portion of the pouch forms a recess in the floor of the third ventricle known as the median eminence.

The neural stalk together with the median eminence forms the infundibular stalk and this, together with the posterior lobe, is collectively termed the neurohypophysis. The cleft-like remnant of the Rathke pouch demarcates the boundary between the anterior and posterior lobes of the pituitary gland. The hypothalamo–pituitary axis is established by week 20 of gestation. The development of different types of hormone-secreting cells in adenohypophysis involves sequential expression of transcription factors coded by number of genes.

Physiology of the hypothalamic and pituitary glands

Functions of the hypothalamus include the control of the autonomic nervous system and the regulation of body temperature, hunger and thirst; it also has a role in memory, behaviour and emotional responses. In this chapter, we restrict discussion to the regulation of the endocrine system.

ANTERIOR PITUITARY GLAND

The anterior pituitary gland is regulated by three interacting elements: hypothalamic input (releasing and inhibitory factors), feedback effects of circulating hormones and paracrine and autocrine secretions of the pituitary gland itself. From a clinical perspective, the anterior pituitary gland synthesizes and secretes six major hormones: growth hormone (GH, also called somatotrophin), thyroid-stimulating hormone (TSH, also called thyrotrophin), adrenocorticotrophin (ACTH), follicle-stimulating hormone (FSH), luteinising hormone (LH) and prolactin (PRL).

The physiological control of TSH and ACTH is described in Chapter 17.

Growth hormone

GH is synthesised and secreted by cells called somatotrophs in the anterior pituitary gland. Somatotrophs constitute 40–50% of the total cells in the anterior pituitary gland. GH is a single-chain polypeptide containing 191 amino acids and shares structural homologies with PRL and human chorionic gonadotrophin (hCG), the latter being a GH variant synthesised exclusively in the placenta. GH predominantly affects growth, metabolism, cell differentiation and lactation. The effects of GH on protein metabolism include increases in amino acid uptake and protein synthesis and a decrease in the oxidation of proteins. GH enhances the metabolism of fats by stimulating triglyceride breakdown and oxidation in adipocytes. In carbohydrate metabolism, GH is one of the hormones that maintain blood glucose levels within the normal range. It suppresses insulin-mediated glucose uptake in peripheral tissues and insulin-mediated glucose synthesis in the liver. Somewhat paradoxically, GH stimulates insulin secretion and GH administration can lead to hyperinsulinaemia.

GH exerts its effects directly and indirectly through the family of insulin-like growth factors (IGFs). The IGF family consists of three members (insulin, IGF-I and

FIGURE 16.2 **Actions and regulation of growth hormone and PRL**

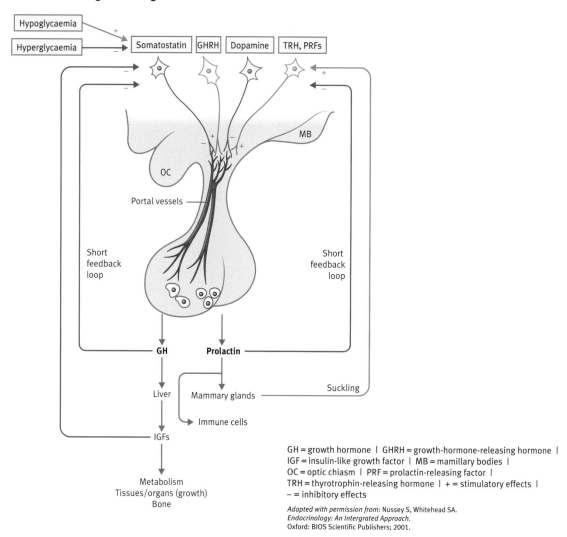

GH = growth hormone | GHRH = growth-hormone-releasing hormone |
IGF = insulin-like growth factor | MB = mamillary bodies |
OC = optic chiasm | PRF = prolactin-releasing factor |
TRH = thyrotrophin-releasing hormone | + = stimulatory effects |
− = inhibitory effects

Adapted with permission from: Nussey S, Whitehead SA.
Endocrinology: An Intergrated Approach.
Oxford: BIOS Scientific Publishers; 2001.

IGF-II) that share common structural similarities. Insulin, IGF-I and IGF-II have metabolic functions, but they also have important roles in cellular proliferation and the functions of differentiated tissues (mediated by the IGF-I receptor). IGF-II is a major fetal growth factor. IGF-I is more important for postnatal growth. Insulin also plays a role in fetal growth. A reflection of this role is the development of fetal macrosomia in pregnancies associated with maternal diabetes. Synthesis and secretion of GH is stimulated by GH-releasing hormone (GHRH) and inhibited by somatostatin, both of which are produced by the hypothalamus (Figure 16.2). GHRH is released from nerve terminals in the median

eminence and transported to the anterior pituitary gland via the hypophyseal portal capillaries. Somatostatin is a 14-amino-acid peptide that is synthesised in hypothalamic neurons mainly located in the anterior periventricular nuclei. Factors affecting GHRH and somatostatin secretion include sleep, exercise, stress and blood glucose levels. In addition, IGF-I provides negative feedback to the pituitary glands and hypothalamus. Finally, estradiol acts to increase the sensitivity of tissues to GH.

GH production begins early in fetal life and continues throughout life, although at a progressively lower rate. Mean daily GH secretion is pulsatile. It is high in childhood with a peak at puberty and secretion falls during adulthood. In the adult human, approximately five pulses of GH are secreted during a 24-hour period with a larger peak occurring at the onset of sleep at night. The half-life of GH in the circulation is about 20 minutes.

Prolactin

PRL is produced and secreted by the lactotrophs in the anterior pituitary gland. Lactotrophs constitute 10–15% of the anterior pituitary cells. PRL is a single-chain protein made up of 199 amino acids with three disulphide bridges. It shares strong structural homologies with GH and the cell surface receptors of PRL and GH are also similar. Estrogen stimulates the proliferation of pituitary lactotroph cells, resulting in an increased quantity of these cells in premenopausal women, especially during pregnancy.

In animals, PRL has a plethora of actions but in humans it is mainly involved in preparation of the female breast for lactation. PRL also binds to specific receptors in the gonads, lymphoid cells and liver. Other roles are poorly understood, although there is widespread tissue expression of PRL receptors. It is also notable that men have the same circulating concentrations of PRL as nonlactating women. PRL has effects on the hypothalamo–pituitary–gonadal axis, it can inhibit pulsatile secretion of GnRH from the hypothalamus and it can alter the activity of certain steroidogenic enzymes.

PRL secretion is regulated by a dual hypothalamic inhibitory and stimulatory system. In addition, it can regulate its own secretion through a short feedback loop.

PRL secretion is pulsatile and increases with sleep. The control of PRL release by the hypothalamus is unique in that the predominant hypothalamic influence is inhibitory, whereas it is stimulatory for all other hormones. Thus, damage to the hypothalamic control causes increased PRL levels. Dopamine, released into the hypophysial portal veins from nerve terminals in hypothalamus is the main neurohormone inhibiting PRL secretion. Somatostatin also has an inhibitory effect. Stimulatory factors include TRH, other releasing factors, pregnancy, lactation (suckling), estrogen, opioids, dopamine D_2 receptor antagonists, sleep and stress.

Gonadotrophins

The gonadotrophins, such as FSH, LH and hCG, are glycoproteins (molecular weights approximately 30 000 Dalton) made up of a gonadotrophin-specific alpha subunit and a beta subunit that confers biological specificity to each hormone. LH and FSH are secreted from gonadotrophs in the anterior pituitary gland. These cells make up 10–15% of the anterior pituitary cells (Figure 16.3). Their receptors are typical G-protein-linked proteins. Receptor activation by gonadotrophin binding stimulates adenylate cyclase, resulting in a rise in cyclic adenosine monophosphate (cAMP) levels. FSH and LH are important regulators of steroidogenesis in the gonads. In the testis, LH acts on the interstitial or Leydig cells, whereas FSH acts on the Sertoli cells. In the ovary, each hormone acts on more than one cell type. There are numerous isoforms of circulating LH and FSH and biological potency depends on the degree and

FIGURE 16.3 **Actions and regulation of gonadotrophins**

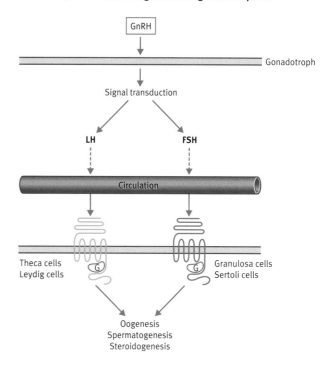

FSH = follicle-stimulating hormone | G = G-protein-linked receptor | GnRH = gonadotrophin-releasing hormone | LH = luteinising hormone

Adapted with permission from: Nussey S, Whitehead SA. Endocrinology: An Intergrated Approach. Oxford: BIOS Scientific Publishers; 2001.

sites of glycosylation and the electrical charge of the molecule. Thus, different assays of LH and FSH concentrations may not always give a true index of biological activity.

POSTERIOR PITUITARY GLAND

AVP and OXY are small peptides with strong structural homologies. They consist of nine amino acids arranged in a ring structure with a short 'tail'. AVP is mainly synthesised in the supraoptic nuclei and to a lesser extent the paraventricular nuclei, whereas the reverse is true for OXY. The hormones synthesised in the large (or magnocellular) neurosecretory cells of these nuclei are transferred to the posterior pituitary gland, whereas those synthesised in the smaller (or parvocellular) neurons control the hormone secretions of the anterior pituitary gland.

Like all other peptide and protein hormones, AVP and OXY are synthesised as large prohormones. Once packaged into secretory granules, the AVP and OXY prohormones pass by axonal flow to the nerve terminals (Herring bodies) in the neurohypophysis. During this passage, the prohormones are cleaved into the biologically active AVP or OXY molecules and a larger polypeptide fragment. Neurophysin II is the product cleaved from the vasopressin prohormone, neurophysin I is cleaved from the OXY prohormone. Both neurophysins are co-secreted with the active hormones upon electrical activation of the neurosecretory cells.

Arginine vasopressin

AVP derives its name from the first action ascribed to it nearly 100 years ago: an increase in systemic blood pressure (it is a pressor agent). The actions of AVP on water balance in the kidney (where it is effective in very low concentrations) gave rise to an alternative name, antidiuretic hormone, and the two names tend to be used interchangeably. AVP has three known receptors and acts in concert with aldosterone and atrial natriuretic peptide to control blood volume and pressure. However, this chapter will consider exclusively the actions of AVP.

In the kidney, AVP acts on the G-protein-linked V_2 receptors on the capillary (basal) side of the distal convoluted and collecting ducts and stimulates the synthesis of cAMP (Figure 16.5) cAMP activates a kinase on the luminal (apical) side of the ducts, which initiates a series of events culminating in the insertion of water channels, known as aquaporins, into the luminal membrane. Water passes into the collecting-duct cells and, by osmosis, across the basal membrane into the interstitial fluid and hence back into the circulation. There is also an osmotic gradient (set up by the counter-current activity of the loop of Henle) from the cortex to the medulla of the kidney. Thus, as the collecting ducts pass through the cortex to the medulla, increasing amounts of solute-free water (also termed free water) can be reabsorbed by the osmotic gradient. This is governed by the aquaporins and hence AVP.

Increased osmolality of the extracellular fluids stimulates AVP release (Figure 16.5). Changes in osmolality are detected by osmoreceptors. Osmotically sensitive cells were first described in the hypothalamus, but it is now known that there are additional osmoreceptors in the circumventricular organs and in systemic viscera. These are not only important in regulating AVP secretion but also in stimulating thirst. As a result, AVP induces an increase in water retention and a reduction in serum osmolality.

Another potent stimulus to AVP secretion is a reduction in effective blood volume; in fact, AVP secretion is stimulated by a volume reduction of just 5–10%. This is controlled by so-called stretch receptors that detect changes in blood volume or pressure. These include the baroreceptors and other receptors in the cardiovascular system. Thus, for example after a haemorrhage, AVP secretion will be stimulated and water will be retained to increase blood volume. The reverse occurs in response to an increase in blood volume or pressure.

Other stimulants of AVP secretion include emotional stress, pain and a variety of drugs. Nausea and vomiting are also extremely potent stimulators of AVP release. The effects of these stimuli may be important in situations such as the postoperative state, affecting water balance. By contrast, alcohol is a potent inhibitor of AVP release (as little as 30–90ml of whiskey is sufficient) resulting in inappropriate dehydration and some of the symptoms associated with a hangover. The preventative measure is to drink a restorative volume of water after excess ethanol consumption.

Apart from its primary role in water conservation, AVP is also important in maintaining blood pressure after a haemorrhage as a result of its vasopressive effects on arteriolar smooth muscle. Acting on smooth muscle cells, it induces vasoconstriction via calcium and phospholipase-C-generated second messengers. The final established role of vasopressin is the potentiation of CRH action on pituitary corticotrophs.

Oxytocin

OXY is neuropeptide and exerts a wide spectrum of central and peripheral effects as neurohormone, neurotransmitter or neuromodulator. OXY is centrally produced in magnocellular neurons in hypothalamus. OXY is also produced in peripheral tissues; for example, uterus, placenta, amnion, corpus luteum, testis and heart. OXY receptors have also been identified in other tissues, including the kidney, heart, thymus, pancreas and adipocytes. The major action of OXY is in lactation, when, through a neuroendocrine reflex, it initiates the let-down of milk by inducing contractions of the myoepithelial cells surrounding the alveoli of the mammary gland. In animals, there is evidence that OXY has a major role in parturition, but in humans there is much less evidence to support this role. OXY does, however, have a contributing role in that it induces powerful contractions of the uterine muscle. Thus, synthetic OXY is widely used therapeutically in obstetrics, not only to induce labour but also to reduce postpartum bleeding.

OXY can have stimulatory effects at the AVP V_2 receptor in the kidney. There is no naturally occurring disease associated with excess OXY secretion but in obstetric situations, when given in high doses as an intravenous infusion 5% dextrose, it can cause water retention and iatrogenic hyponatraemia.

Hypothalamic and pituitary control of puberty

Puberty is defined as the stage of physical maturation in which an individual becomes physiologically capable of sexual reproduction. It is associated with marked endocrine changes, including an increase in growth rate, skeletal changes (such as increase in hip width in girls),

increase in fat and muscle and profound psychological changes.

PHYSIOLOGY OF PUBERTY

The onset of puberty is characterised by an increase in the secretions of LH and FSH that is driven by GnRH release from the neurons that are diffusely situated in the arcuate nucleus and other nuclei of the hypothalamus. Before the onset of puberty, both LH and FSH are secreted in very small amounts (with low concentrations in peripheral blood) and there is no apparent stimulation of the gonads. However, as puberty approaches, the amplitudes of LH and FSH pulsatile secretions (and hence the mean secretion rates) increase and the nocturnal rise in LH secretion is amplified. It is notable that this nocturnal rhythm is specific to puberty as it disappears in adulthood. The gonad itself does not seem necessary for the changes to occur and thus it must be concluded that the brain is in some way programmed to produce more GnRH and hence LH and FSH.

The increasing circulating concentrations of LH and FSH stimulate pubertal development of the gonads and thus an increase in the output of sex steroids. These, together with adrenal androgens, induce the physical changes that occur at this time (Figures 16.4 and 16.5).

In boys, the earliest sign of increasing LH and FSH secretions is an increase in testicular size (a volume increase of more than 4 ml or a length increase of more than 2.5 cm). In girls, thelarche (breast development) is a sensitive indicator of LH- and FSH-stimulated ovarian steroid secretions. Before the menarche, however, estradiol secretion fluctuates widely, probably reflecting waves of follicular development in which the follicles fail to reach the ovulatory stage. Estrogen stimulates growth of the uterus but menarche does not occur until the estrogens have stimulated sufficient uterine growth such that their withdrawal causes the first menstruation. The onset of menstruation is such a milestone in the development of girls that primary amenorrhoea can be relied upon to indicate underlying pathology. The growth of axillary and pubic hair in both sexes is a consequence of increased concentrations of not only of gonadal steroids (gonadarche) but also of adrenal steroids (adrenarche).

FIGURE 16.4 **Actions and regulation of arginine vasopressin**

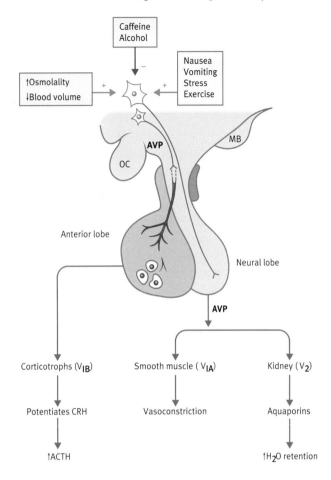

↓ = decrease │ ↑ = increase │ ACTH = adrenocorticotrophin │
AVP = arginine vasopressin │ CRH = corticotrophin-releasing hormone │
V_{1A}, V_{1B} and V_2 = AVP receptor subtypes │ + = stimulatory effects │
− = inhibitory effects

Adapted with permission from: Nussey S, Whitehead SA. *Endocrinology: An Intergrated Approach.* Oxford: BIOS Scientific Publishers; 2001.

PRECOCIOUS PUBERTY

The changes during puberty normally follow a reliable pattern that is sometimes called consonance. If these changes happen early (before the age of 8 years in girls and before the age of 9 years in boys) puberty is considered to be precocious. However, recent studies indicate that signs of early puberty (breasts and pubic hair) are often present in girls (particularly black girls) aged 6–8 years. Central precocious puberty is gonadotropin-dependent, is

the early maturation of the entire hypothalamo–pituitary–gonadal (HPG) axis with the full spectrum of physical and hormonal changes of puberty and is idiopathic in 90% of girls. It can be associated with central nervous system abnormalities such as tumours, brain injury or congenital brain anomalies. Peripheral precocious puberty (pseudo-puberty) is much less common and refers to conditions in which increased production of sex steroids is gonadotropin-independent.

DELAYED PUBERTY

Delayed puberty is defined as an increase in testicular volume of less than 4 ml by the age of 14 years in boys and no breast development by the age of 13–15 years in girls. Boys are much more likely than girls to have idiopathic delay (termed constitutional delay). Constitutional delay affects both growth and puberty and by definition, the investigations are normal. The causes of delayed puberty are given in Table 16.1.

AMENORRHOEA

Amenorrhoea is the absence of a menstrual period in a woman of reproductive age. Physiological states of amenorrhoea are seen during pregnancy and lactation. Outside of the reproductive years there is absence of menses during childhood and after menopause. Primary amenorrhoea is usually defined as no menarche by the age of 16 years. Secondary amenorrhoea is defined as absence of menstruation for at least 3 months in a previously menstruating girl or woman of reproductive age. Primary amenorrhoea can be a feature of delayed puberty.

From a clinical point of view, considerable diagnostic accuracy can be gained from defining the presence of breast development and a uterus. Thus, when a uterus is present and there is no breast development, the cause is probably a failure of the whole hypothalamo–pituitary-ovarian axis; for example, Kallmann syndrome or ovarian failure (for example Turner syndrome) before the onset of puberty. If a uterus is present and the breasts have developed, this indicates that the failure of the axis has occurred after breast development. If breasts have developed and a uterus is absent, the likely cause is androgen insensitivity or congenital absence of the uterus.

FIGURE 16.5 **Tanner stages of puberty**

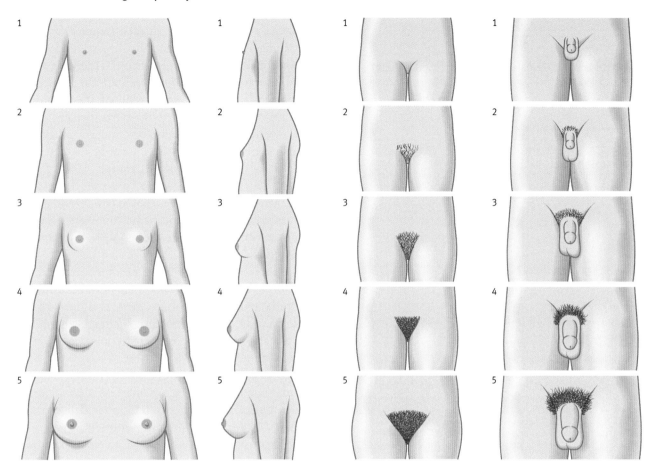

FEMALE

STAGE	BREAST DEVELOPMENT
1	Prepubertal; no breast tissue
2	Areolar enlargement with breast bud
3	Enlargement of breast and areola, which arise as a single mound
4	Projection of areola above breast as a secondary mound
5	Adult; papilla projects out of areola, which is part of breast contour

MALE

STAGE	GENITAL DEVELOPMENT
1	Prepubertal
2	Testes enlarge (4 ml); scrotum enlarges, reddens and develops coarser skin
3	Penis enlarges, initially in length; continued growth of testes and scrotum
4	Penis grows in length and breadth; continued growth of testes and scrotum, which becomes pigmented
5	Testes, scrotum and penis adult size

BOTH SEXES

STAGE	PUBIC HAIR DEVELOPMENT
1	None
2	Few darker hairs along labia or at base of penis
3	Curly pigmented hairs across pubes
4	Small adult configuration
5	Adult configuration with spread onto inner thighs

Adapted with permission from: Nussey S, Whitehead SA. *Endocrinology: An Intergrated Approach*. Oxford: BIOS Scientific Publishers; 2001.

From an endocrine point of view, the causes can be defined in terms of the serum concentrations of the gonadotrophins LH and FSH. High gonadotrophin concentrations indicate a problem in the ovary, whereas low levels indicate hypothalamo–pituitary dysfunction.

Diseases of the hypothalamus and pituitary gland

Endocrine disease of the hypothalamus or pituitary is characterised either by loss of hormone or excess of

TABLE 16.1 Causes of delayed puberty

Cause	Frequency
Constitutional delay	Common (~90%)
HYPOGONADOTROPHIC HYPOGONADISM	Rare (~10%)
GnRH deficiency[a]	
Gonadotrophin deficiency[b]	
HYPERGONADOTROPHIC HYPOGONADISM	Rare (~10%)
Sex chromosome abnormality[c]	
Gonadal dysgenesis with normal karyotype	
Gonadal damage[d]	
Loss-of-function mutation in the beta subunit of LH[e]	
Loss-of-function mutation in gonadotrophin receptors (resistant ovary syndrome)	

[a] May be isolated or associated with other features, for example anosmia (Kallmann syndrome), cognitive impairment or dysmorphic features (Prader–Willi syndrome) | [b] May be isolated (fertile eunuch syndrome resulting from LH deficiency) or more commonly associated with any form of hypopituitarism | [c] For example Klinefelter syndrome (47,XXY) in boys, Turner syndrome (45,X) in girls | [d] May be viral (e.g. mumps orchitis), iatrogenic (surgical, chemotherapy or radiotherapy) or autoimmune (often associated with Addison's disease) | [e] Reduced LH bioactivity but elevated concentrations of LH in immunoassay | GnRH = gonadotrophin-releasing hormone | LH = luteinising hormone

hormone. Excess hormone secretion is usually caused by a pituitary tumour and generally involves over secretion of a single hormone. The vast majority of pituitary tumours are benign adenomas, but these may compress the optic chiasm and adjacent structures. Carcinomas are very rare. These are rapidly growing, may invade locally and may either compress or destroy the adjacent structures.

When the disease affects an end-organ such as thyroid, ovary or adrenal the condition is termed as primary disorder. Secondary disorders arise when function is affected by defective pituitary hormone secretion. Tertiary disorders result from hypothalamic dysfunction that produces both pituitary and target-organ hypofunction.

ACROMEGALY

Acromegaly is a very rare disease (annual incidence approximately three/million). The disease results from a chronic exposure to high levels of GH leading to the classic clinical features outlined in Table 16.2. Exposure to high levels of GH before fusion of the epiphyseal plates results in gigantism. Ninety-five percent of the cases are due to GH-producing pituitary adenomas. These adenomas are often over 1 cm in diameter and described as macroadenomas. Around 15% of GH-secreting pituitary tumours also co-secrete PRL. More rarely, acromegaly may be caused by hypothalamic tumours such as glioma and hamartoma and even less often by peripheral tumours such as adenocarcinoma of the pancreas.

In acromegaly caused by a pituitary tumour, the secretion of GH remains pulsatile but the duration, amplitude and number of secretory episodes are elevated. The characteristic nocturnal surge is absent and there are abnormal responses to physiological suppression and stimulation.

Pregnancy is a state of physiological GH-IGF-I excess. The placenta produces a variant GH that increases through term and rapidly declines after delivery. The placental GH stimulates the production of hepatic IGF-I. The placenta also produces GH-releasing hormone and IGF-I.

Most of the deleterious effects of GH hypersecretion are caused by its stimulation of excessive amounts of IGF-I. IGF-I leads to the proliferation of bone, cartilage and soft tissue and an increase in the size of other organs.

The usual age of onset of acromegaly is in the third or fourth decade of life and it progresses insidiously. The incidence is the same in both sexes. The duration of symptoms before diagnosis is usually 5–10 years.

Soft-tissue proliferation is one of the early manifestations, leading to the classic symptoms of enlarged hands and feet and exaggerated facial features. Local symptoms of pituitary mass effect include headache and visual impairment (usually bitemporal hemianopia with loss of peripheral vision). Hypopituitarism may lead to the additional clinical features of hypothyroidism, hypogonadism and hypoadrenalism. The musculoskeletal abnormalities are generally not reversible but myalgias and arthralgias frequently decrease after treatment.

TABLE 16.2 **Clinical features of acromegaly**

Body system	Symptoms (prevalence among those with acromegaly)	Signs (prevalence among those with acromegaly)
Skeletal	Arthralgia/arthritis (85%) Carpal tunnel syndrome (50%)	Enlarged hands and feet (100%) Jaw protrusion (90%) Dental malocclusion (80%) Osteoarthritis (30%)
Skin	Excessive sweating (85%)	Greasy skin, skin tags (60%)
Cardiovascular	Angina (5–10%)	Hypertension (50%) Cardiomyopathy (5%)
Respiratory	Diurnal drowsiness (30%)	Obstructive sleep apnoea (30%)
Metabolic	Polydipsia and polyuria (5%)	Neuropathy (50%) Retinopathy (15%)
Renal	Renal colic (20%)	Renal stones (20%)
Other endocrine	Menstrual irregularity (50%) Impotence (40%)	Hypogonadism (40%)

There is an increase in the rates of mortality from cardiovascular and cerebrovascular atherosclerosis (36–62%), respiratory disease (0–25%) and malignancies (9–25%). Death rates tend to be higher when diabetes or hypertension is associated.

The confirmatory test to establish the diagnosis of acromegaly is the oral glucose tolerance test. Seventy-five grams of glucose is administered after an overnight fast. Healthy people usually respond with suppression of the serum GH to less than 2 mU/l. In acromegaly, there is failure to suppress GH levels after glucose load; in fact, GH level may increase, described as paradoxical increase.

TRH or GnRH stimulation will increase GH levels in 70–80% of people with acromegaly; this is not the case in healthy individuals. Formal assessment of visual fields should be performed and this may show bi-temporal hemianopia. The imaging modality of choice is magnetic resonance imaging (MRI).

Treatments for acromegaly include medical and surgical approaches and radiotherapy. Surgery may be curative, especially when the tumours are smaller than 10mm in diameter. After radiotherapy, panhypopituitarism develops in 15–20% of people treated with a lag time of a few years.

GROWTH HORMONE DEFICIENCY

GH deficiency in childhood is usually detected rapidly as a result of the effects on growth velocity. The causes of adult GH deficiency include any damage to the hypothalamo–pituitary axis.

The laboratory diagnosis of adult GH deficiency requires a stimulation test to confirm the diagnosis. The insulin tolerance test is the diagnostic test of choice, provided adequate hypoglycaemia is achieved and the individual is not subject to seizures and does not have ischaemic heart disease. A peak GH response of less than 9 mU/l is indicative of GH deficiency.

HYPERPROLACTINAEMIA

Serum PRL concentrations can be elevated for a number of reasons (Table 16.3).

Prolactinoma

Prolactinomas are the most common hormone-secreting pituitary tumours. Based on its size, a prolactinoma can be classified as a microprolactinoma (<10mm diameter) or a macroprolactinoma (>10mm diameter).

TABLE 16.3 **Causes of hyperprolactinaemia**

Cause	Frequency
Drugs, such as neuroleptic agents (e.g. phenotiazine) or dopamine D$_2$ receptor antagonists used as antiemetics (e.g. metoclopramide)	Common (~90%)
Primary hypothyroidism	
Macroprolactinaemia	Uncommon (~10%)
Stalk syndrome[a]	
Pituitary tumour (micro- or macroprolactinoma)[b]	
Renal failure	Rare (<1%)

[a] Interference in the supply of dopamine to the normal lactotrophs; usually associated with moderately elevated circulating concentrations of prolactin (<3000 mu/l) | [b] Usually associated with markedly elevated circulating concentrations of prolactin (>5000 mu/l)

PRL-secreting lactotrophs, normally constitute up to 20% of pituitary cells in men and in nulliparous women. These increase during pregnancy and by the end of pregnancy, they make up as many as 50% of pituitary cells. The number of lactotrophs declines quickly after delivery, especially if lactation is not maintained. However, this regression is not complete, and lactotroph hyperplasia has been demonstrated 11 months postpartum. PRL is also produced by maternal decidua during pregnancy. Decidual PRL is identical to pituitary PRL. There is no inhibition of decidual PRL production by dopamine or dopaminergic agonist drugs.

Prolactinomas are benign tumours and the clinical presentation is different in men and women. Women tend to have smaller tumours that come to light earlier because these tumours cause galactorrhoea or amenorrhoea owing to the inhibitory effects of excess PRL on the pituitary gland and ovaries. Men tend to have larger tumours that come to light late, because of subtle features of hypogonadism resulting in few symptoms.

Treatment is indicated if mass effects from the tumour or significant effects from hyperprolactinemia are present. The natural history of prolactinomas is unclear. Most microprolactinomas (up to 95%) do not progress to macroadenomas. If a patient with a microprolactinoma has minimal symptoms and fertility is not an issue, then such a patient can be monitored closely with serial estimations of serum PRL levels combined with imaging studies at yearly intervals. However, if a patient with a microprolactinoma has significant effects from the hyperprolactinemia, treatment is indicated. Any patient with macroprolactinoma needs treatment.

Dopamine-agonist drugs (including cabergoline or bromocriptine) are recommended as first-line treatment for prolactinomas, even in the presence of visual-field defects. These drugs lower serum concentration of PRL and shrink the tumours. These drugs are also safe in pregnancy. Data on the safety of other dopamine-agonists pergolide and quinagolide during pregnancy are too limited to recommend their use. In people who cannot tolerate these drugs or in whom the drugs fail to shrink the tumours sufficiently, surgery, radiotherapy or temozolomide, a chemotherapeutic alkylating agent may be used. In pituitary apoplexy associated with mass effects, such as visual loss, surgical intervention may be recommended to decompress the optic chiasm.

Given the stimulatory effects of pregnancy on the normal lactotrophs, enlargement of the normal pituitary can be expected. This does not necessarily mean that the adenomatous pituitary may enlarge. Prolactinomas that symptomatically enlarge during pregnancy are uncommon. Symptoms suggestive of growth are headache, visual field changes and diabetes insipidus. The risk of clinically significant enlargement for women with microprolactinoma is 1.3%. The risk of enlargement for a woman with untreated macroprolactinoma is 23.2%, while a macroprolactinoma that has been previously treated with surgery and/or radiation has a 2.8% risk of clinically significant enlargement. Shrinkage of a prolactinoma with bromocriptine is associated with a less likely chance of symptomatic growth during pregnancy.

NONFUNCTIONING ADENOMA

These relatively common pituitary adenomas do not result in excess hormone production. They cause problems because of their size and location. The clinical features are headache, visual-field defects, cranial-nerve palsies and those of hypothyroidism, hypogonadism, hypoadrenalism and GH deficiency detailed elsewhere.

Investigation requires assessment of pituitary function, visual-field assessment and the use of MRI as the imaging modality of choice.

Treatment is usually surgery with or without radiotherapy. The cure rate is generally higher for smaller tumours and those that do not invade the cavernous sinus.

CRANIOPHARYNGIOMAS AND RATHKE CLEFT CYSTS

A craniopharyngioma is a slow-growing, extra-axial, epithelial-squamous, calcified tumour arising from remnants of the craniopharyngeal duct and/or Rathke cleft and occupying the (supra)sellar region. Craniopharyngiomas have benign histology but have malignant behaviour. These lesions have a tendency to invade surrounding structures and to recur after a seemingly total resection.

Rathke cleft cysts (RCCs) are benign, epithelium-lined intrasellar cysts believed to originate from remnants of the Rathke pouch.

Craniopharygiomas cause symptoms in three different ways:

- By increasing the intracranial pressure
- By disrupting the function of the pituitary gland resulting in hypopituitarism and diabetes insipidus
- By compressing optic chiasm resulting in visual field defects.

Craniopharyngiomas are nearly always cystic, sometimes lobulated and filled with oily green fluid that has a characteristic appearance on MRI. They may also calcify and appear as suprasellar calcification on a plain skull X-ray. Craniopharyngiomas are usually picked up in people under the age of 20 years.

The usual treatment for craniopharyngiomas is surgery, with postoperative radiotherapy recommended for any residual tumour. Medical treatment involves the replacement of deficient hormones.

RCCs require surgical treatment only when they become symptomatic. Trans-sphenoidal surgery is the recommended treatment.

DIABETES INSIPIDUS

Central diabetes insipidus is characterised by decreased secretion of AVP. This results in polyuria and polydipsia because the ability to concentrate urine is diminished. Reduced or absent AVP secretion can result from a defect in one or more sites involving the hypothalamic osmoreceptors, the supraoptic or paraventricular nuclei or the supraopticohypophysial tract. Lesions of the posterior pituitary rarely cause permanent diabetes insipidus because AVP is produced in the hypothalamus and can still be secreted into the circulation.

Nephrogenic diabetes insipidus is characterised by a decrease in the ability to concentrate urine owing to a resistance to AVP action in the kidney. It can be observed in chronic renal insufficiency, lithium toxicity, hypercalcaemia, hypokalaemia and tubulointerstitial disease.

There are rare forms of hereditary nephrogenic diabetes insipidus. One potential cause is an X-linked genetic defect that results in failure of the AVP V_2 receptor in the kidney to function correctly. More rarely, a mutation in the gene encoding aquaporin-2 can cause a break in the kidney water channel, which results in the kidney being unable to absorb water. The mutation is inherited in an autosomal recessive manner.

The diagnosis of diabetes insipidus is usually made clinically and laboratory tests provide confirmation. Most people with diabetes insipidus can drink enough fluid to replace their urine losses if the thirst mechanism is intact. The synthetic AVP analogue desmopressin may be used twice a day as subcutaneous, nasal or oral preparation to control symptoms. It is important to avoid hyponatraemia through overuse of desmopressin.

LYMPHOCYTIC HYPOPHYSITIS

Lymphocytic hypophysitis is a rare disease and represents an inflammatory/autoimmune disorder that primarily involves the pituitary gland and, in many cases, the pituitary stalk. It is most commonly diagnosed in women during pregnancy or in the postpartum period, and it can be associated with other types of autoimmune disease. Although most commonly occurring in women during the child-bearing years, lymphocytic hypophysitis is now recognised to affect both men and women of any age. The clinical presentation of this inflammatory condition may mimic that of a pituitary adenoma. It includes headache, nausea, vomiting, fatigue, hypopituitarism and diabetes insipidus. If there is mass effect on the optic chiasm, vision may be impaired, usually with a typical bitemporal hemianopsia, and if the cavernous sinus is involved, patients may have diplopia and orbital pain. Hypophysitis is classified as primary when it is idiopathic. Secondary hypophysitis can be due to sarcoidosis, tuberculosis, Langerhans cell granulomatosis, Wegener's granulomatosis and IgG-IV-related hypophysitis (plasma-cell rich). Diagnosing and differentiating them can be a major challenge.

Medical treatment is the use of corticosteroids to treat the inflammatory process. This is given in the form of high-dose prednisone or equivalent steroids (hydrocortisone or dexamethasone), and tapered depending upon the extent and duration of the response. If there is a strong suspicion of lymphocytic hypophysitis and there is no visual loss, then corticosteroid therapy is usually given as first-line management. A pretreatment assessment of pituitary function is essential, because most patients develop one or more pituitary hormone deficiencies that need replacement. In the presence of diabetes insipidus, desmopressin (DDAVP) is administered and the patient is closely monitored for fluid intake and output, and particularly for serum sodium levels. Medications such as methotrexate, azothiaprine and cyclosporine may be considered in patients who are resistant to corticosteroids or develop relapses after several courses of treatment. It has been reported that more than 72% of patients with lymphocytic hypophysitis will require lifelong hormone replacement therapy. Indications for a surgical procedure include lack of response to a trial of medical treatment and mass effect with visual loss. Stereotactic radiotherapy has been used effectively in intractable cases.

Pituitary diseases in pregnancy

PROLACTINOMA

Excess levels of PRL directly inhibit pulsatile GnRH secretion, resulting in anovulation/amenorrhoea and infertility. Correction of hyperprolactinaemia with dopamine agonists restores ovulation in approximately 90% of women with prolactinoma.

There are two key issues in a woman with a prolactinoma who becomes pregnant. The first is the effect of a dopamine agonist on early fetal development before the pregnancy is discovered. In principle, fetal exposure to dopamine agonists should be limited. Bromocriptine seems to be safe in pregnancy and available data suggest that cabergoline is also safe, although the evidence

regarding cabergoline safety is based on a small number of pregnancies. Data on the safety of pergolide and quinagolide during pregnancy are too limited to recommend the use of these agents. The reported heart valve damage seen with high-dose cabergoline has not been demonstrated with cabergoline at the doses used to treat hyperprolactinaemia, nor with bromocriptine or quinagolide (a non-ergot-based dopamine agonist).

The second issue is the effect of pregnancy on the prolactinoma. Pregnancy stimulates normal lactotrophs and causes enlargement of the normal pituitary. This does not necessarily mean that the adenomatous pituitary gland may enlarge. Prolactinomas that enlarge and become symptomatic during pregnancy are uncommon. Symptoms suggestive of prolactinoma growth are headache and visual field changes. The risk of clinically significant enlargement for women with a microprolactinoma is 1–2%. The risk of enlargement for a woman with untreated macroprolactinoma is about 20%. A macroprolactinoma that has been previously treated with surgery, radiation or both has a 2–5% risk of clinically significant enlargement. Shrinkage of a prolactinoma with a dopamine agonist is associated with a reduced chance of symptomatic growth during pregnancy once treatment is discontinued.

Reinitiation of medical treatment is recommended for pregnant women with prolactinomas that become symptomatic. The symptoms tend to regress quickly. Transsphenoidal surgery or delivery is an alternative if the tumour does not respond to medical treatment or if further visual deterioration occurs. Careful follow-up with monthly visual field examinations is important in pregnant women with a known macroadenoma. MRI is performed on women who develop symptoms of tumour enlargement, visual field defects or both.

Breastfeeding has not been associated with any growth of an underlying prolactinoma. Resolution of hyper-prolactinaemia and regression of the prolactinoma have been reported following the pregnancy. Idiopathic hyperprolactinaemia is even more likely to resolve following pregnancy.

SHEEHAN SYNDROME

Severe haemorrhage, shock or hypotension during or before parturition may lead to postpartum pituitary necrosis or Sheehan syndrome. This results in partial or complete hypopituitarism. The syndrome is now fortunately uncommon owing to improved obstetric practice. The pathogenesis of Sheehan syndrome is still not completely clear. During pregnancy, there is an approximately 50% increase in the volume of the pituitary gland. A sudden fall in blood pressure after an event, such as a postpartum haemorrhage results in hypoperfusion and infarction of the gland causes ischaemia of the gland, cellular damage and oedema. In turn, the oedema results in swelling of the pituitary gland. It is more likely to occur in the presence of a previously known or unknown pituitary mass. Pregnant women with type 1 diabetes, especially those with pre-existing vascular disease, seem to be particularly at risk.

Usually, only anterior pituitary function is affected because the posterior pituitary and hypothalamus are supplied by the inferior hypophyseal artery and the circle of Willis, which makes them less vulnerable to ischaemic necrosis. Some women with Sheehan syndrome have an impairment of AVP secretion that may lead to partial or overt diabetes insipidus.

The clinical presentation of women with Sheehan syndrome is highly variable. Following destruction of 95–99% of the anterior pituitary gland, the disease is characterised by postpartum failure of lactation, secondary amenorrhoea, loss of axillary and pubic hair, genital and breast atrophy, increasing signs of secondary hypothyroidism and adrenocortical insufficiency. Less extensive pituitary destruction (50–95%) is associated with an atypical form of the disease with the loss of one or more hormones. The pattern of loss of trophic hormones is unpredictable but invariably results in hypothyroidism (owing to impaired TSH secretion) and hypoadrenalism (owing to impaired ACTH secretion). Mental disturbances are frequent, and sometimes the patient may have overt psychosis. These changes revert with hormone replacement. Women with type 1 diabetes may present with decreasing insulin requirements.

Imaging with MRI or computed tomography (CT) scanning is indicated to exclude mass lesions. In longstanding Sheehan syndrome, the sella frequently is empty, filled only with cerebrospinal fluid. Occasionally, small remnants of pituitary tissue may be observed.

Treatment is hormone replacement. In some instances, gonadotrophin secretion may be preserved and pregnancy is possible. Spontaneous recovery from hypopituitarism caused by postpartum haemorrhage has also been reported.

Premature ovarian failure

Menopause is defined by the last menstrual period and marks the end of a woman's reproductive phase. The average age of menopause is reported to be approximately 51 years. Ovarian failure is diagnosed when sex steroid deficiency, elevated gonadotrophins and amenorrhoea occur. Premature ovarian failure (POF) is diagnosed statistically when ovarian failure occurs at an age that is more than two standard deviations below the mean age at menopause estimated for reference population or, more arbitrarily, below the age of 40 years.

POF can occur before or after the onset of menarche and affects 1% of women under the age of 40 years and 0.1% under the age of 30 years. The prevalence of POF varies by ethnicity, with women of oriental origin having a lower risk and black women having a higher risk than white women. POF is diagnosed in 10–28% of women with primary amenorrhoea and in 4–18% of those with secondary amenorrhoea.

POF results from either a dysfunction or a depletion of the ovarian follicles. In contrast to normal menopause, half of the women with POF have intermittent ovarian function up to 15 years after the onset of POF. Pregnancies have been documented in those diagnosed with POF even in the absence of follicles on ovarian biopsy.

CAUSES OF PREMATURE OVARIAN FAILURE

In the majority of women with POF, no aetiological factor can be identified. A small initial follicle pool and/or inappropriate luteinisation of Graafian follicles have been suggested as causes of spontaneous POF. Other potential causes include:

- chromosomal and genetic abnormalities involving the X chromosome or autosomes
- autoimmune ovarian damage with positive antiovarian antibodies
- iatrogenic disease following pelvic surgery, radiotherapy or chemotherapy

- environmental factors such as viral infections or toxins, for which no clear mechanism is known.

CLINICAL PRESENTATION

The clinical presentation of POF is variable. Rarely, POF presents as primary amenorrhoea with variable degrees of development of secondary sexual characters. More commonly, POF presents as secondary amenorrhoea. Some women present with symptoms of estrogen deficiency or menstrual disturbance, others present as part of a work-up for infertility and some as part of a syndromic condition, which can be genetic or autoimmune. Women with chromosomal defects commonly present with primary amenorrhoea and absent secondary sex characteristics. Those with mosaicism may have some functioning gonadal tissue. Various degrees of sexual development and transient menstruation may therefore be present.

There are no specific warning signs of approaching POF. Approximately 50% of women with POF have a history of oligomenorrhoea or dysfunctional uterine bleeding, which has been termed prodromal POF. In 25% of affected women, acute onset of amenorrhoea has been associated with pregnancy and delivery or with discontinuation of the oral contraceptive pill. Vasomotor symptoms are only present in women with secondary amenorrhoea and may become apparent while the woman is still having regular periods, suggesting prodromal POF.

In general, women with POF have normal fertility before the disorder starts to develop. A decline in fertility owing to resistant ovaries or an increase in the levels of FSH may be a sign of developing POF.

Women with POF are at high risk of developing a variety of health problems and therefore have nearly twice the age-specific mortality risk. Sex steroid deficiency in young women with POF occurs for longer periods than it does in naturally menopausal women. This results in a significantly increased risk of osteoporosis, which is particularly high in those who have developed POF before achieving peak adult bone mass. Two-thirds of women with normal karyotype and POF have a bone mineral density one standard deviation below the mean for women of similar age, despite having taken standard hormonal therapy. This translates to a 2.6-fold increased risk of hip fracture.

The risk of cardiovascular disease in women with POF is also significantly increased. A significantly increased mortality owing to coronary heart disease, stroke, cancer and other causes has been documented (age-adjusted odds ratio of death: 1.29, 3.07, 1.83 and 2.14, respectively).

AUTOIMMUNE PREMATURE OVARIAN FAILURE

Autoimmune mechanisms may be involved in the pathogenesis of POF in up to 30% of affected women. Autoimmune oophoritis is an important cause (10–30%) of reversible POF. It could be mediated either humorally or cellularly. Antibodies against steroidogenic enzymes (for example 3-hydroxy steroid dehydrogenase), gonadotrophins and their receptors, the corpus luteum, the zona pellucida and the oocyte have been identified but their specificity for the disease is unknown.

Autoimmune lymphocytic oophoritis is commonly associated with an increased activity of peripheral T lymphocytes and may be isolated or associated with other endocrine or non-endocrine disorders, such as Addison disease, diabetes mellitus, myasthenia gravis, systemic lupus erythematosus, rheumatoid arthritis and autoimmune hypothyroidism. Lymphocytic infiltration may also be present in the ovarian hilum, with an accumulation of lymphocytes around neural tissue. Forty percent of women with POF can be positive for at least one organ-specific autoantibody, the most common being antithyroid antibodies (found in about 20% of women with POF).

POF accounts for 25% of young women presenting with amenorrhoea. Some 5–30% of women with POF have another affected female relative. In these women, the mode of inheritance could be X-linked or autosomal, dominant or recessive. The causal mutation tends to be unknown.

Chromosomal and genetic abnormalities associated with POF include Turner syndrome (45,X), triple X syndrome, fragile X syndrome and fragile X premutation. Other causes include Swyer syndrome (pure gonadal dysgenesis with an XY chromosomal constitution), blepharophimosis, Perrault syndrome, Down syndrome and infections such as oophritis following mumps, malaria, varicella and *Shigella* infections.

Radiotherapy and chemotherapy can lead to POF. In general, younger women are more resistant to the effects of chemoptherapy and prepubertal ovaries are least susceptible to the toxicity. Complete ovarian failure occurs with a dose of 20 Gy in women under the age of 40 years and with only 6 Gy in older women.

DIAGNOSIS

The diagnosis of POF is based on the finding of elevated serum FSH concentrations (40 IU/l) on at least two occasions separated by a few weeks. The reason for two samples is that the natural history of POF can be very variable. In many women, the condition follows an unpredictable course of relapse and remission, often given the label fluctuating ovarian function. A pregnancy rate of approximately 1–5% has been reported in women with POF.

Ovarian biopsy adds little to the investigative process because the small samples obtained are not predictive of the natural history of the condition. Pelvic ultrasound is not predictive but may help to define those who may be candidates for oocyte preservation. An autoimmune screen for thyroid and adrenal autoantibodies may be helpful for future surveillance of other autoimmune problems.

A good family history can help to identify other affected members in as many as 30% of women with POF. Genetic screening is increasingly being used in women with a family history of POF, but it can also be used in sporadic POF with a high index of suspicion of a genetic disorder. For example, fragile X premutations occur in 15% of women with POF who have a positive family history of POF and in 3% of sporadic presentations. Karyotype and fragile X premutation screening should be considered in persons with a family history or unusually young onset.

MANAGEMENT

Management of POF will not be discussed in detail but has three main components: medical treatment, fertility advice and psychological support. The major medical issues are quality of life and bone protection. These issues can be addressed by prescribing hormone replacement therapy. Options for addressing infertility include oocyte donation and adoption. Psychological treatment requires personal and emotional support to deal with the impact of the diagnosis on a woman's health and relationships. Long-term follow-up is essential to monitor hormone replacement therapy and to allow surveillance for any emerging associated autoimmune pathology.

CHAPTER 17

Adrenal and thyroid glands and the pancreas

Gul Bano

Adrenal gland

ANATOMY

The adrenal glands rest on the upper poles of the kidneys. Each adrenal gland weighs approximately 4–5 g. The arterial blood supply comes from three sources, with branches arising from the inferior phrenic artery, the renal artery and the aorta. Venous drainage flows directly into the inferior vena cava on the right side and into the left renal vein on the left side. Lymphatics drain medially to the aortic nodes.

Each adrenal gland is composed of two distinct parts: the adrenal cortex and the adrenal medulla. The cortex is divided into three zones. From exterior to interior these are the zona glomerulosa, the zona fasciculata and the zona reticularis.

PHYSIOLOGY OF THE ADRENAL CORTEX

Steroid synthesis

The adrenal cortex secretes three classes of steroid hormones

- glucocorticoids – mainly cortisol, secreted by the zona fasciculate
- mineralocorticoids – mainly aldosterone, secreted by the zona glomerulosa
- androgen precursors – mainly dehydroepiandrosterone (DHEA), secreted by the zona reticularis.

All adrenocortical hormones are steroid compounds derived from cholesterol.

Cortisol binds to proteins in the blood, mainly cortisol-binding globulin or transcortin. More than 90% of cortisol is transported in the blood in this bound form. In contrast, only 50% of aldosterone is bound to protein in the blood. All adrenocortical steroids are degraded in the liver and predominantly conjugated to glucuronides, with lesser amounts of sulfates formed. About 75% of these degradation products are excreted in the urine, and the rest is excreted in the stool by means of the bile.

Control of hormone synthesis

Glucocorticoids and androgens

The synthesis of glucocorticoids and androgens is regulated by the hypothalamo–pituitary axis (Figure 17.1). Approximately 95% of glucocorticoid activity comes from cortisol, with corticosterone, a glucocorticoid less potent than cortisol, making up the rest. The normal cortisol concentration in the blood averages 12 micrograms/dl, with a secretory rate averaging 15–20 mg/day.

Cells in the paraventricular nucleus of the hypothalamus secrete corticotrophin-releasing hormone (CRH). Released from nerve terminals in the median eminence, this 41-amino-acid peptide is transported in the hypophysial portal capillaries to the anterior pituitary corticotrophs to stimulate both the synthesis and the release of adrenocorticotrophin (ACTH).

FIGURE 17.1 **Hypothalamo–pituitary–adrenal axis and control of cortisol secretion**

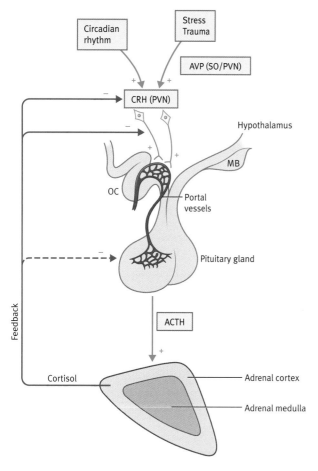

ACTH = adrenocorticotrophin | AVP = arginine vasopressin |
CRH = corticotrophin-releasing hormone | MB = mamillary bodies |
OC = optic chiasm | PVN = paraventricular nucleus | SO = supraoptic nucleus |
MB = mamillary bodies | OC = optic chiasm | + = stimulatory effects |
– = inhibitory effects |

Adapted with permission from: Nussey S, Whitehead SA. *Endocrinology: An Intergrated Approach.* Oxford: BIOS Scientific Publishers; 2001.

ACTH is derived from a large precursor molecule, pro-opiomelanocortin (POMC), which is cleaved by the action of specific peptidase enzymes. The prohormone POMC can give rise to numerous hormones, including opioid peptides and melanocyte-stimulating hormone, but the main product of POMC cleavage in the corticotroph cells is ACTH. (In the brain, other products predominate.)

The main role of ACTH is to stimulate the synthesis and release of glucocorticoids and androgens from the adrenal cortex via a G-protein-coupled receptor. The immediate actions of ACTH in terms of steroid synthesis are:

- increase in cholesterol esterase
- transport of cholesterol into the mitochondria
- binding of cholesterol to CYP11A1.

This all leads to the induction of steroidogenic enzymes and to specific structural changes such as hypervascularisation, cellular hypertrophy and cellular hypertrophy and hyperplasia.

The action of CRH on pituitary corticotrophs is potentiated by arginine vasopressin (AVP), formally known as antidiuretic hormone. AVP is secreted by parvocellular (small) neurosecretory cells into the hypophysial portal capillaries and by magnocellular (large) neurosecretory cells into the general circulation (see Chapter 16).

The production of glucocorticoids is controlled by a classic negative feedback loop in which neurons in the hypothalamus detect circulating concentrations of glucocorticoids and consequently stimulate or inhibit the release of CRH and AVP from the parvocellular neurons (Figure 17.1). The secretion of AVP by the magnocellular neurons is controlled by different stimuli, namely serum osmolality and blood volume.

In normal situations, CRH, ACTH and cortisol secretory rates demonstrate a circadian rhythm, with a peak in the early morning and a nadir in the evening. The negative feedback effect of cortisol on the anterior pituitary and the hypothalamus helps to control these increases and to regulate plasma cortisol concentrations. As ACTH also stimulates the release of androgen precursors by the adrenal gland, the secretion of these hormones parallels that of cortisol.

It should be noted that CRH is also produced in the placenta along with the binding protein CRH-BP. In this organ, CRH/CRH-BP is thought to play a role in the initiation of parturition. CRH synthesis and CRH receptors have also been identified in immune cells, where CRH has both anti-inflammatory and pro-inflammatory effects.

Mineralocorticoids

The secretion of aldosterone is regulated by a number of factors, the most important of which involve the renin–angiotensin system and changes in the plasma K^+ concentration (Figure 17.2). Renin, secreted by the granular cells (also called juxtaglomerular cells) of the afferent arterioles at the juxtaglomerular apparatus, is an enzyme that converts angiotensinogen (produced in liver) to angiotensin 1. In the lung, angiotensin-converting enzyme (ACE) converts angiotensin I to angiotensin II, a potent vasoconstrictor and stimulator of aldosterone release by the adrenal gland.

Actions of adrenocortical steroids

Glucocorticoids

Cortisol has many effects on the body:

- It stimulates gluconeogenesis, the overall result being an increase in serum glucose concentrations.
- It has a catabolic effect, decreasing protein stores in the body.
- It has clinically significant anti-inflammatory effects (for which it is used extensively therapeutically).

FIGURE 17.2 **Control of aldosterone secretion**

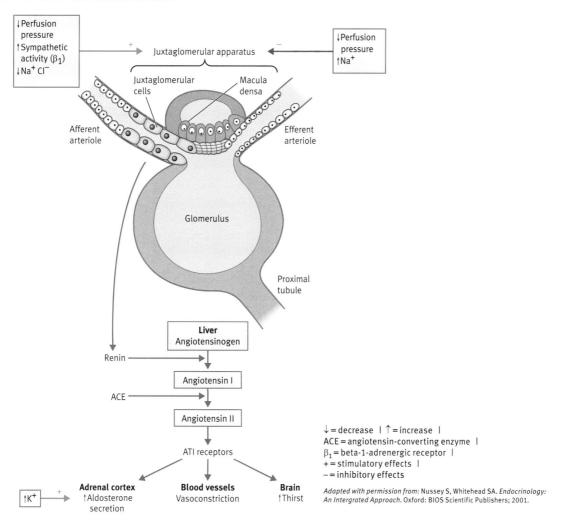

$\downarrow$ = decrease | $\uparrow$ = increase |
ACE = angiotensin-converting enzyme |
β_1 = beta-1-adrenergic receptor |
+ = stimulatory effects |
− = inhibitory effects

Adapted with permission from: Nussey S, Whitehead SA. *Endocrinology: An Intergrated Approach*. Oxford: BIOS Scientific Publishers; 2001.

- It can adversely affect immunity (eosinophil and lymphocyte counts in the blood decrease with atrophy of lymphoid tissue).

Adrenal androgens

The adrenal cortex continually secretes several male sex hormones, including DHEA and its sulphate (DHEAS), androstenedione and 11-hydroxyandrostenedione, as well as small quantities of the female sex hormones progesterone and estrogen. All have weak effects, but in boys they probably have a role in the early development of the male sex organs and in girls they have an important role during puberty and menarche. Most androgenic effects result from extra-adrenal conversion of the androgens to testosterone (see Chapter 6).

Mineralocorticoids

Aldosterone accounts for 90% of mineralocorticoid activity. This hormone promotes Na^+ reabsorption and K^+ excretion by the renal tubular epithelial cells of the collecting and distal tubules. As Na^+ is reabsorbed, H_2O follows passively, leading to an increase in the extracellular fluid volume with little change in the plasma Na^+ concentration. Persistently elevated extracellular fluid volumes cause hypertension. Without aldosterone, the kidney loses excessive amounts of Na^+ and consequently H_2O, leading to fluid depletion.

Steroid transport and metabolism

Cortisol binds to proteins in the blood, mainly cortisol-binding globulin (also called transcortin). More than 90% of cortisol is transported in the blood in this bound form.

Only 50% of aldosterone is bound to protein in the blood. All adrenocortical steroids are degraded in the liver and conjugated predominantly to glucuronides, with lower amounts of sulphates formed. About 75% of these degradation products are excreted in the urine and the rest is excreted in the stool by means of bile.

PHYSIOLOGY OF THE ADRENAL MEDULLA

Catecholamine synthesis and secretion

The adrenal medulla constitutes less that 20% of the adrenal gland and the cells are polygonal and arranged in cords. The medulla receives blood either directly from the medullary arterioles or from the cortical venules, which are rich in cortisol and drain centripetally to the medullary venules. Epinephrine and smaller amounts of norepinephrine are synthesised by, and secreted from, the chromaffin cells of the medulla, in response to stimulation of preganglionic (cholinergic) sympathetic nerves that originate in the thoracolumbar lateral grey matter of the spinal cord. Chromaffin cells are so named because of their affinity for chromium salts, which leads to characteristic staining. As modified postganglionic nerve cells, they are classic neurosecretory cells (that is, neurons releasing hormones into the general circulation).

Like melatonin and thyroid hormones, the catecholamines are synthesised from tyrosine but, in contrast to thyroid hormones, they are made from single tyrosine molecules. These in turn are either synthesised from phenylalanine or imported from the circulation. The rate-limiting step in the synthesis of catecholamines is that catalysed by tyrosine hydroxylase, converting tyrosine to 3,4-dihydroxyphenylalanine (DOPA). The enzyme aromatic-l-amino-acid decarboxylase converts DOPA to dopamine. Hydroxylation of dopamine by dopamine β-hydroxylase leads to the formation of norepinephrine. In some adrenal medullary cells, the synthetic process stops at norepinephrine, but in most cells (particularly those at the corticomedullary junction) norepinephrine is converted to epinephrine by phenylethanolamine N-methyltransferase.

The output of the adrenal gland is controlled from nerve cells within the posterior hypothalamus, which can ultimately stimulate acetylcholine release from preganglionic nerve terminals. This induces depolarisation of the chromaffin cells and exocytosis of the catecholamine-containing granules following a transient rise in intracellular Ca^{2+} concentration. Once secreted, catecholamines have a very short half-life in the circulation (approximately 1–2 minutes).

Actions and metabolism of catecholamines

Catecholamines act on their target tissues through typical G-protein-linked membrane receptors. These receptors are classified as alpha-adrenergic or beta-adrenergic receptors on the basis of the physiological and pharmacological effects induced by hormone binding. The physiological effects of the catecholamines are manifold and summarised in Table 17.1. They have been characterised as preparing us for 'fight or flight', with overall actions comprising an increase in heart rate and stroke volume, an increase in blood pressure, a dilatation of the bronchi, the mobilisation of glucose and the stimulation of lipolysis. These actions are mediated by β-adrenergic receptors. Blood flow to the splanchnic bed is reduced by vasoconstriction of arterioles. This effect is mediated by α-adrenergic receptors and helps to divert blood flow to skeletal muscles.

While most catecholamines released from sympathetic nerves are taken back up into the presynaptic terminal (termed uptake 1), catecholamines released into the circulation are taken up by non-neuronal tissues (termed uptake 2) and are rapidly converted to deaminated products by monoamine oxidase (MAO) or to O-methylated products by catechol O-methyltransferase. The latter enzyme also catalyses the m-O-methylation of the products of MAO action (metanephrine, normetanephrine, epinephrine and vanillylmandelic acid). These may then be conjugated with glucuronide or sulphate and excreted in the urine.

TABLE 17.1 **Effects of catecholamines**

Body system	Effect	Mediator of the effect
Cardiovascular	Increase in heart rate and force	β_1-receptors
	Increase in venous return	α-receptors
	Increase in peripheral resistance	α-receptors, especially those in the subcutaneous, mucosal, splanchnic and renal vascular beds
Autonomic nervous	Smooth muscle relaxation	β_2-receptors
	Smooth muscle contraction	α-receptors
	Modulation of fluid and electrolyte transport in the gut, kidney and gallbladder	α-receptors
Fuel metabolism	Glycogenolysis, lipolysis	β-receptors
	Increase in diet-induced and nonshivering thermogenesis	β-receptors
Fluid and electrolyte balance	Decrease in Na^+ excretion and glomerular filtration	Direct effects on the kidney
	Increase in aldosterone production resulting in enhanced Na^+ retention in the distal tubule	β-receptor-mediated effects on renin secretion
	Increase in serum K^+ levels	α-receptor-mediated effects on the liver
	Decrease in serum K^+ levels	β_2-receptor-mediated effects on muscle
Endocrine	Modulation of the renin–angiotensin–aldosterone system	β_1-receptors
	Increase in the secretion of glucagon and insulin	β_2-receptors
	Inhibition of the carbachol-stimulated synthesis of catecholamines	α_2-receptors

Adapted with permission from: Nussey S, Whitehead SA. *Endocrinology: An Intergrated Approach.* Oxford: BIOS Scientific Publishers; 2001.

TABLE 17.2 Clinical features of Cushing syndrome

Overall frequency	Clinical feature (prevalence among those with Cushing syndrome)
Common	Moon face (with plethora) (100%)
	Weight gain, central obesity (100%)
	Hypertension (80%)
	Mental changes (80%)
	Impaired glucose tolerance/diabetes mellitus (70%)
	Hypogonadism[a] (70%)
	Hirsutism in women (70%)
	Purple striae (60%)
	Acne (60%)
	Osteopenia/osteoporosis (50%)
	Easy bruising (50%)
	Proximal myopathy (50%)
Less common	Poor wound healing (30%)
	Polycythaemia (10%)
	Renal stones (10%)
	Headache (10%)
	Exophthalmos (10%)

[a] Menstrual irregularity/infertility in women, loss of libido in men
Adapted with permission from: Nussey S, Whitehead SA. *Endocrinology: An Intergrated Approach*. Oxford: BIOS Scientific Publishers; 2001.

TABLE 17.3 Causes of Cushing syndrome

Overall frequency	Cause
Common (~99%)	Exogenous therapeutic glucocorticoids
Uncommon (<1%)	Anterior pituitary adenoma
	Ectopic ACTH production
	Adrenal adenoma
Rare (<0.01%)	Adrenal carcinoma
	Ectopic CRH production
	Alcoholism
	Bilateral multinodular hyperplasia

ACTH = adrenocorticotrophin | CRH = corticotrophin-releasing hormone
Adapted with permission from: Nussey S, Whitehead SA. *Endocrinology: An Intergrated Approach*. Oxford: BIOS Scientific Publishers; 2001.

with the loss of other pituitary hormones may also be apparent. These include hypothyroidism, hypogonadism and growth hormone deficiency.

Diagnosis

Screening tests for Cushing syndrome include:

- measurement of 24-hour urinary levels of free cortisol
- measurement of midnight levels of salivary cortisol
- low-dose dexamethasone suppression test.

The latter may be combined with the CRH test to differentiate between pseudo-Cushing caused by obesity, alcoholism or depression, pituitary Cushing due to ACTH excess and Cushing syndrome caused by primary adrenal disease or ectopic ACTH production (Table 17.4).

When investigating solid lesions of the adrenal gland, unenhanced or delayed contrast-enhanced computed tomography (CT) may help in distinguishing benign from malignant lesions by their attenuation. Benign lesions tend to have decreased attenuation because of an increased fat content. Magnetic resonance imaging (MRI) is also useful and its main benefit over CT is its improved ability, with gadolinium enhancement or with chemical shift imaging, to help in differentiating benign from malignant lesions. Ultrasonography is often the first imaging study performed in children who are

DISEASES OF THE ADRENAL GLAND

Cushing syndrome

The term Cushing syndrome is used for an excess of glucocorticoids, however produced. The term Cushing's disease is used when the excess of glucocorticoids is attributable to an ACTH-secreting pituitary tumour. When Cushing syndrome is caused by ectopic ACTH secretion (for example secretion by a lung tumour), the clinical features may not be typical of classic disease and include hypokalaemia and metabolic alkalosis.

The clinical features of Cushing syndrome are given in Table 17.2 and the causes in Table 17.3. When the cause is a pituitary tumour, clinical features associated

TABLE 17.4 **Combined dexamethasone and CRH test**

Condition	Cortisol level at baseline	ACTH level at baseline	Cortisol and ACTH levels after dex administration	Cortisol and ACTH levels after CRH administration	Ratio of ACTH precursors to ACTH
Pseudo-Cushing	Normal or high	Normal or high	Both suppressed	No response	Normal
Pituitary Cushing	High or normal	High	Incomplete suppression	Increase by $\geq$40% in both	Normal
Adrenal adenoma	High	Normal or low	No suppression	No change	Normal
Ectopic ACTH secretion	High	High	No suppression	No change	High

ACTH = adrenocorticotrophin | CRH = corticotrophin-releasing hormone | dex = dexamethasone

suspected to have an ACTH-secreting adrenocortical tumour. It can differentiate cystic from solid adrenal masses and is useful to assess for vascular involvement and liver metastases. Radioisotope scanning is now rarely used.

For lesions of the pituitary gland, MRI is the imaging modality of choice. Visual field examination most often reveals bitemporal hemianopia if a large pituitary tumour is present.

Treatment

The definitive treatment for Cushing syndrome is surgery. This includes transphenoidal surgery for pituitary disease and adrenalectomy (either laparoscopic or conventional) for adrenal disease.

Medical management includes supportive treatment for hypokalaemia with K^+-sparing diuretics and K^+ supplements.

Medications used in the management of Cushing syndrome include the following:

- Somatostatin analogues (e.g. pasireotide)
- Adrenal steroid inhibitors (e.g. metyrapone, ketoconazole, aminoglutethimide, mifepristone.

Primary aldosteronism

An excess of mineralocorticoid steroids results in Na^+ retention in the kidney with loss of K^+. Na^+ retention promotes H_2O retention and expansion in the extracellular volume, resulting in hypertension and a suppression of renin production. This condition is also called Conn syndrome. It accounts for up to 2% of the total incidence of hypertension in the general population. The causes include:

- adrenal adenoma (accounting for 80% of the total incidence)
  - solitary adenoma (65–70%)
  - multiple adenomas (13%)
  - microadenomatosis (6%)
- adrenal gland hyperplasia (20%)
- adrenal carcinoma (less than 1%).

Clinical presentation

The common clinical scenarios in which the possibility of primary aldosteronism should be considered include the following:

- Patients with spontaneous or unprovoked hypokalemia, especially if the patient is also hypertensive.
- Patients who develop severe and/or persistent hypokalemia in the setting of low to moderate doses of potassium-wasting diuretics.
- Patients with treatment-refractory/-resistant hypertension (HTN).

Patients with severe hypokalemia report fatigue, muscle weakness, cramping, headaches and palpitations. They can also have polydipsia and polyuria from hypokalemia-induced nephrogenic diabetes insipidus. Long-standing HTN may lead to cardiac, retinal, renal and neurological problems, with all the associated symptoms and signs.

Diagnosis

The diagnosis is made from the classic biochemical findings of hypokalaemia and metabolic alkalosis associated with hyperaldosteronism.

Random plasma aldosterone/plasma renin activity (PRA) ratio is fairly constant over many physiological conditions. Simultaneous measurement of plasma renin activity (PRA) and plasma aldosterone concentration (PAC), after discontinuation of appropriate antihypertensive medication can be used in screening for hyperaldosteronism. When aldosterone is measured in ng/dL and PRA is measured in ng/mL/h, a plasma aldosterone/PRA ratio of greater than 20–25 has 95% sensitivity and 75% specificity for primary aldosteronism. When aldosterone is measured in pmol/l, a ratio greater than 900 is consistent with primary aldosteronism.

Genetic–familial primary aldosteronism

Three distinct genetic–familial varieties of primary aldosteronism exist:

- type 1 variety of familial primary aldosteronism, glucocorticoid-remediable aldosteronism (GRA)
- type 2 variant of familial primary aldosteronism, which is not glucocorticoid sensitive
- type 3 variant of familial primary aldosteronism, which is due to potassium channel mutations.

Treatment

In 75–90% of people with a solitary aldosterone-producing tumour, surgical adrenalectomy corrects hypertension and hypokalaemia. Surgery should be avoided in bilateral hyperplasia. As a result, it is important to distinguish the two and, as with Cushing syndrome, CT or MRI scans are the best modalities to localise a tumour or establish bilateral adrenal hyperplasia. If

hyperplasia is present, then pharmacotherapy is used to correct hypokalemia and treat hypertension.

Drugs that are commonly used include mineralocorticoid antagonists like spiranolactone. The drug has estrogen-like adverse effects, including impotence and gynaecomastia. Eplerenone is a selective anti-aldosterone agent, which is a specific aldosterone-receptor antagonist that does not have the additional antiandrogen effects associated with spironolactone.

GRA is treated with small doses of glucocorticosteroids (i.e., hydrocortisone, prednisone). At optimal doses, glucocorticosteroids normalise aldosterone and blood pressure.

Phaeochromocytoma

A phaeochromocytoma is a rare catecholamine-secreting tumour of the sympathetic nervous system. The majority (90%) of such tumours arise from adrenal sites, whereas 10% occur elsewhere in the sympathetic chain. Tumours that arise outside the adrenal gland are termed extra-adrenal phaeochromocytomas or paragangliomas.

Most tumours release both epinephrine and norepinephrine, but large and extra-adrenal tumours produce almost entirely norepinephrine. Excessive catecholamine secretion from phaeochromocytomas may precipitate life-threatening hypertension or cardiac arrhythmias. The tumour is malignant in 10% of cases, but may be cured completely by surgical removal. Although phaeochromocytoma has classically been associated with 3 syndromes – von Hippel-Lindau (VHL) syndrome, multiple endocrine neoplasia type 2 (MEN 2) and neurofibromatosis type 1 (NF1) – there are now 10 genes that have been identified as sites of mutations leading to phaeochromocytoma.

Diagnosis

The choice of diagnostic test should be based on the clinical suspicion of a phaeochromocytoma. Plasma metanephrine testing has the highest sensitivity (96%) for detecting a phaeochromocytoma, but it has a lower specificity (85%). In comparison, a 24-hour urinary collection for catecholamines and metanephrines has a sensitivity of 87.5% and a specificity of 99.7%. Localisation of the lesion is usually made with the help of CT or MRI scanning. A scan with iodine-123 (^{123}I)–labelled metaio-dobenzylguanidine (MIBG) is reserved for cases in which a phaeochromocytoma is confirmed biochemically but CT scanning or MRI does not show a tumour.

A somatostatin-receptor analogue, indium-111 (^{111}In) pentetreotide, is less sensitive than MIBG. However, it may be used to visualise phaeochromocytomas that do not concentrate MIBG.

PET scanning with ^{18}F-fluorodeoxyglucose (^{18}F-FDG), which is selectively concentrated as part of the abnormal metabolism of many neoplasms, has been demonstrated to detect occult phaeochromocytomas.

It is important to note the family history because a number of germline mutations have been identified to be responsible for familial forms of phaeochromocytoma.

Treatment

The only form of curative therapy is complete surgical removal of the tumour after initial medical treatment. Careful preoperative management is required to control blood pressure, correct fluid volume and prevent intraoperative hypertensive crises. Preoperative medical treatment reduces the risk of acute catecholamine release in response to anaesthetic drugs and surgical handling. The usual preoperative treatment is initially with α-adrenergic blockade followed by a combination of α-adrenergic and β-adrenergic blockade.

Hypoadrenalism

This condition can occur as a result of primary adrenal insufficiency (also termed Addison's disease) but it can also be secondary to pituitary damage and results in deficient production of hormones by the adrenal cortex. The causes are summarised in Table 17.5.

In autoimmune Addison's disease, the autoimmune destruction of the adrenal glands may be isolated or part of multi-organ involvement. There are two types of autoimmune polyendocrinopathy. Autoimmune polyendocrinopathy syndrome (APS) type 1 is also known as autoimmune polyendocrinopathy, candidiasis and ectodermal dystrophy (APECED) syndrome. APS type 1 occurs in association with autoimmune

TABLE 17.5 **Causes of hypoadrenalism**

Overall frequency	Type of hypoadrenalism	Cause
Common (>99%)	Primary hypoadrenalism (Addison's disease)	Abrupt cessation of exogenous sources of glucocorticoids
Rare (<1%)	Primary hypoadrenalism (Addison's disease)	Autoimmunity
		Infection (e.g. tuberculosis or fungal infections)
		Haemorrhage
		Metastases
		Drugs (e.g. etomidate, ketoconazole, metyrapone)
	Secondary hypoadrenalism	Any pituitary disease causing hypopituitarism
	Tertiary hypoadrenalism	Any hypothalamic disease causing hypopituitarism

Adapted with permission from: Nussey S, Whitehead SA. *Endocrinology: An Intergrated Approach*. Oxford: BIOS Scientific Publishers; 2001.

hypoparathyroidism, chronic mucocutaneous candidiasis and other organ-specific autoimmune disorders. It is a monogenic autoimmune disorder and has autosomal recessive inheritance.

APS type 2 (Schmidt syndrome) is the association of autoimmune Addison's disease with autoimmune thyroid disease and/or type 1 diabetes. APS type 2 has a predilection for women in middle age and the average age of onset is between 35 and 40 years. The genetic basis of isolated autoimmune Addison's disease and APS type 2 is not clearly understood. Other autoimmune disorders can be associated with APS type 2 and these include primary gonadal failure, pernicious anaemia, vitiligo and alopecia. Antibodies to the adrenal cortex mediate autoimmune destruction of the adrenal glands.

The clinical features of Addison's disease are given in Table 17.6. High concentrations of ACTH result in buccal pigmentation and pigmentation of scars and palmar creases.

TABLE 17.6 **Clinical features of Addison's disease**

Overall frequency	Clinical feature (prevalence among those with Addison's disease)
Common	Weakness (100%)
	Weight loss (95%)
	Pigmentation (95%)
	Anorexia (95%)
	Nausea (95%)
Less common	Abdominal pain (30%)
	Postural hypotension (25%)
	Vitiligo (20%)
	Salt craving (15%)
	Aches and pains (10%)
	Hypoglycaemia (in adults <1%)

Adapted with permission from: Nussey S, Whitehead SA. *Endocrinology: An Intergrated Approach*. Oxford: BIOS Scientific Publishers; 2001.

Diagnosis

The diagnosis of hypoadrenalism may be suspected from evidence in routine biochemical tests of hyponatraemia, hyperkalaemia and hypercalcaemia. Biochemical confirmation may be made using a tetracosactrin test. Tetracosactrin is a peptide identical to the 24 amino-terminal amino acids of ACTH. ACTH and cortisol are measured in peripheral venous blood before a single injection of 250 micrograms of peptide and cortisol is assayed again 30 minutes thereafter. Two criteria are necessary for diagnosis: (1) an increase in the baseline cortisol value of 7 micrograms /dl or more and (2) the value must rise to 20 micrograms or more in 30 or 60 minutes, establishing normal adrenal glucocorticoid function. The absolute 30- or 60-minute cortisol value carries more significance than the incremental value, especially in patients who may be in great stress and at their maximal adrenal output. If the cortisol response is impaired and the baseline ACTH level is high, the diagnosis is primary adrenal failure. If the baseline ACTH level is low, the diagnosis is secondary adrenal failure. Stimulation of the adrenal gland in primary disease will not result in the release of cortisol. In secondary insufficiency, the atrophic adrenal glands still produce some cortisol when exposed to ACTH and the serum cortisol level rises to more than 1000 nmol/l.

Imaging studies can be useful in helping to elucidate the cause of hypoadrenalism. Both CT and MRI demonstrate a reduced adrenal gland size in people with autoimmune destruction and an enlarged adrenal gland in people with infection such as tuberculosis. MRI is superior to CT in differentiating adrenal masses but MRI cannot distinguish a tumour from an inflammatory process.

Treatment

In patients in acute adrenal crisis, intravenous access should be established urgently, and an infusion of isotonic sodium chloride solution should be begun to restore volume deficit and correct hypotension. Some patients may require glucose supplementation. The precipitating cause should be sought and corrected where possible. Treatment of acute adrenal insufficiency requires immediate intravenous administration of 100 mg hydrocortisone followed by administration of 100–200 mg hydrocortisone over 24 hours under close monitoring. Individuals with adrenal insufficiency who require long-term replacement usually receive two or three daily doses of hydrocortisone. An extra dose of hydrocortisone may be required before strenuous exercise and doses are usually doubled for intercurrent illness. The standard mineralocorticoid replacement is fludrocortisone acetate at 100–150 micrograms/days. The dose of fludrocortisone acetate is titrated individually on the basis of the clinical examination (mainly the body weight and arterial blood pressure) and the levels of plasma renin activity. As long as the patient is receiving 100 mg or more of hydrocortisone in 24 hours, no mineralocorticoid replacement is necessary. The mineralocorticoid activity of hydrocortisone in this dosage is sufficient. In women, the adrenal cortex is the primary source of androgen in the form of DHEA and DHEAS. Although the physiological role of these androgens in women has not been fully elucidated, their replacement is being increasingly considered in the treatment of adrenal insufficiency. Patient education is important for long-term care of these patients:

- Patients should wear an emergency medical alert bracelet.
- Patients should be instructed to double or triple their steroid replacement doses in stressful situations, such as having a common cold or tooth extraction.
- Patients should be instructed to contact their regular physician or to go to the emergency department in case of illness.
- Patients should be instructed on how to give themselves intramuscular injections. They should be given a prescription for parenteral hydrocortisone for use on occasions when oral intake may not be possible or when marked vomiting or diarrhoea occurs.
- No adjustment needs to be made on the mineralocorticoid replacement dose in stressful situations.

Congenital adrenal hyperplasia

The term congenital adrenal hyperplasia (CAH) encompasses a group of autosomal recessive disorders, each of which involves a deficiency of an enzyme involved in the synthesis of cortisol, aldosterone or both. Deficiency of 21-hydroxylase, resulting from mutations or deletions of *CYP21A*, is the most common form of CAH, accounting for more than 90% of cases.

The clinical phenotype of CAH depends on the nature and severity of the enzyme deficiency. Although the presentation varies according to chromosomal sex, the sex of a neonate with CAH is often initially unclear because of genital ambiguity. If the defect is severe and results in salt wasting, then the presentation is at age 1–4 weeks with failure to thrive, recurrent vomiting, dehydration, hypotension, hyponatremia, hyperkalemia and shock (classic salt-wasting adrenal hyperplasia).

Clinical presentation

- Females with severe CAH due to deficiencies of 21-hydroxylase, 11-β-hydroxylase or 3-β-hydroxysteroid dehydrogenase have ambiguous genitalia at birth (classic virilising adrenal hyperplasia).
- Females with mild 21-hydroxylase deficiency are identified later in childhood because of precocious

pubic hair, clitoromegaly or both, often accompanied by accelerated growth and skeletal maturation (simple virilising adrenal hyperplasia).
- Females with still milder deficiencies of 21-hydroxylase or 3-β-hydroxysteroid dehydrogenase activity may present in adolescence or adulthood with oligomenorrhoea, hirsutism and/or infertility (nonclassical adrenal hyperplasia).
- Females with 17-hydroxylase deficiency appear phenotypically female at birth but do not develop breasts or menstruate in adolescence; they may present with hypertension.
- Males with 21-hydroxylase deficiency have normal genitalia.

Diagnosis

The diagnosis of CAH depends on the demonstration of inadequate production of cortisol, aldosterone or both in the presence of accumulation of excess concentrations of precursor hormones. In 21-hydroxylase deficiency there is high serum concentration of 17-hydroxyprogesterone (usually greater than 1000 ng/dl) and urinary pregnanetriol (metabolite of 17-hydroxyprogesterone) in the presence of clinical features suggestive of the disease. In nonclassical cases, a testacosactrin-stimulation test is used to diagnose CAH. In 11-β-hydroxylase deficiency cases there are excess serum concentrations of 11-deoxycortisol and deoxycorticosterone, or an elevation in the ratio of 24-hour urinary tetrahydrocompound S (metabolite of 11-deoxycortisol) to tetrahydrocompound F (metabolite of cortisol). In addition, in the salt-wasting forms of CAH, there are low serum aldosterone concentrations, hyponatremia, hyperkalaemia and elevated plasma renin activity (PRA), indicating hypovolaemia.

Imaging studies include pelvic ultrasonography in an infant with ambiguous genitalia to demonstrate a uterus or associated renal anomalies. A bone-age study is useful in evaluating for advanced skeletal maturation in a child who develops precocious pubic hair, clitoromegaly or accelerated linear growth. Another useful test is a karyotype, to establish the chromosomal sex. Genetic testing is essential for genetic counselling and prenatal diagnosis of adrenal hyperplasia. Newborn screening programmes for 21-hydroxylase deficiency may be life-saving in an affected male infant who would otherwise be undetected until presentation with a salt-wasting crisis.

Treatment

Patients presenting with a salt-wasting crisis are treated with intravenous sodium chloride to restore intravasular volume and blood pressure. Dextrose must be included in the rehydration fluid after the bolus dose to prevent hypoglycaemia. After samples are obtained to measure electrolyte, blood sugar, cortisol, aldosterone and 17-hydroxyprogesterone concentrations, the patient should be treated with glucocorticoids. After the patient's condition is stabilised, all patients are treated with long-term glucocorticoid or fludrocortisone replacement (or both).

The Endocrine Society's 2010 clinical practice guidelines note the following:

- Prenatal treatment for CAH should be regarded as experimental.
- Glucocorticoid therapy should be carefully titrated to avoid Cushing syndrome.
- Mineralocorticoid replacement is encouraged; in infants, mineralocorticoid replacement and sodium supplementation are encouraged.
- The use of agents to delay puberty and promote growth are experimental.
- Psychiatric support should be encouraged for patients with adjustment problems.
- Medication should be used judiciously during pregnancy and in symptomatic patients with nonclassical CAH.

Surgical care

Infants with ambiguous genitalia require surgical evaluation and plans for corrective surgery. The traditional approach to the female patient with ambiguous genitalia due to adrenal hyperplasia is clitoral recession early in life followed by vaginoplasty after puberty. Some female infants with adrenal hyperplasia have only mild virilisation and may not require corrective surgery if they receive adequate medical therapy to prevent further virilisation.

The Endocrine Society's 2010 clinical practice guidelines note the following:

- Adrenalectomy should be avoided.
- Surgical reconstruction may not be necessary during the newborn period in mildly virilised girls, but may be appropriate in severely virilised girls; it should be a single-stage genital repair, performed by experienced surgeons.

Thyroid gland

PHYSIOLOGY OF THE THYROID GLAND

The thyroid gland synthesises and secretes three hormones:

- follicular cells produce thyroxine (T_4) and triiodothyronine (T_3)
- C cells produce calcitonin.

The discussions in this chapter focus on the hormones produced by the follicular cells (referred to as thyroid hormones). For further information on calcitonin see Chapter 8.

Synthesis of thyroid hormones

Iodine uptake

Iodine is an indispensable component of the follicular cell thyroid. Ingested iodine is absorbed through the small intestine and transported in the plasma to the thyroid, where it is concentrated. Iodide uptake by thyroid cells is dependent on membrane ATPase. The protein responsible for iodide transport is the Na^+–iodide symporter. Passive transport occurs across the apical plasma membrane. The Na^+–iodide symporter is sensitive to iodine availability and stimulation by thyroid-stimulating hormone (TSH, also called thyrotrophin).

Formation of iodotyrosines and iodothyronines

After concentrating iodide, the thyroid rapidly oxidises it and binds it to tyrosyl residues in the protein thyroglobulin, followed by coupling of iodotyrosines to form T_4 and T_3.

The process requires the presence of iodide, a peroxidise (thyroid peroxidase), a supply of hydrogen peroxide

(H_2O_2) and thyroglobulin (the iodine acceptor). This process occurs at the apical plasma membrane–follicle lumen boundary. The final step in hormone synthesis is the coupling of two iodotyrosyl residues to form iodothyronine:

- two diiodotyrosines form T_4
- onc diiodotyrosine and one monoiodotyrosine form T_3.

Hormone storage and secretion

Iodination and hormone formation of thyroglobulin results in mature hormone-containing (T_4 and T_3) molecules. These are stored in the follicular lumen, where they make up the bulk of the thyroid–follicle colloid content. When stimulated by TSH, colloid is taken up into follicular cells and lysosomal enzymes release T_3 and T_4 from thyroglobulin.

Estimates of average normal secretion for euthyroid humans are about 100 micrograms/day of T_4 and 20 micrograms/day of T_3. The thyroid may also convert some T_4 to reverse T_3.

Control of thyroid hormone synthesis

TSH, released from the anterior pituitary gland, is a complex glycoprotein with a molecular weight of about 30 000 Dalton. TSH acts on G-protein-coupled transmembrane receptors on the surface of thyroid follicle cells, thereby increasing cyclic adenosine monophosphate (cAMP) and phosphatidylinositol concentrations. TSH stimulates the expression of the Na^+–iodide symporter, thyroid peroxidise and thyroglobulin and the generation of H_2O_2. TSH also increases the formation of T_3 relative to T_4, alters the priority of iodination and hormonogenesis among tyrosyls and promotes the rapid internalisation of thyroglobulin by thyrocytes. TSH forms part of a negative feedback loop and its release is inhibited by increased T_3 and T_4 serum concentrations, by somatostatin and glucocorticoids and by chronic illness (Figure 17.3). The hypothalamic tripeptide thyrotrophin-releasing hormone (TRH) stimulates the release of TSH from the thyrotrophs in the anterior pituitary and upregulates transcription of the gene encoding TSH. T_3 receptors present in the pituitary

FIGURE 17.3 **Control of thyroid hormone secretion**

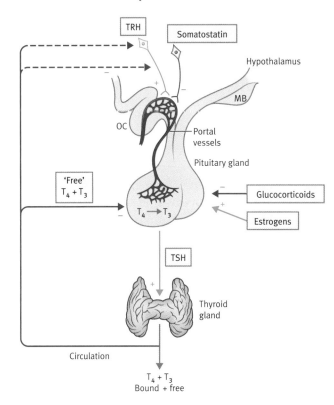

IL-1β = interleukin-1 beta | T_3 = triiodothyronine | T_4 = thyroxine | TRH = TSH-releasing hormone | TSH = thyroid-stimulating hormone | MB = mamillary bodies | OC = optic chiasm | + = stimulatory effects | – = inhibitory effects

Adapted with permission from: Nussey S, Whitehead SA. *Endocrinology: An Intergrated Approach.* Oxford: BIOS Scientific Publishers; 2001.

and hypothalamus inhibit TSH release and transcription of the gene encoding the TRH prohormone. T_3 excess also inhibits TSH release. This negative feedback system helps to maintain serum T_3 concentrations.

Transport and metabolism of thyroid hormones

Thyroid hormones circulate bound to plasma proteins. Approximately 70% are bound to T_4-binding globulin, with the rest being bound to transthyretin and albumin. Only 0.1% of T_4 and 1% of T_3 are unbound or free. Peripheral tissues can regulate local T_3 levels by increasing or decreasing T_3 synthesis. T_4 is converted to T_3 by deiodination. There are three main forms of deiodinase.

Effects of thyroid hormones

Thyroid hormones have effects on virtually every cell in the body, as reflected by the wide range of clinical manifestations caused by their lack or excess. Many actions of thyroid hormones are mediated by nuclear receptors that have a preferential affinity for T_3. Like all steroid hormone receptors, T_3 receptors are members of a family of nuclear transcription factors that, in combination with other transcription factors, regulate gene expression in target cells. Unlike some steroid receptors (such as those for sex steroids and glucocorticoids), thyroid hormone receptors exist in the nucleus, not the cytoplasm, and may remain bound to DNA in the absence of hormone binding. Thyroid hormones were once considered to be lipid soluble and able to readily cross cell membranes. It is now recognised that there are transport mechanisms in the membrane. Once inside the nucleus, T_3 binds to its receptor. This dimerises with another T_3 receptor (to form a homodimer) or with a different receptor, notably the retinoic acid receptor, to form a heterodimer. The dimers then interact with DNA. In most tissues (exceptions include the brain, spleen and testis), thyroid hormones stimulate the metabolic rate by increasing the number and size of mitochondria, stimulating the synthesis of enzymes in the respiratory chain and increasing membrane Na^+, K^+-ATPase concentration and membrane Na^+ and K^+ permeability. As much as 15–40% of a cell's resting energy expenditure is used to maintain its electrochemical gradient (pumping Na^+ out in exchange for K^+). Increasing the Na^+, K^+-ATPase activity therefore increases the resting metabolic rate.

DISEASES OF THE THYROID GLAND

Hyperthyroidism

This is defined as overactivity of the thyroid gland leading to excessive synthesis of thyroid hormones and accelerated metabolism in the peripheral tissues. The terms hyperthyroidism and thyrotoxicosis are frequently used interchangeably but the former refers to hyperfunction of the thyroid gland, while the latter refers to any state characterised by thyroid hormone excess, including ingestion of excess amounts of thyroid hormone and thyroiditis. Hyperthyroidism is a common disorder that

TABLE 17.7 **Causes of hyperthyroidism**

Cause (prevalence among those with hyperthyroidism)	Overall frequency
Graves disease[a] (80%)	Common
Toxic multinodular goitre (15%)	
Toxic adenoma ('hot' nodule) (2%)	Uncommon
Thyroiditis (1%)	
Thyrotoxicosis factitia[b] (<1%)	Rare
TSH-secreting pituitary tumour[c] (<0.01%)	
Thyroid follicular carcinoma (<0.01%)	
Trophoblastic tumour[d] (<0.001%)	

[a] Autoimmune disease with stimulating antibodies to the TSH receptor | [b] Excess T_4 ingestion to achieve weight loss and other perceived benefits associated with hyperthyroidism | [c] Must be distinguished biochemically from thyroid hormone resistance, where TSH secretion is increased because of a loss of negative-feedback effects | [d] Associated with increased concentrations of human chorionic gonadotrophin, which can stimulate the TSH receptor | TSH = thyroid-stimulating hormone

affects approximately 3% of women and 0.5% of men. The causes are given in Table 17.7, and it is noteworthy that they tend to be different at different ages. In young people aged 50 years or less, Graves disease is almost always the cause, whereas in elderly people toxic nodular goitre is a more common cause. The signs and symptoms of hyperthyroidism are summarised in Table 17.8.

Graves disease

Graves disease is an autoimmune disease that is characterised by hyperthyroidism attributable to circulating autoantibodies. In some people, Graves disease represents part of a more extensive autoimmune polyglandular syndrome.

In Graves disease, B- and T-lymphocyte-mediated autoimmunity is known to be directed at four thyroid antigens: thyroglobulin, thyroid peroxidase, the Na^+–iodide symporter and the TSH receptor. The TSH receptor itself is the primary autoantigen of Graves disease and is responsible for the manifestation of hyperthyroidism. The thyroid gland is under continuous stimulation by circulating autoantibodies against the TSH receptor and pituitary TSH secretion is suppressed because of the increased production of thyroid hormones. Antibodies to the Na^+–iodide symporter,

TABLE 17.8 **Clinical features of excess thyroid hormone**

Symptom (prevalence among those with excess thyroid hormone)	Sign (prevalence among those with excess thyroid hormone)	Overall frequency
Anxiety and irritability (>90%)	Tachycardia (100%)	Common
Palpitations (90%)	Goitre (100%)	
Increased perspiration and heat intolerance (90%)	Tremor (95%)	
Fatigability (80%)	Warm moist skin (95%)	
Weakness (70%)		
Increased appetite and weight loss (85%)		
Dyspnoea (65%)	Atrial fibrillation (10%)	Less common
Increased bowel frequency (30%)	'Liver palms' (5%)	
Oligomenorrhoea (25%)	Heart failure (5%)	
Anorexia (10%)	Onycholysis (<5%)	
Weight gain (<5%)		

Adapted with permission from: Nussey S, Whitehead SA. *Endocrinology: An Intergrated Approach*. Oxford: BIOS Scientific Publishers; 2001.

thyroglobulin and thyroid peroxidise seem to have little role in the aetiology of hyperthyroidism in Graves disease and act as markers of autoimmune disease against the thyroid. Graves disease is the most common cause of hyperthyroidism and affects more women than men, with hyperthyroidism due to Graves disease having a female-to-male ratio of 7–8 to 1. Most of the clinical features of Graves disease are related to the hyperthyroid state. Clinical features that are virtually unique to Graves disease and not associated with other causes of hyperthyroidism include ophthalmopathy and dermopathy. The thyroid gland is diffusely enlarged and smooth. A bruit may be heard as a result of increased vascularity. Very rarely gynaecomastia may be present.

Goitre

Goitre is a nonspecific term describing diffuse or nodular enlargement of the thyroid glan goitre is independent of thyroid function. The thyroid gland becomes more nodular with increasing age. In multinodular goitre, nodules typically vary in size and most multinodular goitres are asymptomatic. Multinodular goitre can be toxic or nontoxic. Toxic multinodular goitre occurs when multiple sites of autonomous nodule hyperfunction develop, resulting in thyrotoxicosis.

Diagnosis of hyperthyroidism

Assays have been developed to measure the serum concentrations of total T_4 and T_3, free thyroid hormone and TSH. Assays for TRH are not used. In hyperthyroidism, the concentrations of total and free T_4 and T_3 are elevated and the TSH level is suppressed as a result of negative feedback at the hypothalamus and pituitary gland. Subclinical hyperthyroidism has been defined as the presence of free T_4 or T_3 levels within the reference range with suppressed TSH. Subclinical hyperthyroidism can also be seen when only the levels of free T_3 are elevated, a syndrome known as T_3 toxicosis. This may be associated with toxic multinodular goitre or the ingestion of T_3. Ultrasound, CT and MRI demonstrate the anatomy, size and presence of nodules within the gland. Radioactive isotope scanning and measurements of isotope uptake are useful in differentiating the causes of hyperthyroidism. In Graves disease, the uptake of radioactive iodine is increased and diffusely distributed within the entire gland. In thyroiditis and hyperthyroidism caused by excess iodine ingestion, there is poor radioactive uptake. In multinodular goitre, isotope uptake serves to define the functional characteristics of the gland and shows multifocal areas of varying activity.

TABLE 17.9 **Pharmacological treatment of hyperthyroidism**

Drug	Indication	Advantages	Disadvantages/adverse effects
Thiocarbamides (e.g. carbimazole, propylthiouracil)	People with mild thyroid disease and small goitre People with eye disease or cardiorespiratory disease Pregnant women Children	Cheap Effective	Rash Pruritus Neutropenia Hepatitis Pneumonitis
Beta-adrenoreceptor-blocking drugs (e.g. propranolol)	Symptomatic relief (especially from cardiac symptoms) Hyperthyroid storm	Propranolol inhibits conversion of T_4 to T_3 in the liver	Asthma Heart failure
Glucocorticoids (e.g. prednisolone)	Hyperthyroid storm	Prednisolone inhibits conversion of T_4 to T_3 in the liver	Iatrogenic Cushing syndrome
Iodine (e.g. Lugol's solution)	Hyperthyroid storm Before surgery to reduce blood flow	Rapid inhibition of thyroid hormone synthesis (Wolff–Chaikoff effect)	Becomes ineffective with time
Perchlorate	Iodine-induced hyperthyroidism	Discharge of iodide excess from thyroid gland	Rash Gastric upset Lymphadenopathy Agranulocytosis Aplastic anaemia
Lithium	Second-line alternative to thiocarbamides	Inhibits T_4 and T_3 release	Lithium toxicity (tremour, ataxia, coma) Polydipsia Polyuria

Adapted with permission from: Nussey S, Whitehead SA. *Endocrinology: An Intergrated Approach*. Oxford: BIOS Scientific Publishers; 2001.

Treatment of hyperthyroidism

Treatment of hyperthyroidism involves alleviation of symptoms and correction of the thyrotoxic state. Correction of the high thyroid hormone levels can be achieved with antithyroid drugs, radioactive iodine or surgery, each of which has advantages and disadvantages. Factors to consider in determining the therapeutic modality include the age of the person to be treated, the size of the goitre and the presence of coexisting medical conditions that affect anaesthetic and operative risks. Two types of drugs are used to inhibit thyroid hormone synthesis and release, namely thioamides and iodine

(see also Table 17.9). Thioamides (such as carbimazole and propylthiouracil) inhibit thyroid hormone synthesis by competing with the tyrosyl residues of thyroglobulin for oxidised iodine, thereby inhibiting thyroid peroxidase. Propylthiouracil tends to be prescribed to pregnant and lactating women because it binds to plasma proteins and crosses the placenta or enters the breast milk in smaller amounts. It also has the added advantage of reducing the hepatic conversion of the less active T_4 to T_3. Iodine is the fastest-acting antithyroid agent, reducing thyroid hormone synthesis within 3 days through a presumed autoregulatory mechanism. Perchlorate also reduces thyroid hormone synthesis but this agent is no longer used routinely because it is relatively toxic with adverse effects on bone marrow. Destruction of thyroid tissue is the alternative to drug therapy. This can be done surgically or using radioactive isotopes of iodine. Treatment with iodine-131 (^{131}I) is safe; many clinicians now use a fixed dose of isotope and aim to produce hypothyroidism. Once hypothyroidism is induced, the person can be treated with oral T$_4$, which is cheap, effective and easy to monitor. ^{131}I is also used to treat euthyroid goitres (so as to avoid surgery) and such treatment usually reduces the volume of the thyroid gland. It is contraindicated in children, pregnant women and women who are breastfeeding. Women of child-bearing age should wait for at least 4 months after ^{131}I therapy before becoming pregnant.

Thyroid surgery is usually restricted to large and unsightly goitres that are not treatable medically or with radioactive iodine.

Hypothyroidism

Hypothyroidism is a common endocrine disorder that results from deficiency of thyroid hormone. The causes are given in Table 17.10 and the signs and symptoms in Table 17.11. Worldwide, iodine deficiency remains the foremost cause of hypothyroidism. In areas of adequate iodine intake, autoimmune thyroid disease (Hashimoto thyroiditis) is the most common cause of hypothyroidism. The prevalence of antibodies is higher in women and increases with age. Unlike Graves disease, T-cell mediated actions in Hashimoto thyroiditis result in thyroid gland destruction rather than stimulation.

Chronic autoimmune thyroiditis (Hashimoto thyroiditis)

Hashimoto thyroiditis is similar to Graves disease in that it has an autoimmune aetiology and occurs with about the same incidence and with the same sex bias, peak age of presentation and family history of thyroid disease or related autoimmune diseases. It differs in being associated with cell-mediated destruction of the gland. When a goitre is present, it is the result of diffuse lymphocytic infiltration (which gives it a number of alternative names such as chronic lymphocytic thyroiditis), together with TSH-stimulated hyperplasia of surviving thyroid tissue owing to loss of feedback inhibition from the thyroid hormones.

TABLE 17.10 **Causes of hypothyroidism**[a]

Type of hypothyroidism	Overall frequency	Cause
Primary hypothyroidism	Common (95%)	Hashimoto's disease[b]
		Primary (atrophic) hypothyroidism[c]
		Radioiodine therapy[d]
		Surgery of the thyroid gland
	Uncommon (5%)	Thyroiditis (nonlymphocytic)
		Genetic defect resulting in impaired T$_4$ synthesis
		Antithyroid drugs
	Rare (<1%)	Loss-of-function mutation in the gene encoding the TSH receptor
		Thyroid hormone resistance
Secondary (pituitary) hypothyroidism	1%	Hypopituitarism caused by a tumour, surgery or radiotherapy
		Impaired TSH synthesis
Tertiary (hypothalamic) hypothyroidism	<1%	Hypothalamic damage caused by a tumour, radiotherapy or trauma

[a] In most Western countries, iodine deficiency is not a cause of hypothyroidism; it is a major cause in iodine-deficient areas | [b] Autoimmune thyroid destruction | [c] Probably end-stage Hashimoto disease | [d] Destroys thyroid tissue

TABLE 17.11 **Clinical features of hypothyroidism**

Overall frequency	Symptoms (prevalence among those with hypothyroidism)	Signs (prevalence among those with hypothyroidism)
Common	Fatigue (90%)	Dry, scaly skin (90%)
	Cold intolerance (80%)	Puffy eyes (90%)
	Depression (70%)	Hair loss or dryness (70%)
	Poor concentration (65%)	Coarse, brittle thinning hair (60%)
	Musculoskeletal aches and pains (25%)	Bradycardia (40%)
	Carpal tunnel syndrome (15%)	
Rare	Constipation	Anaemia
	Hoarse voice	Oedema
	Menorrhagia	Cerebellar signs[a]
		Deafness[a]
		Psychosis[a]

[a] Cerebellar ataxia, deafness and myxoedema madness are commonly cited as signs of hypothyroidism but in clinical practice these signs are unusual and only seen in very severe disease

Other features of Hashimoto thyroiditis are antibodies against thyroid peroxidase and thyroglobulin. Some people are affected by a period of hyperthyroidism, which is termed hashitoxicosis, but the degree of hyperthyroidism is usually milder than that in Graves disease.

Diagnosis of primary hypothyroidism

In primary hypothyroidism caused by decreased function of the thyroid gland itself, the total and free concentrations of T_4 and T_3 are low and the levels of TSH are elevated as a result of negative feedback at the hypothalamus and pituitary gland.

Subclinical hypothyroidism has been defined as a free T_4 or free T_3 level within the reference range with an elevated thyrotrophin. The presence of thyroid autoantibodies (antimicrosomal or antithyroid peroxidase antibodies) and antithyroglobulin is typical for autoimmune hypothyroidism. The occurrence of antithyroid peroxidase antibodies has been associated with a higher risk of infertility and miscarriage.

Diagnosis of secondary hypothyroidism

Hypothyroidism can also arise because of a loss of TSH secretion from either pituitary or hypothalamic dysfunction (secondary and tertiary hypothyroidism, respectively). In these situations, TSH concentrations do not increase in appropriate relation to the low T_4 and T_3 concentrations. The absolute levels of TSH may be in the normal or even slightly elevated range but they are inappropriately low for the severity of the hypothyroid state.

Hence, when secondary or tertiary hypothyroidism is suspected, measurement of serum TSH alone is inadequate; the level of free T_4 should also be determined.

Treatment of hypothyroidism

The hypothyroidism treatment of choice is levothyroxine (synthetic T_4). It is chemically stable and T_4 is converted to T_3 in peripheral tissues. Measurement of TSH should be made after 6 weeks and the dose should be adjusted in increments of 25–50 micrograms.

Treatment with T_4 is also recommended in people with subclinical hypothyroidism who are positive for antithyroid microsomal antibodies. Once the appropriate dose is established, it tends to remain constant except in pregnancy, when there is a need to increase the dose by at least 50 micrograms/day to maintain normal TSH concentration.

Altered thyroid function in nonthyroidal illness

A number of changes can occur in the hypothalamo–pituitary–thyroid axis of people who are severely ill with a nonthyroidal disease. Most commonly, serum concentrations of TSH are normal or decreased, total T_4 levels are decreased and total T_3 levels are markedly decreased. This can be confused with secondary hypothyroidism. However, the primary abnormality is the decreased peripheral production of T_3 from T_4. There may be an increase in the level of reverse T_3, the magnitude of which correlates with the severity of illness. During recovery, some people have transient elevations in serum TSH concentrations (up to 20 mU/l). Thyroid function should not be evaluated in a critically ill person unless thyroid dysfunction is strongly suspected. If so, screening with TSH measurement alone is insufficient.

THYROID DISORDERS AND PREGNANCY

Changes in normal pregnancy

During pregnancy, maternal thyroid function is modulated by three factors:

- increase in the concentration of human chorionic gonadotrophin (hCG), which stimulates the thyroid gland
- increase in urinary iodide excretion, resulting in a fall in plasma iodine concentration
- increase in T_4-binding globulin during the first trimester, resulting in increased binding of T_4.

These factors are responsible for the increased demand for thyroid hormones during pregnancy. Women with hypothyroidism therefore require an increased dosage of levothyroxine during pregnancy to maintain the euthyroid state.

There is a structural similarity between hCG and TSH. Therefore, hCG possesses an intrinsic, weak thyroid-stimulating activity. In addition, homology exists between the TSH and luteinising hormone/hCG receptors. As a result, TSH levels fall predictably during the first trimester, mirroring in a reciprocal fashion the concomitant rise in hCG. The overall effect is a degree of thyroid stimulation and TSH suppression. Despite hCG-mediated stimulation of the thyroid gland, serum

concentrations of free T_4 generally remain within, or slightly above, the normal range during the first trimester. The stimulatory effects of hCG are normally confined to the first half of gestation. In certain pathological conditions, including hyperemesis gravidarum and trophoblastic tumours, hCG concentrations may increase into a range sufficient to induce biochemical hyperthyroidism. The maternal plasma concentration of inorganic iodine decreases as a result of increased glomerular filtration during pregnancy. The thyroid gland compensates by enlarging and increasing the plasma clearance of iodine to produce sufficient thyroid hormone so as to maintain the euthyroid state. This mechanism is responsible for an increase in thyroid size in pregnancy, particularly in iodine-deficient areas. Serum concentrations of T_4-binding globulin increase in pregnancy owing to the effects of estrogen. As a result, the serum concentrations of total T_3 and T_4 are elevated between weeks 6 and 12 of gestation, stabilising by midgestation. The concentrations of free thyroid hormone remain within the normal range for nonpregnant women, although they tend to decrease by 10–15% in late pregnancy. During the first trimester, serum TSH values decrease slightly in response to elevations in hCG and its intrinsic thyroid-stimulating activity. During the remainder of a normal pregnancy, serum TSH values increase but remain well within the normal range. There is evidence of maternal transfer of thyroid hormone to the fetus and there are fetal consequences of maternal hypothyroidism. The maternal thyroid provides all thyroid hormone necessary for fetal development until the fetal thyroid is able to produce sufficient amounts of endogenous hormone. Fetal TSH and T_4 are first detectable at week 10 of gestation. In a fetus at risk for thyroid dysfunction, surveillance with ultrasound may be performed, directed at detecting the presence of fetal goitre. This is of clinical relevance as fetal goitre may result in local airway compromise during delivery.

Gestational hypothyroidism

The causes, symptoms and signs of maternal hypothyroidism are the same as those in any woman of reproductive age. The requirement for thyroid hormone replacement therapy is increased during pregnancy. If untreated, hypothyroidism worsens during pregnancy and there is increased risk of fetal loss and psychoneurological deficit in the fetus. There is no evidence for an increased risk of birth defects associated with a history of maternal hypothyroidism. Women diagnosed with hypothyroidism in pregnancy should immediately be given full replacement doses of T_4 regardless of the degree of thyroid dysfunction. This will minimise further fetal exposure to the hypothyroid environment.

Therapy should be titrated rapidly in young pregnant women with no other comorbid conditions. For women on thyroid hormone replacement therapy before conception, the dose of thyroid hormone commonly has to be increased by up to 50% during pregnancy. Such women will require close follow-up during pregnancy to maintain optimal thyroid hormone concentrations. In women who have no previous history of hypothyroidism and in whom the diagnosis is made during pregnancy, thyroid hormone therapy may be discontinued during the postpartum period, with reassessment of thyroid function 5–6 weeks later. Recovery may be delayed because normal thyroid function may remain suppressed for a number of weeks after prolonged thyroid hormone therapy. Most will remain hypothyroid and will ultimately require chronic replacement therapy.

Neonatal hypothyroidism

Neonatal hypothyroidism has a number of causes, including thyroid dysgenesis and thyroid hormone resistance. Prompt identification and treatment of newborn infants with congenital hypothyroidism is vital to ensure their appropriate neuropsychological development. Identification through screening programmes, with immediate institution of replacement therapy, leads to a normal IQ at 5–7 years of age. If left untreated, neonatal and early childhood hypothyroidism results in profound mental and developmental restriction.

Gestational hyperthyroidism

Although menstrual irregularity is frequent in women with mild to moderate hyperthyroidism, fertility does not seem to be impaired. The effects of gestational hyperthyroidism include:

- effects on the mother (premature labour, pre-eclampsia, heart failure)

- effects on the fetus (neonatal mortality, low birth weight).

Mild to moderate thyrotoxicosis is not a contraindication to the continuation of pregnancy and pregnancy does not make thyrotoxicosis more difficult to control. Indeed, hyperthyroidism may be more easily controlled during pregnancy, although relapses tend to occur postpartum. Treatment of hyperthyroidism during pregnancy is similar to that in nonpregnant individuals but limited to antithyroid drugs or surgery because radioactive iodine is contraindicated. Antithyroid drugs include the thioamides (propylthiouracil and carbimazole). Pregnant women tolerate mild degrees of hyperthyroidism without great difficulty and the goal of antithyroid therapy during pregnancy is to maintain the level of free T_4 at, or slightly above, the upper limit of the normal range. Thioamides are transferred into the breast milk of women receiving these drugs but, overall, breastfeeding seems to be safe in mothers taking thioamides. Beta-blockers are not recommended for the long-term treatment of thyrotoxicosis during pregnancy.

Fetal thyrotoxicosis

Fetal thyrotoxicosis is usually caused by the placental transfer of thyroid-stimulating immunoglobulins. Maternal thyroid-stimulating antibodies may be present even when the maternal thyroid has been ablated or when the mother is in remission, as the antibodies can persist. Thus, the possibility of fetal thyrotoxicosis should be considered in all pregnant women with a history of Graves disease regardless of the current thyroid status.

The diagnosis is suggested by clinical features such as persistent fetal tachycardia, growth failure or increased fetal activity. There may be elevated concentrations of maternal thyroid-stimulating immunoglobulins and ultrasonography may detect the presence of a goitre in a thyrotoxic fetus. Fetal thyrotoxicosis is associated with increased fetal morbidity and mortality, so early diagnosis is crucial.

Antithyroid drug therapy directed specifically towards the fetus should be used and close monitoring is mandatory. After delivery, the baby should continue to be treated for thyrotoxicosis, which is usually self-limited

Management of thyroid dysfunction during pregnancy and postpartum: practice guidelines by the Endocrine Society

Management of hypothyroidism: maternal and fetal aspects

- Caution should be taken in the interpretation of serum-free T_4 levels during pregnancy. The nonpregnant total T_4 range (5–12 µg/dl or 50–150 nmol/l) can be adapted in the second and third trimesters by multiplying this range by 1.5-fold. Alternatively, the free T_4 index appears to be a reliable assay during pregnancy.
- Overt maternal hypothyroidism is known to have serious adverse effects on the fetus. Therefore, maternal hypothyroidism should be avoided.
- Subclinical hypothyroidism (SCH; serum TSH concentration above the upper limit of the trimester-specific reference range with a normal free T_4) may be associated with an adverse outcome for both the mother and offspring, as documented in antibody-positive women. In retrospective studies, T_4 treatment improved obstetrical outcome, but it has not been proved to modify long-term neurological development in the offspring. However, given that the potential benefits outweigh the potential risks, T_4 replacement is recommended in women with SCH who are thyroid peroxidase antibody positive (TPO-Ab$^+$).
- For neurological outcome, T_4 replacement is also recommended in women with SCH who are TPO-Ab negative (TPO-Ab$^-$), although evidence is poor.
- If hypothyroidism has been diagnosed before pregnancy, adjust the preconception T_4 dose to reach before pregnancy with a TSH level not higher than 2.5 mIU/l.
- The T_4 dose usually needs to be incremented by 4–6 weeks of gestation and may require a 30% or more increase in dosage.
- If overt hypothyroidism is diagnosed during pregnancy, thyroid function tests should be normalized as rapidly as possible. T_4 dosage should be titrated to rapidly reach and thereafter maintain serum TSH concentrations of less than 2.5 mIU/l (in an assay using the International Standard) in the first trimester (or 3 mIU/l in second and third trimesters) or to trimester-specific TSH ranges. Thyroid function tests should be remeasured within 30–40 days and then every 4–6 weeks.
- Women with thyroid autoimmunity who are euthyroid in the early stages of pregnancy are at risk of developing hypothyroidism and should be monitored every 4–6 weeks for elevation of TSH above the normal range for pregnancy.
- After delivery, most hypothyroid women need to decrease the T_4 dosage they received during pregnancy to the pre-pregnancy dose.

Thyroid nodules and their management in pregnancy

A solitary thyroid nodule during pregnancy is evaluated by ultrasound scan and fine-needle aspiration cytology. An ultrasound scan provides information about the size of the nodule and whether the nodule is solid or cystic. It is also useful in identifying the presence of diffuse thyroid disease and in revealing the presence of previously undetected, nonpalpable nodules. Fine-needle aspiration cytological assessment is indicated in:

- women with nodules that are larger than 1 cm in diameter
- women with enlarging nodules
- women who have nodules associated with palpable cervical lymph nodes.

If the biopsy specimen is adequate and does not reveal suspect cells, TSH suppression with T4 may be instituted for the duration of the pregnancy. If the biopsy is suggestive of malignancy, surgery is indicated.

The diagnosis of thyroid carcinoma during pregnancy is not an absolute indication for termination of the pregnancy. Pregnancy does not have a direct effect on the natural history of thyroid carcinoma. Treatment options for thyroid carcinoma during pregnancy are more limited than in the nonpregnant state as radioactive iodine is contraindicated. Thyroid surgery remains the main option.

Postpartum thyroiditis

Postpartum thyroiditis (PPT) reportedly affects 4–10% of women. PPT is an autoimmune thyroid disease that occurs during the first year after delivery. Women with

PPT present with transient thyrotoxicosis followed by hypothyroidism with return of euthyroid state by 1 year postpartum. This presentation may be unrecognised, but is important because it predisposes the woman to develop permanent hypothyroidism. The thyrotoxicosis always predates hypothyroidism and occurs between 2 and 6 months postpartum. The hypothyroid phase can occur at any time between 3 and 12 months following delivery. Women who express antithyroid peroxidase or antithyroglobulin antibodies in the first trimester of pregnancy have a 33–50% risk of developing PPT. The higher the thyroid antibody titre is, the more likely is the development of PPT. Spontaneous recovery occurs in 90% of women with PPT, but the risk of recurrence after subsequent pregnancies is as high as 25%. In fact, there is an increased risk of developing permanent hypothyroidism, particularly in those with high titres of antithyroid peroxidase antibodies, so follow-up is recommended. The signs and symptoms of PPT are often subtle. Many of them, such as fatigue, irritability and fluctuations in weight, are common in the postpartum period. A painless small goitre is palpable in half the women with postpartum thyroiditis. The laboratory diagnosis of thyrotoxicosis in postpartum thyroiditis is based on high levels of free T_4 with suppression of TSH on thyroid function tests. In contrast to Graves disease, the uptake of radioisotopes such as technetium in PPT is low. Like primary hypothyroidism, the subsequent hypothyroid phase is diagnosed by an increased serum TSH concentration and a decreased serum T_4 concentration.

Symptoms of autoimmune thyroid diseases tend to improve during pregnancy. A postpartum exacerbation is not uncommon and perhaps occurs because of an alteration in the maternal immune system during pregnancy.

Thioamide drugs are the first-line treatment in pregnancy. Propylthiouracil (PTU), methimazole (MMI) and carbimazole (CMI) are the antithyroid drugs (ATD). A controversial association exists between MMI and fetal scalp defects, aplastic cutis and choanal and/or oesophageal atresia. Therefore, PTU tends to be the first choice in this class of drugs.

The US Food and Drug Administration (FDA) had added a boxed warning to the prescribing information for PTU. The boxed warning emphasises the risk for severe liver injury and acute liver failure, some of which have been fatal. It also states that PTU should be reserved for use in those who cannot tolerate other treatments such as MMI, radioactive iodine or surgery.

Doses of ATDs should be maintained at the lowest dose needed to keep the mother's free F_4 level in the high–normal range. Weight gain, pulse rate, free F_4 results and TSH levels should be monitored monthly.

Gestational thyrotoxicosis

Gestational thyrotoxicosis is a transient, mild hyperthyroidism that occurs early in pregnancy and is not due to intrinsic thyroid disease. Human chorionic gonadotropin, which peaks during the first trimester, has the ability to stimulate the thyroid TSH receptor. Women with higher levels or enhanced activity of human chorionic gonadotropin have elevated T_4 levels and suppressed TSH concentrations. Gestational thyrotoxicosis has been documented in up to 10–15% of pregnant women, and it commonly occurs in several situations like multiple gestations, hyperemesis gravidarum, hydatidiform mole and in familial gestational thyrotoxicosis (thyrotropin receptor mutation).

In most cases, the symptoms of gestational thyrotoxicosis are mild, mainly nausea, and sometimes vomiting, resolving spontaneously by 20 weeks of gestation. The most severe form of gestational thyrotoxicosis is hyperemesis gravidarum, known as transient hyperthyroidism of hyperemesis gravidarum, characterised by severe nausea and vomiting, dehydration, weight loss and ketonuria. In very severe cases, hospitalisation and parental nutrition are needed. Distinguishing this condition from Graves hyperthyroidism may be challenging. Treatment with an antithyroid drug is not indicated because the symptoms subside spontaneously with progression of pregnancy, with normalisation of T_4 levels by 14–20 weeks of gestation. In some patients, serum TSH may remain suppressed or below normal after normalisation of serum T_4.

Endocrine pancreas

PHYSIOLOGY OF THE ENDOCRINE PANCREAS

The pancreas has both digestive and hormonal functions. The enzymes secreted by the exocrine tissue in the pancreas help to break down carbohydrates, fats, proteins and acids in the duodenum. The exocrine tissue also secretes bicarbonate to neutralise stomach acid in the duodenum. The hormones secreted by the endocrine tissue in the pancreas include insulin, glucagon, somatostatin, gastrin, vasoactive intestinal peptide (VIP) and pancreatic polypeptide.

Insulin

Insulin is a protein with a molecular weight of about 6000 Dalton and is composed of two chains held together by disulphide bonds. The insulin mRNA is translated into a single-chain precursor protein called preproinsulin. Removal of the precursor's signal peptide during insertion into the endoplasmic reticulum generates proinsulin. Proinsulin consists of three domains: an amino-terminal B chain, a carboxy-terminal A chain and a connecting peptide in the middle known as the C peptide. Within the endoplasmic reticulum, proinsulin is exposed to several specific endopeptidases that excise the C peptide, thereby generating the mature form of insulin. When the beta cell is appropriately stimulated, insulin is secreted from the cell by exocytosis and diffuses into islet capillary blood. Insulin is secreted after an oral glucose load. The early insulin response to glucose (at 30 minutes) is due to neuronal stimulation, whereas the late response (at 120 minutes) is primarily due to elevated blood concentrations of glucose. Glucose is transported into the beta cell by facilitated diffusion via a glucose transporter.

This leads to membrane depolarisation and an influx of extracellular Ca^{2+}. The resulting increase in intracellular Ca^{2+} is thought to be one of the primary triggers for exocytosis of insulin-containing secretory granules. Increased levels of glucose within beta cells also seem to activate Ca^{2+}-independent pathways that participate in insulin secretion.

The receptor for insulin is a tyrosine kinase that is embedded in the plasma membrane. It is composed of two alpha subunits and two beta subunits, which are linked by disulphide bonds.

The major targets for the anabolic actions of insulin are:

- liver
- adipose tissue
- muscle.

In the liver, insulin promotes glycogen synthesis by stimulating glycogen synthetase and inhibiting glycogen phosphorylase. Insulin induces the rapid uptake of glucose in muscle and fat tissue and as a consequence muscle converts glucose to glycogen. In adipose tissue, glucose is converted to fatty acids for storage as triglyceride. Insulin also stimulates the uptake of amino acids into muscle. At the same time, insulin suppresses the mobilisation of fuels by inhibiting the breakdown of glycogen in the liver, the release of amino acids from muscle and the release of free fatty acids from adipose tissue. This partly explains weight loss in people with diabetes, despite normal or increased appetite.

Glucagon

Glucagon is a linear peptide of 29 amino acids that is initially synthesised as proglucagon, which is proteolytically processed within alpha cells of the pancreatic islets to yield glucagon. It is secreted in response to hypoglycaemia. Other stimuli of glucagon secretion include elevated serum concentrations of amino acids and exercise. Glucagon secretion is inhibited by high levels of blood glucose, either as a direct effect of glucose on the alpha cells or as a result of insulin secretion by the beta cells. Glucagon secretion is also inhibited by somatostatin.

Glucagon has counter-regulatory actions to insulin, promoting the mobilisation of fuels, particularly glucose. Its primary action is on the liver, where it stimulates the breakdown of glycogen to glucose and the production of glucose from amino acids (gluconeogenesis). In addition, it stimulates the release of free fatty acids from adipose tissue. Glucagon is both a hyperglycaemic and a ketogenic hormone. By and large, it is the molar ratio of insulin to glucagon in the portal blood that governs the metabolic state of the liver.

Somatostatin

Somatostatin is secreted by a broad range of tissues, including the pancreas, the gastrointestinal tract and regions of the central nervous system outside the hypothalamus. Two forms of somatostatin are synthesised, termed somatostatin 14 and somatostatin 28 in reflection of the length of their amino acid chains. Both forms of somatostatin are generated by proteolytic cleavage of prosomatostatin. Somatostatin 14 is the predominant form produced in the nervous system, whereas the intestine secretes mostly somatostatin 28. The two forms have different biological potencies. Somatostatin 28 is nearly ten times more potent than somatostatin 14 in inhibiting the secretion of growth hormone, but less potent than somatostatin 14 in inhibiting the release of glucagon.

Five somatostatin receptors have been identified, all members of the G-protein-coupled receptor superfamily. Four of the five receptors do not differentiate between somatostatin 14 and somatostatin 28.

Somatostatin acts by both endocrine and paracrine pathways to affect its target cells and inhibit the secretion of many other hormones, including growth hormone, from the pituitary gland.

In the pancreas, somatostatin seems to act primarily in a paracrine manner to inhibit the secretion of both insulin and glucagon. It also suppresses pancreatic exocrine secretions by inhibiting the cholecystokinin-stimulated secretion of enzymes and the secretin-stimulated secretion of bicarbonate.

In the gastrointestinal tract, somatostatin inhibits the secretion of many of the other gastrointestinal hormones. Moreover, somatostatin suppresses the secretion of gastric acid and pepsin, lowers the rate of gastric emptying and reduces smooth muscle contractions and blood flow within the intestine. These activities seem to have the overall effect of decreasing the rate of nutrient absorption.

Vasoactive intestinal peptide

VIP is a peptide hormone that contains 28 amino acids and is produced in many areas of the human body, including the gut, the pancreas and the suprachiasmatic nuclei of the hypothalamus in the brain. In the digestive system, the roles of VIP are stimulation of H_2O and electrolyte secretion, dilatation of peripheral blood vessels, stimulation of pancreatic bicarbonate secretion and inhibition of the gastrin-stimulated secretion of gastric acid. VIP acts via two known VIP-specific receptors, termed VPAC1 and VPAC2.

Gastrin

Gastrin is a linear peptide synthesised as a preprohormone that is cleaved to form a family of peptides. The predominant circulating form is gastrin-34 (big gastrin), but biological activity is present even in the smallest peptide (gastrin-14 or minigastrin). In fact, full bioactivity is preserved in the five carboxy-terminal amino acids of gastrin, known as pentagastrin. Gastrin is synthesised in G cells, which are located in gastric pits found primarily in the antrum of the stomach. The hormone binds receptors that are found predominantly on parietal and enterochromaffin-like cells. These receptors also bind cholecystokinin and are known as gastrin/cholecystokinin type B receptors. They belong to the family of G-protein-coupled receptors. Gastrin is a major physiological regulator of gastric acid secretion and has a growth-promoting influence on the gastric mucosa. The primary stimulus for the secretion of gastrin is the presence of certain foodstuffs (especially peptides, certain amino acids and Ca^{2+}) in the gastric lumen. Secretion of this hormone is inhibited when the lumenal pH of the stomach becomes very low.

ENDOCRINE DISEASES OF THE PANCREAS

Diabetes mellitus

The term diabetes mellitus describes a group of metabolic diseases that are characterised by hyperglycaemia resulting from defects in insulin secretion, insulin action or both. Diabetes mellitus is diagnosed on the basis of symptom history plus fulfilment of one of the following criteria:

- a random venous plasma glucose concentration of at least 11.1 mmol/l
- a fasting plasma glucose concentration of at least 7.0 mmol/l
- a plasma glucose concentration of at least 11.1 mmol/l 2 hours after administration of 75 g anhydrous glucose in an oral glucose tolerance test (OGTT).

In the absence of symptoms, the diagnosis should not be made on the basis of single glucose estimation. At least one additional glucose test result on another day with a value in the diabetic range is essential, with the blood sample taken either randomly, after fasting or 2 hours after a glucose load. The diagnosis should never be based solely on the finding of glycosuria.

In January 2011 the World Health Organization (WHO) recommended that glycated haemoglobin (HbA1c) could be used as an alternative to standard glucose measures to diagnose type 2 diabetes among non-pregnant adults. A normal fasting blood glucose reading is generally defined as a level below 6 mmol/l. Impaired fasting glucose is defined by values between 6.0 mmol/l and 7.0 mmol/l. Impaired glucose tolerance is recognised with serum glucose values between 7.8 mmol/l and 11.1 mmol/l 2 hours after administration of 75 g of oral glucose. HbA1c levels of 6.5% (48 mmol/mol) or above indicate that someone has type 2 diabetes, but there is no fixed point to indicate when someone has 'pre-diabetes'. The WHO recommendation stated that someone with increasing levels of HbA1c, up to the 6.5% (48 mmol/mol) cut-off point, is at increased risk of type 2 diabetes. The report also recognised that there is a continuum of risk across a range of sub-diabetic HbA1c levels.

Type 1 diabetes

Type 1 diabetes mellitus is considered to be a T-lymphocyte dependent autoimmune disease that is characterised by infiltration and destruction of the beta cells in the islets of Langerhans. Studies in twins have clearly established a major genetic element to type 1 diabetes mellitus. However, in fewer than half of instances where one twin of an identical pair has the disease, the other will develop it as well. Currently, autoimmunity is considered to be the major factor in the pathophysiology of type 1 diabetes mellitus. The prevalence is increased in people with other autoimmune diseases, such as Graves disease, Hashimoto thyroiditis and Addison's disease. Approximately 85% of people with type 1 diabetes mellitus have circulating islet cell antibodies and the majority will have detectable anti-insulin antibodies before receiving insulin therapy. Most islet cell antibodies are directed against glutamic acid decarboxylase within pancreatic beta cells. Environmental factors that have been hypothesised to induce an attack on beta-cell function include viruses (for example mumps virus, rubella virus, Coxsackie B4 virus), toxic chemicals, cytotoxins and exposure to cow's milk in infancy.

Type 1 diabetes mellitus is predominantly a disease of white populations. It tends to develop after the age of 20 years. Overall, it occurs with equal frequency in men and women and there are increases in incidence around puberty and before starting school.

Patients with type 1 diabetes mellitus require lifelong insulin therapy to control hyperglycaemia. Most require two or more injections of insulin daily, with doses adjusted on the basis of self-monitoring of blood glucose levels. Long-term management requires a multidisciplinary approach that includes physicians, nurses, dietitians and selected specialists. The goal of insulin treatment is to keep blood glucose levels at normal or near-normal levels. Different types of insulin are available and these vary with respect to onset and duration of action. Careful control of blood glucose levels can help to prevent both the short-term effects of poorly controlled blood glucose, such as diabetic ketoacidosis, and the long-term effects, such as complications of the eye, kidney and cardiovascular system.

Pancreatic transplantation for patients with type 1 diabetes mellitus is a possibility in some referral centers. It is performed most commonly with simultaneous kidney transplantation for end-stage renal disease (ESRD).

Type 2 diabetes

Type 2 diabetes mellitus is characterised by:

- hyperglycaemia
- insulin resistance
- relative impairment of insulin secretion.

It is a common disorder with a prevalence that rises markedly with increasing degrees of obesity. For type 2 diabetes mellitus to develop, both insulin deficiency and defects of insulin resistance must coexist. All overweight individuals have insulin resistance but only those with an inability to increase beta cell production of insulin develop diabetes. About 90% of people who develop type 2 diabetes mellitus are obese. Relative insulin deficiency owing to damaged beta cells also results in a lack of glucagon suppression and this further contributes to hyperglycaemia. People with type 2 diabetes mellitus retain the ability to secrete some endogenous insulin and generally do not develop diabetic ketoacidosis.

Type 2 diabetes is often accompanied by other clinical features, such as hypertension and a dyslipidaemia, including high serum levels of low-density lipoprotein (LDL) cholesterol and low serum levels of high-density lipoprotein (HDL) cholesterol. This constellation of clinical conditions is referred to as metabolic syndrome and is associated with an increased risk of cardiovascular disease.

Treatment of diabetes mellitus

Diabetes is associated with serious complications that are generally divided into:

- microvascular complications (including retinopathy, nephropathy and neuropathy)
- macrovascular complications (including atherosclerotic disease of the coronary, carotid and femoral arteries).

Since the complications of diabetes are, by and large, related to the duration of the disease and the degree of blood sugar control, much effort is made to control blood glucose. A sensible approach to diet, control of body weight and exercise is therefore important in all forms of the disease. It is also important to manage dyslipidaemia and blood pressure. Dietary modification is fundamental to the long-term treatment of all forms of diabetes mellitus. The generally recommended diet, the so-called healthy eating diet, contains more than 55% of carbohydrate, 10–15% of protein and less than 30% of fat (of which less than 10% saturates). In general, no further dietary modification is required other than to reduce sources of simple sugars (less than 25g/day of added sucrose) and replace them with complex carbohydrates. Glycaemic control is judged by measurement of the HbA1c level. An optimal HbA1c value for a person with diabetes lies between 6.5% and 7.0%. The majority of people with type 2 diabetes have inadequate glycaemic control. Monotherapy will fail by the end of 9 years in 75%. To achieve ideal glycaemic control in type 2 diabetes, early aggressive combination therapy is recommended, not allowing the HbA1c level to go above 7.8%. Recommendations for the treatment of type 2 diabetes mellitus from the European Association for the Study of Diabetes (EASD) and the American Diabetes Association (ADA) place the patient's condition, desires, abilities and tolerances at the centre of the decision-making process. The EASD/ADA position statement contains seven key points:

1. Individualised glycaemic targets and glucose-lowering therapies.
2. Diet, exercise and education as the foundation of the treatment programme.
3. Use of metformin as the optimal first-line drug unless contraindicated.
4. After metformin, the use of one or two additional oral or injectable agents, with a goal of minimising adverse effects if possible.
5. Ultimately, insulin therapy alone or with other agents if needed to maintain blood glucose control.
6. Where possible, all treatment decisions should involve the patient, with a focus on patient preferences, needs and values.
7. A major focus on comprehensive cardiovascular risk reduction.

Pharmacotherapy includes the use of:

- Biguanides
- Sulphonylureas
- Meglitinide derivatives
- Alpha-glucosidase inhibitors
- Thiazolidinediones (TZDs)
- Glucagon-like peptide-1 (GLP-1) agonists
- Dipeptidyl peptidase-4 (DPP-4) inhibitors
- Selective sodium-glucose transporter-2 (SGLT-2) inhibitors
- Insulins.

Biguanide

Metformin reduces the release of hepatic glucose and is considered to be a first-line therapy in overweight and non-overweight people. Metformin lowers basal and postprandial plasma glucose level. It reduces cardiovascular outcomes in obese individuals but can cause gastrointestinal adverse effects. It rarely causes hypoglycaemia.

Metformin is contraindicated in patients with impaired renal function. It also should not be used within 48 hours of intravenous iodinated contrast medium.

Sulphonylureas

Sulphonylureas function by stimulating the release of insulin from pancreatic beta cells and can usually reduce

HbA1c by 1–2% and blood glucose concentrations by about 20%. They are effective hypoglycaemic agents, but are associated with weight gain, hypoglycaemia and accelerated beta-cell exhaustion.

Meglitinides

Meglitinides are much more short-acting insulin secretagogues than sulphonylureas. Preprandial dosing potentially achieves more physiological insulin release and less risk for hypoglycaemia. Meglitinide monotherapy has efficacy similar to that of sulphonylureas.

Alpha-glucosidase inhibitors

Alpha-glucosidase inhibitors prolong the absorption of carbohydrates and thus help to prevent postprandial glucose surges. Their induction of flatulence greatly limits their use. Doses of these agents should be titrated slowly to reduce gastrointestinal intolerance. Their effect on glycaemic control is modest, affecting primarily postprandial glycaemic excursions

Thiazolidinediones

TZDs reduce insulin resistance in the periphery (sensitise muscle and fat to the actions of insulin) and to a small degree in the liver. They activate peroxisome proliferator-activated receptor (PPAR) gamma, a nuclear transcription factor that is important in fat cell differentiation and fatty acid metabolism. These drugs may have beta-cell preservation properties. TZDs have moderate glycaemic efficacy. These agents can be used as monotherapy or in combination therapy, but they may be associated with modest weight gain. They must be taken for 12–16 weeks to achieve maximal effect. The side effects include fluid retention, worsening of heart failure, increased risk of fractures and bladder cancer. Rosiglitazone has been banned in Europe and restricted in the USA because of increased cardiovascular morbidity. Pioglitazone has been banned in France and black-box warnings have been applied in the USA because of bladder cancer.

Incretins are gut-derived factors that increase glucose-stimulated insulin secretion. There are two incretin hormones:

- GLP-1 produced in the ileum and colon; and
- gastric inhibitory peptide produced in the jejunum.

GLP-1 analogues

These agonists have a novel mechanism of action: they mimic the endogenous incretin GLP-1, stimulating glucose-dependent insulin release (as opposed to oral insulin secretagogues, which may cause nonglucose-dependent insulin release and hypoglycaemia), reducing glucagon and slowing gastric emptying. These are available as subcutaneous injections.

Dipeptidyl peptidase 4 inhibitors

DPP-4 inhibitors work by blocking the action of DPP-4, an enzyme that destroys the hormone incretin. They increase insulin release and decrease glucagon levels in the circulation in a glucose-dependent manner. GLP-1 action can be enhanced by the use of the oral DPP-4 inhibitor. These are used once daily, orally, and are weight neutral. These drugs can be used as a monotherapy or in combination with other oral hypoglycaemic and insulin treatment.

SGLT-2 inhibitors

SGLT-2 inhibitors reduce glucose reabsorption in the proximal renal tubules and lower the renal threshold for glucose, thereby increasing urinary glucose excretion. They are indicated as an adjunct to diet and exercise to improve glycaemic control in type 2 diabetes mellitus. They are indicated as monotherapy, as initial therapy with metformin, or as an add-on to other oral glucose-lowering agents and insulin.

Insulins

Most newly diagnosed persons with type 1 diabetes can be started on a total daily insulin dose of 0.2–0.4 U/kg. The majority will ultimately require 0.6–0.7 U/kg daily.

Adolescents often need more, especially during puberty. About one in three people diagnosed with type 2 diabetes will require insulin at some stage.

Indications for insulin therapy in type 2 diabetes are:

- symptoms of hyperglycaemia such as polyuria, thirst, recurrent fungal infections or bacterial infections
- pregnancy or planning pregnancy
- oral hypoglycaemic treatments not tolerated or contra-indicated
- weight loss
- painful neuropathy
- foot ulceration and infection.

There are different types of insulins. These are classified by how fast they start to work, when they reach their 'peak' level of action and how long their effects last.

The types of insulin include:

- Rapid-acting insulin, which starts working within a few minutes and lasts for a couple of hours.
- Regular- or short-acting insulin, which takes about 30 minutes to work fully and lasts for 3–6 hours.
- Intermediate-acting insulin, which takes 2–4 hours to work fully, and its effects can last for up to 18 hours.
- Long-acting insulin, which takes 6–10 hours to reach peak levels in the bloodstream, and can keep working for 24 hours.

There are two schemes for insulin treatment:

- Approximately one-half of the total dose should be given as a basal insulin. This can be either as once per-day long-acting insulin or as twice-per-day intermediate-acting insulin (isophane). Long-acting insulin can be given either at bedtime or in the morning.
- The remainder of the total daily insulin requirement is given as short-acting or rapid-acting insulin before meals (sliding scale insulin therapy).

The pre-meal dose is determined before each individual meal, taking into account the carbohydrate content of the meal, the blood glucose level and the activity level.

The treatment targets for diabetes are widely accepted and include a fasting blood sugar level below 7 mmol/l, an HbA1c value of no more than 6.5%, a systolic blood pressure below 130 mmHg, a diastolic blood pressure below 80 mmHg, a total cholesterol level below 4 mmol/l, an HDL cholesterol level above 1 mmol/l, an LDL cholesterol level below 2 mmol/l and a triglyceride level below 1.5 mmol/l.

Insulin pumps

Continuous subcutaneous insulin infusion or 'insulin pump' therapy is recommended as a possible treatment for adults and children 12 years and over with type 1 diabetes mellitus if:

- Attempts to reach target HbA1c levels with multiple daily injections result in the person having disabling hypoglycaemia; or
- HbA1c levels remain high 8.5% or above with multiple daily injections, including long-acting insulin analogues, despite the person and/or their carer carefully trying to manage their diabetes.

Endocrine tumours of the pancreas

The cells in pancreatic endocrine neoplasms are termed amine precursor uptake and decarboxylation (APUD) cells because they have a high amine content, are capable of amine precursor uptake and contain an amino acid decarboxylase. Most pancreatic endocrine neoplasms discovered clinically are functional apudomas and are named after the predominant secreted hormone. Thus, the following apudomas exist:

- insulinoma
- gastrinoma (also termed Zollinger–Ellison syndrome)
- glucagonoma
- VIPoma (Verner–Morrison syndrome)
- somatostatinoma.

The clinical features in people with functional pancreatic endocrine neoplasms reflect the physiological derangements related to the normal action of the hormonal product that the tumours overproduce. By contrast, people with nonfunctional pancreatic endocrine neoplasms typically present later in the course of their disease, when their tumours begin to cause symptoms related to mass effect. To a large extent, investigation of pancreatic endocrine neoplasms consists of demonstrating that the concentrations of circulating hormone are inappropriate to the clinical situation.

Treatment

Endocrine tumours of the pancreas usually grow slowly and have a relatively low metastatic potential. Definitive treatment is surgical removal. Medical treatment with somatostatin analogues may control symptoms in tumours that express somatostatin receptors. Proton pump inhibitors have a major role in providing symptomatic relief in the case of gastrinomas. Embolisation or radiofrequency ablation may be useful for hepatic metastases.

ENDOCRINE PANCREAS AND PREGNANCY

Glucose metabolism during pregnancy

Pregnancy changes both basal and postprandial glucose metabolism as early as by the end of the first trimester. In the nonpregnant state, the liver is the predominant source of endogenous glucose production. Normal pregnancy (especially late pregnancy) is associated with reduced levels of fasting plasma glucose and increased levels of fasting insulin, presumably because of an increase in glucose uptake by the fetal and placental unit. Despite these changes, maternal hepatic glucose production is increased, suggesting reduced hepatic insulin sensitivity or the presence of hepatic insulin resistance to increase glucose availability to the fetus in the fasted state. Postprandial glucose values are slightly elevated in association with maternal postprandial hyperinsulinaemia, especially in the second and third trimester.

The physiological factors responsible for the decrease of insulin sensitivity or the development of insulin resistance in pregnancy are not fully known. The metabolic effects of several hormones (including human placental lactogen, progesterone, prolactin and cortisol) and cytokines (including tumour necrosis factor alpha [TNF-α]) have been implicated; their levels are elevated in the maternal circulation during pregnancy. An increase in TNF-α concentration is associated with decreased insulin sensitivity in a number of conditions, including obesity, ageing and sepsis.

In normal pregnancy, there are progressive increases in insulin concentration with advancing gestation. These increases are more pronounced in lean women than in obese women because lean women tend to begin their pregnancies with better insulin sensitivity. Lean women have a greater total decrease in insulin sensitivity than obese women with normal glucose tolerance. Increased insulin secretion during pregnancy represents compensation for progressive insulin resistance. However, insulin secretion increases by as much as 50% early in the second trimester before insulin resistance of pregnancy becomes manifest. Pregnancy may therefore exert a primary effect to increase insulin secretion independent of the presence of insulin resistance.

Lipid metabolism during pregnancy

Significant alterations during pregnancy also occur in lipid metabolism. Women who are not obese gain approximately 3.5 kg of fat during normal pregnancy, but there is a wide variation both within and between various ethnic and racial groups. Subcutaneous fat mass, primarily centrally distributed, significantly increases in early gestation. There is an increase in both preperitoneal and subcutaneous fat regions by the late third trimester of pregnancy. The increases in visceral fat may relate to the decreases in insulin sensitivity in late gestation.

Lipid metabolism differs between lean and obese women with normal glucose metabolism.

Total triglyceride concentrations increase two- to four-fold and total cholesterol concentrations increase by 25–50% during normal human pregnancy. There is a 50% increase in LDL cholesterol and a 30% increase in HDL cholesterol by midgestation, followed by a slight decrease in HDL cholesterol at term. There is also an increase in the concentration of free fatty acids in late pregnancy.

Fetal endocrine pancreas

The fetal pancreas appears during the fourth week of fetal life. The alpha cells, which contain glucagon, and the delta cells, which contain somatostatin, develop before differentiation of the beta cells. Human pancreatic insulin and glucagon concentrations increase with advancing fetal age and are higher than the concentrations found in the adult pancreas. In maternal diabetes mellitus, fetal islet cells undergo hypertrophy such that the rate of insulin secretion increases.

Diabetes in pregnancy

Abnormal maternal glucose regulation occurs in 3–10% of pregnancies. The prevalence of diabetes mellitus among women of childbearing age is increasing worldwide. This increase is attributable to more sedentary lifestyles, changes in diet, continued immigration from high-risk populations and an epidemic of childhood and adolescent obesity. Gestational diabetes mellitus (GDM) accounts for 90% of the total incidence of diabetes in pregnancy.

Gestational diabetes mellitus

The term GDM refers to carbohydrate intolerance that is first identified during pregnancy. GDM is characterised as follows:

- Women with GDM have increased fasting glucose concentrations. In obese women with GDM, the fasting insulin concentration also rises and is greater than in women without GDM. The increase in circulating glucose concentrations despite increased insulin concentrations suggests an imbalance between the requirements for tissue insulin needed for the regulation of the glucose metabolism and the ability of the pancreatic beta cells to meet those requirements.
- There is an increase in insulin resistance from the time before conception through early pregnancy (weeks 12–14 of gestation), particularly in women with reduced insulin sensitivity before conception.
- There is failure to suppress the hepatic production of free fatty acids.

In GDM, insulin signalling changes do not only occur at the postreceptor level, as seen in a normal pregnancy; tyrosine phosphorylation of the insulin-receptor beta subunit is also impaired. This defect is not found in either pregnant or nonpregnant women with normal glucose tolerance and results in a 25% decrease in glucose transport activity. These receptor defects may

contribute in part to the pathogenesis of GDM and the increased risk of type 2 diabetes later in life.

In addition to the previously mentioned changes, women with GDM also have a decreased serum concentration of adiponectin and this change correlates with decreased insulin sensitivity and impaired glucose disposal. Adiponectin is a hormone that is secreted from adipose tissue and serum concentrations are negatively associated with obesity, hyperinsulinaemia and insulin resistance. Adiponectin and TNF-α produce opposing effects on insulin signalling (adiponectin increases insulin sensitivity whereas TNF-α reduces it).

GDM results from inadequate insulin secretion that arises in women with chronic insulin resistance and is therefore related to type 2 diabetes. The range of beta cell defects in GDM could be similar to the spectrum of beta cell defects that lead to diabetes in nonpregnant people. Women with GDM have a 30–70% decrease in beta cell function relative to women who maintain normal glucose tolerance during pregnancy. As women with GDM tend to have chronic insulin resistance, most beta cell dysfunction in GDM occurs against a background of insulin resistance. Insulin secretion increases in pregnant women with GDM but not to the required extent. GDM therefore represents the detection during pregnancy of chronic metabolic abnormalities that antedate pregnancy but are detected when pregnancy leads to the first evaluation of glucose tolerance in otherwise healthy young women. The risk of type 2 diabetes after GDM ranges from 20% to 50%.

In addition to having abnormalities in their glucose metabolism, women with GDM, like those with pregestational type 2 diabetes, have higher triglyceride and decreased HDL concentrations than pregnant women with normal glucose tolerance.

Screening and diagnosis of gestational diabetes mellitus

GDM is found in 1–4% of evaluated pregnancies. It poses many challenges to screening and diagnosis. The difficulty in diagnosing GDM arises as a result of the fact that there is more than one diagnostic test and no agreed gold-standard. In addition, there are several threshold criteria for the tests that are currently used and there is no agreement on criteria that best identify women at risk of poor outcomes.

Screening for GDM can be accomplished in many ways. Generally, methods of screening comprise risk factor assessment and laboratory glucose measurement.

Factors often evaluated in risk assessment include:

- maternal age
- ethnicity
- obesity
- gestational weight gain
- suspected macrosomia
- polyhydramnios
- glycosuria.

In addition, the family history of diabetes is taken as well as the history of previous GDM, delivery of a macrosomic infant, stillbirth, neonatal death and congenital anomaly. Risk factor screening may also be used to identify a subset of women who are at low risk of GDM and in whom laboratory testing can be avoided.

Risk assessment for GDM should be undertaken at the first prenatal visit. Laboratory testing is usually undertaken at weeks 24–28 of gestation. A fasting plasma glucose level above 7.0 mmol/l or a casual plasma glucose level above 11.1 mmol/l is indicative of diabetes. If confirmed on a subsequent day, there is no need for any glucose challenge.

In the absence of this degree of hyperglycaemia, evaluation for GDM in women with average or high-risk characteristics should follow one of two approaches:

- The one-step approach involves a diagnostic OGTT without prior plasma or serum glucose screening. This strategy may be cost-effective in high-risk individuals or populations.
- The two-step approach involves initial screening for hyperglycaemia by measurement of plasma or serum glucose concentrations 1 hour after a 50-g oral glucose load (glucose challenge test) followed by performance of a diagnostic OGTT on the subset of women who exceed the glucose threshold value on the glucose challenge test.

When the two-step approach is employed, a glucose threshold value of 7.8 mmol/l identifies approximately 80% of women with GDM and the yield is further increased to 90% by using a cutoff level of 7.2 mmol/l.

With either approach, the diagnosis of GDM is based on an OGTT. A glucose load of either 100g or 75g can be used, but the 75g OGTT is not as well validated for the detection of at-risk infants or mothers as the 100g OGTT.

Maternal morbidity associated with diabetes during pregnancy

Women with diabetic microvascular complications at the start of pregnancy may experience a deterioration in their symptoms that may in part result from the rapid induction of glycaemic control in early pregnancy. As a result, current management recommendations include baseline ophthalmology referral for pregnant women with diabetes with follow-up according to the degree of retinopathy. Women with underlying nephropathy can have varying degrees of deterioration of renal function during a pregnancy. The degree of proteinuria also increases but generally pregnancy does not cause progression to end-stage renal disease. Chronic hypertension complicates approximately 1 in 10 pregnancies in women with diabetes, and pre-eclampsia is also more frequent among women with diabetes.

Women with GDM are at increased risk for the development of diabetes (usually type 2 diabetes) after pregnancy. Obesity and other factors that promote insulin resistance seem to enhance the risk of type 2 diabetes after GDM.

Fetal morbidity associated with diabetes during pregnancy

There is a strong association between the degree of glycaemic control before pregnancy and the rate of miscarriage. Women with longstanding (more than 10 years) and poorly controlled (HbA1c exceeding 11%) diabetes have been shown to have a miscarriage rate of up to 44%.

Major birth defects occur in 1–2% of the general population. In women with overt diabetes and suboptimal glycaemic control before conception, the likelihood of a structural anomaly is increased four- to eight-fold. Two thirds of anomalies involve the cardiovascular and central nervous systems. Periconceptional glycaemic control is the main determinant of abnormal fetal development in women with diabetes. Since birth defects occur during the critical 3–6 weeks after conception, nutritional and metabolic intervention must be initiated well before pregnancy begins.

If the maternal pancreatic insulin response is inadequate, maternal, and subsequently fetal, hyperglycaemia results. This typically manifests as recurrent postprandial hyperglycaemic episodes. These postprandial episodes lead to accelerated fetal growth and are accompanied by episodic fetal hyperinsulinaemia. Fetal hyperinsulinaemia promotes excess nutrient storage, resulting in macrosomia.

Macrosomia occurs in 15–45% of pregnant women with diabetes, a four-fold increase compared with the frequency in normoglycaemic pregnant women. Maternal obesity, common in type 2 diabetes, seems to significantly accelerate the risk of infants being large for gestational age. The macrosomic fetus in diabetic pregnancy develops a unique pattern of overgrowth, involving central deposition of subcutaneous fat in the abdominal and interscapular areas. The rates of neonatal morbidity among newborns with macrosomia are excessive.

The energy expenditure associated with the conversion of excess glucose into fat causes depletion in fetal O_2 levels. These episodes of fetal hypoxia are accompanied by surges in adrenal catecholamines, which in turn cause hypertension, cardiac remodelling and hypertrophy, stimulation of erythropoietin, red cell hyperplasia and increased haematocrit. Polycythaemia (haematocrit above 65%) occurs in 5–10% of newborns whose mothers have diabetes. This finding seems to be related to the level of glycaemic control and is mediated by decreased fetal O_2 tension. High haematocrit values in the newborn baby lead to vascular sludging, poor circulation and postnatal hyperbilirubinaemia.

While most fetuses of mothers with diabetes exhibit growth acceleration, growth restriction occurs with significant frequency in pregnancies in women with pre-existing type 1 diabetes. The most important predictor of fetal growth restriction is underlying maternal vascular disease. Pregnant women with diabetes-associated retinal or renal vasculopathies and/or chronic hypertension are most at risk of delivering a growth-restricted baby.

Infants of mothers with diabetes have five-fold higher rates of severe hypoglycaemia and a two-fold increase in neonatal jaundice. Birth injuries are also more common among infants of mothers with diabetes.

Excessive body fat stores, stimulated by excessive glucose delivery during diabetic pregnancy, often extend into childhood and adult life. Glucose intolerance and increased serum insulin levels are more frequent in children of mothers with diabetes than in children of healthy controls. By the age of 10–16 years, children of mothers with diabetes during pregnancy have a 19.3% rate of impaired glucose intolerance. Development of childhood metabolic syndrome includes childhood obesity, hypertension, dyslipidaemia and glucose intolerance. Fetuses of women with diabetes that are born large for gestational age seem to be at the greatest risk. Markers of islet-cell-directed autoimmunity, if present, are associated with an increase in the risk of type 1 diabetes.

Pre-pregnancy counselling for women with diabetes

For women with pre-existing diabetes, pre-pregnancy counselling is a major way of achieving a reduction in diabetes-associated neonatal morbidity. A thorough assessment of cardiovascular, renal and ophthalmological status is required. A regimen of frequent and regular monitoring of both preprandial and postprandial capillary glucose levels is required with the aim of keeping fasting plasma glucose levels at 5.0–5.5 mmol/l, 1-hour postprandial plasma glucose levels below 7.8 mmol/l and 2-hour postprandial plasma glucose levels below 6.7 mmol/l. The HbA1c level should ideally be within the reference range for at least 3 months before conception.

Women with diabetes should be advised to take a vitamin supplement containing at least 1.0 mg/day of folic acid for at least 3 months before conception to minimise the risk of neural tube defects in the fetus. Optimal prepregnancy counselling will also include a review of body weight, smoking, blood pressure control and the use of oral medications such as ACE inhibitors and statins.

Management of diabetes during pregnancy

As in all forms of diabetes, women with GDM should receive nutritional counselling. Individualisation of medical nutrition therapy depending on maternal weight and height is recommended. For women who are obese (body mass index above 30 kg/m^2), a 30–33% calorie restriction (to 25 kcal/kg actual weight per day) has been shown to reduce hyperglycaemia and plasma triglycerides with no increase in ketonuria. Restriction of carbohydrates to 35–40% of calories has been shown to decrease maternal glucose levels and improve maternal and fetal outcomes. Moderate physical exercise has been shown to lower maternal glucose concentrations in women with GDM.

Insulin therapy has most consistently been shown to reduce fetal morbidities when added to nutritional therapy. The selection of pregnancies for insulin therapy is based on measures of maternal glycaemia with or without assessment of fetal growth characteristics. When maternal glucose levels are used, insulin therapy is recommended when the diet fails to maintain self-monitored whole-blood glucose levels below 5.3 mmol/l (fasting), 7.8 mmol/l (1 hour postprandial) or 6.7 mmol/l (2 hours postprandial). Appropriate values for plasma glucose levels are 5.8 mmol/l, 8.6 mmol/l and 7.2 mmol/l, respectively. The goal of insulin therapy during pregnancy is to achieve glucose profiles similar to those of pregnant women without diabetes.

Insulin lispro, insulin aspart, regular insulin and isophane insulin are well studied in pregnancy and regarded as safe and efficacious. Insulin regimens during pregnancy must be continuously modified as the woman progresses from the first to the third trimester and insulin resistance rises. In a select group of women, use of a subcutaneous continuous insulin infusion using a pump may improve control.

Oral glucose-lowering agents have generally not been recommended during pregnancy. The biguanide metformin functions mainly by decreasing hepatic glucose output. It crosses the placenta and cord levels are even higher than maternal levels. Studies of women with polycystic ovary syndrome who used metformin at 1.5–2.5 g/day throughout pregnancy have illustrated the relative safety of the drug in the second and third trimesters. The use of metformin in women with type 2 diabetes in pregnancy to reduce insulin levels needs further investigation.

Glibenclamide, a sulphonylurea, is minimally transported across the human placenta. Several studies have

concluded that it is as safe and efficacious as insulin in type 2 diabetes mellitus. Success rates for achieving glycaemic control with glibenclamide are about 80%. The drug has been shown to be safe in breastfeeding, with no transfer into human milk.

Many women with diabetes take antihypertensives such as ACE inhibitors or statins as part of their treatment. ACE inhibitors are contraindicated in the second and third trimesters of pregnancy as they interfere with normal fetal renal development, causing oligohydramnios and fetal growth restriction. Methyldopa is the drug of choice, although therapeutic doses of atenolol and nifedipine may be considered as safe alternatives in pregnant women. The use of statins is contraindicated during pregnancy.

Monitoring of pregnant women with diabetes

Maternal monitoring is directed at detecting hyperglycaemia that is severe enough to increase risks to the fetus. Women are advised to self-monitor blood glucose levels every day. For women treated with insulin, success depends on the glycaemic targets that are set and achieved. The frequency and timing of home glucose monitoring should be individualised. Good glycaemic control requires attention to both preprandial and postprandial glucose levels. Urine glucose monitoring is not useful in GDM. Blood pressure and urine protein should be monitored to detect hypertensive disorders.

Increased surveillance of pregnancies at risk is appropriate, particularly when fasting glucose levels exceed 5.8 mmol/l or the pregnancy progresses past term. Assessment for fetal growth by ultrasonography, particularly in the early third trimester, may aid in identifying fetuses that can benefit from maternal insulin therapy.

Long-term therapeutic considerations in women with gestational diabetes mellitus

Maternal glycaemic status should be checked after at least 6 weeks have passed since delivery. If glucose levels are normal postpartum, reassessment of glycaemia should be undertaken at least every 3 years. Women with impaired fasting glucose or impaired glucose tolerance in the postpartum period should be tested for diabetes annually. These women should receive intensive dietary and lifestyle advice and be counselled on the need for family planning. Oral contraceptives may be used in those with prior histories of GDM. Women should be advised to seek medical attention if they develop symptoms suggestive of diabetes mellitus.

Children of women with GDM should be followed closely for the development of obesity and/or abnormalities of glucose tolerance.

Management of diabetes and its complications from pre-conception to the postnatal period: NICE guidelines: Key priorities

Pre-conception care

- Women with diabetes who are planning to become pregnant should be informed that establishing good glycaemic control before conception and continuing this throughout pregnancy will reduce the risk of miscarriage, congenital malformation, stillbirth and neonatal death. It is important to explain that risks can be reduced but not eliminated.
- The importance of avoiding unplanned pregnancy should be an essential component of diabetes education from adolescence for women with diabetes.
- Women with diabetes who are planning to become pregnant should be offered pre-conception care and advice before discontinuing contraception.

Antenatal care

- If it is safely achievable, women with diabetes should aim to keep fasting blood glucose between 3.5 and 5.9 mmol/l and 1-hour postprandial blood glucose below 7.8 mmol/l during pregnancy.
- Women with insulin-treated diabetes should be advised of the risks of hypoglycaemia and hypoglycaemia unawareness in pregnancy, particularly in the first trimester.
- During pregnancy, women who are suspected of having diabetic ketoacidosis should be admitted immediately for critical care, where they can receive both medical and obstetric care.
- Women with diabetes should be offered antenatal examination of the four-chamber view of the fetal heart and outflow tracts at 18–20 weeks.

Neonatal care

- Babies of women with diabetes should be kept with their mothers unless there is a clinical complication or there are abnormal clinical signs that warrant admission for intensive or special care.

Postnatal care

- Women who were diagnosed with gestational diabetes should be offered lifestyle advice (including weight control, diet and exercise) and offered a fasting plasma glucose measurement (but not an OGTT) at the 6-week postnatal check and annually thereafter.

Advice and information on

- the risks of diabetes in pregnancy and how to reduce them with good glycaemic control
- diet, body weight and exercise, including weight loss for women with a body mass index (BMI) over 27 kg/m^2
- hypoglycaemia and hypoglycaemia unawareness
- pregnancy-related nausea/vomiting and glycaemic control
- retinal and renal assessment
- when to stop contraception
- taking folic acid supplements (5 mg/day) from pre-conception until 12 weeks of gestation
- review of, and possible changes to, medication, glycaemic targets and self-monitoring routine
- the frequency of appointments and local support, including emergency telephone numbers.

Gestational diabetes

Risk factors for screening:

- BMI above 30 kg/m^2
- previous macrosomic baby weighing 4.5 kg or above
- previous gestational diabetes
- first-degree relative with diabetes
- family origin with a high prevalence of diabetes (South Asian, black Caribbean and Middle Eastern).

Screening and diagnosis

Offer:

- screening for gestational diabetes using risk factors at the booking appointment
- early self-monitoring of blood glucose or a 2-hour 75g OGTT at 16–18 weeks to test for gestational diabetes if the woman has had gestational diabetes previously, followed by OGTT at 28 weeks if the first test is normal
- an OGTT to test for gestational diabetes at 24–28 weeks if the woman has any other risk factors.

Do not offer:

- screening for gestational diabetes using fasting plasma glucose, random blood glucose, glucose challenge test or urinalysis for glucose.

Information and advice before screening and testing

- There is a small risk of birth complications if gestational diabetes is not controlled.
- Gestational diabetes will respond to changes in diet and exercise in most women.
- Oral hypoglycaemic agents or insulin injections may be needed if diet and exercise do not control blood glucose levels.
- Extra monitoring and care may be needed during pregnancy and labour.

Obesity and pregnancy

Obesity is associated with reduced fertility, and negative effects on *in vitro* fertilisation outcomes. Obesity characterised by a hyperinsulinaemic and hyperandrogenaemic state may lead to oligo/amennorhoea, often in association with polycystic ovarian syndrome. The relative risk of anovulatory infertility has been found to be as high as 3 : 1 in patients with a BMI greater than $27\,kg/m^2$.

Obese women have:

- an increased risk of stillbirth or intrauterine fetal death
- a greater risk of preterm labour, miscarriage and fetal chromosomal anomalies, as well as macrosomia

- a greater incidence of dysfunctional labour, caesarean section and associated perioperative morbidity, and postpartum haemorrhage.

Obese women are more likely to suffer from:

- thromboembolism
- gestational diabetes
- pregnancy-induced hypertension
- pre-eclampsia.
- proteinuria after 20 weeks of pregnancy.

Bariatric surgery

Bariatric surgery is being offered as a treatment to young women resulting in a substantial amount of weight loss with a positive change in fertility. Seventy-one percent of women with fertility problems linked to obesity may start ovulating regularly for the first time after the surgery. In women with polycystic ovarian syndrome (PCOS), post surgery weight loss improves fertility and resolves metabolic problems.

Counselling and treating women who become pregnant after bariatric surgery

Outcomes following bariatric surgery are generally good; nutritional and surgical complications can arise. Bariatric surgery appears to have positive effects on fertility and reduces the risk of gestational diabetes and pre-eclampsia. Rates of congenital anomalies after bariatric surgery are not increased compared with the general population. There may be a trend toward lower birth weights in infants of women who have undergone bariatric surgery. Maternal weight gain during pregnancy seems to be a predictor of birth weight. There appears to be a reduced incidence of fetal macrosomia post-bariatric procedure.

Timing pregnancy after bariatric surgery

It is best to avoid pregnancy after weight-loss surgery until weight stabilises – typically at least 12 months and preferably for 18 months after surgery. Rapid or persistent weight loss may deprive baby of important nutrients, leading to low birth weight. This reduces the potential for maternal and fetal malnutrition and small-for-gestational-age infants.

Monitoring nutritional status during pregnancy after bariatric surgery

Protein, iron, folate, calcium, and vitamins B12 and D are the most common nutrient deficiencies after gastric bypass surgery. Evaluation for deficiencies in micronutrients should be done at the beginning of pregnancy. Treatment should be initiated if any deficits are present. Vitamin A and E should be stopped and continue vitamin D, iron, vitamin B_{12} and calcium.

Genetics

CHAPTER 18   Single-gene and chromosome abnormalities

Single-gene and chromosome abnormalities

Shwetha Ramachandrappa and Katrina Tatton-Brown

Chromosomes, genes and cell division

CHROMOSOMES

Each human somatic cell has 23 pairs of chromosomes that are distinguished according to their length and pattern of light and dark bands. Each chromosome has a centromere (a constriction along its length), which divides the chromosome into short and long arms known as the p and q arms, respectively (Figure 18.1). When the short and long arms are of approximately equal length, the chromosome is known as a metacentric chromosome. When the centromere divides the chromosome into two arms where one arm is obviously longer than the other, the chromosome is known as a submetacentric chromosome. When the centromere is situated at the top of the chromosome, the chromosome is known as an acrocentric chromosome.

The first 22 pairs of chromosomes are known as autosomes and have been designated the numbers 1 through to 22 depending upon the decreasing relative length of the chromosome pairs. The composition of the 23rd pair of chromosomes, the sex chromosomes, determines a person's gender with female individuals having two X chromosomes and male individuals having an X and a Y chromosome.

In the creation of germ cells, the number of chromosomes is halved so that each ovum and spermatozoon contains only one chromosome from each pair. Germ cells therefore have 23 chromosomes, known as the haploid number, whereas somatic cells have 46 chromosomes, referred to as the diploid number.

GENES

Each chromosome is composed of tightly coiled threads of DNA organised around proteins called histones (Figure 18.1). A gene is a specific sequence of DNA that carries the instructions for the construction of a protein (see Chapter 5 for further information on the structure of DNA and protein synthesis). The human genome is estimated to contain approximately 20 000 genes.

CELL DIVISION

Mitosis

When somatic cells divide, they go through a process known as mitosis, whereby the cell duplicates its DNA and cleaves to generate two identical daughter cells also with 23 pairs, or the diploid number, of chromosomes (Figure 18.2).

Meiosis

By contrast, when germ cells divide to produce ova or sperm, they undergo meiosis. Meiosis is unique to the

FIGURE 18.1 **Structure of a chromosome**

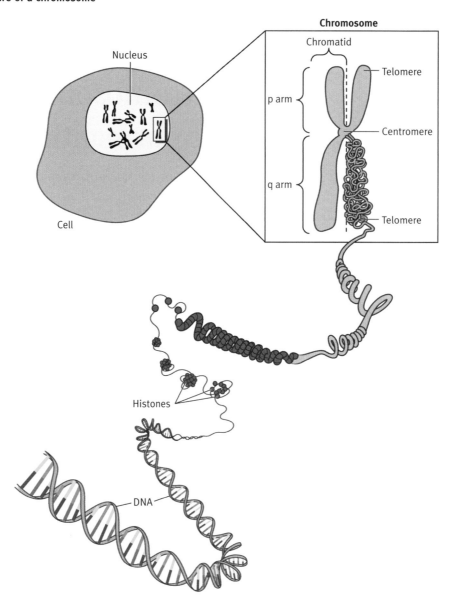

germ cells and is essential to reduce the somatic diploid number of 46 chromosomes to the haploid number of 23 chromosomes (Figure 18.3). This reduction ensures that, when fertilisation occurs, the zygote has 46 chromosomes rather than 92, which would be the result of fertilisation involving two diploid germ cells.

Meiosis consists of two consecutive division cycles that are designated meiosis I and meiosis II.

Meiosis I

Chromosomes duplicate at the beginning of meiosis I. Homologous chromosomes, now consisting of identical sister chromatids, align and reciprocal exchange of genetic material occurs between homologous but non-identical chromatids. This process, known as recombination, enables the mixing of paternally and maternally inherited genes, ensuring that children inherit unique

FIGURE 18.2 **Mitosis**

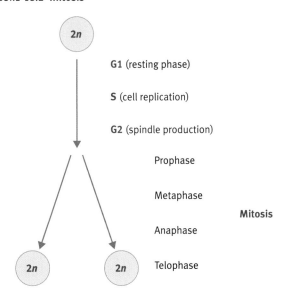

G1 (resting phase)

S (cell replication)

G2 (spindle production)

Prophase

Metaphase

Anaphase   Mitosis

Telophase

2n = diploid chromosome number

FIGURE 18.3 **Meiosis**

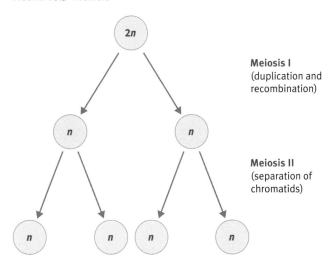

Meiosis I
(duplication and
recombination)

Meiosis II
(separation of
chromatids)

n = haploid chromosome number | 2n = diploid chromosome number

MEIOSIS II

The phases of meiosis II resemble those of mitosis except that, as each chromosome is already duplicated at the beginning of meiosis II, there is no requirement for additional replication. Therefore, the single chromosomes align at the spindle equator, the spindle matrix is generated and sister chromatids are pulled to opposite poles of the cell before cytokinesis.

CHROMOSOMES, GENES AND CELL DIVISION

- There are 46 chromosomes (23 pairs) in each somatic cell; this is the diploid number.
- There are 23 individual chromosomes, one from each chromosome pair, in the ova and sperm; this is the haploid number.
- The chromosomes contain approximately 20 000 genes.
- Genes code for the production of specific proteins.
- Mitosis is the process whereby somatic cells divide. The progenitor cell has 46 chromosomes and each daughter cell has 46 chromosomes.
- Meiosis occurs in the generation of germ cells. It has two distinct phases:
  - During meiosis I, chromosomes duplicate, paternally and maternally inherited chromosomes are recombined and the diploid number is reduced to the haploid number.
  - During meiosis II, splitting of sister chromatids occurs.
  - Therefore, by the end of meiosis, four daughter cells are generated from one dividing germ cell, paternal and maternal genetic material is mixed and each germ cell has only 23 chromosomes.

Thus, by the end of meiosis, four daughter cells are generated from each dividing germ cell. Each of these daughter cells should have 23 individual chromosomes, representing one chromosome from each pair of autosomes in addition to an X chromosome in ova and either an X chromosome or a Y chromosome in sperm. As a result of recombination during meiosis I, each germ cell will have a unique combination of both paternally and maternally inherited genes.

Of note, in female meiosis, three of the daughter cells constitute polar bodies and will not survive; only one daughter cell becomes an ovum. By contrast, all four daughter cells produced from male meiosis develop into spermatozoa.

gene combinations. Following recombination, the pairs of duplicated chromosomes align at the spindle equator and one duplicated chromosome from each pair, consisting of two sister chromatids, is pulled to either pole of the cell before cytokinesis generates two daughter cells. Therefore, at the end of meiosis I each daughter cell has 23 chromosomes, each consisting of two chromatids (Figure 18.3).

Chromosome abnormalities

An abnormality of chromosome number is known as aneuploidy. Aneuploidy can result from various mechanisms, including nondisjunction and translocation.

NONDISJUNCTION

Occasionally, pairs of homologous chromosomes at meiosis I or sister chromatids during mitosis anaphase do not separate and so both chromosomes are passed to one daughter cell and none to the other. One daughter cell therefore has an additional chromosome, a phenomenon known as trisomy, whereas the other is missing one chromosome, known as monosomy.

Common trisomic conditions include Down syndrome (trisomy 21), Edward's syndrome (trisomy 18), Patau syndrome (trisomy 13) and Klinefelter syndrome (47,XXY); Table 18.1 provides an overview of these conditions. Turner syndrome (45,X) is the most common monosomy identified at birth. In addition, mosaic (where only a proportion of cells have the additional chromosome) trisomy 16 and mosaic trisomy 8 are occasionally identified postnatally. Other trisomies and monosomies are rarely seen postnatally as they are not compatible with term development of the fetus.

The risk of chromosome nondisjunction increases with advancing maternal age (Table 18.2).

Down syndrome

Nondisjunction resulting in three separate copies of chromosome 21 accounts for more than 95% of the total incidence of Down syndrome. Alternative causes include Robertsonian translocations and other chromosome rearrangements.

All individuals with Down syndrome have some degree of learning difficulties, usually moderate. In addition, atrioventricular septal defect is 1000 times more common in children with Down syndrome than in the general population. The facial appearance of children and adults with Down syndrome is characteristic and consists of upslanting palpebral fissures, epicanthic folds (folds of skin from the upper eyelid continue down to the nasal corner), a flat midface and brachycephaly

(short anterior–posterior diameter of the cranium). Other associated features are shown in Table 18.1.

Edwards syndrome

Edwards syndrome is associated with a poor prenatal and postnatal outcome. The great majority of occurrences are caused by meiotic nondisjunction but, as with Down syndrome, the syndrome can be attributable to unbalanced Robertsonian translocations and other chromosome rearrangements.

Edwards syndrome is usually detected prenatally either through aneuploidy screening methods or through identification of a combination of many associated prenatal anomalies (Table 18.1). Babies with Edwards syndrome who survive to term are likely to die within the first year of life (usually within the first months). Very rarely, children have survived beyond the first year with profound cognitive impairment and associated anomalies described in Table 18.1.

Patau syndrome

Patau syndrome, caused by an additional copy of chromosome 13, is also associated with a high rate of spontaneous pregnancy loss and, if the baby survives to term, poor postnatal outcome. Most (90%) occurrences of Patau syndrome are caused by nondisjunction of chromosome 13 (the vast majority of which occur during maternal meiosis). The remainder are attributable to unbalanced translocations (primarily Robertsonian translocations).

Klinefelter syndrome

Individuals with Klinefelter syndrome have an additional sex chromosome, with a karyotype of 47,XXY. Many individuals with Klinefelter syndrome are not diagnosed unless as an incidental finding prenatally during chorionic villus sampling (CVS) or amniocentesis or in adulthood during infertility investigations. As Klinefelter syndrome does not, in general, cause an increase in nuchal translucency (NT) thickness and does not result in features that are evident on the second trimester anomaly scan, the condition is usually not identified prenatally.

TABLE 18.1 **Karyotype and clinical features associated with common trisomy conditions**

Syndrome name	Additional chromosome	Clinical features
Down syndrome	21	Moderate to severe learning difficulties (100%)
		Cardiac problems (40–50%, VSD, ASD, AVSD)
		Hypothyroidism (20–40%)
		Dementia (10–15%)
		Acute lymphoblastic leukaemia
Edwards syndrome	18	Profound learning difficulties (100%)
		Congenital heart disease (90%, commonly VSD)
		Facial clefts
		Spina bifida
		Clenched hands
		Rocker-bottom feet
Patau syndrome	13	Profound learning difficulties (100%)
		Congenital heart disease (80%, VSD, ASD)
		Holoprosencephaly (60–70%)
		Microphthalmia/anophthalmia (60–70%)
		Postaxial polydactyly (60–70%)
		Scalp defects
		Cleft lip/palate (60–70%)
		Omphalocele
		Renal anomalies
Klinefelter syndrome	X (in an XY individual)	Slightly decreased IQ but within the normal range
		Tall stature
		Infertility
		Transient gynaecomastia
Triple X syndrome	X (in an XX individual)	Slightly decreased IQ but within the normal range
		Tall stature
		Normal fertility
XYY syndrome	Y (in an XY individual)	Slightly decreased IQ but within the normal range
		Tall stature after puberty
		Behavioural problems

ASD = atrial septal defect | AVSD = atrioventricular septal defect | VSD = ventricular septal defect

TABLE 18.2 **Maternal age versus risk of chromosome nondisjunction**

Age (years)	Risk
20	1 in 1500
30	1 in 900
34	1 in 500
36	1 in 300
38	1 in 200
40	1 in 100
42	1 in 60
45	1 in 30

FIGURE 18.4 **Reciprocal translocation**

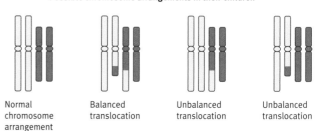

Parents' chromosomes

Chromosomes in parent carrying a balanced translocation

Chromosomes in other parent (normal arrangement)

Possible chromosome arrangements in their children[a]

Normal chromosome arrangement

Balanced translocation

Unbalanced translocation

Unbalanced translocation

[a]Other arrangements occur less frequently

Other sex chromosome abnormalities resulting from nondisjunction

These are illustrated in Table 18.1. The most common examples are a 47,XXX karyotype (triple X syndrome) in female persons and a 47,XYY karyotype in male persons. Triple X syndrome is usually identified incidentally as it causes few problems prenatally or postnatally.

Turner syndrome

In general, girls with Turner syndrome (45,X) have IQ scores 10–15 points lower than their siblings but they attend mainstream school and do not have learning difficulties. Many fetuses with 45,X do not survive to term because of fetal hydrops. Indeed, Turner syndrome should be considered in any fetus with an NT thickness above 4 mm. The attrition rate for conceptions with Turner syndrome is reported to be very high, so if the syndrome is diagnosed in the first trimester, parents should be advised of a high risk of spontaneous miscarriage.

TRANSLOCATIONS

Reciprocal translocations

Chromosome rearrangements involving the transfer of genetic material between two nonhomologous chromosomes are known as reciprocal translocations (Figure 18.4). The most common reciprocal translocation in

humans, t(11; 22)(q 23; q 11), involves chromosomes 11 and 22.

Reciprocal translocations can be either balanced or unbalanced. In general, a balanced exchange of chromosome material does not have phenotypic consequences as the adult or child has a normal amount of genetic material. However, if unbalanced, there will be one chromosome with missing genetic material (a monosomy) and another chromosome with duplicated genetic material (a trisomy), a combination that is usually associated with developmental and other congenital problems.

If a woman with a balanced reciprocal translocation is seen before she conceives, she should be advised that a pregnancy can have four possible outcomes (Figure 18.4):

- A normal pregnancy with a normal karyotype.
- A normal pregnancy with the familial balanced reciprocal translocation.
- A spontaneous miscarriage owing to an unbalanced product of the familial reciprocal translocation.
- A pregnancy that goes to term but the child has a high likelihood of learning difficulties and possibly other congenital anomalies associated with an unbalanced product of the familial reciprocal translocation.

The relative proportion of pregnancies that spontaneously miscarry or go to term with problems depends upon the chromosomes involved and the size of the translocated chromosome segments.

If an unbalanced reciprocal translocation is detected prenatally, it is likely to be associated with fetal anomalies and the parents should be counselled accordingly. If a balanced reciprocal translocation is identified, the parents should be karyotyped to determine whether it is *de novo*. If it is familial and the parent carrying the balanced rearrangement is healthy with no learning or other medical difficulties, the baby is unlikely to have problems related to the translocation. However, if the balanced translocation has arisen for the first time in the fetus (it is *de novo*), it may or may not be associated with problems and it would be recommended to undertake an array comparative genomic hybridisation (aCGH) to investigate for a microdeletion.

Robertsonian translocations

A Robertsonian translocation is a chromosome rearrangement that involves fusion of the long arms of two acrocentric chromosomes and loss of their short arms (Figure 18.5). The genes contained on the short arms are represented elsewhere and so their loss does not result in any phenotypic effect of acrocentric chromosomes.

FIGURE 18.5 **Robertsonian translocation**

Parents' chromosomes

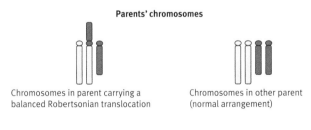

Chromosomes in parent carrying a balanced Robertsonian translocation

Chromosomes in other parent (normal arrangement)

Possible chromosome arrangements in their children

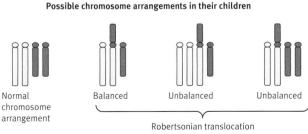

Normal chromosome arrangement

Balanced

Unbalanced

Unbalanced

Robertsonian translocation

By definition, Robertsonian translocations only involve the five acrocentric chromosomes 13, 14, 15, 21 and 22. The most common Robertsonian translocations are rob (13q; 14q), which involves fusion of chromosome 13 to chromosome 14, and rob(14q; 21q), which involves fusion of chromosome 14 to chromosome 21. Occasionally, the long arms of two homologous chromosomes may fuse resulting in an isochromosome.

Individuals who are seen before conception to discuss the implications of a balanced Robertsonian translocation for a future pregnancy should be advised of a number of possible outcomes (Figure 18.5):

- A normal pregnancy with a normal karyotype.
- A normal pregnancy associated with a balanced Robertsonian translocation.
- A spontaneous miscarriage attributable to an unbalanced Robertsonian translocation (the fetus will be trisomic or monosomic for one of the component chromosomes).
- A spontaneous miscarriage owing to an imprinting defect.
- A liveborn child with abnormalities; in all instances, these will be attributable to trisomy rather than monosomy, as the latter will always result in spontaneous miscarriage; in the common rob (13q; 14q) and rob(14q; 21q) translocations, there is a risk of a child with Patau syndrome or Down syndrome, respectively; these risks are higher if the mother carries the balanced translocation (10–15%) than if the father carries it (below 1%).
- A liveborn child with abnormalities associated with an imprinting defect (risk below 0.5%).

Imprinting is the process by which one parental allele is preferentially silenced according to its parental origin. Of the five acrocentric chromosomes, imprinted genes are found only on chromosomes 14 and 15. Imprinting abnormalities associated with Robertsonian translocations are therefore only of concern if one or both of these two chromosomes are involved. Following mitosis, a trisomic conceptus may occur, but this may be 'corrected' through trisomy rescue. This reduction of three copies to two copies leaves the cell with an apparently balanced arrangement. However, if both the remaining chromosomes are of the same parental origin (known as uniparental disomy or UPD) and contain imprinted genes, there may be phenotypic consequences.

Babies with maternal UPD14 generally survive to term and are small, have learning difficulties, hypotonia and relative macrocephaly. By contrast, paternal UPD14 tends to result in spontaneous miscarriage, but if babies do survive to term they have severe problems including profound learning difficulties, feeding difficulties and joint contractures.

Paternal UPD15 and maternal UPD15 cause Angelman syndrome and Prader–Willi syndrome, respectively. These are well described syndromes that are both associated with severe learning difficulties. In addition, children with Angelman syndrome have a characteristic facial appearance and an ataxic gait. Children with Prader–Willi syndrome are characteristically poor feeders in the neonatal period but develop an insatiable appetite from childhood onwards. In addition, they may be hypotonic and of short stature.

CHROMOSOME MICRODELETIONS

Chromosome microdeletions are an important cause of a number of different syndromes illustrated in Table 18.3. Microarray aCGH is now the technique of choice for identifying chromosome microdeletions and microduplications. However, not all microdeletions and microduplications are pathogenic: we now know of a number of clearly nonpathogenic deletions/duplications (designated as benign copy number variants) and a number of possible susceptibility loci, the pathogenicity of which is currently unclear.

Gene abnormalities

The normal functioning of genes can be disrupted through a number of different mechanisms, including intragenic mutations (missense, frameshift, nonsense and splice site mutations), exon deletions, triplet repeat expansions and whole gene deletions.

MISSENSE MUTATIONS

Missense mutations are single-base substitutions that have occurred in a coding, critical region of the gene.

Without performing functional studies it is often difficult to elucidate the pathogenicity of these single-base substitutions.

FRAMESHIFT MUTATIONS

Frameshift mutations occur when one or more bases (but not a multiple of three) are inserted or deleted from the usual genetic sequence so disrupting the normal reading frame. Eventually, a variable number of codons along the sequence, a new stop codon will have been generated and the resulting abnormal protein will be prematurely truncated.

NONSENSE MUTATIONS

A nonsense mutation is a single-base substitution that generates a premature stop codon resulting in a truncated protein. As both frameshift and nonsense mutations result in truncated proteins, they are sometimes referred to together as truncating mutations.

SPLICE SITE MUTATIONS

Splicing is the process by which introns are removed from the primary transcript and consecutive exons joined together. Splice site mutations affect the nucleotides at the splice site, at the junction between the introns and exons.

EXON DELETIONS

Exon deletions, alternatively known as partial gene deletions, can occur when one or more exons within a gene are deleted in a process that does not constitute an alternative splicing event.

TRIPLET REPEAT EXPANSIONS

Triplet repeat conditions result from extensive duplication of a single codon. If such a run of nucleotide triplets increases above a critical threshold, an abnormal phenotype results. Common triplet repeat conditions include fragile X syndrome, Huntington's disease and myotonic dystrophy. Features common to these conditions include variability of phenotype, anticipation (progression in

TABLE 18.3 **Common microdeletion syndromes**

Microdeletion	Syndrome name	Cardinal features
1p36		Severe learning difficulties Seizures Hypotonia Feeding difficulties Characteristic facial appearance with low-set horizontal eyebrows and deep-set eyes
4p15	Wolf–Hirschhorn	Severe learning difficulties Low birth weight and postnatal failure to thrive Characteristic facial appearance with 'Greek helmet' profile
5p15	Cri du chat	Severe learning difficulties Characteristic cat-like cry Characteristic facial appearance with bitemporal narrowing, hypertelorism and downslanted palpebral fissures
7q11	Williams	Mild to severe learning difficulties Cardiac problems, particularly supravalvular aortic/pulmonary stenosis Renal artery stenosis Characteristic facial appearance with short upturned nose, long philtrum, wide mouth, periorbital fullness 'Cocktail party personality' (chatty, interactive behaviour)
8q24	Langer–Giedion	Contiguous gene deletion syndrome characterised by fine sparse hair, brittle nails, bulbous nose and cone-shaped epiphyses on X-ray (owing to deletion of the *TRPS1* gene) in addition to exostoses and mental restriction (owing to deletion of neighbouring genes including *EXT1*)
17p11	Smith–Magenis	Severe learning difficulties Severe behavioural problems with self-injuring Sleep problems Characteristic facial appearance with square-shaped face and heavy eyebrows
17p13	Miller–Dieker	Lissencephaly Characteristic facial appearance with vertical furrowing on the forehead, hypertelorism and short nose with anteverted nares
22q11	DiGeorge/ velocardiofacial/ Shprintzen	Mild to moderate learning difficulties Cardiac anomalies, most commonly tetralogy of Fallot, VSD and interrupted aortic arch Short stature Psychiatric disorders Renal anomalies Cleft palate with or without velopharyngeal insufficiency Hypocalcaemia T cell immune disorder Characteristic facial appearance with tubular nose, narrow palpebral fissures and simple ears

VSD = ventricular septal defect

triplet repeat size and phenotype severity as the repeat is passed on to the next generation) and a parent-of-origin effect (the triplet repeat may expand more if passed on by the mother rather than the father or vice versa).

ABNORMALITIES OF CHROMOSOMES AND GENES

Common chromosome abnormalities include:

- nondisjunction (for example Down, Edward's, Patau, Klinefelter and Turner syndromes)
- translocations
  - ○ Robertsonian translocations
  - ○ Reciprocal translocations
- microdeletions (for example DiGeorge, Wolf–Hirschhorn and Williams syndromes).

Mechanisms that abrogate gene function include:

- missense mutations
- truncating mutations including frameshift and nonsense mutations
- splice site mutations
- partial gene deletions
- whole gene deletions
- triplet repeat expansions.

Principles of inheritance

Genes encode proteins, which are essential to the normal development and functioning of the body. Genes are arranged in pairs, with one gene from each pair being inherited from each parent. Traits determined by a single gene locus generally follow one of four different patterns of inheritance: autosomal dominant, autosomal recessive, X-linked recessive or X-linked dominant inheritance.

AUTOSOMAL DOMINANT INHERITANCE

Autosomal dominant conditions are caused by disruption of only one gene of a gene pair by any of the previously described mechanisms that abrogate gene function. The children of an individual affected by an autosomal dominant condition have a one in two chance of inheriting the disrupted gene and, therefore, the associated condition (Figure 18.6 A). A few more common autosomal dominant conditions are shown in Table 18.4.

FIGURE 18.6 **Autosomal dominant inheritance**

A Pattern of inheritance

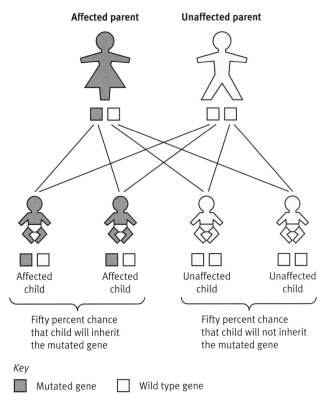

B Pedigree

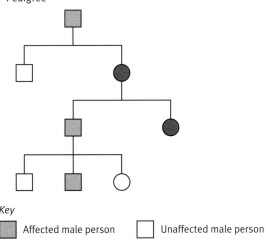

TABLE 18.4 **Common autosomal dominant conditions**

Condition	Gene	Features
Tuberous sclerosis	TSC1/TSC2	Multisystem disorder characterised by cutaneous (angiofibromata, hypomelanotic macules, shagreen patches), neurological (brain hamartomas causing seizures) and renal (angiomyolipomata) abnormalities; should be strongly suspected prenatally if cardiac rhabdomyosarcomas are identified
Marfan syndrome	Fibrillin 1	Tall stature, arm span to height ratio >1.05, long fingers, dolicocephaly, aortic dilatation and other cardiac anomalies
Neurofibromatosis type I	NF1	Combination of café-au-lait spots, neurofibromata, axillary and inguinal freckling and optic glioma
Breast/ovarian cancer susceptibility	BRCA1/BRCA2	Inherited susceptibility to the development of breast cancer (lifetime risk ~80%) and ovarian cancer (lifetime risk 20–40%)
Hereditary nonpolyposis colon cancer	MLH	Inherited predisposition to the development of colon and other cancers including endometrial, gastric and ovarian
Huntington's disease	Huntingtin	Condition characterised by progressive neurological deterioration with dementia, psychiatric disturbance and movement disorder
Autosomal dominant polycystic kidney disease	PKD1/PKD2	Systemic disorder with cysts in the kidneys, liver, pancreas and spleen and cardiovascular anomalies including intracranial aneurysms and mitral valve prolapse
Achondroplasia	FGFR3	Condition characterised by disproportionate short stature with rhizomelic (proximal) shortening and relative macrocephaly

Pedigrees where an autosomal dominant trait has been passed on from generation to generation have several characteristic features (Figure 18.6 B):

- Individuals in each generation are affected.
- Male and female relatives are affected in roughly equal numbers.
- Both men and women can have affected children.

AUTOSOMAL RECESSIVE INHERITANCE

Autosomal recessive conditions (Table 18.5) are caused by disruption of both genes in a gene pair. Where only one gene is disrupted, the individual is known as a carrier and is healthy.

Individuals with an autosomal recessive condition will only have affected children if they mate with another affected individual or a carrier of the condition. If two carriers have children, the chance of their children being affected by the condition is one in four. There is therefore a three in four chance of having healthy children, of whom two would be anticipated to be carriers and one would be anticipated to have

inherited the two normal genes from his or her parents (Figure 18.7A).

Autosomal recessive conditions should be considered in pedigrees with the following features (Figure 18.7B):

- Only one generation is affected.
- Parents of affected children are genetically related (consanguineous).

X-LINKED RECESSIVE INHERITANCE

If a recessive mutation is present within a gene on the X chromosome, male individuals will be affected because they are hemizygous for that gene. However, female individuals who have one mutated copy and one normal copy generally do not manifest features of the disorder. Common X-linked recessive disorders are described in Table 18.6.

Characteristics of X-linked recessive pedigrees include the following:

- Only male individuals are affected, or if female individuals are affected they have a milder phenotype.

TABLE 18.5 **Common autosomal recessive conditions**

Condition	Gene	Features
Cystic fibrosis	*CFTR*	Characterised by chronic pulmonary disease and exocrine pancreatic dysfunction
Spinal muscular atrophy	*SMN*	Characterised by symmetrical proximal muscle weakness; life expectancy ranges from infancy to adulthood depending upon the type of spinal muscular atrophy
Tay–Sachs disease	*HEXA*	A GM2 gangliosidosis characterised by a 'cherry-red spot' on the retina and deteriorating motor and cognitive abilities
Haemochromatosis	*HFE*	Excess absorption of iron with deposition in liver, pancreas and skin leading to cirrhosis, diabetes mellitus and bronzed appearance of skin
α1-Antitrypsin deficiency	*SERPINA1*	α1-Antitrypsin is a proteinase inhibitor that protects the lungs from elastase; without α1-antitrypsin individuals will develop emphysema at a young age; they may also develop cirrhosis owing to a direct effect of the abnormal α1-antitrypsin on the hepatocytes
Congenital adrenal hyperplasia due to 21-hydroxylase deficiency	*CYP21A2*	Attributable to abrogation of 21-hydroxylase, required for the synthesis of cortisol; associated with female virilisation and abnormal puberty (precocious in boys) with or without salt wasting
Deafness due to mutations in connexin 26	*GJB2*	Most common cause of autosomal recessive nonsyndromic deafness

- There is no male-to-male transmission of the condition. If this occurs then the condition cannot be an X-linked recessive condition.
- The condition may seem to skip generations.

X-LINKED DOMINANT INHERITANCE

An X-linked dominant disorder often manifests so severely in male fetuses that it results in a spontaneous loss of pregnancy or early neonatal death. X-linked dominant conditions therefore seem to be restricted to female individuals. Examples of X-linked dominant disorders are shown in Table 18.7.

OTHER FORMS OF INHERITANCE

Occasionally, disorders follow more complex patterns of inheritance including mitochondrial inheritance and imprinting. Disorders resulting from mitochondrial inheritance can only be transmitted through the maternal line. Mitochondrial disorders are caused by a defect in the mitochondrial DNA and include mitochondrial encephalomyopathy with lactic acidosis and stroke-like episodes (MELAS), myoclonic epilepsy with ragged red fibres (MERRF) and Leigh's disease (subacute necrotising encephalomyopathy).

Imprinting is briefly described earlier in this chapter. In summary, it is the process whereby one allele is preferentially silenced according to its parent of origin.

Prenatal genetics

Screening tests available to pregnant women in the first and second trimesters include a combination of NT ultrasound and/or serum screening. These screening investigations will provide the pregnant woman with a statistical risk of having a baby with trisomy 21, 18 or 13. Such investigations do not provide a definitive diagnosis. If the risk is deemed high, women can proceed to a diagnostic test. In practice, CVS or amniocentesis are the only tests offered at the end of the first and beginning of the second trimester.

SCREENING TESTS

An overview is provided in Table 18.8.

FIGURE 18.7 **Autosomal recessive inheritance**

A Pattern of inheritance

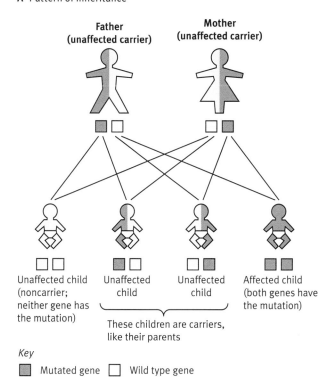

Key

▨ Mutated gene   ☐ Wild type gene

B Pedigree

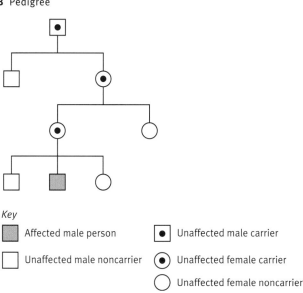

Key

▨ Affected male person

☐ Unaffected male noncarrier

⊡ Unaffected male carrier

⊙ Unaffected female carrier

◯ Unaffected female noncarrier

Nuchal translucency ultrasound

The term NT refers to the sonographic appearance of subcutaneous fluid at the back of the fetal neck between weeks 11 and 14 of gestation (Figure 18.8). An increased NT thickness is associated with chromosomal abnormalities, a wide range of cardiac defects, single-gene defects including Noonan syndrome (syndrome of short stature, cardiac defects, learning difficulties and clotting abnormalities primarily associated with mutations within the *PTPN11* gene) and some skeletal dysplasias.

Chromosome trisomy attributable to nondisjunction occurs more frequently with increasing maternal age (Table 18.2). Many pregnancies are now screened for chromosomal abnormalities by use of an algorithm that combines NT thickness and maternal age. This algorithm will give the pregnant woman the statistical likelihood of her pregnancy being affected with trisomy 21, 18 or 13. It does not provide a statistical risk for abnormalities other than the three trisomies.

Combined test

The combined test uses information derived from the NT scan and two serum biochemical markers: pregnancy-associated plasma protein A (PAPP-A) and beta human chorionic gonadotrophin (β-hCG). Data from prospective studies suggest that use of NT measurement in isolation will detect approximately 70–75% of trisomy 21 pregnancies with a false-positive rate of 5%. By contrast, combining NT scanning with β-hCG and PAPP-A testing increases the trisomy 21 detection rate to nearer 90%.

Other screening tests

Other screening options are shown in Table 18.8 and include the triple test, quadruple test, integrated test (which combines first-trimester and second-trimester risk assessment but with nondisclosure of first-trimester results) and sequential test (which involves disclosure of first-trimester results, which in turn determine whether subsequent serum screening is undertaken).

Some babies with trisomy 21 have recently been shown to have an absent or hypoplastic nasal bone on first-trimester ultrasound. Reverse flow in the ductus

TABLE 18.6 **Common X-linked recessive conditions**

Condition	Gene	Features
Duchenne muscular dystrophy	Dystrophin	Progressive myopathy affecting proximal muscles; causes early loss of ambulation and death in the third decade owing to respiratory failure
Haemophilia A	Factor VIII gene	Attributable to deficiency of factor VIII, an important component of the clotting cascade; affected male individuals have abnormal clotting, with severe haemophilia A leading to spontaneous joint and muscle bleeding
Ocular albinism	GPR143	Hypopigmentation of iris and retina; associated with poor visual acuity, nystagmus, strabismus and abnormal decussation of the optic nerves
X-linked adrenoleucodystrophy	ACBD1	Accumulation of very-long-chain fatty acids in the adrenal glands and brain; results in progressive cognitive deterioration and adrenal failure
Fragile X syndrome	FMR1	Caused by expansion of a CGG repeat; results in learning difficulties and characteristic facial appearance

CGG = cytosine-guanine-guanine trinucleotide

TABLE 18.7 **X-linked dominant conditions**

Condition	Gene	Features
Incontinentia pigmenti	NEMO	Initially presents as blistering lesions following Blaschko lines; these later become hyperpigmented and eventually appear as atrophic streaks
Rett syndrome	MECP2	Associated with cognitive regression and severe learning difficulties; other characteristic features include hand wringing and stereotypical movements

TABLE 18.8 **Aneuploidy risk evaluation**

Test	Effect in trisomy 21 pregnancy	Trisomy 21 detection rate
FIRST TRIMESTER		
NT scan	↑NT	70–75%
NT scan + nasal-bone measurement	Absent or hypoplastic nasal bone	80–85%
NT scan + assessment of blood flow in the ductus venosus	Absent or reversed A-wave	80–85%
COMBINED TEST SECOND TRIMESTER	↑NT + ↑β-hCG + ↓PAPP-A	90%
Triple screen	— α-FP + ↑β-hCG + ↓uE$_3$	70%
Quadruple screen	— α-FP + ↑β-hCG + ↓uE$_3$ + ↑inh	81%
FIRST AND SECOND TRIMESTERS		
Integrated	↑NT + ↓PAPP-A + quadruple screen	86%
Sequential	↑NT + ↓PAPP-A + quadruple screen but quadruple screen is only undertaken if NT scan and PAPP-A indicate a high risk	95%

↑ = increase | ↓ = decrease | α-FP = alpha fetoprotein | β-hCG = beta-human chorionic gonadotrophin | inh = inhibin | NT = nuchal translucency | PAPP-A = pregnancy-associated plasma protein A | uE$_3$ = unconjugated estradiol

FIGURE 18.8 **Nuchal translucency scan showing an increase in subcutaneous fluid behind the baby's neck**

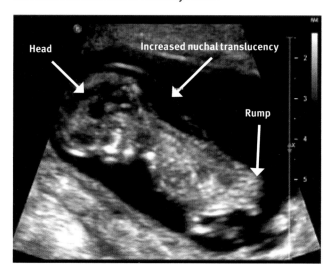

sequence the cell-free DNA in a maternal blood sample and determine the relative proportions of DNA derived from different chromosomes. Provided that there is a high enough fraction of free-fetal DNA in the sample, any chromosomal aneuploidies can be detected with a high degree of accuracy. In some testing protocols the entire complement of cell-free DNA in the sample is sequenced, in others only DNA derived from particular chromosomes of interest is sequenced.

Although at present, analysis of cffDNA is primarily used for fetal sexing, rhesus blood typing and as a highly predictive screening test for chromosomal aneuploidies, in time it is likely to become possible to detect subchromosomal deletions, subchromosomal duplications and sequence variation noninvasively using similar technology.

venosus has also been associated with trisomy 21 (Table 18.8). However, nasal-bone measurement and ductus-venosus blood-flow assessment should be used with caution because they are technically more difficult to perform than NT ultrasound.

Cell-free fetal DNA

New noninvasive screening tests based on the analysis of cffDNA are likely to replace many of the screening tests described above and become part of routine obstetric care in the coming years.

The maternal circulation contains cell-free DNA. The vast majority of this DNA is maternal in origin; however, a small proportion originates from the fetus. Free-fetal DNA is released by apoptotic cells in the placenta; its composition is therefore representative of the nuclear content of cells in the developing fetus. Currently cffDNA can be tested to determine the gender or rhesus D blood typing of the fetus. More recently it has been used for the detection of trisomy 13, 18 or 21. If there is a trisomy of a particular chromosome, there will be more free-fetal DNA in the mother's circulation derived from that chromosome than free-fetal DNA derived from the other chromosomes.

Next-generation sequencing technologies (see below under DNA sequencing) can be used to

DIAGNOSTIC TESTS

Historically diagnostic tests were undertaken if an increased aneuploidy risk was identified through screening, if the maternal age was advanced, if fetal abnormalities were identified on routine screening or if there was a family history of a genetic or chromosomal abnormality. The most commonly used diagnostic tests included CVS and amniocentesis as outlined below. However, more recently, noninvasive prenatal testing on cell-free fetal DNA (cffDNA) allowing detection of the common trisomies (trisomy 13, 18 and 21) in the first trimester has been introduced into routine obstetric care.

Chorionic villus sampling

Following reports of possible fetal-limb abnormalities following early CVS, this investigation is currently performed no earlier than week 11 of gestation. CVS involves the aspiration of placental tissue (Figure 18.9). Chorionic villi consist of two cell layers: the outer rapidly dividing and invading cytotrophoblast and the inner mesenchymal core. As the cytotrophoblast is actively dividing, it can be used in the direct evaluation of metaphases. This 'direct' result is usually available 2–3 days following the procedure. In addition to a direct

FIGURE 18.9 **Ultrasound-guided chorionic villus sampling showing a first-trimester placenta with a chorionic villus sampling needle in place**

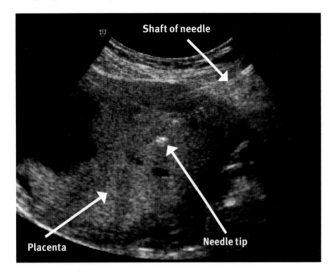

preparation, a culture from the inner mesenchyme is also established. Cultures usually take 1–3 weeks before cells can be harvested and a result obtained. The mesenchymal core is usually considered to be more representative of the fetal cells than the cytotrophoblast as the latter cell line is established earlier in the process of fetoplacental differentiation. If an abnormal result is obtained from the direct preparation, it is therefore wise to wait for the results of the culture as the abnormality may be confined to the cytotrophoblast layer.

Confined placental mosaicism, where a chromosome abnormality is present in placental but not fetal tissue, is observed in a small (approximately 1.5%) number of CVS samples. Confined placental mosaicism should be considered if the CVS karyotype shows only a proportion of the cells to be affected with an abnormal karyotype or if the identified karyotype is not anticipated to be associated with fetal viability. If an abnormal karyotype is present in the placenta but not in the fetus, this may compromise placental functioning, resulting in restricted fetal growth and structural anomalies known to be associated with impaired blood supply.

Amniocentesis

Amniocentesis is performed after week 15 of gestation. The amniocytes, cells derived from fetal skin, urinary tract and gastrointestinal tract, are aspirated and cultured. As the aspirate does not contain any rapidly dividing cells, a direct preparation is not available. Cells cultured from amniocytes are usually available to harvest 1–3 weeks after the procedure has been performed.

Chorionic villus sampling versus amniocentesis

In the past, the miscarriage rate associated with CVS was reportedly higher than that associated with amniocentesis. However, increased use of, and expertise with CVS in recent years mean that the miscarriage rates quoted for amniocentesis and CVS are now more equal (in the order of 1%), although the exact figure depends upon the expertise at the centre where the procedure is undertaken. This equalisation of miscarriage rates has altered prenatal obstetric practice such that, in many centres, CVS is now performed in preference to amniocentesis. This is because CVS can be performed earlier in gestation, whereas amniocentesis cannot be performed until later in pregnancy. An additional advantage that CVS has over amniocentesis is the availability of a rapid result from a direct preparation.

However, cultured amniocytes are fetal cells and as such allow a direct assay of fetal chromosomes/genes. Therefore, if mosaicism is reported following an amniocentesis, this is probably a true reflection of a mosaic state in the fetus. By contrast, CVS involves assaying the placental cells and so there must always be a residual concern that any abnormal result is attributable to confined placental mosaicism, although the risk of this is low.

Cordocentesis

Fetal blood, taken from the umbilical vein, may be sampled from week 18 of gestation. Before week 18, the vein is considered too small for cordocentesis. In addition to genetic/chromosomal investigations, which can be undertaken in cultured lymphocytes, fetal blood sampling is an important means of assessing anaemia and diagnosing prenatal infection. Disadvantages of cordocentesis include the associated miscarriage rate (1–2%) and the technical demands of the procedure.

MOLECULAR GENETIC AND CYTOGENETIC TECHNIQUES IN PRENATAL DIAGNOSIS

An overview of these methods is provided in Table 18.9.

Conventional cytogenetic analysis

Before the advent of molecular techniques, chromosomes were exclusively analysed microscopically. To do this, cells (from blood, amniotic fluid, placenta, tumour or other tissues) are cultured, arrested midmitosis, lysed and then fixed before a specific banding agent is added. Banding techniques include the commonly used Giemsa banding (or G-banding) technique, but alternative banding patterns can be generated using other techniques such as reverse banding (R-banding), quinacrine banding (Q-banding) or centromeric banding (C-banding).

Fluorescence in situ hybridisation

In general, fluorescence *in situ* hybridisation (FISH) is performed on interphase chromosomes and consists of a DNA probe labelled with a fluorophore. The probe is designed to anneal to one specific chromosome region and can be visualised using fluorescent microscopy.

FISH is useful in the following situations:

- detection of whole-chromosome aneuploidies (there will be three or one rather than two signals for a given chromosome)
- investigation of chromosome microdeletions not detectable with conventional G-banding methods (a specific FISH probe will be unable to anneal to the deleted region and so only one signal will be visualised)
- cytogenetic evaluation of structurally abnormal chromosomes such as derivative chromosomes associated with unbalanced or balanced Robertsonian or reciprocal translocations
- characterisation of supernumerary marker chromosomes.

Supernumerary marker chromosomes are identified in less than 1% of pregnancies and without FISH it is often very difficult to determine the origin of the chromosome material.

Quantitative fluorescence polymerase chain reaction

As ultrasound and biochemical screening tests for fetal aneuploidy become more widely available, so the demand for a rapid, cost-effective diagnostic method has increased. Quantitative fluorescence polymerase

TABLE 18.9 **Comparison of the laboratory methods that may be employed in the analysis of chorionic villus sampling/amniocentesis**

Test	Uses	Advantages	Disadvantages
FISH	Rapid aneuploidy detection Evaluation of unbalanced translocations	A good technique for investigating predictable unbalanced chromosome rearrangement	Expensive Labour-intensive
QF-PCR	Rapid aneuploidy detection	Rapid results Cheap	Will usually only identify abnormal dosage involving chromosomes 13, 18 or 21
MLPA	Rapid aneuploidy detection Evaluation of unbalanced translocations	Rapid results	Limited genomic coverage
Array-CGH	Rapid aneuploidy detection Detection of microdeletions Detection of microduplications	Rapid results Information about gene dosage throughout the genome	New assay, so unclear whether abnormal results are pathogenic variants or polymorphisms

Array-CGH = microarray comparative genomic hybridisation | FISH = fluorescence *in situ* hybridisation | MLPA = multiplex ligation-dependent probe amplification | QF-PCR = quantitative fluorescence polymerase chain reaction

chain reaction (QF-PCR) is now commonly used and involves amplification with fluorescent primers that target highly polymorphic short tandem repeats (STRs, consisting of repetitive sequences of one, two, three or maybe four bases) specific to the chromosomes of interest. In most centres, QF-PCR is restricted to investigating trisomy 13, 18 and 21 and possibly the sex chromosomes (primarily to identify 45,X) as abnormalities of these chromosomes account for 80% of clinically significant aneuploidies diagnosed in the prenatal setting.

The main advantages of QF-PCR are the speed with which results are available (1–2 days) and the relative cost-effectiveness compared with conventional cytogenetic techniques. The main disadvantage is that, in general, only STRs from chromosome 13, 18 and 21 are amplified and so other more complex chromosome rearrangements or abnormal dosage of other chromosomes are not identified.

Multiplex ligation-dependent probe amplification

Multiplex ligation-dependent probe amplification (MLPA) is a relatively new technique designed to detect dosage abnormalities (deletion or duplication) of specific genes, chromosome regions or whole chromosomes. It is different from QF-PCR in that it is the probe and not the DNA that is amplified and quantified.

Each MLPA probe consists of two oligonucleotides (short DNA sequences) that are designed to anneal to specific adjacent target DNA sequences. If both target sequences are present, the two annealed probes will be joined with a ligase and amplified using polymerase chain reaction (PCR). A computer program calculates the relative quantities of the PCR products, which are compared with those of a control sample, and the result is presented as a ratio. A ratio of 1.0 indicates that both alleles are present; a ratio of 0.5 indicates that one allele is deleted and a ratio of 1.5 suggests that one allele is duplicated.

Microarray comparative genomic hybridisation

Array-CGH compares DNA from a test subject to that of a control person to detect any areas of deletion or duplication across the genome. The technique uses a prepared chip which comprises many hundreds of different wells.

Each well contains a DNA probe which corresponds to a region of the genome. The probe is either an oligonucleotide (25–85 base pairs long) or a bacterial artificial chromosome (BAC, 80–200 base pairs long). The spacing of the DNA probes varies from chip to chip such that some chips provide denser genomic coverage than others.

Test and reference DNA are labelled with different coloured fluorophores, conventionally green and red respectively, and then combined together in equal quantities, and added to the chip. In each well, complementary DNA hybridises to the DNA probe. If there is an equal amount of complementary DNA in the test and reference samples then equal amounts of green labelled and red labelled DNA are bound and the well emits a yellow signal. If there is more complementary DNA in the test sample than in the reference sample, the well emits a green signal. A green signal indicates that there is an area of duplication at the corresponding genomic locus in the test subject. If there is more complementary DNA in the reference sample than the test sample, the well emits a red signal, suggesting that the test subject harbours a deletion in this region.

The advantage of aCGH is that it can detect DNA dosage imbalance over the whole genome in a single simultaneous assay. The technique is, therefore, well placed to identify aneuploidies, microdeletions and microduplications, but does not detect balanced arrangements, such as a balanced reciprocal translocation, where there is no net loss or gain of genetic material.

DNA sequencing

The techniques which have been described thus far measure gene dosage at particular locations in the genome (FISH, QF-PCR, MLPA) or across the entire genome (aCGH). They are not able to detect anomalies within individual genes. Each gene is encoded by a length of DNA comprising a precise sequence of four different bases, adenine, guanine, thymine and cytosine. DNA sequencing techniques can be used to determine the specific sequence of bases in an individual's DNA; by comparing this with a reference sequence from a control population any sequence variation can be identified.

Until relatively recently, the predominant DNA sequencing technique was the chain termination method, which enables a specific target region of the genome to be sequenced. A DNA primer anneals to the test DNA in the region of interest and an enzyme sequentially adds bases to this primer that are complementary to the test DNA. The reaction contains a mixture of unmodified bases, which can be sequentially added to the growing DNA strand, and bases that have been chemically modified, so that once they are incorporated into the strand it is terminated. Each of the modified bases is labelled with a different radioactive or fluorescent label such that the four bases can be distinguished. This reaction generates DNA strands of varying lengths, which have terminated at different distances from the DNA primer by the random incorporation of a modified base. The DNA sequence of the region of interest can be determined by sorting the strands by their lengths, and analysing each strand in turn to determine which modified base was incorporated at its terminus. The chain termination method can reliably sequence regions of DNA up to 800 bases long and enables the detection of sequence anomalies within a region of interest. This technique is particularly useful in monogenic (single gene) disorders where the region of interest has been well characterised.

The advent of next-generation sequencing technology has revolutionised DNA sequencing in that multiple genes can be sequenced in a single experiment. DNA from an individual is fragmented into short lengths and DNA adaptors are ligated to either end. The short lengths of DNA are immobilised on a surface and a DNA primer anneals to the adaptor. An enzyme attaches a fluorescently labelled base to the DNA primer, which is complementary to the DNA fragment being sequenced. The sequencing apparatus captures a fluorescent image of the surface and is able to determine which base has been added by its unique fluorescent signal. Bases are sequentially added to the growing DNA strand in a stepwise reaction in which the identity of each successive base is determined in real time by fluorescent imaging. Using this technology hundreds of thousands to hundreds of millions of DNA fragments can be sequenced in parallel, making it possible to sequence the entire genome of an individual in a relatively short time-scale.

As sequencing technology has improved, the challenge has shifted from one of obtaining large amounts of sequence information, to that of distilling potentially pathogenic sequence variants from the thousands of benign variants that are an integral part of any genomic

sequence. Next-generation sequencing has transformed the diagnostic pathway in some conditions by enabling the introduction of multi-gene panels in which a large number of potentially causal genes can be sequenced simultaneously. Similar panels may soon replace current prenatal genetic testing strategies.

Pre-implantation genetic diagnosis

Couples in whom one partner has an inherited condition that they want to avoid passing on to their children may wish to consider pre-implantation genetic diagnosis (PGD). In the UK, PGD is tightly regulated by the Human Fertilisation and Embryology Authority (HFEA) to ensure that embryo selection is only undertaken for serious genetic disorders.

The initial stages of PGD are identical to those of a traditional cycle of *in vitro* fertilisation (IVF). The female partner undergoes hormonal treatment to stimulate her ovaries and her eggs are collected by fine needle aspiration when they have reached maturity. Each egg is injected with a single sperm from the male partner by a technique called intracytoplasmic sperm injection (ICSI). If fertilisation is successful, the resultant embryo will begin to divide. One frequently employed technique is to remove one or two cells at the eight-cell blastocyst stage, which are then analysed to determine whether the embryo is at risk of inheriting the genetic condition. Of any of the embryos that are characterised as being at low risk, one is transferred into the uterus of the female partner in the hope that it will give rise to an unaffected pregnancy; any additional low-risk embryos may be frozen for future PGD cycles.

Genetics of gynaecological malignancies

Inherited gynaecological malignancies are rare. However, germline mutations within specific cancer-predisposing genes have been identified in a small minority of families with ovarian cancer or endometrial cancer.

OVARIAN CANCER

The lifetime risk of developing ovarian cancer in the general population is in the order of 1 in 70. A small proportion of ovarian cancers are attributable to a familial predisposition, and the breast cancer susceptibility genes *BRCA1* and *BRCA2* together account for 6–8% of ovarian cancers. To a lesser extent, the mismatch repair genes *MSH2*, *MLH1*, *MSH6* and *PMS2* have been identified in families with ovarian cancer, usually in association with many other cancer types.

BRCA1 and BRCA2

Alterations within the *BRCA1* and *BRCA2* genes are associated with an increased susceptibility to developing breast and ovarian cancer. In general, if a woman is found to have a mutation within the *BRCA1* gene, she has a 60–90% lifetime risk of developing breast cancer and a 40–60% lifetime risk of developing ovarian cancer. A mutation within *BRCA2* is also associated with a high lifetime risk (45–85%) of developing breast cancer but the risk of developing ovarian cancer (10–30%) is lower than that associated with *BRCA1*. However, the overall contribution of *BRCA1* and *BRCA2* to the prevalence of female breast cancer is less than 2%.

Mismatch repair genes

Alterations within the mismatch repair genes *MSH2*, *MLH2*, *MSH6* and *PMS2* are associated with a spectrum of tumour types that most commonly include colorectal, endometrial, gastric and ovarian cancers. Together this tumour predisposition syndrome is known as hereditary nonpolyposis colon cancer (HNPCC). Mutations within one of these mismatch repair genes confer a lifetime risk of developing ovarian cancer in the order of 4%. This is a two- to three-fold increase over the lifetime risk of developing ovarian cancer in the general population.

Surveillance and management of increased ovarian cancer susceptibility

Where a familial susceptibility to ovarian cancer has been identified, it is important to consider what kind of surveillance can be offered to carrier family members. Ovarian cancer screening is currently controversial and while many centres will offer a combination of serum CA-125 measurement and ovarian ultrasonography, there is no consensus of opinion as to how frequently the tests should be undertaken. Some clinicians even argue that no screening would be preferable to that currently on offer, given that both CA-125 and ultrasonography screening are associated with high rates of false-positive results (leading to unnecessary anxiety and possibly surgical intervention) and false-negative results (meaning that ovarian cancers are not being detected).

Indeed, given the limitations of current ovarian cancer screening, some women who are found to have a germline mutation in *BRCA1* or *BRCA2* opt for a bilateral salpingo-oophorectomy (BSO). This has the advantage of nearly eliminating their ovarian cancer risk (there is a small residual risk, equivalent to 1%, of primary peritoneal ovarian cancer) and halving their breast cancer risk, but it also has the disadvantage of precipitating an abrupt menopause. Current practice is to advise carriers of *BRCA* mutations who have completed their family to consider BSO as a method of managing their breast and ovarian cancer risk.

ENDOMETRIAL CANCER

An inherited susceptibility to uterine cancer (lifetime risk approximately 50%) is conferred by the mismatch repair genes associated with HNPCC. Unfortunately, screening (for example by use of Pipelle biopsy) is neither optimal nor universally available and so women are advised to monitor the regularity of periods and act if postmenopausal bleeding occurs. Some women will consider a prophylactic hysterectomy.

In addition, a predisposition to endometrial cancer is associated with Peutz–Jegher syndrome and Cowden disease. Peutz–Jegher syndrome, caused by mutations within the gene encoding serine/threonine protein kinase 11 (*LKB1*), is associated with pigmented macules of the mucous membranes and skin, gastrointestinal polyps and a predisposition to cancers including gastrointestinal cancer (lifetime risk approximately 30%) and endometrial cancer (lifetime risk approximately 40%). Cowden disease is caused by germline mutations within the gene encoding phosphatase and tensin homologue (*PTEN*). It is characterised by multiple hamartomas and an increased risk of breast, thyroid and endometrial cancers. The lifetime risk of endometrial cancer in *PTEN* carriers has not yet been ascertained.

Immunology

CHAPTER 19

Basic immunology

Sharon Cookson and Ian Sargent

Organisation of the immune system

The main function of the immune system is to protect the host from invasion by infectious organisms. Immune responses comprise:

- rapid, nonspecific reactions against foreign invaders (innate immunity)
- antigen-specific reactions that 'recognise' the pathogenic organism both during initial infection and upon subsequent contact with the same organism (adaptive immunity).

The innate immune response is mediated principally by macrophages and neutrophils and by soluble circulating molecules such as complement proteins. The adaptive immune response is mediated by T cells and B cells.

The innate and adaptive arms of the immune system must interact to generate an effective immune response. Cytokines are key molecules that control this interaction.

Table 19.1 and Table 19.2 provide an overview of innate compared with adaptive immunity and of the cells of the immune system, respectively.

Innate immune response

CELLS OF THE INNATE IMMUNE SYSTEM

Phagocytes

Phagocytes are derived from the bone marrow and their primary function is to engulf, ingest and destroy (phagocytose) exogenous or endogenous particles such as infectious agents and cellular debris. Phagocytes are attracted by chemokines and activated by cytokines that have been secreted by antigen-specific T cells. Thus, the innate and adaptive arms of the immune system are intrinsically linked.

There are two basic types of phagocyte:

- the monocyte/macrophage lineage
- granulocytes, which may be subdivided into neutrophils, mast cells, basophils and eosinophils.

Each cell type has distinct effector functions. Monocytes are short-lived cells that circulate in the blood for a few hours before migrating into tissues and differentiating into mature macrophages. They express three distinct

TABLE 19.1 **Comparison of innate and adaptive immunity**

Parameter of comparison	Innate	Adaptive
Response time	Hours	Days
Specificity	Limited	Diverse
Memory	None	Efficient
Response to repeat infection	Identical to primary response	Much more rapid and vigorous than primary response
Cellular components	Phagocytes, natural killer cells	T cells, B cells
Humoral components	Complement	Antibody

TABLE 19.2 Immune cells in adult blood

Type of cell	Proportion of total leucocytes
Neutrophils	50–70%
Lymphocytes	20–40%
T cells	70–85%[a]
B cells	10–15%[a]
Natural killer cells	10%[a]
Monocytes	1–6%
Eosinophils	1–3%
Basophils	<1%
Dendritic cells	<1%

[a] Proportion of total lymphocytes

receptors for the crystallisable fragment (Fc) region of immunoglobulin (Ig) G: Fc gamma receptor I (FcγRI; high affinity), FcγRII (medium affinity) and FcγRIII (CD16; low affinity).

Tissue macrophages are long-lived. They bind to microorganisms via their Fc receptors if the pathogen is coated with antibody or via their complement receptors if the bacteria have been opsonised with complement. Following binding, macrophages phagocytose and kill microorganisms. Internalised microorganisms can be processed and presented as peptides to T cells, thus triggering the adaptive arm of the immune response.

Dendritic cells are an additional phagocytic cell type derived from monocytes or from lymphoid lineages. This is the only cell type whose sole function is to capture, process and present antigen to T cells, that is, they are 'professional' antigen-presenting cells (APCs).

Neutrophils are the most abundant type of circulatory phagocyte, comprising the majority of leucocytes in the blood. These cells recognise and kill invading microorganisms (mainly bacteria), either by phagocytosis or by the release of granules and cytotoxic substances, which can occur when neutrophils are activated through their Fc or complement receptors. Neutrophils are short-lived, surviving only a few days; once they have phagocytosed material and destroyed it, they die.

Mast cells are located in the skin, mucosal surfaces and around blood vessels. They are phagocytic and express Fc receptors specific for the antibody immunoglobulin

(IgE). Activation results in the release of a wide range of mediators including histamine, heparin, prostaglandin and a variety of cytokines and chemokines, which induce or control inflammation in the surrounding tissues.

Basophils are phenotypically similar to mast cells and also have receptors for IgE. They circulate in the blood and may not be phagocytic.

Eosinophils are a highly specialised group of leucocytes. They principally reside in tissues such as the respiratory and gut subepithelia, where they attach to the surface of parasites such as schistosomes. Following attachment, the eosinophils degranulate and release proteins that damage the parasite membrane. Degranulation releases cytokines, which amplify the immune response.

Natural killer cells

Natural killer (NK) cells bridge the innate and adaptive arms of the immune system. NK cells are large granular lymphocytes that represent a morphologically distinct population and display cytotoxic activity against a wide range of tumour cells and virally infected cells. They can distinguish these targets from normal cells by means of two different types of receptor on their surface:

- FcγRIII (CD16) receptors, which attach to specific antibodies bound to tumour cells or virally infected cells in a process called antibody-dependent cell-mediated cytotoxicity
- killer cell immunoglobulin-like receptors (KIRs), a heterogeneous group that includes both activating and inhibitory cell surface receptors that engage class I major histocompatibility complex (MHC) molecules on target cells.

Healthy cells expressing self-MHC class I molecules are protected from NK cell lysis but some disease processes (for example many tumours) cause a downregulation of MHC class I. The cytolytic activity of NK cells is regulated by KIRs that detect the absence of MHC class I expression on target cells.

The mechanisms for NK cell killing resemble those for cytotoxic T cells described later in this chapter. Like phagocytes, NK cells can be activated by cytokines, such as interleukin-2 (IL-2) and interferon gamma (IFN-γ), secreted from activated T cells.

COMPLEMENT SYSTEM

The complement system consists of a series of approximately 20 serum proteins that together constitute almost 10% of the total serum proteins, thereby making it one of the major immune defence systems of the body. The major function of the complement system is to remove or destroy antigen. Activation of complement has three main consequences:

- lysis of microorganisms, enveloped viruses and infected cells by damaging the plasma membrane
- opsonisation, that is, coating of foreign particles with complement protein fragments; phagocytes expressing receptors for these complement components are then able to bind to the target and phagocytose it
- triggering of the complement cascade (forming a bridge between the adaptive and innate immune responses).

Complement components are largely designated by numerals (C1–C9) and activated in a cascade such that a small initial stimulus can rapidly cause a large effect. Many cells express receptors for one or more complement products. When activated, a component is able to cleave the next component in the sequence into two or more fragments:

- the minor fragments (designated the suffix 'a', as in C3a) diffuse from the site of activation and are able to initiate a local inflammatory response by binding to specific receptors
- the major fragment (designated the suffix 'b', as in C3b) binds to the target cell membrane.

Mechanism of complement activation

Complement may be activated by one of three pathways, depending upon composition of the initial stimulus:

- classic pathway
- alternative pathway
- lectin pathway.

Central to all three is cleavage of the most abundant complement protein, C3, followed by activation of the lytic sequence (Figure 19.1).

The classic pathway is initiated by the binding of antibody to antigen, with the antibody being either IgG or IgM bound to the surface of a pathogen. Formation of an antigen–antibody complex causes a conformational change in the Fc portion of the antibody that exposes a binding site for the first complement component, C1q.

The alternative pathway does not require antibody. It is activated by the binding of C3b to hydroxyl and amine groups on the surface of pathogens, including many Gram-positive and Gram-negative bacteria. This pathway is relatively inefficient because its activation requires high concentrations of the various components.

The mannose-binding lectin pathway is more efficient than the alternative pathway. It is initiated by the binding of lectin to glycoproteins or carbohydrates on the surface of pathogens, including Gram-positive and Gram-negative bacteria.

All three pathways of activation converge at the final lytic sequence. Here, C5, C6, C7, C8 and C9 sequentially interact to form a membrane attack complex, which binds to the membrane of the target forming a trans-membrane channel through which salts and water can flow, resulting in lysis of the target cell.

The classic pathway links to the adaptive immune system because its activation requires that the host has previously encountered the target and has generated an

FIGURE 19.1 **Pathways of complement activation**

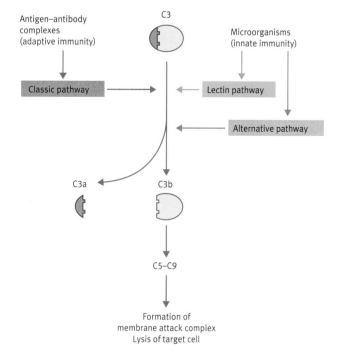

antibody response to it. The alternative and lectin pathways are considered to be part of the innate immune system because they are activated by microorganisms rather than antibody.

The importance of complement is readily apparent in individuals who lack particular components. For example, classic-pathway deficiencies result in tissue inflammation and individuals with C3 deficiencies are subject to overwhelming bacterial infections.

LIMITATIONS OF INNATE IMMUNITY

Although innate immunity can provide a line of defence against many common microorganisms, such as bacteria, yeasts and parasites, there are many more-sophisticated pathogens, such as viruses or intracellular microorganisms, that the cells of the innate immune system cannot recognise or effectively destroy. This limitation has been addressed by the evolution of the adaptive immune system as a more versatile and adaptable means of host defence.

Adaptive immune response

Adaptive immune responses are mediated by lymphocytes that have the capacity to recognise foreign antigens and distinguish them from self-antigens. In many instances this mechanism confers lifelong protective immunity against re-infection with the same pathogen, which can be intracellular or extracellular.

There are two basic lymphocyte categories: bursa-equivalent cells (B cells) and thymus-derived cells (T cells) (Table 19.2).

B CELLS

B cells are so called because of their similarity to lymphocytes found in the bursa of Fabricius organ in birds. B cells develop in the bone marrow, are found in all lymphoid tissues and represent up to 15% of the circulating lymphoid pool. Antibodies on the surface of B cells serve as antigen receptors and binding initiates a series of events whereby antigen is internalised, degraded, complexed with MHC class II molecules and returned to the cell surface. This peptide–MHC complex can then be presented to antigen-specific T cells, which secrete cytokines and induce clonal B cell proliferation and differentiation into antibody-producing plasma cells.

Antibodies

Antibodies, also known as immunoglobulins, are a particularly effective means of combating extracellular organisms such as bacteria, and are efficient at neutralising circulating viruses. In mammals, there are five distinct classes of immunoglobulin (Table 19.3): IgG, IgM, IgA, IgE and IgD. All are made up of a unit comprising two identical light chains and two identical heavy chains but they differ in size, charge, carbohydrate content and amino acid sequence (Figure 19.2). It

TABLE 19.3 **Properties and biological activities of immunoglobulin isotypes**

Property	IgM	IgG	IgA	IgE	IgD
Heavy chain	Mu	Gamma	Alpha	Epsilon	Delta
Normal serum level (mg/ml)	1.5	13.5	3.0	0.0003	0.03
Activates classic complement pathway	+	+	–	–	–
Binds to phagocyte Fc receptors	?	+	–	–	–
Present on membrane of mature B cells	+	–	–	–	+
Transported in mucosal secretions	–	–	+	–	–
Induces mast cell degranulation	–	–	–	+	–
Crosses placenta	–	+	–	–	–

Fc = crystallisable fragment | Ig = immunoglobulin | + = yes | – = no | ? = not known

FIGURE 19.2 **Structure of immunoglobulins**

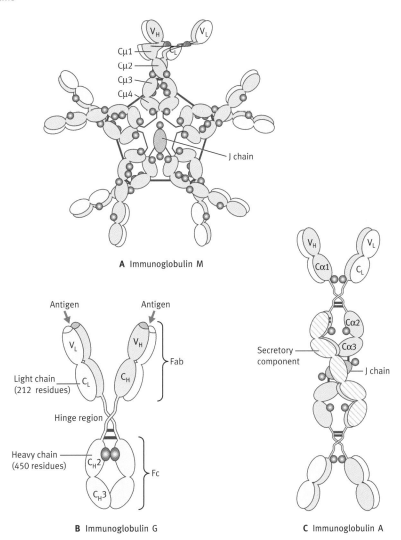

Cμ1
Cμ2
Cμ3
Cμ4

J chain

A Immunoglobulin M

Cα = alpha heavy chain |
Cδ = delta heavy chain |
Cε = epsilon heavy chain |
C_H = heavy chain of the
constant region |
C_L = light chain of the
constant region |
Cμ = mu heavy chain |
Fab = antigen-binding
fragment |
Fc = crystallisable fragment |
V_L = light chain of the
variable region |
V_H = heavy chain of the
variable region

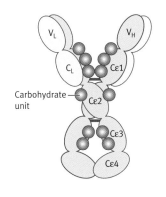

Antigen   Antigen

V_L V_H Fab

Light chain
(212 residues) C_L C_H

Hinge region

Heavy chain
(450 residues) C_H2 Fc

C_H3

B Immunoglobulin G

V_H V_L

Cα1 C_L

Cα2
Secretory
component   Cα3   J chain

C Immunoglobulin A

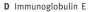

V_L V_H

C_L Cε1

Carbohydrate
unit   Cε2

Cε3

Cε4

D Immunoglobulin E

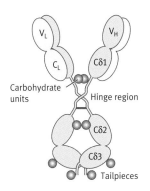

V_L V_H

C_L Cδ1

Carbohydrate
units   Hinge region

Cδ2

Cδ3

Tailpieces

E Immunoglobulin D

is the type of heavy chain that determines the class and subclass of antibody; for example, IgM has a mu heavy chain, whereas IgA1 and A2 have alpha 1 and alpha 2 heavy chains, respectively.

Different parts of an antibody have distinct functions. The antigen-binding fragment (Fab) region comprises the amino-terminal domains of each heavy and light chain (referred to as the variable region) and forms the antigen-binding site, thereby determining the antibody's antigen specificity. The other part of the antibody, the Fc region, comprises the carboxy-terminal domains of each heavy and light chain (referred to as the constant region). The Fc region determines which effector function will be activated.

All immunoglobulin isotypes, with the exception of IgD, are bifunctional in that they do not only recognise and bind antigen but they also exhibit one or more effector functions.

IgM comprises 5–10% of the serum immunoglobulin pool. It is secreted from plasma cells as a pentamer and is largely confined to the intravascular pool. IgM is the first antibody formed in a primary response to an antigen and is also the first antibody to be synthesised by the newborn baby, but it is unable to cross the placenta. This immunoglobulin is a potent activator of the classic pathway of complement owing to its five complement-binding sites.

IgG comprises 70–80% of the serum immunoglobulin pool. It is the predominant antibody of secondary immune responses and equilibrates between the intra-vascular and extravascular pools. There are four sub-classes with unique effector functions:

- IgG1, IgG3 and IgG4 readily cross the placenta and have an important role in protecting the developing fetus.
- IgG1 and IgG3 are extremely efficient in activating complement via the classic pathway, IgG2 less so.
- IgG1 and IgG3 bind with high affinity to Fc receptors on phagocytic cells and thereby mediate opsonisation.

IgA constitutes 10–20% of the serum immunoglobulin pool. It is the predominant antibody in secretions such as saliva, tears and mucus of the bronchial, digestive and genitourinary tracts. Breast milk is also rich in secretory IgA, which protects the newborn against infection

during the first few months of life. IgA participates in secondary immune responses. IgA-containing immune complexes opsonise antigens and induce phagocytosis through Fc receptors. Binding of secretory IgA to micro-bial antigens prevents their attachment to mucosal cells, thus inhibiting infection and colonisation.

IgE achieves very low serum levels. It binds with high affinity to specific receptors on mast cells and basophils. Cross-linkage of bound IgE by antigen causes degranu-lation and release of a range of pharmacologically active mediators. IgE can give rise to a variety of allergic manifestations.

IgD comprises less than 0.5% of the serum immuno-globulin pool. It has no known effector functions as a serum protein; instead, it functions as a transmembrane antigen receptor on mature B cells.

Vaccination

The importance of antibody to host defence comes into play when considering the crucial role it plays during vaccination. During infection, a primary antibody response is launched to eliminate the pathogen. This also leads to the generation of long-lived antigen-specific memory B cells, which are restimulated upon subsequent exposure to the same pathogen, resulting in a faster and much more intense secondary response.

It is important to realise that antibodies do not recog-nise the whole microorganism but particular parts of antigens called epitopes. Successful vaccine develop-ment therefore relies upon modification of a pathogen so that it retains its antigenicity (that is, it is still able to generate a primary antibody response) but is innocuous. In essence then, a vaccine essentially replaces the initial infection but still leads to the generation of memory B cells. This consequently provides immunity to vaccin-ated individuals such that when they are exposed to the microorganism in question, they are able to mount a quick and effective secondary response, leading to pro-tection from and elimination of the pathogen.

T CELLS

T cells are the principal mediators of the adaptive immune response and exhibit a wide variety of effector functions including target-cell lysis and cytokine release, which can cause proliferation, differentiation or activation of many different cells of the immune system. Antigen recognition takes place through the T cell receptor (TCR).

Two types of TCR have been characterised:

- alpha/beta TCRs, which are expressed on more than 95% of circulating T cells
- gamma/delta TCRs, which are rarely expressed on peripheral-blood T cells but are present on populations of T cells in mucosal surfaces (small intestine, pregnant uterus) and liver.

T cell maturation

Alpha/beta T cells are generated in the bone marrow and recognise nonself antigens that are presented by self-MHC class I or class II molecules on the surface of APCs. This specificity is the result of a rigorous selection process.

Following TCR gene rearrangement in the thymus, immature T cells (thymocytes) that recognise self-MHC molecules expressed on cortical epithelial cells with high affinity are positively selected. Those cells that are not selected undergo death by apoptosis.

As the thymocytes migrate to the deeper cortex, they increase their expression of TCR and the cell surface molecules CD3, CD4 and CD8. Those TCRs that recognise self-antigens with high affinity are deleted by a process called negative selection. T cells at this stage of maturation go on to express TCRs at high density and to lose either CD4 or CD8, becoming single-positive (positive for either CD4 or CD8) mature thymocytes.

The mature cells leave the thymus and travel to the secondary lymphoid tissues and periphery, where they have the potential to function as one of the following, depending on whether they express CD4 or CD8:

- T helper (Th) cells, which are CD4-positive and MHC class II restricted
- cytotoxic T (Tc) cells, which are CD8-positive and MHC class I restricted.

T cells that express a gamma/delta TCR are also generated from bone marrow precursors but differ from T cells that express alpha/beta TCRs in their specificity (they are MHC-unrestricted) and expression of CD4 and CD8 (they are predominantly double-negative).

The mechanism by which T cells become committed to one or the other of these two TCR cell types is largely unknown.

CD4-positive T cells

CD4 is a transmembrane protein that is expressed on T cells and macrophages. It serves as a cell adhesion molecule, facilitating TCR/CD3-mediated signal transduction upon binding of MHC class II molecules on APCs.

CD4-positive T cells can be categorised as Th1 or Th2 cells according to the pattern of cytokines they secrete (Figure 19.3A):

- Th1 cells produce IFN-γ and IL-2, which activate macrophages and CD8-positive T cells, promoting cell-mediated immunity.
- Th2 cells secrete IL-4 and IL-5, which stimulate B cells to produce antibody, promoting humoral (that is, antibody-mediated) immunity.

Following stimulation by antigen, naïve CD4-positive T cells produce IL-2 and subsequently polarise towards a Th1 or Th2 phenotype, depending on signals received during and after activation (Figure 19.3A). IFN-γ and IL-12 enhance Th1 development, whereas IL-4 promotes differentiation into Th2 cells. The type of APC and the antigen dose may also have a role. It is likely that the polarisation to a Th1 or Th2 immune response occurs through the complex interaction of various factors, rather than on the basis of any single criterion.

Other CD4-positive T cell types are Th3, Th0 and type 1 regulatory T (Tr1) cells:

- Th3 cells produce high amounts of transforming growth factor beta (TGF-β).
- Th0 cells express both Th1 and Th2 cytokines.
- Tr1 cells secrete high levels of IL-10 (and little or no IL-2 and IL-4) leading to immune suppression.

CD8-positive T cells

CD8 serves as a cell adhesion molecule by binding to MHC class I, thereby stabilising the interaction of a class I restricted T cell with a target cell or APC. CD8 expression predominantly identifies a subset of T cells

FIGURE 19.3 **Generation of Th1 and Th2 CD4-positive subsets**

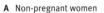

A Non-pregnant women

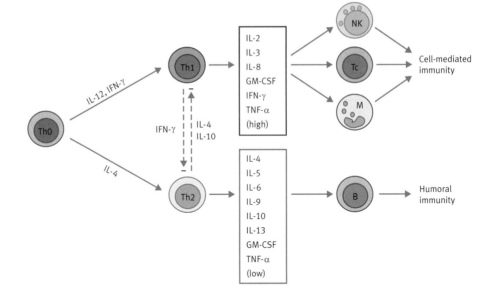

B Pregnant women (normal pregnancy)

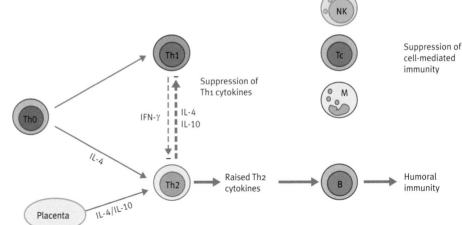

B = B cell |
GM-CSF = granulocyte–macrophage
colony-stimulating factor |
IFN-γ = interferon gamma |
IL = interleukin | M= macrophage |
NK = natural killer cell |
Tc = cytotoxic T cell |
Th = T helper cell |
TNF-α = tumour necrosis factor alpha

called Tc cells. These can kill tumour cells or virally infected cells following appropriate priming and activation.

In addition to their cytotoxic activity, CD8-positive T cells can also secrete distinct patterns of cytokines. As with CD4-positive cells, CD8-positive precursors can be driven toward a type 1 cytotoxic (Tc1) phenotype by IL-12 and IFN-γ, whereas IL-4 induces the generation of Tc2 cells. Both of these phenotypes retain cytolytic function.

CYTOKINES

Cytokines are molecules produced by a variety of cell types, including monocytes, macrophages, lymphocytes, endothelial cells, fibroblasts and tissue epithelia, and provide a link between the innate and adaptive immune responses. Although they are often described as hormone-like, cytokines differ from hormones in that their effects are predominantly exerted at a local level. Cytokines are low-molecular-weight proteins that act at

TABLE 19.4 **Biological activities of the most important interleukins**

Name	Cells secreting this interleukin	Biological function
IL-1	Macrophages and monocytes	Has proinflammatory effects
IL-2	T cells	Acts as a growth factor for T cells
		Stimulates proliferation and differentiation of T cells
		Increases the cytolytic activity of NK cells
IL-4	Th2 cells	Promotes proliferation and differentiation of B cells
		Upregulates B-cell HLA class II expression
IL-10	T cells, B cells, monocytes and mast cells	Has potent anti-inflammatory effects
		Inhibits the synthesis of IL-2 and IFN-γ by Th1 cells
		Regulates growth and differentiation of B cells
		Enhances expression of HLA class II
IL-12[a]	Macrophages, dendritic cells and B cells	Enhances the cytolytic activity of CD8$^+$ T cells and NK cells
		Directs the immune response towards a Th1-type bias by inducing the secretion of IFN-γ, IL-2 and TNF-α

[a] Secretion strongly induced by bacteria, bacterial products and certain parasites. | CD8$^+$ = CD8-positive | HLA = human leucocyte antigen | IFN = interferon | IL = interleukin | NK = natural killer | Th = T helper | TNF-α = tumour necrosis factor alpha

very low concentrations by binding to specific cell surface receptors.

A cytokine may act in one of three ways:

- in an autocrine fashion by binding to receptors on the membrane of the cell that secreted it
- in a paracrine fashion by binding to receptors on cells in the immediate vicinity
- in an endocrine fashion by binding to distant cells.

Cytokines can be subdivided into categories (such as interferons, interleukins, chemokines, growth factors) according to their primary function, although there is considerable overlap between these groups.

Interferons

This family of molecules was first recognised by their ability to inhibit viral replication. They are produced early in infection and are pivotal in controlling the spread of a virus until adaptive immunity has had a chance to develop.

IFN-α and IFN-β are produced by virally infected leucocytes and fibroblasts, respectively.

IFN-γ is a product of activated Th1 and NK cells. It has the following functions:

- antiviral effects
- increasing the expression of both MHC class I and MHC class II molecules
- activating macrophages and NK cells
- promoting cytotoxic susceptibility of target cells
- polarising Th0 cells to the Th1 phenotype.

Interleukins

Interleukins are a large and diverse group of cytokines with a wide range of functions. They are predominantly secreted by lymphocytes. The most important immunoregulatory interleukins are listed in Table 19.4.

Proinflammatory cytokines

Two cytokines are principally responsible for the early inflammatory reaction that occurs in response to microbial invasion:

- IL-1, produced by macrophages and B cells, activates lymphocytes (T cells, B cells and NK cells) and increases the expression of adhesion molecules on endothelial cells.

■ Tumour necrosis factor alpha (TNF-α) exerts similar effects to IL-1 but is primarily produced by macrophages and activated T cells.

Macrophages are stimulated to produce IL-1 and TNF-α by oxidative stress or by endotoxins such as bacterial lipopolysaccharide.

Chemokines

Chemokines are a group of chemotactic cytokines that are involved in cell migration, activation and chemotaxis. They diffuse from the site of production (for example tissue leucocytes, endothelium) to form a concentration gradient along which circulating leucocytes can migrate towards the stimulus.

Specific chemokine receptors are selectively expressed on particular populations of leucocytes and this is what determines which cells a chemokine will attract. Some receptors (for example chemokine C-C motif receptor 5 or CCR5) are expressed preferentially by Th1 cells, while others (such as CCR3 and CCR4) are characteristic of Th2 cells.

Growth factors

Growth factors are required for the differentiation of haematopoietic cells. Granulocyte–macrophage colony-stimulating factor (GM-CSF), released by macrophages, T cells and fibroblasts, induces the development of nonlymphoid cells such as granulocytes and activates macrophages and eosinophils. TGF-β modulates the immune response by inhibiting the proliferation of T and B cells and suppressing the activities of macrophages and NK cells.

MAJOR HISTOCOMPATIBILITY COMPLEX

T cells cannot respond to protein antigens unless they have been processed and presented as short peptides, complexed with MHC molecules, on the surface of an APC. The MHC is conventionally divided into three subregions: class I, class II and class III. Class I and class II molecules are closely related in structure and function, whereas class III molecules show little structural similarity. The genes that encode the human MHC, also known as human leucocyte antigen (HLA), have been mapped to chromosome 6p21.3.

Class I major histocompatibility complex

There are two major groups of class I MHC antigens:

■ 'classic' class I molecules (HLA-A, HLA-B and HLA-C)
■ 'nonclassic' class I molecules (HLA-E, HLA-F and HLA-G).

The classic molecules are constitutively expressed on most nucleated cells. They are highly polymorphic, with over 500 *HLA-A*, over 900 *HLA-B* and over 300 *HLA-C* alleles being described.

The nonclassic molecules have a limited polymorphism and their tissue expression is also limited. HLA-E and HLA-F are expressed on a variety of adult and fetal tissues, while HLA-G is predominantly restricted to the invasive extravillous cytotrophoblast tissue of the placenta.

Class I molecules present peptides of 8–9 amino acids in length, predominantly derived from within the cell cytoplasm (endogenous antigens, such as viruses), to CD8-positive T cells. The Tc cells are then able to kill the infected cells and eliminate the pathogen.

Class II major histocompatibility complex

The MHC class II region encodes more than 30 proteins, including HLA-DR, HLA-DQ and HLA-DP. These antigens are highly polymorphic (with over 800 alleles having been described) and are expressed on specialised APCs including monocytes, macrophages, B cells and dendritic cells.

Compared with the peptide-binding groove of class I molecules, the class II peptide-binding groove is more open-ended, allowing longer peptides of 15–24 amino acids to bind. Class II molecules present antigenic peptides derived from outside the cell (exogenous antigens) to CD4-positive T cells.

Class III major histocompatibility complex

The MHC class III region contains a large number of genes, most of which encode a diverse range of serum and plasma proteins. These include the complement components C2 and C4 and complement factor Bf, some heat shock proteins (HSP70, HSP71 and HSP72) and the proinflammatory cytokine TNF-α.

Transplantation

Transplantation refers to the act of transferring cells, tissues or organs from one site to another. It is the only treatment for end-stage organ failure but its success largely depends upon the level of disparity between graft donor and recipient. There are four main types of transplant:

- An autograft is tissue transferred from one part of the body to another in the same individual, for example skin grafting in people with burns.
- An isograft is tissue transferred between genetically identical individuals, for example monozygotic twins.
- An allograft is tissue transferred between genetically different members of the same species.
- A xenograft is tissue transferred between different species, for example the graft of a pig heart into a human.

Thus, autografts and isografts are usually accepted by the host but allografts and xenografts are recognised as foreign by the recipient's immune system and, unless treated, will be rejected. This latter phenomenon is principally attributable to recipient T cells recognising allogeneic MHC antigens, a process known as allorecognition.

ALLORECOGNITION

The immune response against a transplanted organ is much more vigorous than the response seen against a pathogen. Since isolated MHC antigens in themselves are considered to be poor immunogens that do not induce graft rejection, other factors in addition to MHC incompatibility must be responsible for the allograft response.

The presence of MHC-incompatible dendritic cells (passenger dendritic cells) in a recently transplanted graft has been shown to be of crucial importance in this context. These cells can present donor-derived peptides in the binding groove of donor MHC molecules and, being professional APCs, they are able to activate naïve T cells (that is, T cells that have never encountered antigen before).

In addition, the strength of the alloresponse is attributable to the fact that the normal T cell repertoire contains a high proportion of T cells that are capable of recognising the MHC molecules on the graft as foreign and reacting against them.

It is important to note that minor histocompatibility antigens can also be targets of rejection even when the MHC is identical between donor and recipient. The most important example is the histocompatibility antigen H-Y, which is encoded by the Y chromosome and hence expressed only on male cells.

GRAFT-VERSUS-HOST DISEASE

In certain circumstances, for example during bone marrow transplantation, it is the graft that initiates a rejection response against the recipient. Immune-competent donor T cells that reside in the graft recognise the recipient's MHC and/or minor histocompatibility antigens as being foreign and initiate an immune response against the host. This reaction is known as graft-versus-host disease and can be prevented by careful matching of the donor and recipient, removal of all T cells from the graft and effective immunosuppression.

TYPES OF REJECTION

Hyperacute rejection

Hyperacute rejection occurs within minutes to hours of connecting the host's circulation to the transplanted organ. It is defined as a severe immunological response to the graft, mediated by preformed, naturally occurring antibodies that react against antigens expressed on donor cells. For example, it may occur as a result of ABO blood group incompatibility or because the recipient has been sensitised to the donor MHC (for example by a previous transplant). Antibody binding initiates an immunological cascade, with complement activation, increased vascular leakage, activation of the coagulation process and increased expression of adhesion molecules; the end result is rapid destruction of the graft.

Acute rejection

Acute rejection is normally seen days to weeks after transplantation. It is caused by donor leucocytes (so-called passenger leucocytes) migrating out of the graft and initiating a primary immune response. Activated recipient T cells then migrate to the organ and initiate tissue damage by the induction of delayed (type IV) hypersensitivity reactions and by the generation of Tc cells.

Chronic rejection

Chronic rejection occurs months to years after transplantation. It is less understood than hyperacute or acute rejection. Occlusion of blood vessels, macrophage infiltration and smooth muscle proliferation lead to blockage of the blood vessels and ischaemia of the graft.

METHODS TO PREVENT REJECTION

Two major methods are employed to minimise graft rejection:

- donor and recipient matching
- use of immunosuppressive drugs.

Table 19.5 provides an overview of drugs that are commonly used to prevent graft rejection.

Human leucocyte antigen matching

Human MHC class I and class II antigens display extensive polymorphism and the chances of matching an unrelated donor and recipient at all of the class I and class II gene loci is extremely remote. However, the strength of graft rejection inversely correlates with

TABLE 19.5 **Immunosuppressive drugs**

Drug name	Mechanism of action
Azathioprine	Inhibition of nucleic acid synthesis in all mitotic cells
Corticosteroids (e.g. prednisolone)	Prevention of the generation of cytotoxic effector cells; general anti-inflammatory effects
Ciclosporin A and tacrolimus	Blocking of T cell activation
Sirolimus	Inhibition of T cell proliferation
Anti-CTLA-4 antibodies	Promotion of unresponsiveness in alloreactive T cells

CTLA-4 = cytotoxic T lymphocyte antigen 4

the degree of HLA matching: the better the match, the lower the chance of rejection. Moreover, differences at class II loci are more detrimental to graft survival than differences at class I. Thus, a single class II difference has been shown to have the same effect on the graft as that observed when there are three or four class I mismatches. When both class I and class II antigens are mismatched, rejection is greatly accelerated.

Hypersensitivity

An immune response provides the host with protection from a wide range of pathogens. However, some immune responses can have deleterious effects, resulting in tissue damage. Such an excessive or inappropriate reaction is referred to as hypersensitivity. Hypersensitivity reactions may be distinguished by the type of immune response generated (Figure 19.4). It is important to note that most hypersensitivity reactions involve a range of mechanisms and are not restricted to a single type.

IMMEDIATE (TYPE I) HYPERSENSITIVITY

This is mediated by antigens (allergens) that enter the body via inhalation or ingestion (Figure 19.4A). The allergens bind to and cross-link IgE antibodies that are bound to Fc receptors on the surface of tissue mast cells or blood basophils. This leads to cell activation and the release of histamine (degranulation). The primary effects may be localised ('weal and flare reaction') or systemic depending on the degree of mediator release.

Type I hypersensitivity includes severe anaphylactic reactions to peanuts, bee venom and penicillin as well as the atopic diseases of asthma and hay fever.

ANTIBODY-MEDIATED (TYPE II) HYPERSENSITIVITY

Type II reactions are mediated by IgG or IgM antibodies that react against antigen bound to specific cells or tissues (Figure 19.4B). The antibodies interact with the Fc receptors on a range of effector cells including platelets and neutrophils, causing activation of the complement system and damage to target cells.

Examples include transfusion reactions and haemolytic disease of the newborn.

FIGURE 19.4 **Hypersensitivity reactions**

A Immediate (type I)

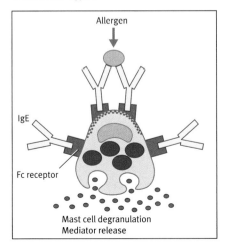

B Antibody-mediated (type II)

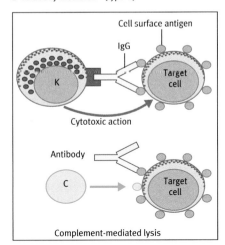

C Immune complex (type III)

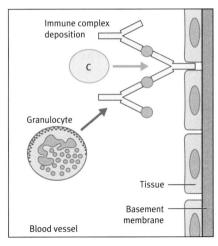

D Delayed-type (type IV)

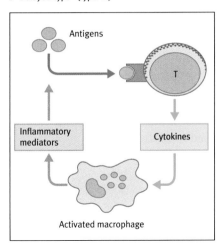

C = complement | Ig = immunoglobulin |
Fc = crystallisable fragment |
K = K cell (responsible for antibody-dependent
cell-mediated cytotoxicity) |
T = T cell

Reproduced by permission: Immunology. 6th ed. Roitt IM, Brostoff J, Male D. St Louis: Mosby; 2002.

IMMUNE COMPLEX (TYPE III) HYPERSENSITIVITY

Type III hypersensitivity is caused by failure of phagocytes to clear immune complexes (Figure 19.4C). The immune complexes then initiate an inflammatory response via complement activation and histamine and proinflammatory cytokine release. The magnitude of the reaction depends upon both the quantity and the location of the immune complexes. Much of the tissue damage stems from the release of lysosomal enzymes by granulocytes as they attempt to phagocytose complexes that are bound to vessel walls.

This type of hypersensitivity is found in persistent infections (for example leprosy and viral hepatitis), autoimmune disease (for example rheumatoid arthritis and systemic lupus erythematosus) and following inhalation of antigen (for example farmer's lung and pigeon fancier's lung).

DELAYED-TYPE (TYPE IV) HYPERSENSITIVITY

This is a localised inflammatory reaction caused by the recruitment of antigen-specific T cells to a site of

305

antigen deposition (Figure 19.4D); it develops over 24–72 hours. There are three variants:

- contact hypersensitivity
- tuberculin-type hypersensitivity
- granulomatous hypersensitivity.

Contact hypersensitivity occurs at the point of contact with an allergen (for example nickel, chromate). It is characterised by an eczema-like reaction within 72 hours.

Tuberculin-type hypersensitivity is induced by soluble antigens from organisms such as *Mycobacterium tuberculosis* and *M. leprae*. It results in a localised inflammatory response in the form of a swelling at the tuberculin injection site.

Granulomatous hypersensitivity develops over 21–28 days. Persistence of antigen leads to chronic stimulation of T cells and the release of cytokines such as TNF-α. This results in the formation of epithelioid cell granulomas. The most important forms of type IV hypersensitivity clinically occur in many chronic diseases including tuberculosis, leprosy and Crohn's disease.

The fetus as an allograft

Pregnancy presents an immune paradox in that half of the fetus's genetic component is derived from the father and therefore the mother would be expected to mount a graft rejection response directed against paternal antigens expressed on the placenta. The fact that this does not happen in normal pregnancy shows that there must be mechanisms that have evolved to prevent rejection of the placenta and hence the fetus by the maternal immune system.

THE TWO IMMUNOLOGICAL INTERFACES OF PREGNANCY

It is the placenta, not the fetus, that forms the interface with the mother. There are two main interfaces (see Figure 19.5).

Interface 1 is formed by the extravillous cytotrophoblast, which invades from the tips of the chorionic villi into the decidua in the early stages of pregnancy to anchor the placenta to the uterine wall. It subsequently invades the spiral arteries that supply maternal blood to the intervillous space, displacing the endothelium and destroying the muscle layer, thereby remodelling the arteries to increase blood flow to the developing placenta (see Chapter 14). This therefore forms a tissue–tissue interface, which plays an important role in the first trimester of pregnancy.

Interface 2 is that between the surface of the chorionic villi (the syncytiotrophoblast) and the maternal blood, across which the exchange of gases and nutrients occurs. This is a tissue–blood interface and is more important in the second and third trimester. The second interface is extended throughout the mother's circulation in two ways. Firstly, there is shedding of cellular and microparticulate syncytiotrophoblast debris, DNA and mRNA from the surface of the placenta into the mother's blood throughout pregnancy and, secondly, there are haemorrhages of fetal blood across the placenta. Thus, fetal red blood cells and leucocytes can be found in the maternal circulation as early as in the first trimester, which has immunological implications.

IMMUNE INTERACTIONS AT INTERFACES 1 AND 2

Interaction between invasive extravillous cytotrophoblast and maternal immune cells in the decidua (interface 1)

The invasive extravillous cytotrophoblast comes into intimate contact with maternal immune cells in the decidua. Some 40% of maternal cells in the decidua are bone-marrow-derived. They comprise T cells (approximately 10%), macrophages (approximately 20%) and dendritic cells (approximately 2%); there are also some reports of T cells that express gamma/delta TCRs. There are virtually no B cells. However, by far the largest immune cell population (up to 70%) are a specialised form of NK cell.

Decidual NK cells stain brightly positive for a marker called CD56 (an adhesion molecule) but are negative for CD16, an Fc receptor found on all other NK cells. The phenotype of these decidual NK cells differs from that of most other NK cells in that, instead of being cytotoxic (for the surveillance of tumours and virally infected cells), activated decidual NK cells produce cytokines, chemokines and angiogenic factors that facilitate trophoblast invasion. The close interaction between the

FIGURE 19.5 **The two immune interfaces of pregnancy**

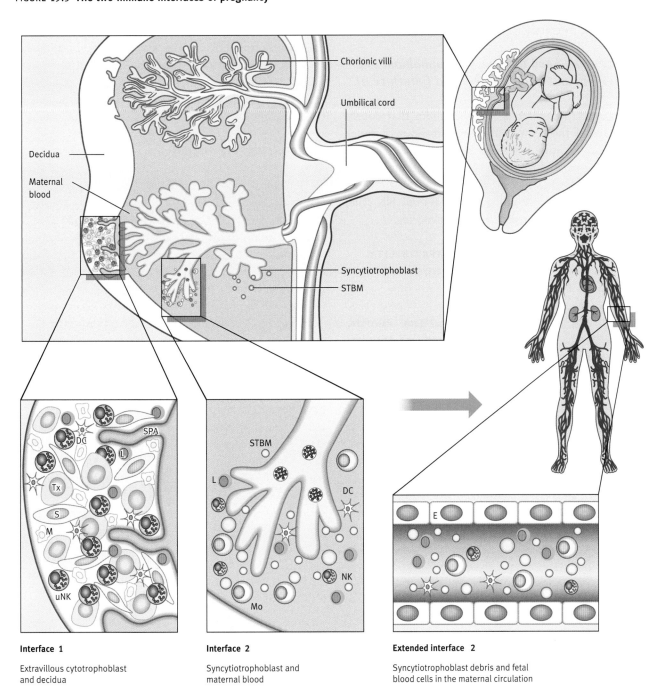

Interface 1

Extravillous cytotrophoblast
and decidua

Interface 2

Syncytiotrophoblast and
maternal blood

Extended interface 2

Syncytiotrophoblast debris and fetal
blood cells in the maternal circulation

DC = dendritic cell | E = endothelial cell | L = lymphocyte | M = macrophage | Mo = monocyte | NK = circulating natural killer cell | S = decidual stromal cell | SPA = spiral artery | STBM = syncytiotrophoblast microparticle | Tx = extravillous cytotrophoblast | uNK = uterine (decidual) natural killer cell

invasive extravillous trophoblast and decidual NK cells suggests that these cells may have a key role in maternal–fetal immune interactions.

Interaction between the syncytiotrophoblast and maternal immune cells in the blood (interface 2)

The syncytiotrophoblast is the epithelium that covers the surface of the human placenta. However, it functions as endothelium as it lines the placental side of the intervillous space through which the maternal blood flows. It is therefore in contact with the full range of maternal blood cells including T cells, B cells, NK cells, monocytes and polymorphonuclear leucocytes.

EXPRESSION OF MAJOR HISTOCOMPATIBILITY COMPLEX ANTIGENS BY THE TROPHOBLAST AT INTERFACES 1 AND 2

Central to the nature of the maternal–fetal immune response is the expression of MHC antigens (the key molecules that stimulate graft rejection) by the trophoblast (see Table 19.6).

Extravillous cytotrophoblast cells are MHC class I positive, but they have a pattern of expression that is unique to this cell type. Unlike any other cell in the body, they do not express the highly polymorphic classic class I antigens HLA-A or HLA-B, which are the principal stimulators of graft rejection. However, they do express the classic class I antigen HLA-C. In addition, they express the nonpolymorphic, nonclassic class I MHC antigens HLA-E and HLA-G.

In contrast to the extravillous cytotrophoblast, the syncytiotrophoblast is completely negative for class I MHC expression, making it almost unique in the human body, with the exception of red blood cells.

The syncytiotrophoblast is therefore unlikely to stimulate the maternal immune system.

Neither the invasive extravillous cytotrophoblast nor the syncytiotrophoblast expresses class II MHC antigens.

Immune interactions in the decidua seem to be predominantly between trophoblast and NK cells rather than T cells, as occurs in graft rejection. The functions of trophoblast HLA-G, HLA-E and HLA-C are as follows.

Human leucocyte antigen G

HLA-G has four different membrane-bound forms (HLA-G1, HLA-G2, HLA-G3 and HLA-G4) and three soluble forms (HLA-G5, HLA-G6 and HLA-G7), which do not contain transmembrane or cytoplasmic domains that would anchor them to the cell surface. Thus, HLA-G can mediate its effects both locally (mainly via the membrane-bound form HLA-G1) and systemically (mainly via the soluble form HLA-G5).

HLA-G is almost always expressed on the extravillous cytotrophoblast, which suggests that it is fundamental to reproduction. In stark contrast to the highly polymorphic HLA-A and HLA-B molecules, HLA-G displays very little polymorphism (only four alleles have been identified that encode slightly modified proteins). Such limited polymorphism ensures that paternal HLA-G molecules are almost identical to the maternal ones and therefore unlikely to induce an alloreactive maternal T cell response during pregnancy.

HLA-G isoforms have a peptide-binding groove and should therefore be able to present peptides in a similar way to polymorphic classic class I molecules; this has indeed been demonstrated for both HLA-G1 and soluble HLA-G5. However, the low polymorphism in HLA-G limits the diversity of peptides it can bind. The binding of peptides might therefore be necessary to

TABLE 19.6 **Major histocompatibility complex antigens expressed by the trophoblast**

Tissue	HLA-A[a]	HLA-B[a]	HLA-C[a]	HLA-E[b]	HLA-G[b]
Adult and fetal tissues	+	+	+	+	–
Extravillous cytotrophoblast (interface 1)	–	–	+	+	+
Syncytiotrophoblast (interface 2)	–	–	–	–	–

[a] Polymorphic | [b] monomorphic | HLA = human leucocyte antigen | + = antigen is expressed | – = antigen is not expressed

FIGURE 19.6 **Interactions between decidual natural killer cells and extravillous cytotrophoblast at interface 1**

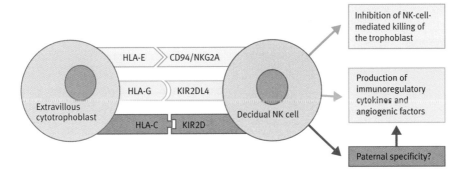

HLA = human leucocyte antigen | KIR = killer cell immunoglobulin-like receptor | NKG2A = natural killer cell receptor group 2A | NK = natural killer

ensure the stability of the HLA-G molecule rather than for it to be involved in antigen presentation.

HLA-G has been shown to interact with both CD4-positive and CD8-positive T cells. Rather than activating the T cells, however, HLA-G induces apoptosis of CD8-positive T cells via a pathway that involves Fas and Fas ligand and suppresses the proliferation of CD4-positive T cells and Tc cells.

HLA-G interacts with NK cells via their KIRs. To date, three KIRs have been identified that interact with HLA-G: KIR2DL4 and the immunoglobulin-like transcripts ILT-2 and ILT-4. These receptors are also expressed on monocytes, macrophages and dendritic cells.

The result of the interaction between HLA-G and the cells of the innate immune system is not the production of an immune response that attacks the placenta but one that facilitates implantation, trophoblast invasion and placentation. On interacting with HLA-G-expressing trophoblast, the decidual NK cells produce a range of immunoregulatory molecules (see Figure 19.6) including:

- cytokines (IFN-γ, IL-10, TGF-β1, metalloproteinase inhibitor 1)
- chemokines (IL-8, IFN-γ-inducible protein 10)
- angiogenic factors (vascular endothelial growth factor, placenta growth factor).

These promote and regulate trophoblast invasion.

Human leucocyte antigen E

HLA-E is also expressed on the invasive cells of the extravillous cytotrophoblast as well as on most other cells

in the body. Like HLA-G, it is virtually monomorphic and only presents a small repertoire of peptides. The primary peptides that HLA-E binds are derived from the leader sequence of other HLA class I molecules, such as HLA-A, HLA-B, HLA-C and HLA-G.

Human leucocyte antigen C

The expression of HLA-C on the extravillous trophoblast is counterintuitive as it is polymorphic and might therefore be expected to stimulate T-cell-mediated graft rejection. Indeed, differences in HLA-C alone between graft and donor are sufficient to trigger a graft rejection response. However, as for HLA-G, the primary interaction of HLA-C seems to be not with T cells but with NK cells (Figure 19.6). This interaction is also believed to stimulate the production of beneficial cytokines, chemo-kines and angiogenic factors.

MATERNAL IMMUNOREGULATION IN PREGNANCY

The extravillous cytotrophoblast and syncytiotrophoblast do not seem to stimulate classic acquired (T cell and B cell) immune responses because of their pattern of MHC expression. However, fetal leucocytes that enter the maternal circulation express HLA-A, HLA-B and HLA-C antigens and therefore have the potential to stimulate both antibody-mediated and cell-mediated immunity.

FIGURE 19.7 **Transport of antibodies across the placenta**

A Passive transfer of immunity

B Placental barrier to antifetal (paternal) antibodies

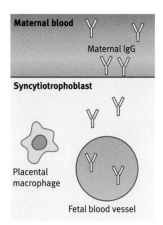

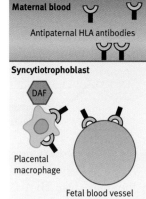

DAF = decay-accelerating factor | HLA = human leucocyte antigen | IgG = immunoglobulin G

Antibody production

The mother is able to make antibodies to paternal HLA-A, HLA-B and HLA-C antigens. This occurs in around 15% of first pregnancies and 60% of subsequent pregnancies by the same father. However, these antibodies do not seem to harm the pregnancy in any way. Harm is a real possibility as one of the major functions of the placenta is to transport maternal antibodies to the fetal circulation (Figure 19.7A). In this process, maternal IgG antibodies in the mother's blood bind to Fc receptors on the surface of the syncytiotrophoblast and are actively transported into the chorionic villus, where they enter the fetal circulation. The maternal antibodies provide immediate protection for the fetus against infections to which the mother has been exposed. Only IgG antibodies are transported in this way; IgM, IgE, IgA or IgD are not.

The potentially harmful antibodies against paternal HLA molecules are filtered out by the placenta before they reach the fetal blood (Figure 19.7B). The antibodies are transported across the syncytiotrophoblast but they then bind to paternal HLA antigens expressed on the macrophages and endothelium of the chorionic villus. Here, the immune complexes formed are cleared by the macrophages, and complement regulatory factors (for example decay-accelerating factor) inhibit complement activation. Thus, none of the harmful antibodies enter the fetal circulation.

One situation where this mechanism breaks down is in haemolytic disease of the newborn or rhesus disease (see Figure 19.8). This occurs when a mother makes IgG

FIGURE 19.8 **Haemolytic disease of the newborn (rhesus isoimmunisation)**

A First birth

B Postpartum

C Subsequent pregnancy

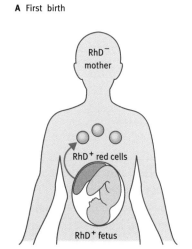

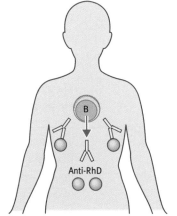

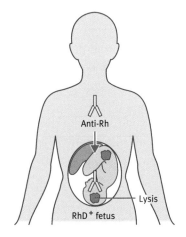

B = B cell | RhD⁺ = rhesus D positive | RhD⁻ = rhesus D negative

Reproduced by permission: Immunology. 6th ed. Roitt IM, Brostoff J, Male D. St Louis: Mosby; 2002.

antibodies to antigens present on the surface of her infant's red blood cells. These antibodies are transferred across the placenta into the fetal circulation and cause the destruction of fetal erythrocytes. The most commonly involved antigen in such a condition is rhesus D (RhD).

During her first pregnancy with an RhD-positive baby, an RhD-negative mother is not exposed to significant numbers of fetal RhD-positive erythrocytes. However, at delivery, separation of the placenta allows fetal blood to enter the mother's circulation (Figure 19.8A). These fetal red blood cells are then recognised by the maternal immune system, leading to the production of RhD-specific memory B cells postpartum (Figure 19.8B).

The first incompatible child is therefore usually unaffected, but activation of such cells during a subsequent pregnancy with an RhD-positive fetus results in the formation of IgG anti-RhD antibodies, which cross the placenta and damage fetal red blood cells (Figure 19.8C). The consequences of this process to the fetus are wide-ranging and sometimes fatal. Symptoms include mild to severe anaemia, impaired platelet function and dysfunction of the liver and spleen.

The incidence of haemolytic disease of the newborn due to RhD incompatibility has fallen dramatically following the introduction of RhD prophylaxis, where anti-RhD antibodies are administered to RhD-negative mothers immediately following the delivery of RhD-positive babies. These antibodies bind to any fetal erythrocytes that may have entered the mother's circulation and destroy them before they can cause sensitisation.

Cell-mediated immunity

In contrast to antibody-mediated immunity, maternal cell-mediated immune responses to paternal antigens during pregnancy are depressed. This is thought to be the result of changes in the Th1/Th2 balance in pregnancy.

As described previously, following stimulation by antigen, naïve CD4-positive T cells polarise to a Th1 or Th2 phenotype depending on the signals they receive during activation. In nonpregnant individuals, responses may go in either direction, allowing them to mount both cell-mediated (Th1) and antibody-

mediated (Th2) responses (Figure 19.3A). However, in pregnancy this equilibrium is altered because the placenta produces Th2-promoting cytokines, such as IL-4 and IL-10, as well as progesterone, which inhibits Th1 responses (Figure 19.3B). Thus, the bias in normal pregnancy is towards Th2 immunity, with suppression of cell-mediated immunity (in particular suppression of IFN-γ production). This leaves the pregnant woman with her antibody-mediated immunity intact and thus she is still able to fight infection.

Clinical evidence for a shift towards Th2 and away from Th1 responses in normal pregnancy includes:

- temporary remission of rheumatoid arthritis (Th1-mediated) during pregnancy
- exacerbation of diseases caused by intracellular pathogens (for example herpes and malaria) during pregnancy
- worsening of systemic lupus erythematosus (Th2-mediated) during pregnancy.

Maternal inflammatory response to pregnancy

While being a useful working model, the Th1/Th2 model is too simplistic to fully explain the immune changes in pregnancy. It has recently been found that during pregnancy there is activation of the mother's innate immune system (monocytes, granulocytes and NK cells) with increased production of Th1 cytokines, IL-12, IL-18 and TNF-α. However, as mentioned previously, IFN-γ production is not stimulated and there is reduced T cell activity. This must be the pivotal point. It is thought that this inflammatory response is triggered by the release of factors, possibly apoptotic microparticulate debris, from the surface of the placenta into the maternal circulation. This material does not express MHC antigens and cannot stimulate T cells.

IMMUNE MECHANISMS IN DISORDERS OF PREGNANCY

If immune mechanisms are important for facilitating trophoblast invasion, then defects in these mechanisms would be expected to lead to disorders such as recurrent implantation failure, miscarriage and pre-eclampsia.

MAJOR HISTOCOMPATIBILITY COMPLEX EXPRESSION AT THE MATERNAL–FETAL INTERFACE

HLA-G is expressed as early as at the two-cell embryo stage in humans. Embryos that produce soluble HLA-G are more likely to implant than those that do not, as shown by studies that measured soluble HLA-G secreted into the culture supernatant by embryos obtained through *in vitro* fertilisation. In addition, HLA-G expression has been reported to be reduced on the invasive extravillous cytotrophoblast in women with recurrent spontaneous abortions and in pre-eclampsia.

HLA-C may also have an important role in miscarriage and pre-eclampsia. HLA-C is polymorphic and individuals express one of two major subtypes: HLA-C1, which mediates the activation of NK cells, or HLA-C2, which mediates their inhibition. Similarly, individuals have KIR receptors belonging to one of two different subtypes: KIR-A receptors, which inhibit NK cells, or KIR-B receptors, which activate NK cells. Thus, a pregnancy where the trophoblast expresses an HLA-C1 subtype and the maternal decidual NK cells express KIR-B receptors will result in activation of the decidual NK cells to produce the cytokines, chemokines and angiogenic factors required for trophoblast invasion (Figure 19.9A). However, a combination of the HLA-C2 and KIR-A subtypes would lead to inhibition of the decidual NK cells and poor trophoblast invasion (Figure 19.9B). The latter two subtypes have been found to be more common in pre-eclampsia and recurrent miscarriage.

Whether there is altered trophoblast HLA-E expression in these conditions is not known.

Balance between type 1 and type 2 T helper cells and inflammatory responses

If a shift to Th2-type immune responses is important for the success of normal pregnancy, then it might be expected that this shift does not occur to the same extent in recurrent miscarriage and pre-eclampsia. This is indeed the case, with IFN-γ production being significantly increased compared with normal pregnancy. The maternal systemic inflammatory response is also significantly increased in pre-eclampsia, as defined by a range

FIGURE 19.9 **Interaction between trophoblast and decidual natural killer cells**

A Normal pregnancy

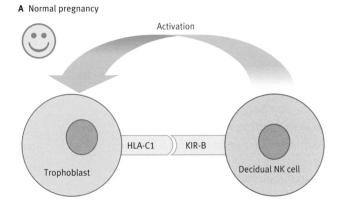

B Pre-eclampsia

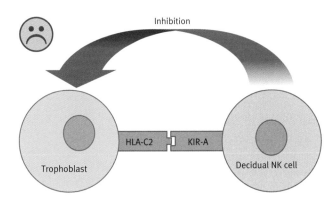

HLA = human leucocyte antigen | KIR = killer cell immunoglobulin-like receptor | NK = natural killer

of markers (including IFN-γ, C-reactive protein). This exaggerated inflammatory response leads to endothelial dysfunction in the mother, which is the cause of the maternal syndrome (including hypertension, proteinuria, oedema and disseminated intravascular coagulopathy). This inflammatory response seems to be centred on NK cells rather than T cells.

Antiphospholipid antibodies

The presence of lupus anticoagulant and anticardiolipin antibodies in maternal blood is closely related to the risk of miscarriage. Lupus anticoagulant antibodies inhibit coagulation by inhibiting the conversion of prothrombin to thrombin. They are present in 2–5%

of the normal obstetric population but have an 85–95% risk of fetal mortality. Anticardiolipin antibodies develop against certain phospholipid components (β2-glycoprotein) of cell membranes and are found in 15% of women with a miscarriage. During differentiation into syncytiotrophoblast, trophoblasts express cell membrane phospholipids that can bind anti-β2-glycoprotein antibodies. These interfere with trophoblast cell maturation, resulting in defective placentation. Low-dose heparin and aspirin, alone or in combination, may improve pregnancy outcome. These antibodies can also be transferred to the fetus, where they may cause transient autoimmune thyroiditis, myasthenia gravis and autoimmune thrombocytopenia.

IMMUNOTHERAPY

The possibility that immune mechanisms may be involved in implantation failure, recurrent miscarriage and pre-eclampsia has lead to the use of immunotherapy as a possible way of preventing these disorders. Three main approaches have been used.

Paternal and third-party leucocyte immunisation

This treatment is based on the premise that in women with implantation failure or recurrent miscarriage, exposure of the maternal immune system to paternal antigens during implantation and early pregnancy fails to trigger the necessary facilitating immune response. By analogy with the finding that pretransplant blood transfusions significantly increase renal allograft survival, it has been argued that injection of a preparation of paternal or third-party leucocytes into the mother on one or more occasions before conception will stimulate the appropriate immune response and lead to successful pregnancy. This is a controversial area. There is little

scientific basis for this treatment and meta-analysis of the published studies has shown little benefit.

Intravenous immunoglobulin therapy

Given the controversies surrounding leucocyte immunotherapy, treatment with intravenous immunoglobulin (IVIg) has been used as a safer alternative. IVIg is produced from pooled human plasma obtained from multiple donors and is used as an immunomodulator in many diseases including autoimmune conditions, transplantation and cancer. It is proposed that it contains antibodies that are beneficial to pregnancy survival by downregulating B-cell and NK-cell function. However, data regarding its ability to prevent miscarriage are conflicting and a number of adverse effects have been reported. This area requires further study.

Treatment with antibodies against tumour necrosis factor alpha

Anti-TNF-α antibodies are used to treat inflammatory conditions such as rheumatoid arthritis and ankylosing spondylitis. It has therefore been proposed that the risk of implantation failure and miscarriage might be modulated by anti-TNF-α antibodies, provided these events are indeed attributable to an excessive Th1 response.

While good success rates for this treatment are claimed, there is no strong scientific support and anti-TNF agents have been reported to be associated with the development of granulomatous disease, lymphoma, systemic lupus erythematosus and congestive cardiac failure.

A Cochrane review has concluded that immunotherapy provides no significant beneficial effect over placebo in improving the livebirth rate.

FURTHER READING

HIBY S E, WALKER J J, O'SHAUGHNESSY K M, REDMAN C W, CARRINGTON M, TROWSDALE J, et al. Combinations of maternal K I R and fetal HLA-C genes influence the risk of preeclampsia and reproductive success. J Exp Med 2004;200:957–65.

HVIID T. HLA-G in human reproduction: aspects of genetics, function and pregnancy complications. Hum Reprod Update 2006;12:209–32.

KINDT T J, GOLDSBY R A, OSBORNE B A. Kuby Immunology, 6th ed. New York: W H Freeman; 2007.

MOFFETT A, LOKE C. Immunology of placentation in eutherian mammals. Nat Rev Immunol 2006;5:584–94.

Microbiology

CHAPTER 20

Microbiology

Susan Hopkins and Daniel Brudney

General bacteriology

CLASSIFICATION AND IDENTIFICATION OF MICROORGANISMS

A systematic approach is required to classify the different forms of microorganisms that can cause disease. A variety of methods can be used but a clinically useful classification is as follows:

- viruses (covered in Chapter 21)
- bacteria
  - Gram-positive bacteria
  - Gram-negative bacteria
  - spirochetes
  - mycobacteria
  - 'unusual' bacteria
- fungi
- protozoa.

Gram staining of bacteria

The majority of clinically important pathogenic bacteria can be visualised under a light microscope with the aid of the Gram stain (named after the Danish bacteriologist Hans Christian Gram). The Gram stain is the most widely used stain in medical microbiology and remains the bedrock of laboratory diagnosis. It allows rapid division of bacteria into two categories, namely Gram-positive and Gram-negative, according to the degree of staining.

The process of Gram staining is illustrated in Figure 20.1. First, the clinical specimen is placed on a slide and dried (Figure 20.1A). Crystal violet, which stains bacterial cell walls, is added to the slide (Figure 20.1B), followed by the addition of Gram's iodine solution as a fixative (Figure 20.1C). The iodine forms a complex with the crystal violet, binding it more tightly to the cell wall. A decolouriser (a mixture of acetone and ethanol)

FIGURE 20.1 **Gram-stain procedure**

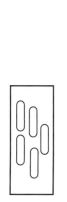 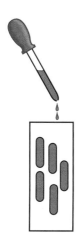 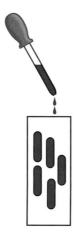 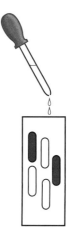 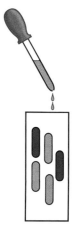

A Specimen preparation   B Staining with crystal violet   C Fixation with Gram's iodine solution   D Decolourisation   E Staining with safranin

is then added (Figure 20.1D). This washes the crystal violet–iodine complex out of Gram-negative cell walls. Gram-positive cell walls have a thicker peptidoglycan layer and lack an outer lipopolysaccharide layer. These properties allow Gram-positive bacteria to retain the crystal violet–iodine dye and to resist washing with the decolouriser. Gram-positive bacteria therefore appear purple. Now, a counter stain such as safranin is added (Figure 20.1E). The decolourised Gram-negative bacteria take up this stain, making them appear pink. Figure 20.1E shows a mixture of Gram-positive (purple) and Gram-negative (pink) bacilli, which can be viewed under the light microscope.

Taxonomic classification of bacteria

Gram-positive and Gram-negative bacteria can be further subdivided according to their morphological and biochemical characteristics. The principal subdivisions include:

- morphology (shape) on microscopy
  - cocci (spherical)
  - bacilli (rod-shaped)
- Oxygen (O_2) requirements
  - aerobes (grow in the presence of O_2)
    - obligate aerobes require O_2 to grow
    - facultative anaerobes can grow in the presence or absence of O_2
  - anaerobes (require the exclusion of O_2 to grow).

By combining the appearance on microscopy after Gram staining with the growth characteristics (aerobic/anaerobic), a rapid initial putative identification may be made as shown in Table 20.1.

Biochemical properties and growth characteristics can also help to further subdivide related bacteria. For example, Gram-negative bacteria can be broadly divided upon their ability to ferment glucose:

- Enterobacteriaceae are glucose fermenters
- pseudomonads and related organisms are glucose non-fermenters.

TABLE 20.1 **Identification of bacteria on the basis of their morphology, Gram stain and O_2 requirements**

O_2 requirements	Gram-positive bacteria		Gram-negative bacteria	
	Cocci	Bacilli (rods)	Cocci	Bacilli (rods)
Obligate aerobes (require the presence of O_2 to grow)	*Micrococcus* spp.	*Nocardia* spp. (*Mycobacterium tuberculosis*)[a]	*Neisseria meningitidis* *N. gonorrhoeae*	*Pseudomonas aeruginosa* *Bordetella pertussis*
Facultative anaerobes (can tolerate aerobic and anaerobic conditions)	*Staphylococcus* spp. (e.g. *S. aureus*) *Streptococcus* spp. *Enterococcus* spp.	*Corynebacterium* spp. (e.g. *C. diphtheriae*) *Listeria monocytogenes* *Bacillus* spp.	There are no common pathogens within the facultative anaerobic Gram-negative cocci group	*Escherichia coli* *Klebsiella* spp. *Enterobacter* spp. *Citrobacter* spp. *Haemophilus influenzae* (coccobacillus)
Obligate anaerobes (require the exclusion of O_2 to grow)	*Peptostreptococcus* spp.	*Clostridium* spp. (e.g. *C. tetani*, *C. difficile*) *Actinomyces israelii* *Lactobacillus* spp. *Propionibacterium* spp.	*Veillonella parvula*	*Bacteroides* spp. *Fusobacterium* spp.

[a] Weakly Gram-positive, stains better with Ziehl–Neelsen stain | spp. = two or more species

Gram-negative organisms will grow well on the majority of laboratory media, but they are best identified on MacConkey agar. MacConkey agar contains bile salts and is selective for enteric bacteria. It is also an indicator medium, allowing differentiation between lactose fermenters (which produce a pink colour, e.g. *Escherichia coli*, *Klebsiella* spp.) and lactose nonfermenters (which produce a pale yellow colour, e.g. *Pseudomonas aeruginosa*, *Serratia* spp.).

New methods of identifying microorganisms

Molecular methods

Molecular techniques have had a direct influence on the clinical practice of medical microbiology. In many cases where traditional phenotypic methods (using enzyme reactions and characteristics) of microbial identification and typing are insufficient or time-consuming, molecular techniques can provide rapid and accurate data, potentially improving clinical outcomes.

Polymerase chain reaction (PCR) is used in microbiology to amplify (replicate many times) a single DNA sequence.

Gel electrophoresis is used routinely in microbiology to separate DNA, RNA or protein molecules using an electric field by virtue of their size, shape or electric charge.

Southern blotting, Northern blotting, Western blotting and Eastern blotting are molecular techniques for detecting the presence of microbial DNA sequences (Southern), RNA sequences (Northern), protein molecules (Western) or protein modifications (Eastern).

DNA sequencing and genomics have been used for many decades in molecular microbiology studies. Due to their relatively small size, viral genomes were the first to be completely analysed by DNA sequencing. A huge range of sequence and genomic data is now available for a number of species and strains of microorganisms. Increasingly, this is becoming the gold standard for identifying species, typing organisms and identifying antimicrobial resistance. It also allows the production of a genetic tree looking at relatedness of organisms to predict whether a transmission event could have occurred.

Specific examples of clinical use include identifying organisms through their molecular sequence when phenotypical methods have failed, rapid detection of organisms (e.g. influenza, methicillin-resistant *Staphylococcus aureus* [MRSA]), typing to review the relatedness of strains (e.g. Spa typing of *Staphylococcus aureus*), detection of resistance (e.g. rifampicin resistance in Mycobacterium tuberculosis).

Matrix-assisted laser desorption/ionisation/time of flight (MALDI/TOF)

MALDI/TOF is an ionisation technique used in mass spectrometry, allowing the analysis of biomolecules. The type of a mass spectrometer most widely used with MALDI is the TOF (time-of-flight mass spectrometer), mainly due to its large mass range.

MALDI/TOF spectra are used for the identification of microorganisms such as bacteria or fungi. A colony of the microbe in question is smeared directly on the sample target and overlayed with matrix. The mass spectra generated are analysed by dedicated software and compared with stored profiles. Species diagnosis by this procedure is much faster, more accurate and cheaper than other procedures based on immunological or biochemical tests. MALDI/TOF may become the standard method for species identification in medical microbiological laboratories over the next few years. It can also be used to determine resistance profiles of organisms where certain proteins are expressed.

Toxin-mediated effects of bacteria

The pathogenic potential of several bacteria is enhanced by the production of either exotoxins or endotoxins. Exotoxins are proteins secreted by bacteria. Some important exotoxins are listed in Table 20.2. The properties of exotoxins and endotoxins are compared in Table 20.3.

Important pathogenic bacteria and associated disease states

This section considers bacterial pathogens of the female urogenital tract and a variety of other bacterial infections that are of relevance to obstetrics or gynaecology.

TABLE 20.2 **Important exotoxins**

Organism	Exotoxin	Action	Clinical significance
Staphylococcus aureus	Toxic shock syndrome toxin 1	Polyclonal T cell activation Cytokine release Fever and shock	Toxic shock syndrome
	Enterotoxins A–E	Vomiting	Food poisoning
	Epidermolytic toxin	Intraepidermal blisters and desquamation	Scalded skin syndrome
	Panton–Valentine leucocidin	Lysis of leucocytes	Invasive, pyogenic and necrotising infections
Streptococcus pyogenes	Streptococcal pyrogenic exotoxins A and B	Endothelial damage Fever	Tissue oedema
	Streptolysin O	Lysis of erythrocytes and leucocytes	Poststreptococcal rheumatic fever
Clostridium spp.	*C. tetani* toxin	Sustained neuronal discharge	Motor spasms
	C. botulinum toxin	Neuromuscular blockade	Botulism (food poisoning, wound botulism)
	C. difficile toxins A and B, binary toxin	Cytotoxicity	Pseudomembranous colitis (association with the use of broad-spectrum antibiotics)
Corynebacterium diphtheriae	Diphtheria toxin	Inhibition of protein synthesis	Diphtheria
Vibrio cholera	Cholera enterotoxin	Activation of adenylate cyclase and gastrointestinal water loss	Cholera (torrential diarrhoea)
Shigella dysenteriae	Shiga toxin	Inhibition of protein synthesis and cell death	Bacterial dysentery
Verocytotoxigenic *Escherichia coli*	Verocytotoxin	Inhibition of protein synthesis and cell death	Bacterial dysentery Haemorrhagic colitis

TABLE 20.3 **Comparison of exotoxins and endotoxins**

Parameter of comparison	Exotoxins	Endotoxins
Producing organisms	Mostly Gram-positive organisms (and a few Gram-negative organisms)	Only Gram-negative organisms
Chemical composition	Proteins	Lipopolysaccharide
Site of production	Manufactured in the bacterial-cell cytoplasm	Bacterial outer-membrane component
Release	Secreted from cell	Released from membrane as vesicles (blebs) during bacterial cell death
Biochemical properties	Heat-labile Denatured by formaldehyde	Heat-stable Not denatured by formaldehyde
Antigenicity	Neutralised by specific antibodies; therefore immunity can be developed	Poorly antigenic; only partially neutralised by specific antibodies

STREPTOCOCCACEAE

These are Gram-positive cocci that are facultative anaerobes. They typically grow in chains or pairs. Streptococci can be distinguished from other Gram-positive cocci biochemically by a negative catalase test (failure to hydrolyse hydrogen peroxide to O_2 and H_2O).

There are numerous genera within the Streptococcaceae. Most pathogens fall into two main genera:

- *Streptococcus*
- *Enterococcus.*

Classification of Streptococcaceae

The classification of streptococci is complicated by the presence of three overlapping methods of subdividing the group, namely on pattern of haemolysis, on serologic (Lancefield) group and on biochemical reactions (Table 20.4).

Haemolysis is visualised by culture of streptococci on blood agar:

- clear zones of haemolysis surrounding the colonies indicate complete haemolysis (beta haemolysis)
- green zones around the colonies indicate partial haemolysis (alpha haemolysis)
- lack of zones around the colonies (also referred to as gamma haemolysis) indicates the presence of a nonhaemolytic strain.

Lancefield serotyping (developed by Rebecca Lancefield) is based on the fact that different streptococci have different cell-wall antigens (polysaccharides). This allows rapid differentiation of streptococci by agglutination. The method is very useful for subdividing beta-haemolytic streptococci. Although some alpha-haemolytic streptococci also possess Lancefield group antigens, this method is not recommended for these organisms.

Finally, streptococci can be subdivided on the basis of biochemical properties. For example, enterococci hydrolyse bile salts (as detected by use of the aesculin test), whereas most streptococci do not.

Streptococcus pyogenes (Lancefield group A)

This *Streptococcus* species possesses a variety of virulence factors, including exotoxins (see Table 20.2), that make it a significant pathogen. Some of the infections and clinical syndromes associated with *S. pyogenes* are described in Table 20.4.

Skin and soft-tissue infections

S. pyogenes is highly infectious and virulent and can be spread by contact with an infected person or with fomites. Persons with a microbiological diagnosis of *S. pyogenes* skin infection should be isolated at least until they have received 48 hours of intravenous antibiotic treatment.

Necrotising fasciitis

This is an important invasive streptococcal infection. It is characterised by necrosis spreading through the fascia and fat, with rapid progression to systemic toxicity, shock and death unless aggressively managed. Bacteria gain entry to the subcutaneous layer often through minor, and sometimes unnoticed, trauma but this may also occur as a postsurgical complication. Characteristically, the site of infection is erythematous or purple with marked pain, often progressing to bullae formation and skin necrosis. Affected persons may show features of an associated toxic shock syndrome.

Two types of necrotising fasciitis have been identified; they are classified according to the organisms involved:

- necrotising fasciitis type 1 is polymicrobial; typical organisms include anaerobes, Gram-negative bacteria (Enterobacteriaceae), streptococci and staphylococci
- necrotising fasciitis type 2 is caused by group A streptococci (with/without a concomitant staphylococci infection).

Treatment should be prompt and aggressive and requires a multidisciplinary approach between physicians, surgeons and microbiologists that involves:

- resuscitation
- immediate surgical debridement (pus and necrotic tissue should be sent for microscopy and culture)
- broad-spectrum intravenous antibiotics (including streptococcal cover):
  - intravenous benzylpenicillin 1.2 g every 4 hours
  - intravenous clindamycin 600 mg four times a day
  - intravenous ciprofloxacin 400 mg twice a day.

TABLE 20.4 **Classification and diseases of Streptococcaceae**

Type of haemolysis	Species	Distinguishing microbial tests	Normal habitat	Disease
Alpha haemolysis	Viridans-type streptococci, e.g. *Streptococcus mitis, S. mutans, S. anginosus, S. bovis*	Optochin-resistant Not bile-soluble	Normal flora of oropharynx, gastrointestinal tract and genitourinary tract	*S. mitis*: endocarditis *S. mutans*: dental caries, endocarditis *S. anginosus* (also known as *S. milleri*): deep-tissue abscesses *S. bovis*: association with colonic carcinoma
Alpha haemolysis	*Enterococcus* spp., e.g. *E. faecalis, E. faecium*	Aesculin-positive	Part of bowel flora	Urinary tract infection Biliary/abdominal sepsis Endocarditis (rare)
Alpha haemolysis	*S. pneumonia*	'Draughtsman' appearance of colonies Lancet-shaped diplococci on Gram stain Optochin-sensitive Bile-soluble	Commensal of the oropharynx	Pneumonia Meningitis Otitis media Sinusitis
Beta haemolysis	*S. pyogenes*	Lancefield group A	Asymptomatic carriage in the oropharynx	Pharyngitis/tonsillitis ('strep throat') Cellulitis/erysipelas Necrotising fasciitis Toxic shock syndrome Poststreptococcal phenomena (rheumatic fever, glomerulonephritis, scarlet fever)
Beta haemolysis	*S. agalactiae*	Lancefield group B	Normal flora of lower gastrointestinal tract and female genital tract; 30% of pregnant women are carriers	Early-onset neonatal infection (bacteraemia, meningitis, pneumonia) Late-onset neonatal infection (meningitis) Maternal infection (urinary tract infection, chorioamnionitis, septic abortion)
Beta haemolysis	*S. equisimilis* *S. dysgalactiae*	Lancefield groups C and G	May be mucosal commensals	As for group A streptococci but usually less virulent
Gamma haemolysis	Viridans-type streptococcia	Optochin-resistant Not bile-soluble	Normal flora of oropharynx, gastrointestinal tract and genitourinary tract	*S. mitis*: endocarditis *S. mutans*: dental caries, endocarditis *S. anginosus* (also known as *S. milleri*): deep-tissue abscesses *S. bovis*: association with colonic carcinoma
Gamma haemolysis	*Enterococcus* spp.[a]	Aesculin-positive	Part of bowel flora	Urinary tract infection Biliary/abdominal sepsis Endocarditis (rare)

[a] Strains from this species may in fact be alpha- or gamma-haemolytic | any one strain will show only one type of haemolysis but there may be variation among different strains of the same species; other clinical characteristics are as for the alpha-haemolytic strains | spp. = two or more species

Repeated surgical exploration and debridement may be required. Treatments such as hyperbaric O_2 therapy and intravenous immunoglobulin may have a role, although convincing evidence of their effectiveness is currently lacking.

People with necrotising fasciitis should be isolated until cultures are negative for *S. pyogenes*.

Toxic shock syndrome

Persons with invasive streptococcal disease, including necrotising fasciitis, may also develop toxic shock syndrome. This is mediated by toxins produced by *S. pyogenes,* particularly streptococcal pyogenic exotoxins A and C. Affected people are unwell with evidence of a marked systemic inflammatory response and shock, often with few superficial signs of infection. Rapid identification and antibiotic treatment is required to avoid progression to organ failure and death.

Streptococcus agalactiae (Lancefield group B)

S. agalactiae (commonly referred to as group B streptococcus or GBS) is part of the normal flora of the lower gastrointestinal tract, the throat and, most importantly, the female genital tract. Carriage of GBS occurs in up to 30% of women during pregnancy but may be intermittent.

Neonatal group B streptococcal disease

About 60% of babies born to mothers colonised with GBS will themselves become colonised during passage through the vagina. Several factors increase the probability of the baby acquiring GBS:

- premature birth (before week 37 of gestation)
- prolonged rupture of membranes (lasting for more than 18 hours)
- intrapartum fever (over 38 degrees C)
- previous infant with GBS disease
- heavy maternal carriage of GBS.

GBS infection in babies can be divided into early-onset and late-onset disease. Early-onset neonatal disease occurs in infants of women colonised with GBS, either during delivery or by retrograde spread of GBS from the vagina into the amniotic fluid. Onset of disease may be a few hours to a few days postpartum. It may present as bacteraemia, meningitis or pneumonia. The incidence of early-onset neonatal GBS disease in the UK is estimated to be 0.5 in 1000 births.

Prompt treatment of the infant is required, including antibiotics active against GBS, such as intravenous benzylpenicillin. However, there remains a significant morbidity amongst survivors, with neurological sequelae such as blindness and mental retardation reported in those with meningitis.

In disease occurring in older infants (late-onset neonatal disease), GBS is usually not acquired at delivery but through another source (for example contact with other children, relatives, hospital staff who are carriers of GBS). The most common presentation is meningitis with bacteraemia.

In pregnant women, ascending infection with GBS can result in urinary tract infection. Infection of the amniotic fluid may result in chorioamnionitis and abortion. Invasive GBS may also cause postpartum sepsis with bacteraemia.

Group B streptococcal disease in other groups of people

In healthy men and nonpregnant women, GBS rarely causes infection. However, it may cause invasive disease in elderly people with other underlying conditions or a degree of immunosuppression. Presentations include septicaemia, pneumonia, cellulitis, osteomyelitis and septic arthritis.

Maternal screening for group B streptococci and peripartum prophylaxis

Current UK guidelines on the peripartum prophylaxis of GBS disease, published by the Royal College of Obstetricians and Gynaecologists, differ from those in the USA in that they do not advocate the routine antenatal screening of all pregnant women for carriage of GBS. This is because the current evidence base is insufficient to determine with certainty its clinical and cost-effectiveness in the UK population. Therefore, a risk-based approach is used to determine which women should receive prophylactic antibiotics peripartum.

Women with one or more of the following risk factors should receive antibiotics:

- GBS disease in a previous baby or pregnancy
- GBS found incidentally in the vagina or urine at any time during pregnancy
- prolonged rupture of membranes at term (more than 18 hours)
- preterm rupture of membranes in labour (before week 37 of gestation)
- preterm rupture of membranes with known GBS (whether in labour or not)
- intrapartum temperature (more than 38 degrees C).

The following antibiotic regimen are used for prophylaxis during labour:

- intravenous benzylpenicillin 3 g at onset of labour or with any of the above risk factors followed by intravenous benzylpenicillin 1.5 g every 4 hours until delivery

- intravenous clindamycin 900 mg every 8 hours until delivery is used in people with penicillin allergy.

STAPHYLOCOCCACEAE

These are facultatively anaerobic Gram-positive cocci that typically appear as clusters, like bunches of grapes, when viewed using a Gram-stain technique. In Table 20.5, the features of staphylococci are compared with those of streptococci.

The genus *Staphylococcus* contains a number of species that are classified mainly upon their ability to clot plasma, which signifies the presence of the extracellular enzyme coagulase:

- *S. aureus* is coagulase-positive
- coagulase-negative staphylococci include *S. epidermidis, S. haemolyticus, S. capitis* and *S. saprophyticus.*

TABLE 20.5 **Comparison of staphylococci and streptococci**

Parameter of comparison	Staphylococci	Streptococci
Gram stain and morphology	Gram-positive cocci in clusters	Gram-positive cocci in pairs or chains
Catalase test (hydrolysis of hydrogen peroxide)	Positive	Negative
Colonisation site	Skin and mucous membranes	Oropharynx, oral mucosa, gastrointestinal tract, genitourinary tract
Infections	*S. aureus* Skin and soft-tissue infections Bacteraemia Endocarditis Osteomyelitis and septic arthritis Coagulase-negative staphylococci Device-associated infections	Streptococci Skin and soft-tissue infections Bacteraemia Endocarditis Osteomyelitis and septic arthritis Pharyngitis ('strep throat') Pneumococci Pneumonia Meningitis Sinusitis Enterococci Urinary tract infections Abdominal/biliary sepsis
First-line antibiotics	Meticillin-sensitive strains Flucloxacillin	Streptococci/pneumococci Penicillin
	Meticillin-resistant strains Vancomycin	Enterococci Amoxicillin, teicoplanin

Staphylococcus aureus

The following features aid the differentiation of *S. aureus* from the other (coagulase-negative) staphylococci in the laboratory:

- positive coagulase test
- positive DNase test, indicating the production of a nuclease enzyme that can break down DNA
- presence of surface protein A (detected by agglutination).

S. aureus may form part of the normal flora of the nose, skin and perineum. It may be spread from person to person by direct contact (for example on unwashed hands) or via fomites. *S. aureus* may, however, also cause disease. Its virulence may be enhanced by the production of exotoxin (see Table 20.2).

Meticillin-resistant S. aureus

S. aureus can gain resistance to all beta-lactam antibiotics by mutations in their cellular targets (the penicillin-binding proteins). This is referred to as meticillin-resistant *S. aureus* (MRSA); meticillin is a beta-lactam antibiotic used previously in laboratory testing but not in clinical practice. MRSA is a major problem in hospitals, where the pressure of antibiotic therapy helps select out meticillin-resistant strains. Like all strains of *S. aureus*, MRSA may be spread from person to person by direct contact or by fomites. People may be asymptomatic carriers of MRSA or develop the same range of infections caused by meticillin-sensitive *S. aureus*.

MRSA infections will not respond clinically to any of the beta-lactam antibiotics (flucloxacillin, other penicillins, cephalosporins, carbapenems). It may, however, still be sensitive to other antibiotics, such as glycopeptides (vancomycin, teicoplanin), tetracyclines, rifampicin and fusidic acid. However, the pharmacokinetic and pharmacodynamic properties of these antibiotics render them suboptimal when compared with flucloxacillin.

Measures for the prevention of MRSA carriage are therefore important to reduce the number of MRSA infections. Several measures can be adopted:

- prevention of spread between persons
  - spacing hospital beds adequately
  - handwashing/use of alcohol hand gels between patients
  - cleaning of equipment (e.g. stethoscopes) between patients
- identification of patients colonised with MRSA screening of patients for MRSA carriage
- decolonisation of patients with known carriage of MRSA (especially before elective surgical procedures)
  - body washes containing chlorhexidine gluconate
  - shampoo containing chlorhexidine gluconate
  - mouthwash containing chlorhexidine gluconate
  - nasal mupirocin.

Although MRSA infection remains more common in hospitals, an increasing proportion of infections are found in the community, sometimes in people with little history of contact with healthcare facilities. This trend emphasises the need to screen asymptomatic patients for MRSA.

National guidelines recommend a risk factor (e.g. frequent hospital attenders, people from nursing or residential homes, intravenous drug users) approach to MRSA screening with screening of high-risk patients for MRSA carriage with swabs of the nose and perineum favoured. However, recent national policy (from the Department of Health, 2008) states that all elective admissions (including day surgery) and emergency admissions should be screened for MRSA carriage with at least a nasal swab.

Coagulase-negative staphylococci

This large group of related staphylococci is part of the normal flora of human skin and mucosal surfaces. In general, these species are of low pathogenicity and are largely opportunistic pathogens. They are frequent contaminants of microbiological specimens and are only associated with disease in a few specific circumstances, particularly device-associated infections such as central venous catheters or prosthetic heart valves.

LISTERIA

The genus *Listeria* comprises six species, of which *L. monocytogenes* is the most significant pathogen of humans and the cause of listeriosis. *L. monocytogenes* bacteria are short, nonsporing, Gram-positive rods that are facultative anaerobes. They produce beta haemolysis on blood agar. Certain groups of people are at increased risk of listeriosis, namely newborn babies, the elderly, people with an underlying immunosuppressive condition and pregnant women.

Pathogenesis and transmission of L. monocytogenes

L. monocytogenes is a common environmental organism found in soil, water and the faeces of many animals. Because it can tolerate wide pH and temperature ranges, it is capable of multiplying in foods that have been refrigerated for a prolonged period. Food-borne outbreaks have been associated with contaminated milk and soft cheese, undercooked meat and unwashed, uncooked vegetables.

L. monocytogenes is an intracellular pathogen. This allows it to 'hide' within phagocytic cells and evade the host immune responses.

Clinical presentations of Listeria infection

Infection during pregnancy

During pregnancy, infection with *L. monocytogenes* is frequently asymptomatic in the mother or may produce a mild febrile illness with associated conjunctivitis, headache and sore throat. The incubation time varies from 3 to 30 days and is occasionally even longer. Colonisation of the mother's bowel and genital tract with *L. monocytogenes* may occur.

However, maternal listeriosis during gestation may result in fetal infection. Infection can occur at any point during pregnancy. In early gestation, infection may result in spontaneous abortion. In later gestation, fetal infection may cause premature labour and stillbirth. The infant may go on to develop neonatal listeriosis. However, about 5% of maternal infections occur without fetal infection.

Diagnosis of maternal disease may be made by cultures of blood, high vaginal swabs, midstream urine and stool samples. Amniotic fluid may be discoloured or contain meconium and may also be culture-positive for *L. monocytogenes*.

Neonatal infection

Early neonatal listeriosis occurs soon (less than 2 days) postpartum and represents infection contracted *in utero*. The infant is usually septicaemic with evidence of disseminated disease and multisystem involvement. The mortality is high (up to 60%).

Late neonatal listeriosis occurs more than 5 days postpartum and is probably the result of infection during delivery from the maternal genital tract or of hospital cross-infection (for example via healthcare workers). It typically presents as meningitis. Examination of the cerebrospinal fluid may show a predominance of lymphocytes or monocytes. Gram staining of the cerebrospinal fluid may show the organisms. The mortality rate is approximately 10%.

Listeriosis in nonpregnant people

In adults and children older than 1 month, listeriosis is rare and is usually associated with an underlying immunosuppressive condition or old age. A number of presentations are recognised, including meningitis and bacteraemia.

People with meningitis may actually have little evidence of meningism and may present with focal brainstem signs. Progression of infection is more rapid in people with an underlying immunosuppressive condition. As with newborn babies, the cerebrospinal fluid may show a mostly lymphocytic picture.

Primary bacteraemia presents most often in people with underlying haematological malignancy or immunosuppression secondary to organ transplant. Bacteraemia may occur secondary to *L. monocytogenes* endocarditis.

Treatment of listeriosis

The antibiotic of choice in the treatment of listeriosis is intravenous amoxicillin at high doses. Long courses of up to 3 weeks are required. Gentamicin is also active against *L. monocytogenes*, but does not cross the blood–brain barrier well enough to treat meningitis. *L. monocytogenes* is intrinsically resistant to cephalosporins.

ENTEROBACTERIACEAE

The Enterobacteriaceae are Gram-negative rods that ferment glucose. The clinically relevant Enterobacteriaceae belong to one of two groups:

TABLE 20.6 Clinically important Enterobacteriaceae

Gastrointestinal commensals	Overt pathogens
Escherichia coli	*Salmonella typhi*
Klebsiella oxytoca	*Salmonella paratyphi*
Klebsiella pneumoniae	*Salmonella enteritidis*
Proteus mirabilis	*Shigella* spp.
Enterobacter spp.	*Campylobacter* spp.
Citrobacter spp.	

spp. = two or more species

- Commensal bacteria form part of the normal bowel flora and some may form part of the flora of the vaginal tract.
- Overt pathogens produce virulence factors making them capable of severe invasive infection. The discovery of these in clinical specimens should always be considered significant. *Salmonella typhi* and *S. paratyphi* are the causative organisms of typhoid fever. Other members of this group (for example *Shigella*, other *Salmonella* species) cause gastroenteritis.

Clinically important Enterobacteriaceae are listed in Table 20.6.

Infections associated with commensal Enterobacteriaceae

Urinary tract infections

Escherichia coli is the most common cause of acute, uncomplicated urinary tract infection in the community. Women are more susceptible to urinary tract infections than men owing to the short length of the urethra. Organisms may be transferred from the perianal region to the vulval region and then spread in a retrograde manner back up the urethra into the normally sterile urinary tract.

In hospitals, a number of other Enterobacteriaceae in addition to *E. coli* may cause urinary tract infection, especially in people who are catheterised or have undergone instrumentation of the urinary tract.

Diagnosis is best made on a clean-catch, midstream urine to culture the organisms. A urine dipstick is a useful screening test, with the presence of leucocytes and nitrites being specific for urinary tract infection. Simple urinary tract infections may be treated with an appropriate oral antibiotic (such as trimethoprim or nitrofurantoin). Urinary tract infections associated with catheterisation require removal of the infected catheter.

During pregnancy, women may be at increased risk of urinary tract infection. In addition, urinary infection may be asymptomatic (asymptomatic bacteriuria). Asymptomatic bacteriuria is estimated to occur in 2–5% of pregnant women. This is important, as untreated urinary tract infection may progress to pyelonephritis (infection of the kidneys) and increases the risk of preterm birth. Therefore, current guidelines recommend screening of asymptomatic women in early pregnancy with midstream urine and treatment of women with infection.

Biliary tract infections

The bowel Enterobacteriaceae may also cause infection of the biliary tree, such as cholangitis or cholecystitis. This is by retrograde spread from the gut, usually in the presence of a structurally abnormal biliary tract (for example obstructed by tumour) or a nidus for infection (for example biliary calculi).

Neonatal sepsis and meningitis

E. coli is also an important cause of neonatal sepsis. Like GBS, neonatal infection with *E. coli* is acquired during passage through the maternal genital tract. Bacteraemia may present quite nonspecifically in newborn babies, with fever, drowsiness and poor muscle tone ('floppy' child). Likewise, meningitis may present without classical signs of meningism.

Prompt antibiotic treatment of suspected neonatal sepsis should be initiated, with antibiotics to cover GBS and Enterobacteriaceae, for example intravenous benzylpenicillin and gentamicin. Cultures of blood, urine and, if indicated, cerebrospinal fluid should be taken before antibiotic therapy to guide future management.

Wound infections

The Enterobacteriaceae may be responsible for wound infections in people who have undergone abdominopelvic surgery, especially those procedures involving the gastro-intestinal or genitourinary tracts. People with impaired immunity, including those with diabetes, are particularly at risk.

Septicaemia

Finally, the Enterobacteriaceae are an important cause of bacteraemia and sepsis syndrome, the most common causative agent being *E. coli.* Gram-negative organisms may produce endotoxins, which are responsible for many of the pathological effects of Gram-negative sepsis, as previously listed.

Blood cultures are important to identify the causative organism and guide antimicrobial therapy. Imaging and culture of other sites may identify the source of sepsis. Management involves initial resuscitation and support-ive measures. Empirical antibiotics should be started while awaiting the results of cultures. Empirical broad spectrum antibiotics should include Gram-negative cover, such as co-amoxiclav or a third-generation cephalosporin such as ceftriaxone. New resistance pat-terns are emerging in Gram-negative organisms, such as extended spectrum beta-lactamase production, therefore consideration should be given to use of

aminoglycosides (for example gentamicin or amikacin) or carbapenems (for example ertapenem or merope-nem) in patients with prior exposure to co-amoxiclav or cephalosporins.

PSEUDOMONADS AND OTHER NONFERMENTERS

This group comprises a mixture of non-glucose-fermenting, non-lactose-fermenting, Gram-negative rods. Some of the clinically important members of this group are shown in Table 20.7.

The members of this group are mostly environmental organisms, being widely found in the soil, water and hospital environment. However, they are largely of low pathogenicity and, with a few exceptions, normally only cause infections in the hospital setting. Infections usually occur in people who have an underlying immunosuppressive condition (for example diabetes, leukaemia), an indwelling device (for example a cath-eter, an intravenous line) or an underlying chronic disease (for example bronchiectasis) and in those who are severely unwell (for example people in intensive care). Members of this group of bacteria do not usually cause infection in otherwise healthy persons.

TABLE 20.7 **Principal pseudomonads and nonfermenters**

Organism	Associated infections
Pseudomonas aeruginosa	Hospital-acquired pneumonia
	Ventilator-associated pneumonia
	Pneumonia in people with chronic respiratory disease (e.g. bronchiectasis)
	Cellulitis (in people with burns, ulcers or underlying immunosuppressive condition)
	Catheter-/device-associated urinary tract infection
	Otitis externa
Stenotrophomonas maltophilia	Rare cause of hospital-associated infections, especially associated with indwelling devices
Burkholderia cepacia	Lower respiratory tract infection in cystic fibrosis
Burkholderia mallei *Burkholderia pseudomallei*	Glanders / Melioidosis
Acinetobacter baumannii	Ventilator-associated pneumonia
	Wound infections (in people with underlying immunosuppressive condition)
	Device-associated urinary tract infections

NEISSERIA

This genus comprises two significant pathogens, namely *N. meningitidis* (also called meningococcus) and *N. gonorrhoeae* (also called gonococcus). Bacteria of the *Neisseria* genus are aerobic Gram-negative diplococci (cocci found in pairs). They are often seen within neutrophils on the Gram stain but extracellular organisms may also be seen. They do not grow on plain agar and may need richer media, such as chocolate agar (containing heated horse blood). All *Neisseria* species give positive catalase and oxidase tests. The various species can be differentiated on the basis of the different sugars they ferment.

Neisseria meningitidis (meningococcus)

Meningococci are part of the normal flora of the nasopharynx in about 10% of the population. They can be divided into 13 serogroups. The most common serogroups associated with disease are serogroups A, B, C and W135. The most common disease-associated serogroup in the UK is serogroup B. Many factors determine whether carriers will go on to develop disease, including bacterial factors (virulence of the strain), host factors (differing immunity) and environmental factors (overcrowding).

Clinical presentations include bacteraemia and meningitis.

Bacteraemia

After usually a quite short incubation period (2–5 days), affected people develop fever. They may develop a petichial or purpuric rash (nonblanching), which often spreads rapidly and indicates underlying disseminated intravascular coagulation. People with bacteraemia rapidly progress to septic shock, which is driven by the production of bacterial endotoxin. Mortality is high and rapid diagnosis and appropriate management are paramount.

Meningitis

Affected persons may present with signs and symptoms of meningitis without septicaemia, although one may rapidly progress to the other. People with meningitis are febrile, with a subacute onset of headache, photophobia, nausea, vomiting and neck stiffness. Inflammatory markers in the blood are raised. Lumbar puncture helps to confirm the diagnosis. The cerebrospinal fluid will show a raised protein count, a low glucose level and a raised white blood cell count, with neutrophils being the predominant cell type. The Gram-negative diplococci may be visible within the neutrophils on the Gram stain. *N. meningitidis* may be cultured from the cerebrospinal fluid.

Management of meningococcal infections

Early diagnosis and the rapid administration of appropriate antibiotics are key to ensure the best possible outcome. In the community, general practitioners should administer intramuscular benzylpenicillin upon suspicion of meningococcal infection. In the hospital setting, high-dose intravenous benzylpenicillin may be used. However, in practice, intravenous ceftriaxone is more commonly given as empirical treatment as this has better activity against other organisms that may cause a similar presentation.

People with meningococcal septicaemia deteriorate rapidly and often require management in the intensive care unit. Contacts of an affected person (including healthcare workers) should be traced and offered prophylaxis with ciprofloxacin or rifampicin.

Neisseria gonorrhoeae (gonococcus)

N. gonorrhoeae is the causative organism of gonorrhoea. Gonorrhoea is the second most common sexually transmitted bacterial infection in the UK and is rising in incidence in younger age groups. Unlike meningococcus, gonococcus does not form part of the normal flora in humans and is always considered a pathogen when found in clinical samples. Accurate laboratory diagnosis is required to differentiate it from other *Neisseria* species as a diagnosis of gonorrhoea has important public health implications in terms of informing and screening potential contacts.

Sample collection and incubation

N. gonorrhoeae rapidly undergoes autolysis if incubated in unfavourable conditions. Therefore, clinical samples should be inoculated directly onto appropriate incubation media at the bedside. Where this is not possible, use of special transport media is required while the specimen is taken to the laboratory.

The organism should be incubated on selective media, such as Thayer–Martin agar, to prevent overgrowth of vaginal or rectal flora from clinical samples. It is a fastidious organism that requires a humid atmosphere and supplementation with CO_2.

The clinical aspects of this infection are covered in Chapter 22.

CHLAMYDIA, MYCOPLASMA AND UREAPLASMA

Bacteria of these genera lack a standard bacterial cell wall and therefore are not stainable by the Gram method. They are mainly intracellular pathogens and contain both DNA and RNA. Diagnosis is predominantly by serology, cell culture or nucleic acid amplification techniques. However, *Mycoplasma hominis* can grow on blood agar plates and in blood culture media.

Table 20.8 provides an overview of infections caused by these three genera. Infection with *C. trachomata* is discussed in detail in Chapter 22.

SPIROCHAETACEAE

These are long and slender bacteria that are between 0.1 and 0.6 micrometres in diameter and 5–250 micrometres long. They are not usually visible by Gram stain microscopy because of their size but may be visualised on dark ground or phase-contrast microscopy as spiral or spring-like organisms. This key feature is attributable to axial filaments that run lengthwise and allow the bacteria to rotate lengthwise. Table 20.9 outlines key species and their disease states.

Syphilis

Syphilis is caused by *Treponema pallidum* subspecies *pallidum*. These are spirochetes, or spiral rod-shaped bacteria, that do not stain by Gram staining, and are difficult to culture in the laboratory. They must therefore be identified by use of special staining techniques and by serology to detect host antibodies against the organism. Several other treponemal species cause nonvenereal infections in humans, including *T. pallidum* subspecies *pertenue* and *T. pallidum* subspecies *endemicum*, the causative agents of yaws and bejel, respectively.

TABLE 20.8 **Overview of *Chlamydia*, *Mycoplasma* and *Ureaplasma***

Genus	Species	Route of transmission	Manifestations
Chlamydia	*C. trachomatis* A–C	Hand to eye, fomites	Ocular trachoma (blindness)
	C. trachomatis D–K	Sexual	Urethritis, cervicitis, pelvic inflammatory disease, epididymo-orchitis
	C. trachomatis L1–L3	Sexual	Lymphogranuloma venereum
	C. pneumoniae	Aerosol	Pneumonia
	C. psittaci	Birds, cats	Pneumonia, abortions, endocarditis
Mycoplasma	*M. pneumoniae*	Aerosol	Pneumonia, Raynauds disease, monoarticular or migratory arthritis, aseptic meningitis
	M. hominis[a]	Human reservoir/ endogenous from urogential tract	Vaginitis, urethritis, pelvic inflammatory disease, arthritis, postpartum fever
	M. genitalium[a]	Human reservoir/ endogenous from urogential tract	Urethritis
Ureaplasma	*U. urealyticum*[a]	Human reservoir/ endogenous from urogential tract	Urethritis, prematurity

[a] Variably implicated in genitourinary disease, abortion, chorioamnionitis and low birth weight

TABLE 20.9 **Overview of spirochaetal organisms**

Genus	Route of transmission	Species	Disease	Manifestations
Treponema	Person to person	*T. pallidum* ssp. *pertenue*	Yaws	Papillomatous skin lesions, periostitis, gummas
		T. carateum	Pinta	Papulosquamous skin lesions, achromic skin lesions
		T. pallidum ssp. *endemicum*	Bejel, nonvenereal or endemic syphilis	Oral mucosal lesions, mucus patches, condylomata lata, gummas
		T. pallidum ssp. *pallidum*	Syphilis	Primary, secondary, cardiovascular, neurological, gummatous (see Chapter 22)
Leptospira	Soil and water, excreted in urine from animal reservoirs	*L. interrogans*	Weil disease	Jaundice, hepatosplenomegaly, renal failure, fever, meningitis
Borrelia	Tick, louse	*B. burgdorferi*	Lyme disease (ixodid ticks)	Erythema migrans, meningitis, arthritis, pancarditis, splenomegaly, lymphadenopathy, myelitis
		B. hermsii *B. recurrentis*	Relapsing fever (tick/louse)	Fever, headache, myalgia, constitutional symptoms

ssp. = subspecies

Epidemiology of syphilis

Syphilis is now relatively uncommon in developed countries, owing to the advent of effective antimicrobial therapy. However, it remains a very important disease worldwide with high prevalences in some countries, and increased prevalences in particular social groups including homosexual men and prostitutes. The long latent course and social stigma associated with infection mean that many of those infected are not tested and diagnosed, leading to underestimation of the true incidence.

The clinical aspects of this infection are covered in Chapter 22.

MYCOBACTERIACEAE

Mycobacteria are obligately aerobic, nonmotile, nonspore-forming, rod-shaped bacteria between 2–4 micrometres in length. Their cell wall is made up of 60% lipids and also contains peptidoglycan. With the exception of tuberculosis, disease by mycobacteria occurs predominantly in people with underlying immunosuppression, as outlined in Table 20.10. The reservoir of tuberculosis is humans and spread is from person to person through droplet inhalation. Other mycobacteria are ubiquitous in nature, particularly in soil and water.

Tuberculosis

Myocobaterium tuberculosis complex is composed of five distinct species: *M. tuberculosis*, *M. bovis*, *M. ulcerans*, *M. microti*, *M. africanum*. However, any disease caused by these organisms is referred to as tuberculosis.

Epidemiology

The prevalence of tuberculosis continues to rise in the UK and recent reports state that approximately 15 out of 100 000 people are infected in England, Wales and Northern Ireland. Nearly half the burden of disease occurs in London with rates approaching 50 per 100 000 population. The rates peak in the 25–29-year-old age group and are approximately three times higher in those not born in the UK. Approximately 60% of people reported to be infected have pulmonary disease.

TABLE 20.10 **Overview of mycobacteria**

Species	Risk factors for infection	Manifestations	Treatment
Mycobacterium tuberculosis complex (*M. tuberculosis*, M. bovis, M. ulcerans, M. microti, M. africanum)	Immunosuppressive condition, HIV, arrival in the UK from countries of high prevalence (sub-Saharan Africa, Asia)	Pulmonary disease, lymphadenopathy, osteomyelitis, meningitis, cerebral tuberculomas	Rifampicin and isoniazid for a minimum of 6 months; ethambutol and pyrazinamide for 2 months if drug-sensitive disease
M. avium complex (*M. avium* and *M. intracellulare*)	COPD, emphysema, smoking, alcoholism, previous granulomatous disease, HIV infection, immunosuppressive condition, children	Pulmonary disease; Disseminated or lymphadenitis disease (immunosuppressed, HIV infection or children)	Clarithromycin, ethambutol, rifamycin (rifampicin/rifabutin) 12 months or until culture-negative
M. kansasii, M. chelonae, M. fortuitum	Immunosuppressive condition, HIV infection, presence of central venous catheter, nosocomial outbreak related to contaminated fluids	Pulmonary, bacteraemic, disseminated, cutaneous, bone and joint disease	As for tuberculosis; treatment for at least 12–18 months
M. abscessus		Pulmonary, disseminated or localised cutaneous	Amikacin, cefoxitin, clarithromycin
M. marinum	Swimming pool and fish tank environments	Cutaneous	As for M. avium complex; treatment for 3 months
M. leprae	Endemic in Asia, Africa, Latin America	Skin, upper respiratory system, eyes, testis, peripheral nerves (destructive lesions)	Dapsone, clofazimine and rifampicin for 6 months to 2 years

COPD = chronic obstructive pulmonary disease

Only 60% of infections reported in 2005 were confirmed by culture. Of those that were culture-positive, 8.7% were resistant to at least one first-line drug; however, less than 1% were multidrug-resistant (defined as resistance to isoniazid and rifampicin).

Diagnosis

Laboratories identify the organism by use of fluorochrome (e.g. auramine) stains and confirm the result by use of the traditional Ziehl–Neelsen stain (staining *Mycobacteria pink* with carbol fuchsin). A positive smear is indicative of 10^5 organisms/ml.

Culture is performed either in liquid culture media, where the organisms are detected owing to the metabolism of substances, or in solid media such as Löwenstein–Jensen slopes, where the organisms appear as small buff-coloured colonies.

Nucleic-acid amplification techniques allow identification of *M. tuberculosis* DNA directly from clinical or cultured specimens. These techniques can also be used to assess the relatedness of organisms through DNA fingerprinting and to identify common mutations related to drug resistance.

Histology findings include caseating granulomas with multinucleate giant cells. Staining of formalin-fixed tissues may also demonstrate the organisms.

Clinical features

The clinical features are predominantly related to the organ involved. Pulmonary disease presents with cough, haemoptysis and evidence of consolidation, nodules or fibrosis on chest radiograph. Genitourinary disease may present from a primary haematogenous focus in the endosalpinx and result in a granulomatous mass (mimicking cancer), chronic pelvic inflammatory disease or primary infertility related to pyosalpinx. Chronic peritonitis may also develop. Miliary disease is the traditional term (pathological 'millet seeds') for disseminated haematogenous disease. Lymphadenopathy, hepatosplenomegaly, skeletal disease and meningitis are other manifestations of disease. Systemic features such as fever, weight loss and night sweats may occur with any presentation.

Treatment

Studies demonstrate that 6 months of treatment with rifampicin, isoniazid and pyrazinamide is effective. However, with rising resistance, particularly to isoniazid, standard treatment in the UK is now recommended to be four drugs (rifampicin, isoniazid, pyrazinamide and ethambutol hydrochloride) for 2 months, de-escalating to rifampicin plus isoniazid for a further 4 months if the strain is known to be sensitive to these drugs and de-escalating to rifampicin, isoniazid and ethambutol hydrochloride for a further 7 months if drug sensitivities are unknown; and to rifampicin and ethambutol if the strain is resistant to isoniazid.

Adverse effects include orange colouring of body secretions (urine, tears, sweat) and hepatotoxicity for rifampicin; hepatotoxicity and peripheral neuropathy (reduced in high-risk groups by the addition of pyridoxine hydrochloride) for isoniazid; hepatotoxicity, arthralgia and raised levels of uric acid/gout for pyrazinamide; and optic neuritis (colour vision) and renal impairment for ethambutol hydrochloride.

Infection control

People with pulmonary tuberculosis and positive smears are moderately infectious. Pragmatic contact tracing should be performed among close contacts, including hospital contacts who spent approximately 8 hours in the same environment. Contact tracing involves tuberculin skin testing and/or the use of interferon gamma testing in certain groups, obtaining a clinical history for tuberculosis symptoms and performing a chest radiograph. People with suspected open tuberculosis (pulmonary) should be admitted to isolation rooms usually for the first 2 weeks of treatment.

Actinomycosis

Actinomycosis is an indolent, slowly progressive infection caused by anaerobic or microaerophilic bacteria. It is most commonly caused by the Gram-positive rod *Actinomyces israelii*. Other *Actinomyces, Arcanobacterium, Actinobaculum* and *Propionibacterium* species are also implicated. Evidence suggests that many infections are polymicrobial in nature.

Epidemiology

Infection may occur at any age and most series have reported more infections in men than in women. The incidence has diminished in the last 50 years owing to better antimicrobial therapy and better dental hygiene.

Risk factors

Disease requires disruption of the mucosal barrier. Oral and cervicofacial disease is associated with dental procedures, oral surgery and head and neck radiotherapy. Abdominal disease is often preceded by diverticulitis or appendicitis. There is a strong association between pelvic actinomycosis and intrauterine contraceptive devices. Immunosuppression owing to steroid use, haematological cancers, transplants or HIV infection is also associated with disease.

Clinical disease

The clinical presentation is sub-acute with fever, weight loss and night sweats.

Orocervicofacial disease presents as a soft-tissue swelling or mass lesion, often in association with recent surgery or manipulation. Extension to any contiguous structure may occur including to carotid vessels, cranium, cervical spine or trachea. Lymphatic spread and associated lymphadenitis are uncommon.

Perimandibular disease is the commonest presentation. It is often associated with dental infection. The fascial planes in this area are contiguous allowing unrestricted growth, although osteomyelitis is rare.

Thoracic disease accounts for about 15% of the total incidence of actinomycosis, with aspiration from the oropharynx being the most common source. Haemoptysis and a productive cough as well as the generic symptoms may occur. There are no specific radiographic changes with mass lesions, hilar adenopathy, pneumonia, pleural effusions or thickenings or cavitatory disease (multiple small rather than large) may occur. Extension to a soft-tissue chest wall mass or a sinus is classic evidence of actinomycosis. Mediastinal or bony extensions are rare.

Abdominal disease presents either as an abscess or as a firm tumour-like lesion. Enterocutaenous or intra-abdominal sinuses may occur and adenopathy is rare. Perforated appendicitis is the most common predisposing event (65% of abdominal infections). It rarely presents as a complication of Crohn disease or ulcerative colitis. All intra-abdominal organs may be affected.

Pelvic disease is most commonly associated with ascending uterine infection associated with intrauterine devices (30% in a recent series). On average, an intrauterine device is in place for 8 years in pelvic-associated disease. A pelvic mass or a 'frozen pelvis' mimicking malignancy or endometriosis is most commonly present. Disease frequently results in hydroureter or hydronephrosis.

Central nervous system, musculoskeletal and disseminated disease are rare but have all been reported.

Diagnosis

The presence of sulphur grains on histopathology specimens is diagnostic. Gram staining shows nonspore-forming, branching, filamentous Gram-positive rods. Culture of an organism associated with actinomycosis from a sterile site is also diagnostic, although they are slow growing and usually take 5–7 days to grow in anaerobic conditions. The use of molecular techniques, particularly 16S ribosomal polymerase chain reaction, is useful.

Treatment

Ideally, treatment is with penicillin (intravenously then orally) for a prolonged period (6–12 months). Erythromycin, doxycycline and clindamycin are reasonable in penicillin-allergic people. Percutanous drainage and appropriate surgical debulking are useful adjuncts to antibiotic treatment.

Mycosis

Table 20.11 provides an overview of diseases caused by yeast-like fungi. Box 20.1 lists important mycology terms for clinicians.

CANDIDA

There are more than 150 species of *Candida* but less than a dozen are considered to be frequent human pathogens. *C. albicans* is the most frequent organism isolated in human disease.

Clinical manifestations

Mucus membrane infection

Candida species can affect all mucus membranes and most commonly affect the oral or vaginal mucosa. It can also affect the oesophagus and the gastrointestinal tract.

Risk factors for oral candidiasis include treatment with inhaled steroids, cancer and severe HIV-related immunosuppression (AIDS). Those for vaginal candidiasis include diabetes mellitus, antibiotic therapy, pregnancy and, according to some studies, the oral contraceptive pill. Estimates are that the majority of women will have at least one episode of vaginal thrush during their lifetime, often in association with recognised risk factors.

Cutaneous syndromes

Cutaneous syndromes most commonly occur in warm moist areas such as intertriginous zones, with examples including balanitis, perianal rash and diaper rash. However, *Candida* species can also affect nails, causing paronychia, and hair follicles, causing folliculitis.

Invasive disease

Deep-organ involvement, such as hepatosplenic candidiasis, endocarditis, pneumonia, intracerebral disease and involvement of the bone and joints, is extremely rare in immunocompetent individuals. However, these syndromes may occur in immunocompetent persons in intensive care, particularly postoperatively after extensive intra-abdominal surgery.

Treatment of Candida infections

Mucus-membrane and limited cutaneous disease can be treated by use of oral nystatin, topical clotrimazole or

TABLE 20.11 **Yeast-like fungi: diseases and diagnostic methods**

Organism name	Geographical site	Diseases	Diagnostic methods
Candida albicans and other *Candida* spp.	Worldwide	Oral thrush, vaginitis, cutaneous candidiasis, invasive and disseminated disease (including eye, heart, bone, joint, hepatosplenic disease)	Gram stain, calcifluor white stain, germ-tube formation, chromogenic agar, PCR
Histoplasma capsulatum	Endemic in Ohio and Mississippi valleys (but has been found worldwide)	Acute pulmonary disease (similar to influenza), cavitatory pulmonary disease, disseminated disease (in people with impaired immunity)	Histoplasma antigen, histoplasma antibody, PCR
Penicillium marneffei	Southeast Asia (particularly in people infected with HIV)	Skin, lung, disseminated	Gram stain, galactomannan antigen
Cryptococcus neoformans	Worldwide (in people with impaired immunity)	Meningitis, cryptococcoma, pulmonary, skin (umbilicated lesions)	India ink stain, cryptococcal antigen
Blastomyces dermatitidis	Endemic in southeastern and central US states	Pneumonia, reactivation pneumonia, chronic skin nodules, osteomyelitis, arthritis, CNS disease	KOH wet mount preparation Gömöri methenamine–silver stain Serology, PCR
Coccidioides	Southern US states, Central and South America	Pneumonia, chronic skin nodules, osteomyelitis, arthritis, CNS disease	KOH wet mount preparation PAS stain Serology, skin testing
Paracoccidioides	Central and South America	Most infections subclinical; skin, lymphadenitis, mucosal, adrenal lesions	KOH wet mount preparation Gömöri methenamine–silver stain Serology
Pneumocystis jirovecii (previously *P. carinii*)	Worldwide (particularly in people with impaired immunity, esp. those infected with HIV)	Predominantly pulmonary disease, rarely disseminated	Grocott methenamine–silver stain in tissue Giemsa stain, immunofluorescence, PCR
Aspergillus spp.	Worldwide (in people with impaired immunity)	APBA, infection associated with foreign body/surgery (e.g. catheter-associated, burns-related, prosthetic-valve endocarditis), infection associated with impaired immunity (invasive pulmonary aspergillosis, rhinosinusitis, disseminated and cerebral aspergillosis)	Gram stain, calcifluor white stain Galactomannan antigen, Aspergillus antibody PCR
Agents of mucormycosis (many species, most frequently *Rhizopus* spp. and *Rhizomucor* spp.)	Worldwide, but predominantly related to severely impaired immunity	Rhinocerebral, pulmonary, gastrointestinal, CNS, cutaneous	KOH preparation Grocott methenamine–silver stain or PAS stain in tissue

ABPA = allergic bronchopulmonary aspergillosis | CNS = central nervous system | KOH = potassium hydroxide | PAS = periodic acid–Schiff stain | PCR = polymerase chain reaction | spp. = two or more species

Protozoal disease

TRICHOMONIASIS

Infection with *Trichomonas vaginalis* is covered in Chapter 22.

MALARIA

There are four species of *Plasmodium*, the protozoan that causes malaria: *P. falciparum*, *P. vivax*, *P. ovale* and *P. malariae*. The majority of deaths are caused by *P. falciparum*. Mixed infection can occur.

Life cycle of *Plasmodium* species

The parasite enters the host's bloodstream as a *Plasmodium* sporozoite after a bite from an infected *Anopheles* mosquito. The *Plasmodium* sporozoites then migrate to the liver, where they multiply in the hepatocytes and mature to schizonts, each containing hundreds of merozoites. They are then released as merozoites into the blood. Within red blood cells, the merozoites first become ring trophozoites and then mature to red blood cell schizonts. The red blood cell schizonts then burst and release further merozoites to infect further red blood cells. Some of these merozoites may develop into male and female gametocytes and circulate in the blood until taken up as a blood meal by the biting mosquito. The male and female gametocytes then complete their lifecycle in the midgut of the *Anopheles* mosquito, where they develop into sporozoites.

Epidemiology

Approximately 40% (2.5 billion) of the world's population is at risk of malaria. More than 500 million become ill and 1 million die from the disease each year. One in five childhood deaths in Africa is related to malaria. Malaria occurs in over 100 countries and large areas of Central and South America, Africa, the Middle East, the Indian subcontinent and southeast Asia are considered to be endemic malaria zones.

HIV infection has no effect on frequency or severity of malaria.

BOX 20.1 **Important mycology terms for clinicians**

Anamorph: a fungus forming only asexual spores

Asexual spores: spores formed by mitosis

Blastospore: an asexual spore formed by budding (e.g. *Cryptococcus neoformans*, *Candida* species)

Conidium (plural: conidia): an asexual spore usually produced at the tip or side of a hypha

Dimorphic: capable of producing both hyphae and yeast (e.g. the agents of coccidioidomycosis, blastomycosis, histoplasmosis, sporotrichosis and chromoblastomycosis)

Germ tube: a hypha emerging from a yeast-like structure, characteristic of *C. albicans* cells placed on specialised culture medium

Hypha (plural: hyphae): the tubular element that forms the body of a fungus

Mould: filamentous fungus; a colony on agar generally appears fuzzy, rather than smooth

Mucormycosis: infection by moulds of the order Mucorales

Pseudohyphae: a string of budding cells (e.g. those formed by most *Candida* species)

Yeast: technically, a fungus of the family Saccharomycetaceae, including *Saccharomyces cerevisiae* (baker's yeast); the terms yeast-form and yeast-like are generally used to denote fungi that reproduce by budding

Zygyomycosis: this term includes mucormycosis, basidiobolomycosis and entomophthoramycosis

---

miconazole. Deep or recurrent disease requires oral azole therapy (for example fluconazole, itraconazole). Invasive disease or nonresponsive disease usually requires intravenous amphotericin.

Nearly all *C. albicans* strains are sensitive to azole therapy. However, azole therapy may fail where resistance has developed or where other *Candida* species (for example *C. glabrata*) are present that are commonly resistant to azoles. If persons are nonresponsive to standard therapy, consideration should be given to culturing the pathogen, identifying which species is present, performing sensitivity testing and consulting a fungal expert.

TABLE 20.12 **Genetic traits that alter the risk of malaria**

Genetic trait	Effect on malaria risk
Sickle-cell trait	In children under 5 years, significantly reduced risk of *Plasmodium falciparum* infection, reduced parasite densities and reduced number of hospital admissions
Alpha thalassaemia	Increased susceptibility to *P. vivax* and significantly reduced *P. falciparum* multiplication
Beta thalassaemia	Reduced parasite multiplication within red blood cells
Absence of Duffy factor	No invasion of *P. vivax*
Ovalocytes	Diminished invasion, poor intraerythrocytic growth and diminished cytoadherence

Genetic traits and malaria

Several genetic traits alter the risk of malaria, as outlined in Table 20.12.

Malaria and pregnancy

Malaria occurs more frequently in pregnant women than in age-matched nonpregnant women. Pregnant women are more likely to have recurrent malaria, develop severe complications and die from the disease.

Malaria makes a large but unquantifiable contribution to the incidence of low birth weight in the developing world and is a major cause of morbidity and mortality in infants and children. Malaria occurs more frequently in women who have had one or two pregnancies than in women who have had more than two pregnancies (multigravida). Younger maternal age and the second trimester of pregnancy carry the highest risks of acquisition. The prevention of malaria in pregnancy reduces the incidence of severe maternal anaemia by 38%, that of low birth weight by 43% and that of perinatal mortality by 27%. Placental malaria occurs when erythrocytes infected with *P. falciparum* accumulate in the intravillous spaces; there can be minimal parasites in peripheral blood, making diagnosis difficult.

It is important to obtain a travel history in all pregnant women with unexplained fever and anaemia. Fever may also be absent or low-grade and is unlikely to follow the typical quartian or tertian cycle. Splenomegaly tends to regress in the second half of pregnancy.

Treatment of malaria

Classification of malaria according to disease severity is used to guide treatment decisions, with severe malaria defined by the World Health Organization as parasitaemia of more than 2% or evidence of complications. The following complications are commonly seen in severe malaria:

- severe anaemia (haemoglobin concentration below 7 g/dl)
- acute pulmonary oedema
- hypoglycaemia (aggravated by parenteral quinine)
- cerebral malaria presenting as impaired consciousness and seizures that may be misdiagnosed as eclampsia
- disseminated intravascular coagulation
- acute renal failure (blackwater fever due to intravascular haemolysis).

Drug treatment and pregnancy

Drugs should be used at adequate doses and according to the clinical condition and local resistance patterns:

- Chloroquine can be used safely at any time during pregnancy but resistance is common. It should not be used to treat *P. falciparum* malaria.
- Quinine can be used in all trimesters of pregnancy. Resistance is rare but can occur in South East Asia and parts of Africa. Intravenous quinine should be used in severe malaria. Side effects are more frequent with parenteral administration and include hypoglycaemia and cardiac arrhythmias (during infusion the person therefore should be placed on a cardiac monitor).
- Artemisinins seem to be safe in the second and third trimesters. They are not commonly available in the UK and treatment with quinine should be initiated while consulting an expert.
- Mefloquine and pyrimethamine with sulfadoxine are safe during the second and third trimesters.

- Clindamycin may have a role as an adjunct treatment in *P. falciparum* malaria.
- Primaquine, tetracycline, doxycycline and halofantrine are contraindicated.

Recurrence of malaria is common in pregnancy and resistance frequently reduces the usefulness of antimalarials. Primaquine (for eradication of *P. vivax* or *P. ovale* hypnozoites) is contraindicated in pregnancy, so a woman who becomes pregnant following treatment should take weekly chloroquine prophylaxis until after delivery.

Travel to malaria zones in pregnancy

Pregnant women should be strongly discouraged from travelling to malaria zones owing to the high risk of infection and complications. If travel is unavoidable, pregnant women should be advised to take clothing precautions, to use the insect repellent *N,N*-diethyl-*m*-toluamide (DEET) at a concentration of up to 50% and to use impregnated nets to avoid mosquito bites.

Chemoprophylaxis during pregnancy

Chloroquine and proguanil hydrochloride are safe in all trimesters of pregnancy but give poor protection in many geographical areas owing to the presence of drug-resistant *P. falciparum* strains. Proguanil hydrochloride in pregnancy should be supplemented with 5 mg/day of folic acid.

With mefloquine, caution is advised. While it seems unlikely that mefloquine is associated with adverse fetal outcomes in the second and third trimesters, there is a lack of data surrounding its use in the first trimester. Its use may be justified in the first trimester where there is a high risk of resistant *P. falciparum* malaria; expert advice should be sought.

Doxycycline is contraindicated in pregnancy.

Evidence on the safety of atovaquone and proguanil hydrochloride in pregnancy is lacking.

Women of childbearing age should be advised to allow time following the completion of certain antimalarials before seeking to conceive:

- mefloquine: 3 months
- doxycycline: 1 week
- atovaquone and proguanil hydrochloride: 2 weeks.

Infection control

Table 20.13 provides examples of infections that require special precautions, listing their means of transmission and appropriate isolation procedures.

TABLE 20.13 **Summary of the aetiology and pathogenesis of common postsurgical infections**

Focus of infection	Pathogenesis	Common causative organisms	Preventative strategies
Surgical site infections	Organisms enter the wound from the skin and environment, or from bowel and perineal flora in the case of abdomino-pelvic surgery	Any site: – *S. aureus* – *S. pyogenes* Abdomino-pelvic surgery: – Enterobacteriaceae (e.g. *E. coli*)	– Appropriate perioperative care – Prophylactic antibiotics – Surgical technique
Hospital-acquired pneumonia	Prolonged periods of bed-rest perioperatively prevent full tidal breathing. This may be exacerbated by pain following abdomino-pelvic surgery	– Enterobacteriaceae (e.g. *E. coli*, *K. pneunioniae*) – *Pseudomonas aeruginosa* – *S. aureus*	– Early mobilisation post-surgery – Physiotherapy – Adequate analgesia – Avoidance of sedative agents that may suppress ventilation
Catheter-associated urinary tract infections	Prolonged catheterisation postoperatively in bed-bound individuals, leads to colonisation of the catheter and ascending infection	– Enterobacteriaceae (e.g. *E. coli*, *Proteus* species) – *Pseudomonas aeruginosa*	– Early removal of catheter postoperatively and use of alternative devices (e.g. convenes, incontinence pads, bedside commodes) – Prophylactic antibiotics for catheter insertion in high-risk patients

Antimicrobial stewardship

Evidence demonstrates that the inappropriate use of broad-spectrum antibiotics is associated with the selection of antimicrobial resistant (AMR) organisms, such as extended-spectrum beta-lactamase (ESBL)-producing Gram-negative bacteria3,4, as well as the specific acquisition of MRSA, the precipitation of *Clostridium difficile* infection (CDI). Antimicrobial stewardship is coordinated intervention designed to improve the selection of the optimal antimicrobial drug dose, duration of therapy and route of administration to reduce antimicrobial resistance; to minimise toxicity; and to improve clinical outcomes from infections. Antibiotic prophylaxis should be single dose unless the operation is prolonged or there is more than 500 ml of blood loss. The UK Department of Health Advisory Committee on Antimicrobial Resistance and Healthcare associated infections 'Start Smart Then Focus' principles should be followed for every prescription.

The UK have recently released an Antimicrobial Resistance Strategy which aims to both monitor AMR and develop metrics to support improved antimicrobial stewardship.

Postsurgical infections

Surgery places individuals at risk of infection from several possible sources as summarised in Table 20.14.

Pneumonia and urinary tract infections are discussed elsewhere in this chapter. This section will now focus on surgical site infections.

SURGICAL SITE INFECTIONS

Surveys have revealed that surgical site infections contribute up to 9% of all hospital-acquired infections, making them important causes of morbidity and mortality amongst hospitalised individuals. The risk of surgical site infection varies according to a number of factors:

- Patient factors
  - Older age
  - Immunocompromise
  - Diabetes mellitus
  - Smoking
  - Poor nutritional state
- Operative factors
  - Preoperative skin preparation (including shaving and antisepsis)
  - Length of operation
  - Design of the theatre (including ventilation)
  - Type of surgery (clean, clean-contaminated, contaminated, dirty)
  - Adequate sterilisation of instruments
  - Surgical technique
  - Presence of foreign material at operative site.

The common causative organisms include *Staphylococcus aureus* and *Streptococcus pyogenes* (Group A

TABLE 20.14 **Interventions to reduce surgical site infections**

Stage	Intervention	Rationale
Preoperative	MRSA screening and decolonisation	See section on MRSA
	Hair removal – using a clipper with a disposable head (not shaving)	Reduces skin trauma and microabrasions, reducing bacterial colonisation and infection
Perioperative	Antimicrobial prophylaxis	See text
	Glucose control (<11 mmol/l)	Reduces wound infections in diabetic individuals
	Maintain normothermia (temperature >36°C)	Reduces infection rates
Postoperative	Good wound care and dressing	Physical barrier to gross contamination. Allows early detection and treatment of infection

MRSA = methicillin-resistant *Staphylococcus aureus*

Streptococcus), which enter the wound from the surrounding skin or from the environment. The bacteriology of these organisms is discussed under the relevant subheadings of this chapter. In abdominal and pelvic surgery, the integrity of the bowel may be compromised, and the wound may become contaminated with perineal and bowel flora, including Enterobateriaceae.

DIAGNOSIS AND TREATMENT OF SURGICAL SITE INFECTIONS

Surgical site infections may present with erythema, pain and purulent discharge from the operative site. In wounds closed by primary intention, there may be dehiscence of the wound. Patients may display signs of a systemic inflammatory response, such as fever, tachycardia and in severe infections hypotension. In severe infections, or infections that fail to respond rapidly to appropriate antibiotics, the possibility of an abscess either superficially under the wound, or deeper within the abdomino-pelvic cavity, should be considered. Imaging may be required to diagnose an abscess.

Wound swabs for culture and sensitivities should be taken prior to commencement of antibiotics. Empirical antibiotics should be targeted against the likely organisms. Therefore an anti-staphylococcal antibiotic, such as **flucloxacillin** is an appropriate first-line agent. If the individual is colonised at other sites with MRSA, then an antibiotic with activity against MRSA, such as **teicoplanin** or **doxycycline** should be used. Both of these agents are also appropriate in individuals with a history of penicillin allergy. In abdomino-pelvic surgery, the presence of a broader range of possible pathogens, means that an antibiotic with broader Gram-negative activity should be used, such as **co-amoxiclav**. Oral antibiotics may be appropriate in the outpatient setting for mild infections, if the individual has no systemic compromise. In severe infections, associated with a systemic inflammatory response, prompt intravenous antibiotics should be given.

Consideration should be given to adjunctive therapies. For example, in necrotic, poorly healing wounds, local debridement will remove infected tissue leaving well-vascularised tissue, aiding antibiotic delivery and the treatment of the infection. If an abscess is present, drainage should be performed, either in theatre, or percutaneously via a radiologically inserted drain.

PRINCIPLES OF ANTIMICROBIAL PROPHYLAXIS AND PERIOPERATIVE CARE

A number of strategies are available to reduce rates of surgical site infections. National campaigns, such as *Saving Lives*, have brought these together into care bundles. The principal interventions are best considered during three stages of an individual's hospital admission, namely preoperative, perioperative and postoperative, as summarised in Table 20.15.

Prophylactic antimicrobials have been shown to reduce the incidence of surgical site infections, deep abscesses, pelvic infection and bacteraemias postoperatively. The antibiotic(s) given should have an adequate spectrum of activity to cover the expected pathogens at the surgical site. For example, in abdomino-pelvic surgery, **co-amoxiclav** would cover the pathogens listed in the previous section. However, a number of other factors may influence the antibiotic choice, including:

- Patient drug allergies (e.g. history of beta-lactam allergy)
- Local resistance patterns
- Previous colonisation of an individual with resistant organisms (e.g. MRSA, when an antibiotic such as **teicoplanin** with activity against MRSA should be included in the regimen).

An initial dose of antibiotic should be given intravenously, ideally no more than 30 minutes prior to the skin incision. The aim is to achieve optimal tissue concentrations of the antibiotic to maximise efficacy. If an antibiotic is administered more than 3 hours before surgery, tissue levels may have declined, significantly reducing its effectiveness. A single dose of antibiotic should therefore be administered at induction of anaesthesia. For most surgical procedures, additional doses of antibiotics, or prolonged courses postoperatively, do not offer any increased benefit over a single-dose regimen. Furthermore, prolonged prophylactic antibiotics significantly increase the risk of *Clostridium difficile* colonisation and infection, and the subsequent carriage of multiresistant organisms. Therefore single-dose antimicrobial practice is advocated. Although strong evidence is lacking, re-dosing of prophylactic antibiotics is advised:

TABLE 20.15 **Infection control in practice**

Route of transmission	Example organisms	Infection-control precautions
Droplet (e.g. coughing)	*Mycobacterium tuberculosis* Influenza virus	Isolation in negative-pressure room (sucks air into room, preventing 'escape' of pathogens) Face mask when seeing patient
Aerosol (e.g. from nebulisers, ventilators, air conditioners)	Gram-negative bacilli (hospital-acquired pneumonia) *Legionella pneumophilia*	Equipment design and maintenance (closed systems) Sterilisation/disposal of equipment between uses Sterilisation and surveillance of ventilation systems
Contact (e.g. person to person on hands)	MRSA Group A streptococci *Clostridium difficile* Multidrug-resistant Acinetobacter *Pseudomonas aeruginosa* Norovirus	Isolation in side room or cohort bay Sleeves rolled up and watches off wrists (arms 'bare to the elbows') Barrier nursing (apron and gloves when entering patient room; disposal after use) Alcohol gel after seeing patient (wash with soap and water if diarrhoeal illness) Disinfection of equipment after use on patient Disinfection and decontamination of room once patient discharged
Inoculation (e.g. sharps injury)	HIV Hepatitis B virus	Universal precautions Disposal of equipment in sharps bins Clearly defined procedures and responsibilities in case of a needlestick incident

MRSA = meticillin-resistant *Staphylococcus aureus*

- prolonged surgery – additional doses should be administered after two half lives of the initial prophylactic antibiotic
- major intraoperative blood loss (>1500 ml) – additional doses of antibiotic after fluid replacement should occur.

PRINCIPLES OF WOUND CARE

Wound care postoperatively aims to reduce the likelihood of surgical site infection, and to detect an infection early, allowing prompt treatment. Dressings offer a physical barrier, protecting the wound from gross environmental contamination until granulation has begun. If the wound is discharging, then regular inspection and changing of the dressing should be performed. A wet, dirty dressing may encourage infection. If non-absorbable sutures are used, timely removal is essential. A suture represents foreign material in the wound and a possible nidus of infection. Delayed removal may precipitate infection.

The wound should remain dressed for the first two days after surgery unless the dressing is visibly wet. Various tools have been developed to aid nursing care of the postsurgical wound, and trigger prompt antibiotic therapy when appropriate.

CHAPTER 21

Viral infections in pregnancy

Philip Rice

Introduction

Viral infections in pregnancy present significant problems in respect of diagnosis, management and prevention, despite all the advances in diagnostic techniques, antiviral agents and vaccinations to try and mitigate their impact. This chapter provides a broad overview of the current state of knowledge in all of these areas.

Varicella zoster virus

The general characteristics of the virus are:

- Herpesvirus; single serotype, minor genotypic differences; lifelong immunity.
- Global distribution but with geographically different epidemiologies.
- Enveloped; dsDNA
- Spread by droplet and person-to-person contact.
- Incubation period 10–21 (median = 14) days.
- Preventable by vaccination (live attenuated; Oka strain).
- Treatable with antivirals (aciclovir, valaciclovir, famciclovir).

NATURAL HISTORY, EPIDEMIOLOGY AND TRANSMISSION

Varicella or chickenpox is the name given to the primary infection with varicella zoster virus (VZV). One attack confers lifelong immunity; re-infection is extremely rare. Zoster or shingles is the clinical manifestation of virus reactivation with 30–50% of people experiencing zoster in their lifetime.

Chickenpox is a clinical diagnosis. A widespread rash restricted principally to the central region of the body and upper parts of the limbs, so-called centripetal distribution, it appears in crops of fresh lesions (macule, papule, vesicle, pustule and scab) every 8–12 hours over 3–5 days. Once lesions have crusted the patient is no longer infectious – normally 5 days for a child, longer for an adult.

Zoster is restricted to one side of the body and very often to one or, occasionally, two dermatomes. Lesions are generally all at the same stage of development when the patient presents and are often associated with pain or altered sensation of the affected area. Occasionally, a rash does not appear, this is referred to as zoster sine herpete.

The epidemiology of primary VZV infection is very different depending on what part of the world one lives in. In temperate climates it is a disease mainly of childhood, such that greater than 95% of adults are immune, and with the increased use of nursery-based child-care it is increasingly being seen at even younger ages. In tropical countries, however, it is far less common in childhood and, as a result, adult susceptibility can be 30–50%; for example, in Sri Lanka, the Caribbean and the Philippines. The most parsimonious reason for this unusual epidemiology is higher levels of ultra-violet radiation inactivating virus in skin lesions so reducing case infectivity.[1]

Congenital infection

The largest and most definitive study of the risk that varicella poses to the developing fetus was a UK–German

343

TABLE 21.1 **Rate of infection and affection by trimester of infection**

Gestation at which varicella developed	Fetuses infected n/n (%)	Fetuses affected n/n (%)	Fetuses affected (CI%)
0–12 weeks	15/339 (4.4)	2/472 (0.4)	(0.05–1.5)
13–20 weeks	28/334 (8.4)	7/351 (2.0)	(0.8–4.1)
>20 weeks	55/277 (19.9)	0/468 (0)	–

From Enders *et al.*[2]
CI = clearance interval

project that examined 1373 and 366 pregnant women with varicella or zoster in pregnancy respectively.[2]

The risk of giving birth to an affected baby was highly dependent on the trimester and the period within that trimester at which the woman developed the rash.

Although the serological assays were imperfect, the best estimates of infection risk were based from this study (Table 21.1).[2]

Rare case reports have been described after the 20th week of gestation.

In order to have a confirmed diagnosis of varicella embryopathy the following are required:

1. A confirmed maternal diagnosis of varicella in pregnancy.
2. The presence of features consistent with varicella embryopathy.
3. Immunological evidence of *in utero* infection.

LABORATORY CONFIRMATION OF THE DIAGNOSIS

When a woman presents with a rash suspicious of chickenpox, VZV-specific immunoglobulin (Ig) G will normally be undetectable, as most present within three days after onset; from day four this antibody becomes detectable. Thus, the diagnosis of chickenpox can be confirmed with acute and convalescent (>7 days) sera, or by taking a current blood sample and collecting some vesicle fluid and cell scrapings for detection of VZV antigens by immunofluorescence or polymerase chain reaction (PCR). Clearly, the detection of virus in the absence of the antibody confirms a primary infection. It is always good practice to confirm what may appear to be a straightforward clinical diagnosis; there may be potential problems which may occur later in pregnancy and the difficulties associated with prenatal diagnosis and an extended period of follow-up ultrasound scans.

With regard to management of maternal chickenpox, a large prospective study of varicella pneumonia demonstrated that it developed in only 5% but that the risk was increased 5- and 15-fold respectively dependent on whether the woman was a current smoker or had greater than 100 lesions. However, the risk of pneumonia was not significantly different according to trimester.[3] With early and high-dose aciclovir treatment and attention to Intensive Treatment Unit treatment, if necessary, there were no fatalities.

PRESENCE OF FEATURES CONSISTENT WITH VARICELLA EMBRYOPATHY

These features include skin scarring and/or hypo/hyper/depigmentation, limb hypoplasia, rudimentary digits, muscle atrophy, chorioretinitis, cortical atrophy and multiple areas of echogenicity of the liver. The rationale for the cutaneous, limb and neurological features is thought to be because VZV reactivated as zoster *in utero*.

The extent of fetal affection is then dependent upon the degree of virus reactivation, such that if the fetus develops disseminated zoster the prognosis is very poor; this is, however, very rare. It is these types of malformations seen in affected babies which has led to theory shown in Figure 21.1 regarding the pathogenesis of varicella embryopathy.

Immunological evidence of in utero infection

This may be by one of two ways: persistence of VZV-specific IgG at one year of age or the detection of VZV-specific immunoglobulin (Ig) M in the neonate or infant. As VZV IgM assays generally lack sensitivity, the former is used. Alternatively, if the child presents within the first two years of life with zoster but without a

FIGURE 21.1 **The pathogenesis of varicella embryopathy**

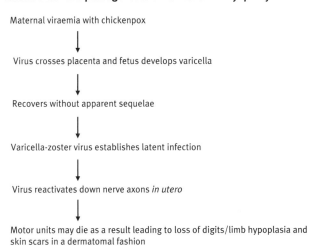

Maternal viraemia with chickenpox

↓

Virus crosses placenta and fetus develops varicella

↓

Recovers without apparent sequelae

↓

Varicella-zoster virus establishes latent infection

↓

Virus reactivates down nerve axons *in utero*

↓

Motor units may die as a result leading to loss of digits/limb hypoplasia and skin scars in a dermatomal fashion

history of clinical chickenpox, *in utero* infection must have occurred.

PREVENTION OF INFECTION

In order to prevent varicella in pregnancy any woman in contact with chickenpox or uncovered zoster who does not have a history of previous infection should have blood taken and tested within 48 hours for VZV-specific IgG. If shown to be antibody negative and the last contact is within the previous 10 days, varicella zoster immune globulin (VZIG) should be administered. Whilst this may not prevent maternal infection, especially if given late (>96 hours after contact), it should at least ameliorate the woman's illness. This is especially important as life-threatening varicella pneumonia is more common in pregnancy, in particular in the third trimester. It is important to remember, however, that if a woman has a very good history of previous chickenpox, or indeed zoster, antibody testing is not necessary and may be misleading, as the tests lack the required sensitivity to detect every individual who has been infected with VZV. This could lead to the overuse of VZIG.

One of the most significant outcomes from the UK–German study was to demonstrate that, even if given as late as 10 days after a virus exposure, VZIG may still be effective in preventing fetal infection even if the woman goes on to develop chickenpox.[2] This is because it is the maternal rash which signals the viraemia that infects the placenta. The presence of intravascular VZV IgG at this time should therefore mitigate against this and so reduce the proportion of fetuses which are infected. This was indeed borne out by the Enders study, which demonstrated that no cases of varicella embryopathy occurred in 97 fetuses in which maternal varicella developed despite post-exposure prophylaxis with VZIG.[2] Indeed, with the caveats of the sensitivity of VZV-specific IgM assays set aside, it was also found that the proportion of these fetuses with VZV IgM was significantly lower compared with asymptomatic infants whose mothers did not have prophylaxis. Finally, there were no cases of varicella embryopathy in the 366 mothers who developed zoster in pregnancy as would be expected, because there is rarely any viraemia with zoster and, even if it were to occur, maternal VZV IgG would quickly neutralise it.

PRENATAL DIAGNOSIS

Prenatal diagnosis is difficult because the virus is restricted largely to nervous tissue and is not often shed in urine or does not always reactivate to produce skin lesions. This makes detection of viral DNA by PCR in amniotic fluid (AF) less sensitive than it is for other herpes viruses, e.g. cytomegalovirus (CMV). Given a transmission rate of VZV of 20–50% depending on the trimester during which maternal infection takes place, the sensitivity of AF by PCR is relatively low. Virus transmission to the fetus was seen in only 9/107 (8.4%) in cases of chickenpox before the 24th week.[4,5]

Varicella developing at the end of pregnancy potentially exposes the fetus to infection without the benefit of passive maternal antibody. Thus, if maternal infection occurs either seven days before or after delivery the newborn will not have sufficient antibody to prevent a severe infection, so is recommended to receive VZIG; consideration should also be given to giving prophylactic, post-exposure aciclovir, especially if the maternal rash developed up to four days before birth. Reports of mortality of *c.* 30% are exaggerated, but the mortality is not insignificant and probably lies at *c.* 1–5%.

Several unresolved problems with the management of pregnancy-related chickenpox remain, however. As the defects may be severe and potentially disabling due to viral reactivation with variable timing and extent, it is important that the value of prenatal diagnosis is explored more extensively and whether or not treating pregnant women with aciclovir has any effect on the risk of transplacental infection.

It has been suggested that antenatal screening for VZV IgG should be considered in order to vaccinate susceptible women postpartum, though because of the low risk of adverse outcomes and low incidence of varicella in pregnancy (*c.* 0.3–0.7/1000/year) this may not be necessary if varicella vaccine is added to the childhood immunisation schedule. What should not be forgotten, however, is to re-test women for VZV IgG who do not develop chickenpox at least eight weeks after receiving VZIG to exclude asymptomatic infection. This will allow those women who escaped infection, and who would, therefore, benefit from postpartum vaccination, to be identified.

Cytomegalovirus

The general characteristics of the pathogen are:

- Herpesvirus; multiple strains; partial immunity – re-infection common
- Global distribution
- Enveloped dsDNA
- Spread by person-to-person contact through contact with infected bodily fluids
- Incubation period *c.* 3 – 4 weeks
- Vaccination in clinical trials
- Treatable with antivirals (ganciclovir [GCV], valganciclovir, foscarnet).

Cytomegalovirus (CMV) is the commonest congenital infection and complicates *c.* 0.5% of all pregnancies.[6] Both primary infection and recurrent infection (a mixture of reactivation of the woman's endogenous strain or re-infection with a different one) are capable of leading to congenital infection.[7]

EPIDEMIOLOGY, TRANSMISSION AND VIRUS SURVIVAL

The women at highest risk of primary infection are those who already have their first child attending a day-care nursery. By the same token, nursery-care

workers who do not adopt good infection control are at substantial risk, as are teenagers. The reasons behind these high-risk groups are principally to do with how the virus is acquired and where it is shed. Approximately 30–40% of nursery-aged children shed virus in urine and transmission depends on good personal hygiene and attention to environmental decontamination. This is because CMV remains viable on metal/wooden surfaces or glass/plastic for one or three hours respectively, though drying of such surfaces reduces the infectivity considerably. This explains why the annual sero-conversion rate can be as high as 10–20% in day-care nursery workers. Teenage pregnancies are at increased risk because of their young age, making it more likely that they are susceptible. Teenagers can become infected as a result of sexual exposure. This group mostly experiences primary infection. However, African and Asian women are mostly at risk of re-infection as the prevalence of past infection at childbearing age is greater than 95% among these ethnic groups compared with a prevalence of approximately 40–50% in Caucasian women. This difference may be due to differences rates of breastfeeding, since the most effective mode of transmission is via breastfeeding. This mode of transmission simply results in an asymptomatic infection of the infant takes place to be followed shortly afterwards by urinary excretion.

It is important to remember that there is no such thing as CMV immunity, and in fact that the level of protection that a previous infection affords against infection with a different strain is only *c.* 60–70%. Finally, there is an increased risk of placental transmission is if conception occurs within 6–12 months of a primary infection.

Table 21.2 shows the sources and routes of transmission of CMV infection.

CLINICAL FEATURES OF MATERNAL INFECTION

Often a primary or recurrent CMV infection is asymptomatic. If symptoms do occur, however, the classical syndrome of a glandular-fever illness akin to Epstein–Barr virus infection is actually much less common than an illness comprising vague lethargy and malaise associated with a moderate fever of *c.* 1–3 weeks duration. Often, if such patients are investigated a biochemical

TABLE 21.2 **Sources of virus and routes of transmission of CMV infection**

Sources of virus	Route of transmission
Breast milk	Breast feeding
Urine	Changing nappies and poor hand-washing
Saliva	Socially
Genital secretions	Sex Peri-/intra-partum
Blood/organs	Iatrogenic

hepatitis with an alanine transaminase (ALT) level of up to 5–8 times normal and a lymphocytosis or lymphopaenia are seen. The monospot test is very often negative.

CLINICAL FEATURES OF CONGENITAL INFECTION

The clinical features of congenital CMV infection are almost always not apparent at birth and reveal themselves later in infancy as failure to thrive, or because of a failure to reach milestones at the appropriate times. If the baby is symptomatic at birth, seen only in 7–10% of cases, it is often small for its gestational age and has microcephaly, hepatitis, splenomegaly and thrombocytopaenia. A chronic respiratory illness may also be a presenting feature.

Table 21.3 shows the range of clinical findings in babies symptomatic at birth with congenital CMV.

TABLE 21.3 **The range of clinical findings in babies symptomatic at birth with congenital CMV**

Clinical feature	Prevalence at birth (%)
Petechiae	76
Jaundice	67
Hepato-splenomegaly	60
Sensorineural hearing loss	56
Microcephaly	53
Small for gestational age	50
Hypotonia	27
Retinitis	10

In 7–10% of babies clinically affected at birth, half will have cytomegalic inclusion disease (CID), with multi-organ involvement of the reticulo-endothelial system and the central nervous system (CNS) – namely hepatosplenomegaly, jaundice, petechiae, microcephaly, seizures, hypotonia and intra-cerebral calcification. Less common manifestations include pneumonitis, dental defects and ocular problems (retinitis, cataracts, strabismus). The overall mortality in this group is 15–30%, mainly in the first weeks of life. Of the survivors, 90% will have long-term problems caused by the CNS involvement – sensori-neural hearing loss (SNHL), language delays, microcephaly, visual impairment and psychomotor retardation.

However, the majority (90–95%) are asymptomatic at birth and in this group the prognosis is much better, but still 15% will go on to develop sequelae, principally SNHL. Globally, congenital CMV is the cause of 10% of SNHL. There is a wide range of hearing loss from bilateral to unilateral high-frequency loss only. Overall, between 2% and 10% develop mental retardation with 1–2% developing retinitis, and less than 1% show signs of cerebral palsy in later life. Therefore, given the risk of placental transmission of 30–60% depending on gestational age at which maternal infection occurs, the overall risk of having an affected baby to a greater or lesser degree is *c.* 20–30% in a woman with a primary infection.

GESTATIONAL AGE AND RISK TO THE FETUS

In women experiencing a primary infection, the principal determinant of the degree of damage to the developing fetus is the trimester at which infection takes place. For a preconceptual or periconceptual infection, the risk of a bad outcome is not always low, however. Daiminger *et al.* found no infections in 3 women with infections 2–8 weeks before the last menstrual period (LMP), but among 20 women with infections closer to the LMP (1–5 weeks before), 9/20 (45%) suffered fetal infections with 5 fetal losses and of the 4 infected, 2 were severe.[8] Revello *et al.* also demonstrated a rate transmission rate of 10% (2/25) for preconceptual transmission – both cases being subclinical, but of the 13 women with periconceptual infection transmission was seen in 4/13 (30%).[9] Other authors have noted an increasing rate of transmission as the pregnancy advances, with approximate transmission rates of 30–40% first trimester, 40–50% second trimester and 70% third trimester.

It is well established that the risk of a poorer outcome is increased if infection occurs before 20 weeks, with approximately 25–30% having CNS abnormalities compared with just 6% where infection occurred after 20 weeks.

Whilst recurrent CMV infection is thought to pose a lower risk of transmission, in communities and ethnic groups where childhood infection is common and recurrent infection in pregnancy is responsible for 90% of maternal infections, the rates of CMV-induced SNHL are no different from countries where primary infection is the principal type of infection.

LABORATORY DIAGNOSIS OF MATERNAL INFECTION

If infection is suspected in the woman because of a compatible clinical illness and/or ultrasound features in the fetus, close liaison between the obstetrician and microbiologist is essential as the diagnosis of CMV infection is often complicated and time critical as the gestation advances. One of the complications is because the available tests for CMV IgM are unreliable as they lack both sensitivity and specificity; low-level IgM may be significant and high-level IgM may be seen to persist for many months and even more than a year. If abnormal findings are present at the anomaly scan at 20 weeks, demonstrating a CMV IgG sero-conversion, whilst definitive, is an unusual event even with recourse to a booking blood sample as most often both IgG and IgM are present at booking. Thus, as CMV IgM may persist it is essential that maternal serum samples be tested by a CMV IgG avidity assay.[10] This is a much more specific and sensitive test for primary infection, and because it can distinguish primary from nonprimary infections, it very often helps to resolve low-level IgM, which often proves to be of no significance.

CMV IGG AVIDITY ASSAY

This assay looks at the maturation of virus-specific IgG. This is always a time dependent process and takes a set time in any individual assay, but is often on average

three months, and is ideally no longer than four months, to show the development of high-avidity IgG. The exception to this is in immune-compromised patients in whom the maturation of the IgG response is significantly prolonged. The assay compares the reactivities of a single serum sample in an enzyme immunoassay (EIA) in two individual wells after incubation and the binding of the patient's CMV-specific IgG to virus antigen, which in one well is followed by a normal wash and in the other by the addition of a denaturating agent. The agent most often used is 6–8 M urea and it breaks the weak bonds between antigen and immature or low-avidity antibody compared with a control. An avidity index is then obtained by comparing the reactions in the two wells where, always, a low avidity indicates a current primary infection whilst high avidity indicates a past infection (at least 3–4 months old) or, at worst, a recurrent infection.

Assessing maternal viraemia is often performed, though diagnostically is of dubious value. Whilst a viraemia in a pregnant women with suspected CMV infection may be present, it requires a highly sensitive nested PCR to be used. With these assays the virus may be detectable, but often only at the limit of sensitivity of the assay and up to three months after diagnosis or symptom onset. Thus, serology is very often able to establish the diagnosis on its own. Furthermore, when used retrospectively and/or in samples with low IgM, the diagnostic utility is limited as no use as a negative PCR result does cannot exclude maternal infection.

LABORATORY DIAGNOSIS OF CONGENITAL/ FETAL INFECTION

The diagnosis of congenital CMV infection after birth is very straightforward if the syndrome is suspected within the first three weeks of life, but this is an unusual event in ordinary clinical practice. In this example, a urine or blood specimen may be tested for virus, either by cell culture or, more likely, PCR. As the maximum incubation period of CMV is three weeks, a positive result must indicate that *in utero* infection has occurred. However, as most babies are not suspected clinically at birth, the often used approach to confirm or refute a congenital infection is to test the newborn blood spot taken within seven days of life for CMV DNA by PCR and to test current and booking maternal blood samples for CMV IgM, IgG and IgG avidity. The sensitivity of PCR in the newborn-dried blood spot is c. 70–90%. It may also be possible to make a diagnosis by detecting a maternal primary CMV infection by either a sero-conversion or by finding low-avidity CMV IgG at booking, or perhaps a re-infection by detecting a rise in IgG titre with or without CMV IgM. Congenitally infected newborns, whilst often shedding large quantities of virus in urine, should be treated in exactly the same manner as other babies on the ward or neonatal unit. Suffice to say that adherence to normal hand washing is extremely effective in preventing transmission to healthcare workers. Indeed, healthcare workers are at no greater risk of acquiring CMV compared with the general public if they adhere to good infection-control practices.

PRENATAL DIAGNOSIS

The types of ultrasound findings in fetuses where virus transmission has occurred include: ventriculomegaly; increased periventricular echogenicity or pseudocysts; microcephaly; intra-cranial calcification; abnormalities of cortical development/cerebellum; echogenic bowel; intrauterine growth restriction (IUGR); splenomegaly; cardiomegaly; pericardial/pleural effusion; and hydrops.

Prenatal diagnosis of CMV is now relatively straightforward, providing that there is clear communication between the obstetrician and the microbiologist. Once maternal infection has been diagnosed and the ultrasound scan (USS) is normal, sufficient time must be allowed to elapse to allow transplacental transmission, fetal infection and replication of virus to take place, such that the virus is detectable in AF. It may be possible to attempt an amniocentesis early at c. 16–18 weeks of gestation if more than 6 weeks has elapsed after maternal diagnosis even though urinary production will not be guaranteed. This would allow an earlier termination if recommended or desired. Nevertheless, at this stage, CMV DNA PCR on AF at 16 weeks is only approximately 50% sensitive.[11]

Despite waiting for urine production to occur (>21st week), occasional false negative results occur, which may necessitate a repeat sample; of these a quarter may be due to early sampling whilst the rest are due to

late transmission of the virus. Approximately 4% of babies with negative PCR results excrete virus at birth so the sensitivity of AF PCR is c. 95%.

The magnitude of the CMV viral load in AF is most closely related to the timing of the maternal infection and amniocentesis, it has no significance for the severity of the fetal damage. Even when the fetus is infected as shown by AF CMV PCR, it is possible that fetal blood sample may still assist in decision-making; thrombocytopenia is an independent predictor of a poorer outcome with regard to CNS development.

It is nevertheless important to remember that if suspicious fetal ultrasound findings (echogenic bowel, small for gestational age, microcephaly, etc.) are seen in a pregnant woman with a confirmed CMV infection, the two are almost always linked.

USS FINDINGS AND THEIR SPECIFICITY FOR PREDICTING OUTCOME

Farkas et al. found that a normal CNS USS in infected fetuses, in whom the mean gestational age at which infection occurred was 18 weeks (range 7–31 weeks), predicted a normal early neuropsychological outcome.[12] However, this was only in 17 patients out of a group of greater than 100 patients originally examined. In terms of longer-term follow-up, the overall development in congenitally infected newborns with normal USS and magnetic resonance imaging (MRI) results in utero is favourable, although false positive MRI findings have been seen.

TREATMENT AND PREVENTION OF INFECTION

There are currently no antiviral treatments licensed to treat either mothers with an active CMV infection or of babies in utero with confirmed infection. One trial examined the efficacy of valaciclovir in ameliorating disease in infected fetuses. There were no differences in outcomes between mothers who received antivirals compared with those who remained untreated. With regard to postnatal treatment, intravenous GCV has been shown to terminate virus replication in the inner ear after birth, which is the underlying mechanism of continued sensorineural hearing loss; some short-term benefits have been shown, but the treatment has not been taken up more widely because of the side-effect profile of GCV, primarily neutropaenia.

Prevention of fetal infection with CMV specific hyper immune globulin was shown to be ineffective in a randomised placebo-controlled trial.

Finally, vaccination of CMV-susceptible women of child-bearing age with a recombinant glycoprotein vaccine has shown an efficacy of 50% for infection prevention over a 3-year period.

Parvovirus B19

The general characteristics of the pathogen are:

- Global distribution
- Parvovirus; single strain; three genotypes; cross-protective immunity
- ssDNA
- Spread by droplet and person-to-person contact
- Incubation periods: 7 days from exposure to infectious
- 18–21 from exposure to symptoms
- Not preventable by vaccination
- Not treatable with antivirals
- Hydrops treatable with *in utero* treatment with blood transfusion
- Animal parvoviruses in dogs and cats, which do not cross the species barrier.

CLINICAL FEATURES AND EPIDEMIOLOGY

Parvovirus B19 infection, so called after it was discovered by accident in well B19 in an EIA plate whilst conducting investigations into the hepatitis B virus, is an infection of childhood and occurs in winter–spring epidemics in temperate areas with a periodicity of 3–6 years. Typically it attacks children aged 5–15 years, but is also seen commonly as outbreaks in primary school-aged children.[13] It has several synonyms, namely fifth disease, slapped cheek syndrome and erythema infectiosum. It is unique among viral exanthems in that once the individual presents with the typical rash and joint pains that are its hallmark,

that individual is no longer infectious. This is because the symptoms result from antigen–antibody complexes deposited in the skin and synovial tissues. Those who were in close contact with the case prior to presenting with symptoms are now infectious and potentially transmitting the virus to tertiary cases. With that as background, one would probably conclude that it is very infectious virus but in fact only 60–70% of adults are immune.

The clinical features are usually a mild febrile illness followed by a rash, which may appear as slapped cheeks on the face or as lacy reticular on other parts of the body. Very often it is itchy and exacerbated by washing in hot water. A cardinal feature is the arthralgia, which typically affects the small joints (fingers and wrists) as well as ankles, elbows and knees. The arthralgia occurs in 80% of women but in only 10% of children. It resolves in a few weeks but can occasionally persist for many months.

TRANSMISSIBILITY

When parvovirus does occur in outbreaks as in schools and healthcare settings the attack rates are often high, approximately 25–50%, but, because of the nature of the illness, the vast majority (>75%) of cases have either occurred or those individuals have already been infected by the time an outbreak is recognised. In addition, attack rates in outbreaks are also high, probably because 20–30% of cases are symptomless even in adults and more so in children. Infection-control precautions are therefore actually of little use, though hand washing may reduce the risk to an individual who has escaped infection during a localised outbreak. In schools, susceptible staff are as much at risk as children. Thus, you can advise a pregnant woman to wash her hands, but whether or not to send her off work until the outbreak is over is a difficult decision because most of the transmission has already taken place by the time the outbreak has been noticed. By furloughing a woman from school until an outbreak is deemed over may put her at increased risk, since she will now be spending time mixing with people she would not normally have been in contact with; indeed, in large community-wide epidemics the attack rate in the susceptible general population can be 10%.

In a household infection an attack rate of 45% has been described, but it was noteworthy that in the four families with two children infected, all had secondary cases in the adults, compared with seven families with only one child infected where only one adult became infected.[12] This underlies the lower infectivity of parvovirus B19 compared with varicella where the household attack rate would be 90%.

INFECTION IN PREGNANCY

Infection in pregnancy shows some variability in different countries dependent upon maternal age and childcare arrangements. Poland appears to have the highest incidence of 1.58%, possibly related to younger maternal age in the first pregnancy, compared with 0.61% in Belgium, possibly as a consequence of widespread daycare provision leading to a decreased age at infection in childhood.

The risk that acute parvovirus B19 poses to pregnancy is one of fetal loss or the development of hydrops. The general understanding is of infection by parvovirus of red blood cell precursors via attachment to a blood group antigen common throughout the world, the P globoside; the 'P' designation is purely coincidental. This receptor is expressed on fetal erythroid cells, the placental trophoblast and cardiac myocytes. Once infected, red blood cell production is shut down and the fetus develops anaemia with appropriate cardiac compensation, though cardiac contractility may also be directly compromised. If infection occurs in the first trimester there is an excess fetal loss of c. 10–12%; later, in the first 8 weeks of the 2nd trimester, the risk of miscarriage progressively reduces to be replaced by a 3–4% risk of fetal hydrops.[14] However, more recent data estimate the fetal hydrops rate to be 10.6% (95% clearance internal [CI], 5.2–18.7%) if infection is acquired between the 9th and 20th weeks.[15] In epidemic years the risk of parvovirus infection in pregnancy may be increased 10-fold.

If a pregnant woman reports a contact with suspected parvovirus infection below the 20th week of gestation, she should be appropriately counselled to have a test for past infection. If IgG is detected and the IgM assay is negative she may be reassured that she is immune; if susceptible, however, she should have a further sample tested four weeks later. If sero-conversion is shown, additional ultrasound scans should be performed for the next 10–12 weeks.[15]

Should a woman experiences acute parvovirus B19 infection after the 20th week there is very little risk to the fetus. In two of the largest studies of B19 infection in pregnancy, fetal loss was not seen when the woman had infection after completing the 20th week of gestation (0%; 95% CI 0–3.1%). However, the fetus may still become infected *in utero* but survive unharmed. This is due partly to the development of a fetal immune response as well as the transfer of maternal IgG to neutralise virus infectivity; however, as some have reported, infection may actually be less likely in the third trimester due to the lack of expression of the P globoside in the placenta at this time. The overall chances of fetal virus transmission is 30%.

LABORATORY DIAGNOSIS

Laboratory confirmation of acute parvovirus B19 infection is made by detection of virus-specific IgM and IgG. However, in cases of suspected fetal hydrops the diagnosis is achieved by a combination of maternal serology and virus detection in AF and/or fetal blood. It is very important to remember that as parvovirus B19 IgM persists for only 2–3 months; by the time a woman presents with an hydropic fetus the virus-specific IgM has often disappeared, and very often the maternal serology is useful only to exclude parvovirus as cause if the virus specific IgG test is negative. Even if IgM is undetectable it may still be possible to demonstrate a sero-conversion by comparison with the booking blood if maternal parvovirus IgG is present at the time fetal hydrops is diagnosed. B19 IgG avidity testing may also be available in reference laboratories. However, if fetal blood is being sampled for the purposes of confirming or refuting anaemia this should also be tested for parvovirus DNA by PCR; thrombocytopenia is also a sensitive marker of fetal infection. If infection is confirmed, the viral load is very often high ($>10^9$ virus particles/ml of either AF or blood). The treatment involves an intrauterine blood transfusion, which is often successful at the first attempt (c. 60–70%), although approximately 20–25% of cases of fetal hydrops will recover spontaneously. Finally, babies who are born to mothers with parvovirus B19 infection in pregnancy suffer no long-term harm.

Herpes simplex virus

The general characteristics of herpes simplex virus (HSV) are:

- Herpesvirus; two types HSV-1 and HSV-2
- Global distribution
- Enveloped dsDNA
- Spread by person-to-person contact through contact with infected bodily fluids.
- Incubation period *c.* 1–2 weeks
- Not preventable by vaccination
- Treatable with antivirals (aciclovir, valaciclovir, penciclovir, famciclovir, foscarnet).

EPIDEMIOLOGY AND TRANSMISSION

Both HSV-1 and 2 are spread through intimate contact. Whilst HSV-2 continues to be the type most commonly encountered in the genital tract, HSV-1 now accounts for approximately 30% of new cases of genital infection presenting to genitourinary medicine clinics. This is due to the increased rates of susceptibility in childhood and exposure in teenage and later years to the virus shed orally. The prevalence of HSV-2 infection is also different depending on country of origin and ethnic group. For example, in the USA and UK the prevalence of HSV-2 antibody is 21% and 5% respectively in the general population.[16] However, the risk is greatest in black ethnic and lower socio-economic groups.

Asymptomatic genital or oral infection is the norm as less than 10% of seropositive individuals report symptoms at the time of primary infection. In addition, the majority of infections are acquired in the asymptomatic phase of a reactivation just before lesions appear.

HSV infections should be regarded as latent virus infections primarily of nervous tissue which, upon reactivation, the virus then passes down the axon to the sensory nerve endings in the skin where a lytic infection is set up and the virus is shed to the exterior and, potentially, to another susceptible host.

HSV infection in pregnancy very rarely causes a disseminated intrauterine infection leading to fetal death. The major clinical problem encountered with HSV infection in pregnancy relates to intrapartum transmission and to the type of infection that a woman may be experiencing in the last six weeks of her confinement.

TYPES OF MATERNAL HSV INFECTION

These fall into three types:

- Primary infection: this is where genital tract infection takes place in an individual who has not been infected with either type of HSV.
- Initial infection: this is infection of the genital tract with one HSV type in the presence of antibody to the opposing type. For example, a woman may already have antibody to HSV-1 and experience cold sores on her lips but is now having an initial genital infection with HSV-2 because she lacks antibody to that virus type.
- Recurrent infection: this is where virus of one type is detected at the same time as its antibody.

INFECTION IN PREGNANCY

In the largest study to date examining the risk of HSV infection in pregnancy it was demonstrated that infection occurs throughout pregnancy, divided equally between all three trimesters, and that the incidence was 94/7046 (1.3%), with one third of infections due to HSV-1. The incidence varied when stratified by antibody status at booking. Among women who were seronegative to both HSV-1 and HSV-2 at booking the incidence was 3.7%, compared with 1.3% who were already HSV-1 antibody positive and 0% in women with pre-existing antibody to HSV-2.[17] This indicates an important phenomenon, namely virus interference. It is likely that women with HSV-2 antibodies have had previous genital infection and, as such, their sacral plexus is already latently infected. Such a state renders it extremely difficult for another virus, in this case HSV-1, from setting up another latent infection in already infected tissue.

In women who had fully sero-converted by the onset of labour, however, there were no cases of illness among their neonates, indicating that passive antibody transfer is protective. There were no differences in the rates of intrauterine death, stillbirth, neonatal death, spontaneous abortion or early delivery between women who completely sero-converted during the pregnancy and those that remained uninfected.[17]

However, in this study a Western blot was used to detect antibody. This is much less sensitive than an EIA, so it is not possible to extrapolate these findings if EIAs are used in the setting of a suspected acute infection.

The situation is very different, however, among women who are actively sero-converting during the last six weeks of pregnancy, since this presents a much higher risk to the neonate.

The approximate incidence of neonatal HSV infection varies between countries; for example, the incidence is 1 : 2500 and 1 : 60 000 live births in the USA and UK respectively. The transmission rate is approximately 40% with a primary or initial infection with genital herpes at time of delivery, but is less than 1% with recurrent attacks of infection.

The incubation period is between 3 and 21 days (median 12 days); most mothers have no lesions at delivery as the majority of primary or initial infections are symptomless or missed.

A nonmaternal source is identified in one third of cases – father, grandparent, sibling or healthcare worker, and in this group the incubation period may be prolonged up to 28 days because of acquisition after birth. Importantly, as the prevalence of HSV-1 antibody is decreasing in women of child-bearing age, hygiene advice about other family members who may have cold sores should be given. Moreover, any healthcare workers with an herpetic whitlow must be barred from working on postnatal and labour wards.

Neonatal disease

Neonatal disease is classified broadly into three distinct disease syndromes depending on the extent of the disease and spread of the virus, namely:

- Skin/eye/mouth lesions
- Neurological disease
- Disseminated infection – sometimes presenting as hepatitis and/or multi-organ failure.

The mortality is extremely high if neonates are not treated because the diagnosis is not suspected, but even in those that are treated promptly the morbidity is still significant. The highest risk pregnancies are where the woman is antibody negative to both HSV types at booking, where the incidence is 54/100 000 (20–120) live births compared with 12/100 000 (0.3–70) live births among women who are antibody positive to both types, a greater than four-fold difference.[18] Clearly, it is essential that the management of women in labour with suspected active HSV infection is in favour of reducing the risk to the neonate, but it is now generally accepted that women with confirmed reactivation of genital HSV in labour or during the last six weeks of pregnancy do not need to have a caesarean section unless there are other considerations. Indeed, an American cost–benefit study estimated that if all women with HSV lesions had caesarean sections, then 1583 such procedures would have to be performed to prevent 1 neonatal death at a cost of $2.5 million and 0.57 (range 0.23–2.28) maternal lives expended.[19]

Management of infection in late pregnancy

If an episode cannot be confirmed as reactivation then a caesarean section should be performed because of the poor neonatal outcomes if virus transmission occurs. There is a slight caveat to this in that if the reactivation of genital infection is with HSV-1 this appears to transmit more efficiently than HSV-2 for reasons that are currently unknown.[18] If the episode is a reactivation then a vaginal delivery is advised; swabs and other bodily samples from the newborn are not necessary. The neonate is watched for any signs of infection, and if these develop and/or the laboratory reports detection of HSV then intravenous aciclovir is commenced immediately. The management of a primary or initial infection is very different. If a primary or initial genital HSV infection is confirmed in the last six weeks of pregnancy the women should receive suppressive aciclovir until and during labour to reduce the likelihood of shedding the virus or to reduce the quantity of the virus in the genital tract. If delivered by caesarean section, the neonate is managed normally. If the membranes have been ruptured for greater than four hours, or a vaginal delivery is unavoidable and primary/initial genital HSV infection is suspected, swabs are taken and post-exposure intravenous aciclovir is started as soon as possible after birth. Babies who develop CNS disease and who survive should receive a 6-month course of suppressive aciclovir, as this has been shown to improve neurological outcome at 12 months of life. It also reduces skin recurrences in neonates with skin, eye and mouth (SEM) neonatal herpes.

What to do with sero-discordant couples remains contentious. Prophylactic aciclovir to the uninfected partner reduces the risk of acquisition by *c.* 75%, but if the woman is pregnant and her partner suffers from genital HSV, the usual advice is to use condoms or, preferably, to abstain from sexual intercourse for the last six weeks of the pregnancy.

To date all trials of candidate prophylactic vaccines have failed to provide any measure of protection.

Rubella virus

The general characteristics of the pathogen are:

- Togavirus; single strain
- ssRNA, enveloped
- Inactivated by detergents, etc.
- Spread by droplet spread and close person-to-person contact
- Incubation period 13–20 days
- Preventable by vaccination (Live attenuated)
- Not treatable with antiviral agents.

CONGENITAL RUBELLA SYNDROME

Congenital rubella syndrome (CRS), as published by McAlister Gregg in 1941, was the first virus to be described to be the cause of a congenital infection syndrome.[20] In Australia in the early 1940s there had been an extensive outbreak of rubella, and many babies that McAlister Gregg saw in his ophthalmology clinics had unilateral and bilateral cataracts in association with other, mainly cardiac, defects. Many of the mothers gave a history of rash/rubella in early pregnancy and so the study of congenital virus infections was born. Because of the severity of this syndrome, it was one of the defining moments of vaccine preventable diseases when, in the 1970s, rubella vaccine was introduced into childhood vaccine programmes. It has been hugely successful in countries with well-developed vaccine programmes at reducing the incidence of CRS, such that now it has

TABLE 21.4 Rubella susceptibility in women booking at St George's Hospital London by country of birth (1999)

Country	Percentage
Africa	10
India/Pakistan	10
Sri Lanka	17
UK	1.2

been all but eliminated from these countries. However, from a global perspective CRS is an enormous problem with approximately 250 000 such babies born annually in association with large epidemics, and this figure may be increased 10-fold during a large epidemic. This is because rubella is not very infectious and, with a reproductive rate of *c.* 3–4, it still leaves 10–15% of adults susceptible. This is borne out by studies of the prevalence of rubella antibody in pregnant women when they have their booking bloods taken. Stratified by country of birth, it is clear that countries without rubella vaccine in their childhood immunisation schedules have a much higher rate of adult susceptibility (Table 21.4).

A clinical illness of rubella should be considered and appropriate investigations performed in any pregnant woman who presents with a viral-type exanthem.

It is very important to remember also that a pregnant woman who gives a history of contact with possible rubella should have blood taken to check for rubella IgG even if a previous positive IgG result is available. The rationale for this is that when screening large numbers of serum samples, in an antenatal setting for example, an error may be made in result transcription or sample identification and a false positive result may have been previously issued. Only if the woman has two previous positive tests or a documented sero-conversion to rubella vaccine is it not necessary to screen for the antibody.

CLINICAL FEATURES OF RUBELLA

A typical clinical illness of rubella is of a viral upper respiratory tract infection with coryzal symptoms associated with fever and malaise. This is quickly followed by lymphadenopathy (occipital/cervical/post-auricular) and a maculo-papular rash over the entire body. Akin to parvovirus B19 infection, joint pains are a prominent feature in up to 70% female infections. These may persist for days to a month or more and are due to antigen–antibody complex deposition in the synovial membranes. Rubella may be so mild, however, or asymptomatic in up to 25%, so it may go unnoticed by the woman and her doctor/midwife. In the mid 1990s in the UK outbreaks of rubella were reported in universities and army camps, with some spill over into pregnant women. It is essential that countries with the rubella vaccine in their childhood vaccination schedule maintain a high (>90%) uptake as the World Health Organization (WHO) recommends, otherwise there is a risk of creating a cohort of young girls who, when they reach child-bearing age, have a much greater chance of being susceptible and also being exposed to the virus. Exactly this scenario occurred in Greece, and the UK is now having to run a nationwide catch-up campaign with the measles, mumps and rubella (MMR) vaccine to counteract the decade-long period of suboptimal uptake secondary to the irrational fears over MMR being linked to autism.

LABORATORY DIAGNOSIS: MATERNAL AND PRENATAL

The laboratory diagnosis of maternal rubella is based on the serological response. Normally, because the rash is so abrupt in onset, the patient presents to their doctor or midwife within one or two days of its appearance. At this stage, if the rubella IgG is negative, acute rubella is almost certainly the diagnosis as there has been insufficient time for it to develop. In addition, rubella-specific IgM is often also negative at this time; convalescent serology from c. 5 days after rash onset is therefore necessary. If there are ultrasound findings compatible with a possible diagnosis of congenital rubella, then rubella IgG avidity may also be employed if there are no earlier samples from the woman.

CRS is characterised by a first-trimester infection where, if the fetus does not miscarry (20% risk), of the remaining fetuses, 80% will have hearing loss, 60% will develop a neurological deficit, 60% will have heart defects (e.g. patent ductus arteriosus, pulmonary valve stenosis, ventricular septal defect), 40% will have purpura and 30% will have or will develop cataracts and/or glaucoma. In later life bony abnormalities become apparent as does diabetes mellitus.

Prenatal diagnosis is really only useful if infection occurs after 12 weeks but before the 20th week, because maternal infection prior to the 12th week almost always results in a badly affected fetus with multiple abnormalities as detailed above, whilst infection after the 20th week only very rarely leads to an affected fetus. It is between these two times that rubella transmission *in utero* carries a c. 15–20% risk of retinopathy (not necessarily sight threatening) and sensorineural hearing loss. However, neither of these are detectable ultrasonographically and so PCR on AF may be attempted. This has a greater than 90% sensitivity and specificity, but the testing of chorionic villous samples may give false positive results due to the persistence or maternal rubella virus RNA.

Even if the rubella virus RNA is detected, however, whilst this proves fetal infection it does not prove affection. Prior to the advent of rubella virus PCR, the diagnosis of fetal infection was only possible by measuring the fetal IgM response at 23 weeks. Whilst this was very reliable, it still does not inform about whether the fetus has a hearing or vision deficit and is clearly a later diagnosis for the purposes of a potential termination.

REFERENCES

1. RICE P S. Ultra-violet radiation is responsible for the differences in global epidemiology of chickenpox and the evolution of varicella-zoster virus as man migrated out of Africa. *Virol J* 2011;8:189.

2. ENDERS G, MILLER E, CRADOCK-WATSON J, BOLLEY I, RIDEHALGH M. Consequences of varicella and herpes zoster in pregnancy: prospective study of 1739 cases. *Lancet* 1994;343:1548–51.

3. HARGER JH, ERNEST JM, THURNAU GR, et al. Risk factors and outcome of varicella-zoster virus pneumonia in pregnant women. *J Infect Dis* 2002;185:422–7.

4. KUSTERMANN A, ZOPPINI C, TASSIS B, et al. Prenatal diagnosis of congenital varicella infection. *Prenat Diagn* 1996;16(1):71–4.

5. MULY F, MIRLESSE V, MÉRITET J F, et al. Prenatal diagnosis of fetal varicella-zoster virus infection with polymerase chain

reaction of amniotic fluid in 107 cases. *Am J Obstet Gynecol* 1997;177(4):894–8.

6. PECKHAM C S, STARK O, DUDGEON J A, MARTIN J A, HAWKINS G. Congenital cytomegalovirus infection: a cause of sensorineural hearing loss. *Arch Dis Child* 1987;62:1233–7.

7. ROSS S A, FOWLER K B, ASHRITH G, *et al.* Hearing loss in children with congenital cytomegalovirus infection born to mothers with pre-existing immunity. *J Pediatr* 2006;148:332–6.

8. DAIMINGER A, BADER U, ENDERS G. Pre- and periconceptional primary cytomegalovirus infection: risk of vertical transmission and congenital disease. *BJOG* 2005;112:166–72.

9. REVELLO M G, ZAVATTONI M, FURIONE M, FABBRI E, GERNA G. Preconceptional primary human cytomegalovirus infection and risk of congenital infection. *J Infect Dis* 2006;193:783–7.

10. WREGHITT T G, TEARE E L, SULE O, DEVI R, RICE, P. Cytomegalovirus infection in immunocompetent patients. *Clin Infect Dis* 2003;27(12):1603–6.

11. ENDERS G, BÄDER U, LINDEMANN L, SCHALASTA G, DAIMINGER A. Prenatal diagnosis of congenital cytomegalovirus infection in 189 pregnancies with known outcome. *Prenat Diagn* 2001;21:362–77.

12. FARKAS N, HOFFMANN C, BEN-SIRA L, *et al.* Does normal fetal brain ultrasound predict normal neurodevelopmental outcome in congenital cytomegalovirus infection? *Prenat Diagn* 2011;31:360–6.

13. RICE P S, COHEN B J. A school outbreak of parvovirus B19 infection investigated using salivary antibody assays. *Epidemiol Infect* 1996;116:331–8.

14. MILLER E, FAIRLEY C K, COHEN B J, SENG C. Immediate and long term outcome of human parvovirus B19 infection in pregnancy. *Br J Obstet Gynaecol* 1998;105:174–8.

15. ENDERS M, KLINGEL K, WEIDNER A, *et al.* Risk of fetal hydrops and non-hydropic late intrauterine fetal death after gestational parvovirus B19 infection. *J Clin Virol* 2010;49: 163–8.

16. FLEMING D T, MCQUILLAN G M, JOHNSON R E, *et al.* Herpes simplex virus type 2 in the United States, 1967 to 1994. *N Engl J Med* 1997;337:1105–11.

17. BROWN Z A, SELKE S, ZEH J, *et al.* The acquisition of herpes simplex virus during pregnancy. *N Engl J Med* 1997;337: 509–15.

18. BROWN Z A, WALD A, MARROW R A, *et al.* Effect of serologic status and cesarean delivery on transmission rates of herpes simplex virus from other to infant. *J Am Med Assoc* 2003;289:203–9.

19. RANDOLPH A G, WASHINGTON A E, PROBER C G. Cesarean delivery for women presenting with genital herpes lesions. Efficacy, risks, and costs. *JAMA* 1993;270(1):77–82.

20. GREGG N M. Congenital cataract following German measles in the mother. *Trans Ophthalmol Soc Aust* 1941;3:35–46.

Infections in obstetrics and gynaecology

Phillip E Hay

Spectrum of genitourinary infections in women

Genitourinary infections are among the most common medical presentations in women. The most common symptomatic infections are bacterial vaginosis, vulvovaginal candidiasis (thrush) and urinary tract infections. Sexually transmitted infections such as chlamydia and gonorrhoea may be symptomatic or asymptomatic but, if causing pelvic inflammatory disease (PID), are a threat to a woman's future fertility. Viral infections can persist for long periods of time, with human papillomavirus (HPV) causing cervical, vulval and anal cancers and herpes simplex virus (HSV) persisting for life. Worldwide, HIV infection is predominantly sexually acquired and in some parts of the world as many as a third of pregnant women are now infected. Clinicians need to be aware of the way that HIV alters the manifestations of, and host susceptibility to, other infections.

Infections can adversely affect the mother during pregnancy, lead to congenital abnormality in the fetus, prematurity or neonatal infection and cause morbidity in the mother in the postnatal period. As in nonpregnant women, many infections can be silent or present with few symptoms.

The spectrum of infections that are important in pregnancy can be summarised by the acronym STORCH[5]:

- S – syphilis
- T – toxoplasmosis
- O – other
  - bacterial vaginosis
  - *Trichomonas vaginalis*
  - group B streptococcus
  - *Escherichia coli*
  - *Ureaplasma urealyticum*
  - *Haemophilus influenzae*
  - varicella zoster virus
  - *Listeria monocytogenes*
- R – rubella
- C – cytomegalovirus
- H[5] – HSV, HIV, hepatitis B virus, HPV
- and human parvovirus.

Lower genital tract infections

The changes in physiology that occur during a woman's lifetime affect the susceptibility to, and site of, infection. At birth, the newborn girl is exposed to high levels of estrogen and progesterone from the mother and the vagina of the newborn is lined with stratified squamous epithelium. It is possible for *T. vaginalis* to be transmitted at birth but the infection usually clears spontaneously. In children, the vagina is lined with a simple cuboidal epithelium. The pH is neutral and the vagina is colonised by organisms similar to skin commensals. Under the influence of estrogen at puberty, stratified squamous epithelium develops and lactobacilli become the predominant organisms. This is accompanied by a drop in pH to a level of approximately 3.5–4.5. Following the menopause, atrophic changes occur with a return to bacterial flora similar to that of the skin. The pH again rises to 7.0.

PHYSIOLOGICAL DISCHARGE

Normal vaginal discharge is white, becoming yellowish on contact with air owing to oxidation. It consists of desquamated epithelial cells from the vagina and cervix, mucus originating mainly from the cervical glands, bacteria and fluid formed as a transudate from the vaginal wall. More than 95% of the bacteria present are lactobacilli. The acidic pH is maintained through the production of lactic acid by the vaginal epithelium metabolising glycogen and by the lactobacilli. Physiological discharge increases in midcycle owing to increased mucus production from the cervix. It also increases in pregnancy and sometimes when women start a combined oral contraceptive pill. Sometimes, a cervical ectropion is associated with excess mucus production causing persistent discharge. This can be treated with cervical cautery.

An overview of the differential diagnosis of abnormal vaginal discharge is provided in Table 22.1.

Vaginal candidiasis

Over 75% of women have at least one episode of vaginal candidiasis in their lifetime. At any time, 25% of women are colonised with *Candida* species in the vagina and a minority get symptoms. The organism is carried in the gut, under the nails, in the vagina and on the skin.

C. albicans is found in more than 80% of affected women. *C. glabrata*, *C. krusei* and *C. tropicalis* account for most of the remaining 20%. Sexual acquisition is rarely important, although the physical trauma of intercourse may be sufficient to trigger an episode in a predisposed person. Vaginal candidiasisis is estrogen-dependent and therefore rarely seen in prepubertal girls or postmenopausal women.

Factors predisposing to vaginal candidiasis include the following:

- immunosuppression
  - HIV infection
  - immunosuppressive therapy, e.g. steroids
- diabetes mellitus
- vaginal douching, bubble bath, shower gel, tight clothing, tights
- increased estrogen levels
  - pregnancy
  - high-dose combined oral contraceptive pill
- underlying dermatosis, e.g. eczema
- broad-spectrum antibiotic therapy.

It should be noted that the role of tight clothing is anecdotal, described before the era of evidence-based medicine.

Clinical features

Vaginal candidiasis is characterised by the following symptoms:

- itching, soreness and redness of the vagina and vulva

TABLE 22.1 **Differential diagnosis of the principal causes of abnormal vaginal discharge**

Symptoms and signs	Candidiasis	Bacterial vaginosis	Trichomoniasis	Cervicitis
Itching or soreness	++	–	+++	–
Smell	May be 'yeasty'	Offensive, fishy	May be offensive	–
Colour	White	White or yellow	Yellow or green	Clear or coloured
Consistency	Curdy	Thin, homogeneous	Thin, homogenous	Mucoid
pH	< 4.5	4.5–7.0	4.5–7.0	< 4.5
Method of confirmation	Microscopy and culture	Microscopy	Microscopy and culture	Microscopy, tests for *Clamdia trachomatis* and *Neisseria gonorrhoeae*

++ = moderate to severe | +++ = severe | – = none

- curdy white discharge, which may smell yeasty but not unpleasant
- may be accompanied by fissures and excoriations.

Not all vaginal *Candida* infections present in the same way; in some women there may be itching and redness with a thin watery discharge. The pH of vaginal fluid is usually normal (between 3.5 and 4.5). The diagnosis can be confirmed by microscopy and culture of the vaginal fluid. Asymptomatic women from whom a *Candida* species is grown on culture do not require treatment.

Recurrent *Candida* infection or *Candida* infection not responding to treatment is relatively uncommon. If the clinical picture suggests the presence of treatment-resistant *Candida* infection, the correct diagnosis is often HSV infection, vulvodynia or a dermatological condition such as eczema or lichen sclerosis.

Treatment

As a general rule, it is better to use a topical treatment than a systemic therapy. This minimises the risk of systemic adverse effects. Vaginal creams and pessaries can be prescribed at a variety of doses and for variable durations. However, some women have a preference for oral therapy, particularly if required at the time of menstruation. Treatment options include the following:

- clotrimazole pessary 500 mg given as a single dose
- oral fluconazole 150 mg tablet given as a single dose (only active against *C. albicans* strains).

Longer courses of treatment are needed when there are predisposing factors that cannot be eliminated, such as steroid therapy.

In pregnancy, treatment with a topical agent such as clotrimazole 100 mg/day for 7 days gives superior cure rates. Oral azoles are not recommended in pregnancy.

Complications and pregnancy

Genuine recurrent infection with a *Candida* species can be suppressed with weekly fluconazole 150 mg for a 6-month period. If resistance to treatment is shown clinically and *in vitro*, new antifungal agents such as voriconazole can be administered. Alternatively, boric acid applied intravaginally can be used.

Complications are uncommon. In some women, a severe episode of vaginal candidiasis can trigger long-term vulvodynia. Candidiasis has not generally been associated with complications in pregnancy, although in one study treatment of asymptomatic vaginal candidiasis was associated with fewer preterm births.

BACTERIAL VAGINOSIS

Bacterial vaginosis is the most common cause of abnormal vaginal discharge in women of childbearing age. Its reported prevalence has varied widely from as low as 5% in a selected group of asymptomatic college students to 50% of women in a large study in Uganda. Studies in antenatal clinics and gynaecology clinics show a prevalence of approximately 12% in the UK.

Bacterial vaginosis is more common in black women and those who have an intrauterine contraceptive device (IUCD). In addition, it is probably more common in women with sexually transmitted infections, although bacterial vaginosis has also been reported in virgin women and may be particularly common in lesbian women. The condition often arises spontaneously around the time of menstruation and may resolve spontaneously in midcycle.

Previously, a variety of names had been used for this condition, including nonspecific vaginitis, *Gardnerella* vaginitis and anaerobic vaginosis. When bacterial vaginosis develops, the predominantly anaerobic organisms that may be present at low concentration in the vagina increase in concentration up to a thousand-fold. This is accompanied by a rise in vaginal pH to between 4.5 and 7.0 and ultimately the lactobacilli may disappear.

The organisms classically associated with bacterial vaginosis are:

- *Gardnerella vaginalis*
- *Bacteroides* (*Prevotella*) species
- *Mobiluncus* species
- *Mycoplasma hominis*.

Novel organisms such as *Atopobium vaginae* have been identified by use of molecular techniques and a biofilm consisting predominantly of *Gardnerella* species and *A. vaginae* has been described.

Clinical features

The typical symptom of bacterial vaginosis is an offensive fishy-smelling discharge that is characteristically thin, homogenous and adherent to the walls of the vagina. It may be white or yellow. The smell is particularly noticeable around the time of menstruation or following intercourse. However, semen itself can give off a weak fishy smell.

In clinical practice, the diagnosis is commonly made using the composite (Amsel) criteria:

- vaginal pH above 4.5
- release of a fishy smell on addition of alkali (10% potassium hydroxide)
- characteristic discharge on examination
- presence of 'clue cells' on microscopy.

Clue cells are vaginal epithelial cells so heavily coated with bacteria that the border is obscured.

Bacterial vaginosis can also be diagnosed from a Gram-stained vaginal smear. Large numbers of Gram-positive and Gram-negative cocci are seen, with reduced or absent large Gram-positive bacilli (lactobacilli). Culture of a high vaginal swab yields mixed anaerobes and a high concentration of *G. vaginalis*. However, *G. vaginalis* can be grown from up to 50% of women with normal vaginal flora. Its presence is not, therefore, diagnostic of bacterial vaginosis.

Treatment

Bacterial vaginosis will resolve on treatment with antibiotics with good antianaerobic activity such as the following:

- metronidazole 400 mg twice/day for 5 days or metronidazole 2 g as a single dose
- metronidazole vaginal gel (0.75%) 5 g/night for 5 nights
- clindamycin cream (2%) 5 g/night for 3–7 nights.

Initial cure rates are greater than 80% but up to 30% of women relapse within 1 month of treatment.

Complications

It is now established that women with bacterial vaginosis are at increased risk of second-trimester miscarriage and preterm delivery during pregnancy. This may result in perinatal mortality or cerebral palsy. Studies in which bacterial vaginosis in pregnant women has been treated with metronidazole or clindamycin have produced conflicting results, so current guidelines do not recommend routine screening and treatment in pregnancy.

Treatment of bacterial vaginosis with metronidazole before termination of pregnancy has been shown to reduce the number of subsequent incidents of endometritis and PID.

In some women, the vaginal flora is in a dynamic state, with bacterial vaginosis developing and remitting spontaneously. Women with symptoms of recurrent bacterial vaginosis can become frustrated as the condition responds rapidly to treatment with antibiotics but may also relapse rapidly. Our inability to alter this process reflects our current lack of knowledge of the factors that trigger bacterial vaginosis. Regular treatment with 0.75% metronidazole gel twice week reduces the rate of recurrence.

TRICHOMONIASIS

Trichomonas vaginalis is a sexually transmitted infection that can be carried asymptomatically for several months before causing symptoms. It is diagnosed in approximately 1% of women attending genitourinary medicine clinics but is highly prevalent in many tropical countries, with a 25% prevalence rate reported in rural Uganda. In men, trichomoniasis is often carried asymptomatically but may present as nongonococcal urethritis.

Clinical features

Trichomoniasis is characterised by the following symptoms:

- vulvovaginitis, which can be severe, with inflammation sometimes extending out onto the vulva and adjacent skin
- purulent green or yellow discharge, sometimes with an offensive smell
- punctate haemorrhages can occur on the cervix, giving the appearance of a 'strawberry cervix'.

Many affected women also develop bacterial vaginosis.

The diagnosis is confirmed by culture, preferably in a specific medium such as Feinberg–Whittington medium. Nucleic acid amplification tests (NAATs) promise a greater diagnostic sensitivity once they become available. Microscopy of vaginal secretions mixed with saline has a 60% sensitivity for detecting the organism. Numerous polymorphonuclear cells are seen and the motile organism is identified from its shape and the presence of four moving flagellae.

Treatment

Treatment of trichomoniasis involves the following antibiotics:

- metronidazole either 2g as a single dose or 400mg twice/day for 5 days
- tinidazole 2g as a single dose, which is more expensive but occasionally works when metronidazole has failed.

The woman should be advised to send her sexual partner(s) for treatment before resuming intercourse together.

Complications

T. vaginalis has occasionally been identified in the upper genital tract of women with PID but the organism is probably not an important cause of upper genital tract pathology. It can also be isolated from the bladder.

Fortunately treatment failure with standard doses of metronidazole is uncommon. This may be attributable to poor compliance with medication, poor absorption, re-infection or, rarely, a treatment-resistant organism. The usual approach is to use higher doses of metronidazole, initially 400mg three times/day orally, increasing to 1g twice/day given per rectum or intravenously. Only a limited number of alternatives are available, including arsphenamine pessaries and clotrimazole, which has an inhibitory effect on *T. vaginalis*.

Pregnancy

Pregnant women symptomatic for trichomoniasis should be treated with a 5-day course of metronidazole. Although *T. vaginalis* infection is a risk factor for preterm birth, treatment of asymptomatic infection has not been shown to improve outcome.

OTHER CONDITIONS AFFECTING THE LOWER GENITAL TRACT

Occasionally, one encounters a true bacterial vaginitis that is caused by a *Streptococcus* strain or another organism not classically associated with this condition. It responds to appropriate antibiotic therapy such as co-amoxiclav 375mg three times/day for 7 days.

The retention of tampons or foreign bodies in the vagina is rarely associated with toxic shock syndrome. An overgrowth of toxin-producing staphylococci causes systemic shock with fever, diarrhoea, vomiting and an erythematous rash. There is a 10% mortality rate. More frequently, a foreign body or retained tampon merely causes an offensive discharge.

Bartholin abscess

The Bartholin glands are situated on either side of the vagina and open into the vestibule. Cysts can develop if the opening becomes blocked. These present as painless swellings. If they become infected, a Bartholin abscess develops. Examination reveals a hot, tender abscess adjacent to the lower part of the vagina. Surgical treatment is required. This is usually done by marsupialisation. Culture may yield a variety of organisms including *Neisseria gonorrhoeae*, streptococci, staphylococci, mixed anaerobic organisms and *E. coli*.

Infestations

Pubic lice and scabies are transmitted by close bodily contact. Pubic lice (*Phthirus pubis*) attach their eggs to the base of the pubic hair. Their claws only attach to thick body hair, so that they can also colonise the axillae and eyelashes. Infected individuals may report small itchy papules or notice debris from the lice in their underwear. Lice are treated by application of topical agents such as malathion, carbaryl or permethrin. Treatment should be repeated after 7 days and be supplied for partners to use simultaneously.

Scabies (*Sarcoptes scabiei*) causes an intensely itchy papular rash. It may be confined to the genital area initially if acquired during intercourse. It responds to applications of malathion or permethrin. Symptoms may take up to 6 weeks to resolve completely.

Upper genital tract infections

Ascending infection of the female upper genital tract is broadly termed pelvic inflammatory disease (PID) and includes endometritis, parametritis, salpingitis and oophoritis. These infections usually spread from the vagina or cervix through the uterine cavity. Lymphatic spread may also occur, either parametrially or along the surface of the uterus. Although rare, salpingitis has occurred in women who have been sterilised. Infection can also spread from the bowel or be blood-borne.

PID is an important condition because it results in tubal damage producing ectopic pregnancy and tubal factor infertility. As many as 20% of affected women may be left with chronic pelvic pain. PID is common. Approximately 12.5% of a cohort of women born in the 1950s in Sweden had at least one episode of PID before the age of 25 years. The symptoms and signs may be mild and subtle, with many women being unaware of the significance of mild pelvic pain for their future fertility. On the other hand, many women are now aware of these complications and seek reassurance about their future fertility when they receive a diagnosis of PID. The best information available is from a study in Lund, Sweden, that was started in the 1960s. In that study, 8% of women had tubal factor infertility following a single episode of PID, rising to approximately 50% after three episodes.

Many different organisms have been cultured from women with PID but the condition is often triggered by either *Chlamydia trachomatis* or *Neisseria gonorrhoeae*. *Mycoplasma genitalium* has also been implicated in PID (in men it causes nongonococcal urethritis) and, like *C. trachomatis* and *N. gonorrhoeae*, it is probably sexually transmitted. Tests for detecting *M. genitalium* are not available routinely but NAATs are being developed. The organism is difficult to culture and requires a specialised medium for growth. Endogenous anaerobes such as *Bacteroides* species or *Mycoplasma hominis* often come in as secondary invaders and are responsible for subsequent tubal abscess formation.

INFECTIONS ASSOCIATED WITH CHLAMYDIATRACHOMATIS AND NEISSERIA GONORRHOEAE

Chlamydia

Infection with *C. trachomatis* is the most common sexually transmitted bacterial infection in industrialised countries. As many as 10% of women of childbearing age are infected in inner cities in the UK. The prevalence is highest among women under 25 years.

The infection is asymptomatic in approximately 50% of men and 80% of women. In men, *C. trachomatis* is the most important cause of nongonococcal urethritis. In women, it causes cervicitis and PID as well as other complications that will be discussed later on. The organism can infect the rectum but severe proctitis is only caused by lymphogranuloma venereum (LGV) strains. In addition, genital strains can colonise the throat and can also cause conjunctivitis.

There is now a national chlamydia screening programme in the UK targeting women below the age of 25 years with the aim of reducing the incidence of PID and tubal factor infertility.

Bacteriology

C. trachomatis is an obligate intracellular pathogen. The species has been subdivided into several serovars:

- serovars A–C cause trachoma, infecting the conjunctiva
- serovars D–K cause genital infections
- serovars L1–L3 cause LGV.

C. trachomatis has a complex life cycle. The infectious form is known as an elementary body. This gains entry to host cells by binding to specific cell surface receptors. Once inside the cell, the elementary bodies differentiate into so-called reticulate bodies. These are the metabolically active form of the organism and can be detected within inclusion bodies. Heavily infected cells die. Damage to the epithelial surface is mainly caused by the inflammatory response to infection and can manifest as cervicitis and PID.

Diagnosis

Chlamydial infection is now diagnosed by NAAT. Self-collected vaginal swabs provide sensitivity equivalent to clinician-collected endocervical swabs, allowing the use of self-collected swabs for screening. In women, first-pass urine testing has a lower sensitivity than vaginal swab testing but in some settings urine samples are obtained more easily. Serological tests are insensitive and nonspecific but high levels of antibody are found in 60% of women with tubal factor infertility.

Treatment

The following treatments are effective for an uncomplicated chlamydial infection:

- azithromycin 1g as a single dose
- doxycycline 100mg twice/day for 7 days
- ofloxacin 400mg once/day for 7 days
- erythromycin 500mg twice/day for 14 days(used in pregnancy).

The partner(s) should also receive treatment for *C. trachomatis* and be screened fully for sexually transmitted infections before sexual intercourse is resumed.

Gonorrhoea

In developed countries, the incidence of gonorrhoea has declined in the last two decades; the prevalence in women of childbearing age is now less than 1%. The spectrum of disease in women is similar to that associated with *Chlamydia* infection. However, chronic asymptomatic infection is common, with 50% of affected women having no symptoms or signs of infection. By contrast, approximately 90% of affected men are symptomatic. The most common presentation in men is severe urethritis with green urethral discharge and dysuria. Women and homosexual men may also present with proctitis, characterised by purulent discharge, bleeding and rectal pain.

N. gonorrhoeae may also be carried in the throat or cause an exudative tonsillitis. In addition, it can cause conjunctivitis in adults.

Bacteriology

N. gonorrhoeae colonises columnar or cuboidal epithelia. In chronic infection, there is a complex interaction with the host immune system. In the presence of an effective antibody response, the expression of antigenic cell surface proteins changes over time, preventing the development of protective immunity.

Diagnosis

Reliable serological tests for *N. gonorrhoeae* have not been developed. In genitourinary medicine clinics, a presumptive diagnosis is made on observation of typical Gram-negative intracellular diplococci on smears of urethral, cervical or rectal swabs. *N. gonorrhoeae* is a fastidious organism that requires a CO_2 concentration of 7%, specific media such as blood agar and antibiotics to inhibit the growth of other organisms. It may fail to grow on culture, especially if transport to the laboratory is delayed. NAATs are available but may have poor specificity. Obtaining a culture remains essential to allow testing for antibiotic sensitivity.

Treatment

Due to increasing major histocompatibility complexes (MICs) to cephalosporins seen worldwide, combination treatment using higher doses of ceftriaxone than used previously are now recommended for treating gonorrhoea: a single dose of azithromycin 1g orally with ceftriaxone 500mg intramuscularly. The azithromycin covers any concomitant chlamydial infection as well as having some synergy with ceftriaxone against *N. gonorrhoeae*. If doxycycline is preferable to azithromycin for other reasons, such as treating pelvic inflammatory disease it can replace the azithromycin.

When ceftriaxone resistance emerges, gentamicin 250mg may be effective.

Because of resistance 'blind' treatment with single doses of ciprofloxacin 500mg, amoxicillin 3g with probenecid 2g, cefixime 400mg orally, can no longer be recommended, although ciprofloxacin may be used if cultures show sensitivity in an untreated patient.

A test of cure with culture, and/or a NAAT test should be performed after two weeks. Sexual intercourse should only be resumed a week after treatment of the patient and her partner.

Cervicitis

Mucopurulent cervicitis is a clinical diagnosis made on detection of purulent mucus at the cervical os, which is often accompanied by contact bleeding. It can be confused with a benign ectropion but the latter does not usually bleed heavily unless swabbed very vigorously. Women with cervicitis may present with postcoital bleeding or complaining of a purulent vaginal discharge. Many, however, are asymptomatic. The condition is often caused by a sexually transmitted agent, with the male partner having nongonococcal urethritis. Tests for *C. trachomatis* and *N. gonorrhoeae* should be performed. If ulceration is present, an HSV test should be obtained.

The treatment is the same as for chlamydial infection, unless a specific organism is detected.

Chronic cervicitis produces scarring. In addition, nabothian follicles (mucus-containing cysts of up to 1 cm in diameter) are often present following chronic cervicitis.

Pelvic inflammatory disease

As infection ascends into the uterus, endometritis develops. Plasma cells are seen on endometrial biopsy and, in women with chronic chlamydial infection, germinal centres may develop.

The first stage of salpingitis involves mucosal inflammation with swelling, redness and deciliation. Polymorphonuclear cells invade the submucosa, followed by mononuclear cells and plasma cells. Inflammatory exudate fills the lumen of the tube and adhesions develop between mucosal folds. Inflammation extends to the serosal surface and pus exudes from the fimbriae to the ovaries and their adnexae. At laparoscopy, the tubes in mild salpingitis are swollen and red. In more severe forms of salpingitis, they are fixed to adjacent structures by fibrin exudate and adhesions. With pelvic peritonitis, all the organs are congested with multiple adhesions producing an inflammatory mass. The omentum usually confines the infection to the pelvis. The infection causes considerable tissue destruction. Tubal or tubo-ovarian abscesses may develop.

Subsequent scarring may lead to the fimbriae being drawn into the ends of the fallopian tubes, with the result that they adhere to and seal the ends of the tubes. The uterus and tubes may be pulled back into the pelvis by adhesions, becoming fixed and retroverted. Accumulation of fluid within the tube causes a hydrosalpinx; the affected tube expands and swells. If infected, a pyosalpinx results. Pelvic adhesions organise, matting together the pelvic organs. Some recovery of the ciliated epithelium within the tubes usually occurs.

Clinical features

As infection extends into the uterus, the fallopian tubes and the ovaries, it causes pelvic pain and deep dyspareunia. Endometritis may cause intermenstrual bleeding and it is common for women with PID to have an associated urinary tract infection.

The diagnosis of PID is made on the basis of the following findings:

- a history of pelvic pain and deep dyspareunia
- cervical motion tenderness (often called cervical excitation) on examination, with or without uterine and adnexal tenderness
- a lower genital tract infection such as bacterial vaginosis, trichomoniasis or cervicitis
- pyrexia, a raised neutrophil count and a raised erythrocyte sedimentation rate (in more severe forms of PID)
- an adnexal mass (present in 20% women, usually those who are most unwell systemically).

At best, the clinical diagnosis is 70–80% accurate. Laparoscopy is regarded as the gold-standard for diagnosis. In early salpingitis, however, the inflammation may not be visible from the serosal surface of the tubes. The important differential diagnoses are shown in Table 22.2. The most important diagnosis to exclude acutely is ectopic pregnancy.

When PID is suspected, endocervical swabs should be taken for detection of *C. trachomatis* and *N. gonorrhoeae*. A high vaginal swab should be taken for detection of *T. vaginalis* and bacterial vaginosis. Laparoscopy

TABLE 22.2 **Findings at laparoscopy in women with suspected pelvic inflammatory disease**

Diagnosis at laparoscopy	Proportion of women (%)
Salpingitis/pelvic inflammatory disease	65
Normal findings	22
Appendicitis	3
Endometriosis	2
Bleeding corpus luteum	2
Ectopic pregnancy	2
Miscellaneous	4

should be performed if the clinical diagnosis is uncertain, if drainage of an abscess might be required or if there is no improvement after 24–48 hours of intravenous antibiotic treatment in a systemically unwell woman.

Treatment

Ambulant women with mild symptoms can be treated as outpatients. The antibiotic regimen should cover both *C. trachomatis* and *N. gonorrhoeae* as well as anaerobic organisms.

Current guidelines recommend the following two oral regimens:

- a single dose of intramuscular ceftriaxone 500 mg, doxycycline 100 mg twice/day for 14 days and metronidazole 400 mg twice/day for 14 days
- ofloxacin 400 mg twice/day for 14 days and metronidazole 400 mg twice/day for 14 days.

However, with increasing quinolone resistance of *N. gonorrhoeae*, it is advisable to include ceftriaxone in any treatment regimen.

Women who are systemically unwell or in whom a tubal abscess is suspected should be admitted for intravenous antibiotic treatment and may require laparoscopy to definitely establish the diagnosis. One recommended regimen comprises intravenous cefoxitin and doxycycline followed by oral doxycycline and metronidazole for 14 days. Another uses intravenous clindamycin and gentamicin followed by 14 days of oral doxycycline and metronidazole or 14 days of oral clindamycin. It is essential that sexual partners are screened for *C. trachomatis* and *N. gonorrhoeae* and prescribed appropriate antibiotic treatment before intercourse is resumed.

Other complications of chlamydia and gonorrhoea

Intra-abdominal spread of *C. trachomatis* or *N. gonorrhoeae* can cause periappendicitis (which mimics appendicitis) or perihepatitis; the latter is termed Fitz-Hugh–Curtis syndrome. Women and, rarely, men with this syndrome present with pyrexia and right hypochondrial pain and tenderness. They are frequently misdiagnosed as having cholecystitis. Careful examination usually elicits signs of salpingitis. At laparoscopy, fine 'violin string' adhesions are seen between the liver capsule and the visceral peritoneum. Treatment is a 3-week course of antibiotics for chlamydia and gonorrhoea depending on the identified cause.

Disseminated infection with *C. trachomatis* may cause Reiter syndrome (sexually acquired reactive arthritis) in about 1% of infected individuals. There is usually an asymmetrical oligoarthritis affecting large joints of the lower limb. In Reiter syndrome, the arthritis is accompanied by uveitis and a rash that, if florid, may be similar to psoriasis. It is associated with the presence of human leucocyte antigen haplotype B27 and there is overlap with other seronegative spondarthritides.

Disseminated infection with *N. gonorrhoeae* presents as a septic oligoarthritis that usually affects the small joints of the hand or wrist, often accompanied by a scanty papular rash. It is rare but occurs more often in women than men because of the larger proportion of asymptomatic and untreated infections in women.

Pregnancy and vertical transmission of chlamydia and gonorrhoea

Genital infection with *C. trachomatis* or *N. gonorrhoeae* during pregnancy can cause chorioamnionitis and women with such infections probably have a two- to three-fold increased risk of preterm birth. Although data on the safety of azithromycin in pregnancy are limited, this drug is now commonly used for the treatment of chlamydia because it is better tolerated than erythromycin. Cephalosporins should be used for gonorrhoea. Quinolones, doxycycline and tetracyclines are contraindicated in pregnancy. Because of altered drug pharmacokinetics in pregnancy, a test of cure should be performed 6 weeks after treatment. If performed earlier, DNA from dead organisms may be detected, leading to unnecessary concern about treatment failure.

Newborn babies usually acquire infection as they pass through an infected birth canal. Both *C. trachomatis* and *N. gonorrhoeae* cause ophthalmia neonatorum. Affected infants develop keratoconjunctivitis, which can progress to corneal scarring and blindness if not treated promptly. The diagnosis of ophthalmia neonatorum is confirmed by taking conjunctival swabs for the detection of *C. trachomatis* by direct fluorescent antibody assay or DNA amplification assay and for the detection of *N. gonorrhoeae* by culture. The mother and her sexual partner(s) should also be screened and receive appropriate treatment. *C. trachomatis* may cause pneumonitis in the first few months of life. Babies with ophthalmia neonatorum should therefore receive systemic therapy with erythromycin.

OTHER CAUSES OF ENDOMETRITIS

Tuberculosis

Mycobacterium tuberculosis can spread through the genital tract via the blood or lymphatics. Nearly always, another organ is also affected by tuberculosis, usually the lung. Granulomata develop in the fallopian tubes and subsequently in the other genital organs. Infection may remain subclinical, presenting ultimately with amenorrhoea, infertility or chronic low-grade pelvic pain. The endometrium is involved in up to 80% of affected women and the ovaries in 20–30%. Abnormal uterine bleeding is a presenting symptom in 10–40% of affected women. The examination is often normal, but an adnexal mass or fixing of the pelvic organs may be detected. The diagnosis can be confirmed by obtaining endometrial tissue from biopsy or from dilatation and curettage. The detection rate is greatest towards the end of the menstrual cycle. Even so, endometrial biopsy does not have a 100% sensitivity.

As the presentation may be subtle, a high index of suspicion is essential. A Mantoux test or Heaf test should be reactive in women with active tuberculosis unless they have an immunosuppressing condition. A chest X-ray should be performed to look for evidence of pulmonary tuberculosis. Bilateral tubal calcification may be seen on abdominal X-ray after chronic infection. Treatment should be supervised by a physician with expertise in tuberculosis.

Actinomycosis

This infection is almost exclusively seen in women with an IUCD. It can be detected on cervical cytology and careful monitoring is required if there are no clinical features to suggest PID. If there is any history of pelvic pain, the IUCD should be removed and antibiotic treatment with penicillin initiated. If undetected, actinomycosis can progress to widespread pelvic involvement with an inflammatory mass and fixing of the pelvic organs. For further information on the clinical features, diagnosis and treatment of actinomycosis see Chapter 20.

Genital ulcer disease

The diagnosis of genital ulcers can be a considerable challenge for the clinician. The following list provides an overview of potential infectious and noninfectious causes of genital ulcer disease:

- Infectious causes
  - Herpes simplex virus
  - Primary syphilis
  - Lymphogranuloma venereum
  - Chancroid
  - Donovanosis
  - HIV
- Noninfectious causes
  - Aphthous ulcers
  - Trauma
  - Skin disease, e.g. lichen sclerosus et atrophicus
  - Behçet syndrome
  - Other multisystem disorders, e.g. sarcoidosis
  - Dermatitis artefacta.

In the UK, HSV infection (discussed in Chapter 21) is by far the most common cause. It is essential, however, to take an adequate sexual and travel history as there are many other sexually transmitted causes of genital ulcers that are common in tropical countries.

Among the noninfectious causes, malignancy, particularly squamous cell carcinoma, may arise on a background of lichen sclerosus et atrophicus or vulval intraepithelial neoplasia. In addition, multisystem disorders such as Behçet syndrome, systemic lupus erythematosus and sarcoidosis may be associated with genital ulceration. It is therefore advisable to arrange for a biopsy if there is any doubt about the diagnosis.

Simple aphthous ulcers can occur on the genital mucosa in the same way as in the mouth. HIV infection may present with genital ulceration, particularly in the form of persistent atypical herpetic ulcers. The presentation of other infections is modified by immunosuppression.

SYPHILIS

At present, the incidence of syphilis is rising in European countries including the UK. The disease is most common in the tropics and in homosexual men. The correct microbiological diagnosis can be difficult and referral to an appropriate specialist may be required.

Syphilis is a systemic sexually transmitted infection caused by *Treponema pallidum*. *In vitro*, *T. pallidum* subspecies *pallidum*, the causative organism of venereal syphilis, cannot be distinguished from *T. pallidum* subspecies *pertenue*, which causes yaws, *T. pallidum* subspecies *endemicum*, which causes endemic syphilis (also called bejel), and *T. pallidum* subspecies *carateum*, which causes pinta. These three tropical treponematoses are not sexually transmitted but are spread by skin-to-skin contact or fomites, often affecting children and household contacts. A description of them is beyond the scope of this chapter. Clinicians in the UK must be aware that they occur in sub-Saharan Africa, in the Caribbean and most of the humid tropics (yaws), in desert regions (endemic syphilis) and in isolated parts of Central and South America (pinta). Following such an infection, the serological tests for syphilis may remain positive for life, causing diagnostic confusion. The tropical treponematoses have become less common following mass treatment campaigns in the 1950s and 1960s, but they still occur.

Clinical features

The first manifestation of venereal syphilis is the chancre, a painless ulcer that arises at the entry site of *T. pallidum*.

Some people have multiple chancres. In addition, the regional lymph nodes become enlarged. The time between infection and appearance of the chancre is usually 3–6 weeks and it heals without treatment after a few weeks. Many women do not notice chancres because these often develop on the cervix.

Secondary syphilis can arise as the primary chancre is healing or up to 6 months thereafter. It is a systemic disease that most often manifests as a nonitchy maculopapular rash. The rash is symmetrical and often involves the palms of the hands and soles of the feet. Intertriginous areas, particularly the perianal area, may show more florid, wart-like lesions called condylomata lata. On mucosal surfaces, mucous patches and lines of ulcers (snail track ulcers) may develop. There may also be generalised lymphadenopathy. Other manifestations include alopecia, arthritis and meningitis. A sensorineural deafness can occur early in the infection owing to destruction of the hair cells in the inner ear.

Resolution of secondary syphilis is followed by a period of latency. The infection can only be detected on serological testing as there are no outward manifestations. There is a potential for lesions of secondary syphilis to recur for up to 2 years and during such a relapse the infection can be transmitted to a sexual partner. This period is therefore called early latent syphilis.

Primary and secondary syphilis are not generally life-threatening. The importance of timely diagnosis rests on the risks of late tertiary syphilis (neurosyphilis or cardiovascular syphilis) and transmission from a mother to a fetus.

Approximately 10% of men and 5% of women develop neurosyphilis if not treated in the early stages. Neurosyphilis can manifest within 5 years of infection in the form of meningovascular syphilis, the presenting symptom often being a stroke. Meningovascular syphilis may subsequently progress to tabes dorsalis or general paresis of the insane. Approximately 20% of people with syphilis will develop cardiovascular syphilis, presenting with thoracic aortic aneurysm or aortic regurgitation often many years after the primary infection.

Vertical transmission may severely affect the new-born baby and even cause fetal death. Surviving babies at risk should be fully evaluated (this should include a lumbar puncture) and receive intravenous penicillin. Less severe congenital infection may present during late childhood with symptoms including eighth-nerve deafness, interstitial keratitis and abnormal teeth. The risk of congenital infection is greatest (as high as 70%) in mothers with primary and secondary syphilis during the pregnancy but vertical transmission can even occur in pregnancies where the primary infection of the mother dates back 5–10 years. The effects of late congenital syphilis are not prevented unless the mother is treated before week 20 of gestation.

Diagnosis

The diagnosis of primary syphilis is traditionally made by visualising the spirochaetes with dark-field microscopy. Polymerase chain reaction (PCR) tests are becoming available. Serological tests for syphilis (Table 22.3) should be requested but these can be negative in early primary syphilis, so repeat serological testing should be performed if clinical suspicion is high. Most laboratories routinely perform an enzyme immunoassay, which detects both immunoglobulin (Ig) G and IgM antibodies against *T. pallidum*. If this screening test is positive, specific treponemal tests such as the *T. pallidum* haemagglutination (TPHA) test or the *T. pallidum* particle agglutination (TPPA) assay are performed. A test for nonspecific treponemal antibodies, such as the venereal disease research laboratory (VDRL) test or the rapid plasma reagin (RPR) test, is used in addition. These tests are diluted serially to report a titre such as 1 in 64. Chancres on the cervix may be misdiagnosed as cervical carcinomas. If there is any doubt, biopsies must be taken.

In secondary syphilis, the VDRL test is usually positive at a titre of one to 32 or greater. Dark-field microscopy of material from mucosal patches or condylomata lata can also be performed.

Owing to the possibility of false-positive test results or labelling errors, it is traditional to start treatment only after a second confirmatory test. However, in pregnancy it is better not to risk a treatment delay while waiting for a repeat test if the serological tests are unequivocally positive. Following treatment of primary or secondary syphilis, the VDRL titre should fall two-fold every 3 months, becoming negative within 2 years.

Treatment

The antibiotic of choice for the treatment of syphilis is penicillin. In early syphilis (primary, secondary and early latent syphilis), the following formulations can be used:

- benzathine benzylpenicillin 2.4 megaunits as a single dose (intramuscularly)
- procaine benzylpenicillin 1.2 megaunits/day to 600 000 units/day for 10 days (intramuscularly).

Alternatives to penicillin are:

- azithromycin 2g single dose or 500mg/day for 10 days
- ceftriaxone 500mg/day for 10 days (intramuscularly)
- doxycycline 100mg two times/day for 14 days
- erythromycin 500mg four times/day for 14 days.

However, erythromycin is rarely used because macrolide resistance has been documented in several outbreaks.

If the infection has been present for more than 2 years, the treatment duration is extended to 21 days for penicillin regimens (benzathine benzypenicillin given as 3 injections at 7-day intervals) and 28 days for oral

TABLE 22.3 **Syphilis serology: interpretation of results**

EIA	TPPA	RPR	IgM	Interpretation
Positive	Positive	Titre >1:8	Positive	Early syphilis
Positive	Negative	Negative	N/A	Biological false-positive reaction
Positive	Positive	Titre <1:8	Negative	Late or treated treponemal infection[a]

[a] IgM assays have a poor sensitivity and specificity, so the diagnosis could also be one of incubating early syphilis
EIA = enzyme immunoassay | IgM = immunoglobulin M | RPR = rapid plasma reagin | TPPA = *Treponema pallidum* particle agglutination

regimens. Only intravenous penicillin or high doses of procaine benzylpenicillin (2.4 megaunits/day) combined with probenecid (500 mg four times/day) produce acceptable levels of penicillin in the central nervous system to treat neurosyphilis.

In the first 24 hours after treatment, fever, malaise and exacerbation of symptoms (including rash) may occur. This is the Jarisch–Herxheimer reaction, which has been attributed to the release of proinflammatory cytokines following death of the infectious organisms. Paracetamol is usually sufficient to reduce the symptoms.

Partner notification is essential to prevent the spread of syphilis. In addition, the sexual history should be reviewed. In some cases, partners from a few years previously should be contacted if possible. Children may also need to be tested for syphilis, as well as siblings of individuals with suspected congenital infection. This may be arranged most easily with the help of a genitourinary medicine clinic.

Treatment in pregnancy

In pregnancy, the absorption of erythromycin is unreliable. In penicillin-allergic pregnant women, intravenous treatment with erythromycin or desensitisation to penicillin should be considered.

Treatment after week 20 of gestation will not necessarily prevent occurrence of the late sequelae of congenital syphilis, as inflammation in the teeth, inner ear and cornea can already occur *in utero*. Therefore, treatment of pregnant women should be initiated after one positive test without delay. In a mother with a high load of organisms, a Jarisch–Herxheimer reaction can precipitate preterm labour. These women should be advised to attend a labour ward if contractions start. When preterm birth occurs, the fetus is usually severely affected by congenital syphilis.

TROPICAL GENITAL ULCER DISEASE

Sexually transmitted infections causing genital ulcer disease present considerable diagnostic difficulty. Sometimes, more than one infecting agent may be present. Most of the aetiological agents cannot be cultured in standard microbiological media. Histological examination of tissue is sometimes the only means of confirming the diagnosis. In many resource-poor tropical countries, a syndromic approach is taken to the treatment of genital ulcers. Recommended treatments are shown in Table 22.4.

Lymphogranuloma venereum

Lymphogranuloma venereum (LGV) is caused by serovars L1–L3 of *C. trachomatis*. It is found in the Far East, sub-Saharan Africa and South America. In the early stages of infection, a small superficial ulcer may appear that slowly increases in size but often remains undetected. More obvious is the enlargement of lymph nodes, forming buboes. In the groin region, such buboes may become compressed by the inguinal ligament, leading to a characteristic finding called the groove sign. The buboes can also become matted together and discharge pus. Women may develop a severe proctocolitis that can progress to fistulae and strictures. Rectal infection presenting as proctocolitis has also become common in homosexual men in Europe and the USA.

The diagnosis of LGV can be confirmed serologically by a complement fixation test.

Chancroid

Chancroid is an infection caused by *Haemophilus ducreyi*. The geographical distribution is similar to that of LGV. The illness starts with small shallow ulcers that are usually multiple and painful. The edges are irregular and there is localised lymphadenopathy. The sores may persist for several months and the glands can suppurate through the skin.

It may be difficult to obtain a positive culture. The organism requires a specialised culture medium, which should ideally be inoculated directly from the person under investigation. NAATs are not commercially available but are offered by many reference laboratories. They are more sensitive than culture. Identification of the Ducreyi bacillus in biopsy tissue confirms the diagnosis if it cannot be done microbiologically.

Granuloma inguinale

Granuloma inguinale (donovanosis) is an infection caused by *Klebsiella granulomatis* (previously known

TABLE 22.4 **Treatment for bacterial genital ulcers**

Antibacterial agent	Primary syphilis	Lymphogranuloma venereum	Chancroid	Donovanosis
Azithromycin	Active but resistance occurs	Active but resistance is common	1g single dose	Not recommended
Ceftriaxone	Active but not fully evaluated	Not recommended	250mg single dose	Not recommended
Ciprofloxacin	Not active	Not reliable	500mg twice/day for 3 days	750mg twice/day for ≥21 days
Co-trimoxazole	Not active	Not recommended	May be used but resistance is common in some areas	960mg twice/day for ≥21 days
Doxycycline	100mg twice/day for 14 days	100mg twice/day for 21 days	Not recommended	100mg twice/day for ≥21 days
Erythromycin	500mg four times/day for 14 days[a]	500mg four times/day for 21 days	500mg four times/day for 7 days	500mg four times/day for 21 days minimum
Penicillin	Procaine benzylpenicillin 600 000 units/day for 10 days or single-dose benzathine benzylpenicillin 2.4 mega units	Not recommended	Not recommended	Not recommended

[a] Rarely used – macrolide resistance has been documented in several outbreaks

as *Calymmatobacterium granulomatis*). It is endemic in India, Papua New Guinea and southern Africa. The disease course is usually slowly progressive, starting with the formation of discrete papules on the skin or vulva. The papules can enlarge to form 'beefy red' painful ulcers, which slowly spread around the genitalia and perineum. As they heal, fibrosis can ensue and cause genital lymphoedema and elephantiasis. The diagnosis is best confirmed by biopsy or tissue crush preparation. Donovan bodies are visible as intracellular 'safety pin' bacteria with bipolar distribution of chromatin.

Other viral infections

HUMAN PAPILLOMAVIRUS INFECTION

More than 100 different types of HPV have been described, with around 20–30 infecting the anogenital tract. These strains are mainly sexually transmitted through skin-to-skin contact and penetrative intercourse is not necessary for infection to occur. Infection with

genital HPV is the most common sexually transmitted infection in Europe and developing countries, with a lifetime risk of 80% such that almost everyone is at risk of a genital HPV infection at some point in their lives. It is therefore not possible to define high-risk groups for HPV infection. Infection is often asymptomatic (80%) and transient, in the majority (80%) being cleared spontaneously after 9–18 months by the immune system.

Genital HPV types can be divided into high-risk and low-risk types according to oncogenic potential. Low-risk types cause genital warts and low-grade lesions. HPV-6 and HPV-11 are the most common low-risk types found in over 90% of genital warts. High-risk HPV types cause anogenital neoplasia. HPV-16 and HPV-18 are the most common high-risk types and are found in over 70% of cervical cancers. Other high-risk types also found in genital cancers include HPV-45, HPV-31, HPV-33, HPV-35, HPV-52 and HPV-58. Only persistent infections with high-risk types may become malignant.

In one study, genital warts developed in nearly two-thirds of people within 3 months of starting a relationship with a partner who had visible genital warts. There is less information on the role of asymptomatic shedding of HPV in those with subclinical lesions. The virus can infect the skin of the vulva and perineum, the vagina, cervix and rectum. Orogenital contact possibly leads to warts developing in the mouth or lips. Warts are frequently multiple and slowly increase in size. They can spread directly to the perianal skin without anal intercourse being practised. The same strains can affect the larynx of a newborn baby (rarely) but do not usually spread to normal skin.

The majority (99.7%) of squamous cell carcinomas of the cervix contain DNA sequences from oncogenic HPV strains. It is thought that the viral proteins E6 and E7 bind to the tumour suppressor proteins p53 and pRB. This leads to dysregulation of the cell cycle and cell proliferation.

Most women infected with HPV-16 or HPV-18 do not develop cancer. It is estimated that 5% of high-risk infections result in cervical cancer in unscreened populations and 1–2% in screened women. The real burden of HPV-related neoplasia is borne by developing countries without cervical screening programmes. Worldwide, there are over 500 000 new cases of cervical cancer annually, 80% of which occur in the developing world.

Other risk factors for anogenital neoplasia exist, such as smoking, but by far the greatest risk is posed by high-risk HPV infection. Vaccines against HPV are now licensed, with a bivalent vaccine targeting HPV-16 and HPV-18 (this vaccine also provides a degree of protection against several other oncogenic strains) and a quadrivalent vaccine targeting HPV-6 and HPV-11 in addition to HPV-16 and HPV-18. In clinical trials, these vaccines were highly effective in preventing high-grade cervical intraepithelial neoplasia associated with the target viruses.

Treatment of genital warts

The following approaches are available for the treatment of genital warts:

- physical methods such as weekly cryotherapy
- podophyllotoxin applied twice/day for 3 days, repeated after 4 days as needed for up to four courses
- imiquimod applied three times/week for up to 16 weeks

- surgical treatment employing lasers, electrocautery or scissor excision; this is used for intractable cases.

People with impaired immunity such as those with HIV infection or underlying malignancies are particularly difficult to treat.

Women with warts on the cervix should be referred for colposcopic assessment. Recent sexual partners should be examined for evidence of genital warts and also other infections. Traditionally, people with warts have been advised to use barrier methods of contraception during treatment and for the subsequent 3 months. We do not know enough about the risks of transmission from asymptomatic carriers of HPV to allow evidence-based recommendations to be made. The role of condoms can be discussed in the general context of protecting against both acquisition and transmission of sexually transmitted infections with new partners.

Immune-based therapies with interferon or topical application of imiquimod, a cream that stimulates local cytokine release, may be helpful for people with genital warts. Nucleotide analogues, a new class of antiviral drugs, are active against HPV and may become useful for its treatment.

MOLLUSCUM CONTAGIOSUM

Molluscum contagiosum virus is a poxvirus that produces painless lesions of up to 5 mm in diameter. The lesions have a pearly appearance and a dimple in the centre. They can be mistaken for genital warts and affected people should be warned not to pick at them because the fluid from the vesicles is infectious. Molluscum contagiosum is common in childhood and clears after a few months. Adults may acquire the virus during sexual intercourse. The infection resolves with cryotherapy or following curettage and application of phenol. In individuals with suppressed immunity, widespread large confluent lesions may develop. In HIV-infected individuals, these resolve with immune restitution following initiation of antiretroviral treatment.

AIDS

AIDS is caused by infection with HIV, a retrovirus. It is a particularly devastating disease because of the stigma of sexual transmission and the risk of vertical transmission to children. Even if a child is not infected, the death of one or both parents threatens his/her development and survival in many parts of the world. The prevalence is greatest in sub-Saharan Africa, where in several cities as many as a third of pregnant women are infected. A resurgence in tuberculosis has occurred hand in hand with the AIDS epidemic.

HIV-related immunodeficiency can manifest itself in any organ system; in people with HIV infection, a high index of suspicion is therefore required because the infection can alter many other disease processes.

Natural history of HIV infection

In 20% of those infected with HIV, an acute seroconversion illness develops within a few weeks of infection. The clinical features include fever, generalised lymphadenopathy, a macular erythematous rash, pharyngitis and conjunctivitis. A steady decline in immune function over the first few years may manifest itself in the form of opportunistic infections that are not life-threatening, including recurrent oral and vaginal candidiasis, single-dermatome herpes zoster (shingles), frequent and prolonged episodes of oral or genital herpes and persistent warts. Furry white patches on the sides of the tongue, termed oral hairy leucoplakia, may come and go. This is pathognomonic of immunodeficiency. Persistent generalised lymphadenopathy may be present. Skin problems include seborrhoeic dermatitis, folliculitis, dry skin, tinea pedis and a high frequency of allergic reactions.

Without antiretroviral treatment, the median time to the development of AIDS is 10 years. Essentially, AIDS is defined by the onset of life-threatening opportunistic infections or malignancies associated with immunodeficiency. The most common presentations are listed in Table 22.5.

Virology

HIV is a retrovirus that contains two single strands of RNA. The world pandemic is predominantly caused by HIV-1. HIV-2 infection originating in West Africa tends to progress to AIDS more slowly and is less infectious. To gain entry into a human cell, the viral outer membrane protein gp120 binds to the CD4 receptors that are present on T helper lymphocytes, macrophages,

TABLE 22.5 **Common AIDS-presenting illnesses**

Affected body system	Presenting illness
Pulmonary	*Pneumocystis* pneumonia
	Tuberculosis (pulmonary or extrapulmonary)
Neurological	Cerebral toxoplasmosis
	Cryptococcal meningitis
	AIDS dementia
Gastrointestinal	Diarrhoea and wasting syndrome[a]
	Oesophageal candidiasis
Ophthalmic	Cytomegalovirus retinitis
Malignancy	Kaposi sarcoma
	Non-Hodgkin lymphoma
Systemic	*Mycobacterium avium* complex infection

[a] May be attributable to infection with Cryptosporidium, Microsporidium or Isospora species

dendritic cells and microglia. Coreceptors, such as the chemokine C-C motif receptor 5 (CCR5), are also used to enhance viral entry. The enzyme reverse transcriptase carried within the virus particle enables the production of proviral DNA in infected cells. Once proviral DNA has been integrated into the host genome, viral peptides are transcribed. Specific viral protease enzymes cleave these before the daughter virus particles are assembled.

Diagnosis

HIV infection is diagnosed by detection of antibodies to gp120. During seroconversion, p24 antigen is detectable in the serum before antibodies are produced. Rapid tests using a fingerprick of blood or a buccal sample are increasingly being used for diagnosis, particularly in outreach settings.

The disease is monitored by measuring the level of CD4 lymphocytes in peripheral blood. A normal lymphocyte count lies above 500 cells/mm^3. There is a 10% risk of AIDS developing within 1 year when the CD4 lymphocyte count drops to 200 cells/mm^3. This is the level at which primary prophylaxis against *Pneumocystis jirovecii* pneumonia is recommended. Using PCR technology, it is also possible to measure the concentration of viral RNA in the plasma. A high level of more than 100 000 particles/ml predicts rapid disease progression.

Where there is access to effective antiretroviral therapy, treatment is now highly successful with a near-normal life expectancy predicted. Widespread testing with minimal pretest discussion is now advocated because failure to test and diagnose early increases the risk of late presentation with potentially irreversible complications.

Treatment

Two treatment strategies are used:

- antiretroviral therapy
- prophylaxis against opportunistic infections in individuals with suppressed immunity.

Antiretroviral drugs targeting reverse transcriptase or viral proteases were the first classes to be developed and are most widely used in initial treatment. Newer drugs, including fusion inhibitors, entry inhibitors and integrase inhibitors, target other stages of the viral lifecycle. The aim of therapy is to reduce the level of virus in the plasma to zero with a combination of antiretroviral agents. First-line regimens usually comprise two nucleoside or nucleotide reverse transcriptase inhibitors (NRTIs) combined with a nonnucleoside reverse transcriptase inhibitor (NNRTI). Protease inhibitors are used instead of the NNRTI if there is resistance or another reason not to use an NNRTI.

If treatment is successful, the immune system partially recovers with a rise in the CD4 count and the risk of opportunistic infection is decreased. If total suppression of viral replication is not achieved, resistant strains of virus will inevitably arise within the treated person over the course of a few months. This is because reverse transcription is inherently inaccurate, leading to a high rate of mutation. With each cycle of replication of the virus, which takes 48 hours, single point mutations arise that will confer reduced sensitivity to antiviral agents.

Unfortunately, HIV infects long-lived memory cells from which the virus can rapidly reseed the body on cessation of therapy. Eradication, and thus cure, is unlikely even after several years of treatment.

If immunodeficiency has already occurred, treatment and prevention of opportunistic infections are needed.

This may include co-trimoxazole to prevent *Pneumocysis* pneumonia and, in individuals with severely suppressed immunity and CD4 counts below 50 cells/mm^3, azithromycin and valganciclovir to prevent disseminated *Mycobacterium avium* complex infection and cytomegalovirus infection, respectively. Regular administration of antifungal agents may be necessary to control oral and vaginal candidiasis.

The prognosis has improved dramatically for those with access to treatment. AIDS is now regarded as a treatable chronic disease with a near normal life expectancy. Increased morbidity and mortality from cancers other than the traditional AIDS-related ones and cardiovascular disease are starting to be recognised.

Of note, antiretroviral drugs, particularly some of the protease inhibitors, have many potential interactions with other drugs through effects on the cytochrome P450 enzymes. This includes an increase in the rate of breakdown of the synthetic estrogens present in oral contraceptive pills.

Transmission

In most developing countries, HIV is principally spread through vaginal intercourse, with approximately equal numbers of men and women being infected. In developed countries, the majority of infections have been acquired through homosexual sex or intravenous drug use, although the incidence of heterosexual transmission is increasing. Genital infections, including genital ulcer disease, chlamydia and gonorrhoea, are risk factors for HIV transmission and acquisition. Bacterial vaginosis may also be a risk factor and is very common in some African countries, with a prevalence of 50% or greater. Good control of sexually transmitted infections should reduce the incidence of HIV infection.

HIV infection in pregnancy

Vertical transmission occurs in 25–40% of affected pregnancies if no interventions are used to reduce the risk. It is thought that a minority of fetuses are infected during gestation. These babies can present with AIDS in the neonatal period. The majority are infected during parturition. Transmission through breastfeeding occurs in up to 15% of pregnancies. Transmission by this route may occur even after several months of breastfeeding. The risk of vertical transmission is increased if there is a high HIV viral load or a preterm delivery. The role of genital infections in vertical transmission is still being assessed. Many children infected with HIV will survive into adolescence.

Combined interventions that have been shown to reduce the risk of vertical transmission of HIV include:

- avoidance of breastfeeding (or continuation of maternal antiretroviral therapy if breastfeeding)
- elective caesarean section
- prescription of antiviral medication during the latter half of the pregnancy and to the newborn for 4 weeks.

If pregnant women with a viral load of less than 50 copies/ml start combination antiretroviral therapy at week 20 of gestation, the risk of transmission is below 1% even with a vaginal delivery, so this option is increasingly being taken up. Efavirenz is a first-line treatment prescribed to more than 50% of those treated in the UK. Its use was associated with neural tube defects in rhesus macaque monkeys; so, hitherto, it had been avoided in women of childbearing potential. Because of a lack of excess malformations in the prospective database, the 2012 British HIV Association (BHIVA) guidelines now allow efavirenz use in women of childbearing potential and its initiation in pregnancy. The dose of some protease inhibitors may need to be modified owing to altered pharmacokinetics in the second and third trimesters of pregnancy.

In many developing countries, the risk of infant death from gastroenteritis in formula-fed infants is greater than the risk of HIV acquisition from breastfeeding. Transmission is more likely if breastfeeding is mixed with bottle-feeding or if juice is added as this can induce damage to the gut, increasing the likelihood of virus penetrating the mucosa. Studies report low rates of transmission from breastfeeding mothers who continue to take antiretroviral therapy during lactation.

Impact of HIV infection on gynaecological health

HPV infection flourishes in individuals with suppressed immunity. Genital warts often persist despite aggressive surgical treatment. Chronic HPV infection can result in the development of cervical carcinoma, anal and vulval intraepithelial neoplasia and Bowen's disease. Because of these risks, most physicians perform cervical cytology annually in women with HIV infection. Persistent atypical warty lesions of the skin or vulva should be biopsied.

Other infections can also be more persistent in HIV-infected individuals. There is limited evidence that PID requires longer courses of antibiotics in women with HIV. Careful follow-up is certainly indicated. Postpartum endometritis is common in this group of women and HSV infection has been implicated occasionally. Eruptions of secondary genital herpes may become widespread, severe and persist for weeks if not diagnosed and treated. Genital herpes often presents as deep, painful ulceration.

Although all HIV-infected women are urged to use condoms to prevent transmission of the infection to others, they should also be advised to use a more reliable form of contraception if they do not wish to become pregnant. Only depot medroxyprogesterone acetate and IUCDs are known to work reliably in women receiving antiretroviral drugs.

Preconceptional advice is important for women with HIV. Antiretroviral medication may need modifying. If the partner is HIV-negative, the couple should use artificial insemination. Infertility treatment is available at a limited number of centres.

Urinary tract infection

Most women experience urinary tract infections at some point in their lives. They are considerably more common in young women than young men. This is generally attributed to the urethra being so much shorter in women, allowing organisms easier access to the bladder. Older men develop more infections as a consequence of prostatic enlargement. Urinary tract infections occurring in childhood require investigation to exclude congenital abnormality. If not detected, chronic pyelonephritis causes renal failure in adulthood.

The majority of infections in sexually active women are benign. It is thought that the vagina and, particularly, the periurethral area become colonised by pathogens, most often *E. coli*. During intercourse, the organisms can be pushed into the urethra, which is also traumatised, and from there ascend into the bladder. A short course of antibiotics will eliminate the infection from the bladder but does not usually stop periurethral colonisation. Broad-spectrum antibiotics such as amoxicillin, which are active against lactobacilli, disturb normal vaginal flora further and it is therefore preferable to use trimethoprim, nitrofurantoin or quinolones, which have less effect on lactobacilli.

Women with a urinary tract infection (cystitis) present with dysuria, suprapubic pain and urinary frequency. The differential diagnosis involves the distinction between internal dysuria, arising from the bladder or urethra, and external dysuria, in which urine causes stinging on contact with the vagina and vulva. The latter is usually attributable to vaginitis or HSV infection. Cystitis may be accompanied by an offensive smell from the urine, nocturia and, in severe cases, haematuria. Unilateral or bilateral loin pain and tenderness indicate pyelonephritis. Systemic features include fever, rigors, vomiting and malaise. Gram-negative septicaemia may ensue. Hospital admission is required in severe or systemic infection for close monitoring and treatment with intravenous antibiotics.

DIAGNOSIS AND TREATMENT

Urine should be tested initially with a dipstick that incorporates tests for leucocyte esterase and nitrite. If both of these are positive, a presumptive diagnosis of urinary tract infection can be made in symptomatic women and treatment can be initiated while the culture is being performed. A pure growth of at least 10^8 organisms/l is interpreted as confirming an infection. Polymorphs are usually present.

Subsequent treatment will of course depend on antibiotic sensitivities reported. The majority of urinary tract infections are caused by *E. coli*. Other common pathogens include *Proteus mirabilis*, *Staphylococcus saprophyticus* and *Klebsiella* species. All these organisms have the potential to develop resistance to antibiotics. The choice of treatment therefore depends on local sensitivity patterns, which usually reflect local antibiotic prescribing, and resistance patterns of previous isolates from the person to be treated. Optimal antibiotic treatment for uncomplicated infections is a 3-day course of antibiotics.

Investigation is indicated if infections are persistently recurring or if complications such as pyelonephritis

occur. A plain abdominal X-ray, requested as a kidney, ureter and bladder (KUB) X-ray, and ultrasound examination of the renal tract are usually sufficient for screening.

Women who experience frequent urinary tract infections in relation to sexual intercourse can be prescribed treatment for 3–6 months with low-dose antibiotics. Those that are used most commonly are trimethoprim 100 mg at night, ciprofloxacin 125 mg at night or nitrofurantoin 100 mg at night. These can be taken every night or only following sexual intercourse. Such long-term treatment should enable periurethral colonisation to disappear. Postmenopausal women benefit from treatment with topical estrogen to reverse atrophic change.

Self-help measures include attention to hygiene and wiping front to back after defaecation. Regular drinking of cranberry juice, which inhibits adherence of coliform bacteria to epithelial cells, might also be of benefit.

Puerperal sepsis/postpartum endometritis

In the 19th century, sepsis accounted for 50% of maternal deaths. Improvements in hygiene, aseptic techniques and our understanding of socio-economic status and appropriate use of antibiotics mean that it is now uncommon in industrialised countries. However, it remains a major cause of maternal morbidity and mortality in developing countries, accounting for 10% of maternal deaths.

After delivery, the uterus and genital tract contain blood and products of conception – an environment highly conducive for the growth of microorganisms. The risk of infection is increased in the following scenarios:

- preterm birth associated with chorioamnionitis
- emergency caesarean section
- prolonged rupture of membranes.

A single dose of prophylactic antibiotics should be given before a caesarean section to reduce the risk of postpartum infection.

Infection is usually polymicrobial, influenced by bacteria colonising the vagina (*E. coli*, beta-haemolytic group B and group G streptococci, *Staphylococcus aureus* and *Citrobacter* and *Fusobacterium* species). Fortunately, the classic puerperal fever associated with group A streptococcus is now a rare event. The organism is often identified in severe infections. Invasive group A streptococcus infection associated with necrotising fasciitis and fulminant streptococcal toxic shock syndrome carries the highest risk of maternal mortality.

Postpartum endometritis may present with fever, purulent discharge and uterine tenderness, usually within a few days of delivery. Septicaemia and septic shock can occur if the early signs of infection are neglected.

TREATMENT

A structured approach to management, as in the Surviving Sepsis Campaign, is associated with improved outcomes. This includes the use of broad-spectrum antibiotics, intravenous fluids and low-dose steroids. Before starting antibiotic treatment, cultures should be obtained from the vagina, urine and blood. Occasionally, uterine evacuation may be required. The choice of antibiotic depends on local guidelines and liaison with microbiologists. Initial therapy is often with clindamycin and an aminoglycoside, or with metronidazole and an aminoglycoside with or without ampicillin.

FURTHER READING

British Association for Sexual Health and HIV (BASHH) [www.bashh.org.uk]. *Includes link to Clinical Effectiveness Group for latest guidelines*

British HIV Association (BHIVA) [www.bhiva.org]. *Includes links to latest guidelines including management of HIV in pregnancy*

Centers for Disease Control and Prevention (CDC); Treatment Guidelines for Sexually Transmitted Diseases [www.cdc.gov/std/treatment].

HOLMES K K, SPARLING P F, STAMM W E, PIOT P, WASSERHEIT J N, COREY L, *et al. Sexually Transmitted Diseases*, 4th ed. New York: McGraw Hill; 2007. *The most comprehensive reference source on sexually transmitted infections*

Royal College of Obstetricians and Gynaecologists (RCOG) [www.rcog.org.uk].

Pathology

CHAPTER 23

Cellular response to disease

Raji Ganesan

The normal cell maintains a steady state termed *homeostastis* in which the internal milieu of the cell is kept within physiological parameters. The response of a cell to any change in its internal or external environment constitutes the pathophysiological basis of clinical symptoms.

Inflammation and healing of tissues

Cells show a number of reactions to injury. These changes are collectively termed as **adaptation**. When the capacity of the cell to adapt is exceeded then the cell undergoes a series of changes referred to as **cell injury** (Table 23.1). The degree of the injury dictates whether the cell will recover or progress to **cell death**.

The causes of cell injury can be interrelated; for example, physical injury can result in hypoxic damage secondary to loss of blood. Whatever the cause of injury,

TABLE 23.1 **Causes of cell injury and examples**

Cause	Example
Hypoxia	Vascular insufficiency
Physical injury	Burns
Chemical injury	Drug overdose
Infectious agents	Viral agents
Immunological reactions	Graft versus host disease
Genetic derangements	Cystic fibrosis
Nutritional imbalances	Scurvy

the main biochemical changes are release of oxygen derived free radicals, increases in cytoplasmic calcium, depletion of adenosine triphosphate (ATP) and defects of permeability of cell membranes.

PATTERNS OF CELL DEATH

Apoptosis This is a regulated event designed for cell death in embryogenesis and physiological events such as ovarian follicular atresia in menopause. It is also termed programmed cell death. A cell undergoing apoptosis shows condensation of chromatin followed by fragmentation of the nucleus. Proinflammatory mediators are not released during the process of apoptosis, and, thus, there is no inflammation in relation to apoptosis.

Necrosis This is the death of cells in living tissue and is characterised by swelling of cells, death of cell organelles and release of mediators of the inflammatory response. Necrosis is, therefore, accompanied by inflammation. The cytoplasm appears more eosinophilic and the nucleus can show karyolysis (dissolution), pyknosis (shrinkage) and karyorrhexis (fragmentation). Necrosis can result in morphological changes in the tissue (Table 23.2).

Autolysis The death of cells post-mortem or after removal from the body at surgery is termed autolysis.

Inflammation Is the response of vascularised tissue to injury. It is composed of a complex series of events that start with tissue injury and progress to vascular, chemical and systemic responses; all aimed at restoration of the tissue to normalcy. The earliest response is *vascular constriction* followed by *dilatation* and the resultant slowing of blood flow (Figure 23.1). As a consequence, the red blood cells aggregate, the white cells adhere to

TABLE 232 **Types of necrosis and examples**

Type of necrosis	Example	
Coagulative necrosis	Myocardial infarction	Outline of tissue preserved
Colliquative necrosis	Cerebral infarction	Liquefaction, tissue morphology lost
Caseous necrosis	Tuberculous lymphadenitis	Cheesy material, tissue morphology preserved
Gangrene	Clostridial infection	Gaseous/frothy, tissue morphology lost
Fat necrosis	Acute pancreatitis	Outline of tissue preserved

FIGURE 23.1 **Mechanisms of increased vascular permeability**

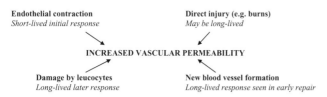

endothelial cells (*margination*) and increase in the gaps between endothelial cells. White cells emigrate (*transmigration*) actively through the vessel wall by a process termed *diapedesis*, where the neutrophils exit the vessels followed by mononuclear cells. Chemical substances released in this process are referred to as *chemical mediators* that may originate either from the plasma or the cells.

Chemical mediators Broadly speaking, the chemical mediators of inflammation originate either from plasma or from cells (Table 23.3). The production of active chemical mediators is triggered by microbial products or by products of the complement, kinin and coagulation systems. The mediators are generally short-lived and removed by phagocytes. This system of balances and checks generally results in avoidance of the possible excess damage by these chemicals.

TABLE 23.3 **Main chemical mediators of inflammation**

Chemical mediator	Source
Histamine	Mast cells, platelets
Serotonin	Platelets, mast cells
Prostaglandins	Leucocytes, platelets, endothelium
Cytokines, nitric oxide	Macrophages, endothelium
Kinins	Plasma

Chronic inflammation Acute inflammation may resolve completely, heal by fibrosis, result in abscess or progress to chronic inflammation (Figure 23.2). Although difficult to define precisely, chronic inflammation is considered to be inflammation of prolonged duration. Chronic inflammation can be a continuation of acute inflammation or start *de novo*. Chronic inflammation is characterised by concurrent tissue destruction and inflammation. The tissue changes include mononuclear cell infiltration, small vessel proliferation and fibrosis.

Granulomatous inflammation Is a specific type of chronic inflammation characterised by the presence of granulomas in the diseased tissue. Granulomas are collections of macrophages referred to as epithelioid cells. When the granulomas show loss of cellular detail with cheese-like material centrally, it is termed caseating granulomas of which tuberculosis is the classical example. Giant cells (multinucleate cells) are seen and when they have nuclei arranged peripherally in a horseshoe shape they are termed Langhans type of giant cells. Sarcoidosis is the prototypical example of noncaseating granuloma. Sarcoid granulomas can occur anywhere in the body with lymph node, lung and skin being commoner sites. Kveim test, where granulomas are induced by injection of sterile sarcoid tissue homogenate is a

FIGURE 23.2 **Outcomes of acute inflammation**

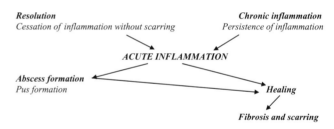

positive response indicative of sarcoidosis. In nearly a third of patients with sarcoidosis, the serum level of angiotensin-converting enzyme is raised.

EFFECTS OF INFLAMMATION

The effects of inflammation are sometimes referred to as the cardinal signs. These include redness (rubor), heat (calor), pain (dolor), swelling (tumour) and loss of function (function laesa). The nonspecific systemic effects of inflammation include raised erythrocyte rate (ESR), raised C-reactive protein (CRP), leucocytosis and fever.

Wound healing

Replacement of dead tissue by living cells or fibrous tissue is known as **wound healing**. Cells with great capacity for renewal are **labile cells** exemplified by surface epithelial cells. **Stable cells** are generally slow at regeneration but can renew nearly completely, for example liver and renal tubular cells. **Permanent cells** lack regenerative capacity and include the cells constituting the central nervous system.

Wound healing is adversely affected by extremes of temperature, persistence of foreign material, infection, early movement or trauma, poor glycaemic control as well as lack of minerals such as zinc.

The sequence of events in wound healing is the formation of granulation tissue followed by growth of new vessels and myofibroblasts into injured tissue. Collagen then accumulates to form a scar. Sometimes the fibroblast proliferation is excessive and results in a hypertrophic scar or a keloid.

Clean surgical incisions with approximated wound margins heal by **first intention**. When there is larger tissue loss, the healing process is referred to as healing by **secondary intention**. The latter differs from the former mainly by the phenomenon of wound contraction.

Adaptive responses

When cells are faced with physiological or pathological stress then they respond in several ways. These include:

Hypertrophy: Increase in cell size without cell replication

Physiological: Muscle hypertrophy in athletes

Pathological: Cardiac muscle hypertrophy in hypertension

Hyperplasia: Increase in cell numbers by cell division

Physiological: Uterine muscle in pregnancy

Pathological: Bone hyperplasia in Paget's disease of bone

Atrophy: Decrease in the size of cells or organs.

Physiological: Involution of the thymus with age

Pathological: Muscle atrophy in paralysis secondary to loss of innervations

Metaplasia: Reversible replacement of one differentiated cell type with another type of differentiated cell

Physiological: Squamous metaplasia in the uterine cervix in response to change in pH of the vagina.

Pathological: Squamous metaplasia in the bronchus secondary to cigarette smoke.

Disturbance in blood flow, shock, infarction

Oedema Refers to an abnormal accumulation of fluid in tissues. This may occur due to alteration of haemodynamic forces as in oedema secondary to cardiac failure; or due to changes in plasma osmotic pressure such as in nephrotic syndrome. Obstruction may also cause oedema. In inflammation, oedema results from increased vascular permeability and is one of the cardinal features of inflammation.

Thrombosis Is the pathological process by which blood clot forms within the uninterrupted vascular system by a complex process involving the endothelium lining the vessels, the platelets and the coagulation or clotting cascade. The three factors needed to effect a thrombus are referred to as Virchow's triad. They are endothelial injury, stasis or turbulence of blood flow and hypercoagulability. Congenital causes of hypercoagulability include Factor V Leiden mutation, which increases the risk of clotting in pregnancy. Acquired causes include prolonged immobilisation. The thrombus formed can undergo dissolution by fibrinolytic activity and then organisation, and recanalisation of vessels occurs with reestablishment of blood flow. Thrombi can also extend and block the vessel further. They can detach from the site of original formation embolise to distant sites.

Embolus This is a detached fragment of material – solid, liquid or gas – that is seen in a blood vessel distant from its site of origin or entry. Examples are:

Pulmonary embolus: Usually from deep venous thrombosis of the limbs

Amniotic fluid embolus: Amniotic fluid in maternal vessels following a tear in placental membranes

Air embolism: In deep-sea divers from sudden decompression

Fat embolism: From fatty marrow of long bones following fractures.

Infarction Is necrosis following ischaemia secondary to occlusion of arterial supply or venous drainage.

Shock This is a condition of circulatory failure that results in hypoperfusion of vital organs. This can result in irreversible neuronal injury, acute renal tubular necrosis, cerebral damage and eventual death. Shock can be:

Cardiogenic shock: Secondary to myocardial infarction

Hypovolaemic shock: Secondary to traumatic haemorrhage

Toxic shock: Secondary to Gram-negative septicaemia

Benign gynaecological pathology

Raji Ganesan

Non-neoplastic disease of the female genital tract can be the underlying cause of morbidity. Common gynaecological symptoms include vaginal discharge; bleeding – irregular periods, heavy periods, postcoital bleeding and postmenopausal bleeding; pelvic pain and prolapse. The benign pathological conditions underlying some of these symptoms are endometriosis, infections, fibroids and polyps. There are some abnormalities that are peculiar to pregnancy. This chapter concentrates on some of these conditions.

Pathology of sexually transmitted infections and tubal damage

A number of organisms can be transmitted through sexual contact (Table 24.1). Some of these organisms are usually spread by sexual contact for example *Chlamydia trachomatis* and others are typically spread by other routes but can also be spread by sexual contact; for

example, *Entameoba histolytica*. Sexually transmitted diseases (STIs) can be the cause of damage after the initial inflammation subsides, can increase the risk for other STIs and can cross the maternal–fetal barrier and affect the unborn fetus.

STI-like gonorrhoea results in pelvic inflammatory disease (PID). The infection usually begins in the Bartholin gland or other glands in perineum, and then the organism spreads upward to involve to the tubes with persistent inflammation (pyosalpinx) or chronic damage (hydrosalpinx). The alterations in the tube can result in infertility and ectopic pregnancy. *Tuberculous salpingitis* is common in areas of the world where the disease is prevalent and is an important cause of infertility in these populations.

ENDOMETRIOSIS

Endometriosis is defined as the presence of endometrial glands and stroma outside of the endometrial cavity.

TABLE 24.1 **Sexually transmitted infections**

Organism	Disease caused	Other effects
Trichomonas vaginalis	Vaginitis	None
Treponema pallidum	Syphilis	Congenital syphilis in fetus
Neisseria gonorrhoeae	Gonorrhoeal cervicitis	Endometritis, bartholinitis, salpingitis with sequelae like infertility, ectopic pregnancy
Chlamydia trachomatis	Urethral syndrome	Bartholinitis, salpingitis with sequelae like infertility
Human Papillomavirus (HPV)	Genital wart or condyloma	Cervical intraepithelial neoplasia and cervical carcinoma
HIV	AIDS	Other infections and unusual malignancies

The commonest sites (in descending order of occurrence) are ovaries, rectovaginal septum, pelvic peritoneum, laparotomy scars and, rarely, the umbilicus or appendix. The presence of endometrial glands and/or stroma in the uterine wall is termed adenomyosis. The theories to explain the presence of endometrial tissue outside the uterus are:

1. The retrograde menstruation theory, which postulates that during menstruation endometrial tissue passes through the fallopian tube and implants in the peritoneal cavity.
2. The metaplastic theory, which implies that the lining of the peritoneal cavity can change to endometrial tissue.
3. The vascular dissemination theory, suggesting that endometrial tissue is disseminated by blood and lymphatic vessels. This could explain endometriosis in distant sites like the lung and nasal cavities.

Endometriosis and adenomyosis can be the underlying cause of pelvic pain, menstrual irregularities and infertility. Endometriotic cysts of ovaries can be filled with altered blood (fancifully likened to liquid chocolate) and are called chocolate cyst of the ovary. Malignancies, notably clear cell carcinoma and endometrioid carcinoma, can arise in endometriosis.

POLYPS

Polyps can be seen commonly in the cervix and endometrium. They are localised protrusions of the lining and include glands and stroma. They can be removed by simple surgery but tend to recur.

Pathology of pregnancy

DISORDERS OF EARLY PREGNANCY

Spontaneous abortion Nearly 10–15% of all recognised pregnancies end in spontaneous loss. The causes include defective implantation, genetic or acquired abnormality of the fetus and maternal viral infections like toxoplasmosis.
Ectopic pregnancy This term is applied to implantation of the fetus in any location other than the uterine cavity. The commonest site is the fallopian tube and this is usually secondary to tubal damage. The ectopic pregnancy can end in tubal rupture, or extrusion of the contents through the fimbrial end of the tube (tubal abortion).

Trophoblastic disease

Tumours of villous trophoblast

Molar pregnancy Hydatidiform mole is a disorder of pregnancy that occurs in about 1 in 1000 pregnancies in the West with significantly higher occurrence in the Far East. There are two kinds of mole and their differences are shown in Table 24.2.
Invasive mole or chorioadenoma destruens This is a rare condition where the chorionic invades the myometrium.

TABLE 24.2

Feature	Complete mole	Partial mole
Karyotype	46,XX (46,XY)	Triploid
DNA	Paternal DNA only	Maternal and paternal DNA
Villous morphology	Scalloped outline of villi	Fjord-like outline of villi
	Villous oedema	Vessels present contain nucleated RBCs
	Lack of vessels	Less prominent trophoblast
	Circumferential trophoblastic hyperplasia	Maternally expressed gene product p57 is positive
Serum human hCG	Elevated	Less elevated
Risk of choriocarcinoma	About 2%	Rare

hCG = human chorionic gonadotrophin I RBC = red blood cells

There is vascular involvement and, although the villi can be transported to distant sites, they are not capable of growing at the distant sites.

Choriocarcinoma This is a very rare malignancy with a marked propensity to vascular dissemination and the favoured sites of metastases are lungs, vagina and brain. The malignancy is very sensitive to chemotherapy.

Tumours of extravillous or placental site trophoblast

Placental site nodule This is a benign condition where hyalinised nodules of intermediate type or placental site trophoblast continue to remain in the endometrial lining. It can result in persistent bleeding.

Placental site trophoblastic tumour This is a rare malignant tumour of placental site or intermediate trophoblast. About 10% of these tumours result in metastases and death. In contrast to diseases of villous trophoblast where the serum human chorionic gonadotrophin (hCG) was raised, the marker is human placental lactogen (HPL).

DISORDERS OF LATE PREGNANCY

Pathology of toxaemia of pregnancy

Pre-eclampsia of pregnancy is a symptom complex characterised by hypertension, proteinuria and oedema. The exact mechanism of disease is still uncertain, but the toxic effects of oxygen-free radicals and lipid peroxides on endothelial cells are important factors. The initial pathology seems to be an abnormality of placentation that results in placental ischaemia. This then simulates the release of vasoconstrictor agents and the inhibition of vasodilator agents. There is reduced uteroplacental perfusion, systemic hypertension and disseminated intravascular coagulation.

Morphological changes in organs

There is no correlation of severity of the disease with the magnitude of pathological changes. The liver shows subcapsular and intraparenchymal haemorrhages. Haemorrhages can also be seen in the brain, heart and, typically, in the anterior pituitary. Placental infarcts and retroplacental haematomas are seen more often than in normal full-term placentas.

On microscopy, the characteristic feature is fibrinoid necrosis of uterine spiral arteries with intramural infiltrates of foam cells. This is termed acute atherosis. In the liver, fibrin thrombi are seen in portal capillaries with peripheral haemorrhagic necrosis. In the kidney, diffuse glomerular lesions are noted with fibrin in glomeruli.

Abnormalities of placentation

Disorders of implantation

Placenta accreta is a disorder of implantation where the chorionic villi go up to or into the myometrium without interposed decidua. This may be a primary disorder or secondary to implantation on an area of endometrial scarring. Postpartum bleeding may result as a failure of separation of this abnormal placenta. Very rarely, when the chorionic villi penetrate through the full thickness of the uterine wall (placenta percreta), hysterectomy may be the only method of control of bleeding.

Discordant implantation

When the interface of the fetal surface of the placenta (chorionic plate) is smaller than the maternal surface (basal plate) there is a discordance of placentation referred to as extrachorial placenatation. This is of two types – circum-marginate and circum-vallate – depending on whether the margin is flat or raised.

Disorders of the umbilical cord

The umbilical cord is inserted centrally or eccentrically in the placenta. When the insertion is at the edge it is referred to as a battledore placenta. If the insertion is beyond the edge into the membranes it is referred to as velamentous insertion of the cord. Nodules on the fetal surface of the placenta, particularly around the cord insertion, are amnion nodosum and this is associated with oligohydramnios.

Inflammation of placenta

When the infection is through the maternal blood stream, as in infections like listeriosis, cytomegalovirus and toxoplasmosis, the chorionic villi are affected and result in villitis. Ascending infections more commonly result in the inflammation of extraplacental membranes – chorioamnionitis.

FURTHER READING

KUMAR V, ABBAS A K, FAUSTO N, MITCHELL R. *Robbins Basic Pathology.* 8th ed. Philadelphia: Elsevier Saunders; 2007.

KURMAN R J. *Blaustein's Pathology of the Female Genital Tract.* 5th ed. Springer-Verlag; 2002.

UNDERWOOD J C E *General and Systemic Pathology.* 2nd ed. Edinburgh: Churchill Livingstone; 1996.

CHAPTER 25

Gynaecological neoplasia

Raji Ganesan

General aspects of neoplasia

Neoplasia has been best defined by the eminent British oncologist Sir Rupert Willis as 'A neoplasm is an *abnormal* mass of tissue, the growth of which *exceeds* and is *uncoordinated* with that of the normal tissues and *persists* in the same excessive manner *after the cessation* of the stimuli which evoked the change'. Tumours can be benign or malignant.

CHARACTERISTICS OF BENIGN TUMOURS

- Slow, expansile growth
- Presence of a limiting capsule
- Microscopic features similar to that of the tissues from which it arises
- Inability to spread beyond the tissue of origin
- Clinical symptoms are related to their size and position
- Ability to function like tissue of site of origin.

CHARACTERISTICS OF MALIGNANT TUMOURS

- Rapid growth
- Invasion of surrounding tissue
- Ability to metastasise
- Degree of differentiation on similarity to the parent tissue
- Anaplasia – variation of cell and nuclear size
- Abnormal mitotic activity with aberrant mitotic forms.

SPREAD OF NEOPLASMS

Benign tumours can compress surrounding tissues. Malignant tumours spread locally by direct invasion and infiltration of surrounding tissues. Distant spread is lymphatic and vascular spread as well as spread across serous cavities. Typically carcinomas spread to lymph nodes. Tumours have preferred modes of spread: osteosarcomas and renal cell carcinomas spread through blood vessels; lobular carcinoma of the breast and ovarian carcinoma spread to serous cavities. Some malignant tumours, like basal cell carcinomas and gliomas, have limited or no capacity to metastasise, whilst intravenous leiomyomas are benign tumours that can spread through vascular channels.

PATHOGENESIS OF TUMOURS

Genetic causes There are well-defined cancers in which inheritance of a single mutant gene increases the risk of developing a tumour. These are referred to as *inherited cancer syndromes* and these include familial retinoblastomas, familial adenomatous polyps of the colon, multiple endocrine neoplasia syndrome and von Hippel Lindau syndrome. Cancers that run in families and are referred to as *familial cancers*. The role of the inherited risk cannot always be clearly defined in an individual case. These include breast, ovarian and colon cancers. A small group of autosomal recessive disorders is collectively characterised by chromosomal or DNA instability and these individuals are predisposed to malignancies. These include xeroderma pigmentosum, ataxia-telangiectasia and Bloom's syndrome.

387

TABLE 25.1 Physical and chemical agents and associated cancers

Carcinogen	Neoplasm
Aflatoxin B$_1$	Hepatocellular carcinoma
Asbestos	Mesothelioma
Aniline dyes	Bladder cancer
Anabolic steroids	Hepatocellular cancer

Oncogenes These are commonly referred to as cancer-causing genes. Normal genes become oncogenic by modification by viruses and other influences (Table 25.1). *Oncogenic viruses* include the human papilloma virus (HPV), associated with cervical cancer; the Epstein–Barr virus (EBV), associated with nasopharyngeal carcinoma and lymphomas; as well as hepatitis B virus, causative for hepatocellular carcinoma.

Tumour markers These are the biochemical indicators of the presence of a tumour and usually refer to a substance that can be detected in blood, plasma or other body fluids (Table 25.2). These substances cannot be the primary modalities for diagnosis of cancer. However, they can be used for screening for cancers, locating the primary in case of disseminated disease, response to therapy and an early indicator of relapse.

Paraneoplastic syndromes These are symptom complexes in cancer patients. They may represent earliest manifestation of an occult neoplasm or mimic metastatic disease. Some of the syndromes are characteristic

TABLE 25.2 Tumour markers used in clinical practice

Tumour markers	Neoplasm
Human chorionic gonadotropin (hCG)	Trophoblastic tumours, e.g. choriocarcinoma
	Nonseminomatous germ cell tumours
Alpha fetoprotein (AFP)	Hepatocellular carcinoma
	Yolk sac tumour
Prostate specific antigen (PSA)	Prostatic carcinoma
CA-125	Ovarian carcinoma
	Primary peritoneal carcinoma

of certain tumours. Hypercalcaemia is probably the most common paraneoplastic syndrome. Others include Cushing's syndrome associated with small cell carcinoma of the lung, polycythaemia associated with renal cell carcinomas and carcinoid syndrome associated with bronchial adenomas.

Neoplasms of the female genital tract

Cervical carcinoma This is a disease that is common in less-developed countries. In developed countries, the incidence of cervical carcinoma is low because of early intervention and treatment of the preinvasive disease. The precursor lesion of cervical squamous cell carcinoma is **cervical intraepithelial neoplasia (CIN)** and of adenocarcinoma is **cervical glandular intraepithelial neoplasia (CGIN)**. Both types of carcinoma are HPV-related lesions. Cervical carcinoma is associated with a number of risk factors, including age at first intercourse, number of sexual partners and frequency of intercourse. All of these are interrelated with the major independent risk factor, which is infection with **HPV**. The other major independent risk factor is cigarette smoking. There are more than 100 subtypes of HPV. Some of these show a predilection for infecting the lower female genital tract, notably HPV 6, 11, 16 and 18. HPV 6 and 11 are implicated in benign condylomata and rarely implicated in malignancy. HPV 16 and, to a lesser extent, 18 are found in CIN and in cervical carcinomas. The area of the cervix where cancers arise is the transformation zone. CIN and CGIN can be recognised in cervical smears and this forms the basis of the cervical screening programme. The aim of the programme is to reduce cervical carcinoma by detection and treatment of the preneoplastic disease. Treatment of preinvasive conditions reduces the incidence of cervical carcinoma. HPV testing is now used to triage low-grade abnormalities detected on cervical smears. It is also used as test of cure of treatment of high-grade abnormalities. A HPV vaccination programme has been introduced in the UK.

Endometrial carcinoma This is emerging as a disease of more affluent populations. Endometrial carcinomas are broadly categorised as Type 1 and Type 2 carcinomas. Type 1 carcinoma occurs in younger perimenopausal women and is associated with unopposed estrogenic stimulation. Other associations include diabetes, hypertension and obesity. The prototypic Type 1 endometrial carcinoma is endometrioid carcinoma, of which early stage and low grade disease has a good prognosis. There is a premalignant state for this cancer that is termed atypical hyperplasia. The other type of hyperplasia is termed non-atypical hyperplasia and includes formerly termed simple and complex hyperplasia. Type 2 cancers occur in older postmenopausal women and has no association with estrogen excess. The prototypic Type 2 endometrial carcinoma is serous carcinoma. Serous carcinoma can present with extrauterine disease even in early stages. The preinvasive condition is known as serous endometrial intraepithelial carcinoma (SEIC).

The commonest tumour of the uterus arises in the uterine wall. These are the benign smooth muscle tumours that are commonly referred to as fibroids. Histologically they are known as **leiomyomas.** Their malignat counterpart l**eiomyosarcoma** is an uncommon malignant neoplasm. Malignant tumours of the endometrial stroma are **endometrial stromal sarcoma.** These tumours tend to spread through vascular channels of the myometrium. They are hormone sensitive and recur locally at the first instance.

Tumours of the ovary A plethora of tumour types are seen in the ovary. These include epithelial tumours, sex cord stromal tumours, germ cell tumours, miscellaneous tumours and metastatic tumours.

Primary ovarian carcinomas These are the commonest ovarian malignancy and can be of many different epithelial types. Ovarian carcinomas are divided into two groups designated Type I and Type II. Type I tumours are slow growing, generally confined to the ovary at diagnosis and develop from well-established precursor lesions that are termed borderline tumours. Type I tumours include mucinous and endometrioid carcinomas. They are genetically stable and are characterised by mutations in a number of different genes including *KRAS* and *BRAF*. Type II tumours are rapidly growing highly aggressive neoplasms for which well-defined precursor lesions have not been described. Type II tumours include high-grade serous carcinoma. This group of tumours has a high level of genetic instability and is characterized by mutation of p53.

Risk factors for ovarian cancers include nulliparity and family history. Women from families with *BRCA* gene are monitored with imaging and serum CA-125 studies because of the definitely increased risk of ovarian cancer. These families also have an increased risk of cancers of the fallopian tube and the peritoneum.

Serous carcinomas of the ovary These are the commonest epithelial tumour. They often present late. Spread to the omentum is common. There is an increasing acceptance that most ovarian serous carcinomas arise in the fallopian tube and spread secondarily to the ovary.

Sex cord stromal tumours The commonest malignant sex cord stromal tumour is the adult type of granulosa cell tumour. They are usually unilateral tumours and can be haemorrhagic. These tumours are characterised by their propensity for late recurrence.

Germ cell tumours Germ cell tumours constitute 15–20% of all ovarian tumours. Benign mature cystic teratomas, also known as ovarian dermoid cysts, are common ovarian neoplasms and occur at all ages. Other tumours in this category are mainly seen in children and young adults.

Metastatic tumours The ovary is a common site for metastatic tumours. Some of these tumours can closely mimic primary ovarian cancers and pose problems for the pathologist. The commonest tumours presenting as metastatic carcinomas are from the uterus, colon, stomach, biliary tract and pancreas. The classic example of metastatic gastrointestinal neoplasia to the ovaries is termed Krukenberg tumour and defines bilateral ovarian enlargement with diffuse infiltrating malignant cells containing intracellular mucin.

Vulva squamous cell carcinoma is the commonest epithelial malignancy of the vulva. The appearances are similar to squamous carcinomas anywhere in the body, and a three-tier grading is done on the basis of resemblance to normal squamous cells. The prognosis is determined by the size, depth of invasion and the degree of differentiation and the presence and extent of nodal metastases. The inguinal lymph nodes are commonly affected. Carcinomas invading to a depth of less than 1 mm are sometimes referred to as superficially invasive and have virtually no risk of metastasis. The preinvasive condition is termed **vulvar intraepithelial neoplasia (VIN).** It is recognised that there are two distinct types of VIN – classical VIN (also sometimes referred to as

TABLE 25.3 **Differences between classical and differentiated VIN**

Classical VIN	Differentiated VIN
Occurs in younger women	Occurs in older women
Associated with HPV high-risk types	Associated with lichen sclerosis
Graded into VIN 1, 2 and 3	No further grading

HPV = human papilloma virus | VIN = vulvar intraepithelial neoplasia

uVIN or usual type VIN) and differentiated VIN (dVIN) (Table 25.3).

Paget disease of the vulva is a rare disease occurring almost exclusively in postmenopausal women and histologically characterised by the presence of mucin containing malignant cells within the epithelium of the vulva. In most cases there is no association with invasion, although rarely it may be a spread from an underlying adnexal malignancy.

Vaginal intraepithelial neoplasia (VaIN) is much less common than CIN or VIN. It is associated with high-risk HPV infection and may coexist with VIN (of classical type) and CIN, reflecting the multicentric nature of the viral-associated disease.

Sarcoma botyroides is the term given to embryonal rhabdomyosarcoma of the vagina that occurs in children before the age of five. The term refers to the macroscopic appearance of a polypoid mass that fills the vagina of the affected child and bears a resemblance to a bunch of grapes (*botyroides* means 'grape like' in Greek).

Pharmacology

CHAPTER 26

Pharmacokinetics, pharmacodynamics and teratogenesis

Kevin Hayes

Drugs are commonly used at all stages of pregnancy. This chapter describes the basic principles of pharmacodynamics and pharmacokinetics and how these are affected by the large physiological changes in pregnancy and breastfeeding. The principles of teratogenesis are also described including patterns of effects that may occur, particular drugs to watch and how to try and avoid the problem by ideal prescribing practice. Special attention is paid to certain clinical conditions treated with known teratogens that present difficult management issues in pregnancy for obstetricians and allied clinicians. Additional sources of information are also provided.

Pharmacokinetics (Pk)

Describe what the body does to the drug and encompasses:

- Drug absorption (from the GI tract)
- Drug distribution (bioavailability + volume of distribution)
- Drug elimination (drug clearance is largely renal and hepatic)

Drug absorption

- Lipid soluble drugs cross membranes and are easily absorbed from the stomach and duodenum
- Water soluble drugs do NOT cross membranes, they need be moved by facilitated diffusion or actively by carriers e.g. ion channels

- Most drugs are given orally unless:
  - Oral intake is not possible e.g. an unconscious patient
  - The drug is not absorbed, altered or digested e.g. insulin

Drug distribution (this describes where the drug goes throughout the body)

Most drugs are designed to reach the systemic circulation but others are deliberately intended to reach other tissues depending upon the desired drug effect (e.g. across the blood brain barrier for meningitis or into the urinary tract for the treatment of UTIs).

- **Bioavailability** is the amount of drug that reaches the systemic circulation unchanged - IV drugs therefore have 100% bioavailability. Oral drugs will lose considerable amounts of bioavailability due to first pass hepatic metabolism – their dosing schedules will reflect this for them to be effective.
- **Volume of distribution (VD)** is the theoretical volume of water in which the amount of drug would need to be uniformly distributed to produce an observed blood concentration. – fat soluble drugs may have an enormous VD and they may have prolonged duration of action as they can have a reservoir in fat tissue.

Whilst principally theoretical concepts they have a practical application as pharmacologists use the above two measures to help calculate doses and timings of drug administration.

Drug elimination

Hepatic metabolism generally changes the original drug and then makes them more water-soluble to aid elimination

- **Phase I** – metabolism is by reduction/oxidation/hydrolysis principally due to the cytochrome p450 enzyme complex. After metabolism drugs can become:
  - **Inactive** – the vast majority of drugs are initially turned into inert biologically non-active chemicals following enzymatic change.
  - **Active** – some compounds do not store well or are best delivered in an alternative chemical format. The cytochrome p450 complex is used to convert the inert form into the desired active chemical e.g. enalapril and diazepam.
  - **Toxic** – occasionally the initial drug is converted to a chemical that can cause harm. This is rare under normal pharmacological conditions but in overdose the drug can be sent down an alternative red-ox pathway e.g. paracetamol overdose.
- **Phase II** – once converted to an alternative chemical the drugs are made more soluble by **conjugation** with another compound. These tend to be:
  - **Glucuronate (for basic drugs)** – e.g. paracetamol, morphine
  - **Acetate (for acidic drugs)** – e.g. hydralazine, procainamide, isoniazid
  - **Sulphate** – e.g. oral contraceptives

Once soluble they are excreted into:

- Urine via filtration from afferent renal blood flow from the liver OR
- Bile if the molecular weight (MW) is greater than 300 Da – the drug is then excreted in the faeces. Some drugs (e.g. combined oral contraceptive) have a recycling via breakdown by colonic bacteria so that some of the chemical is reabsorbed from the lower GI tract before excretion (the enterohepatic circulation).

Renal elimination depends principally upon glomerular filtration rate and renal function:

- Drugs with MW less than 500 Da are filtered, so very large drugs (e.g. heparin) are not renally excreted.
- Filtration is reduced in highly protein bound drugs (e.g. warfarin) as the protein carriers are negatively charged and are repelled from the glomerular basement membrane (GBM). Only "free" non-bound drug will be filtered.
- Excretion can be active in the proximal convoluted tubule (PCT) or by passive diffusion in the descending limb of the Loop of Henle due to drugs concentration gradients between the tubule and the peri-tubular capillaries. It is a dynamic process and depending upon concentration gradients inside or outside the tubule drug will diffuse in or out, particularly if lipid soluble.
- Active transport depends upon the acid-base status of a given drug:
  - Anion transporters are required for acidic drugs e.g. penicillins, cephalosporins, salicylates, frusemide.
  - Cation transporters are required for basic drugs e.g. morphine, pethidine, amiloride, quinine.
- Once a drug reaches the ascending limb of the loop of Henle it will invariably be excreted in the urine

Therapeutic window

All drugs have a dose at which they will be ineffective and a higher dose at which they may become toxic or cause significant side effects. The area between these doses is the therapeutic window. Most drugs have a wide therapeutic window. Some drugs however have a more narrow therapeutic window e.g. gentamicin, cyclosporin.

Drug monitoring

The vast majority of drugs do not need close monitoring as long as recommended doses and timings are adhered to. Certain drugs do however need close level monitoring. Their dosing is often related to individual patient

FIGURE 26.1 **The difference between a wide and narrow therapeutic window**

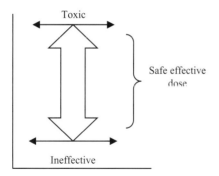

Wide therapeutic window

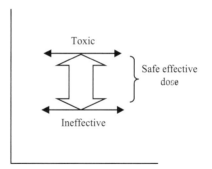

Narrow therapeutic window

weight and or height (e.g. methotrexate). The need for monitoring will be dependent upon the following factors:

- Narrow therapeutic window – the narrower the window the greater the risk of either being ineffective (e.g. increased fit frequency in anti-epileptic drugs (AEDs)) or toxic causing significant side effects (AEDs again).
- Intrinsic toxicity of the drug / how serious its side effects are e.g. gentamicin causing renal impairment and/or oto-toxicity (vestibular component of VIIIth nerve). Minor side effects are clearly less important.
- Impaired renal or hepatic function – these will invariably reduce clearance and increase the risk of toxicity.
- Certain special circumstances affecting Pk or where other harm is possible e.g. pregnancy, breastfeeding, extremes of age – paediatric and very elderly patients handle drugs differently and care is required in dosing.

Pregnancy and pharmacokinetics

Due to the very large physiological changes associated with pregnancy, it is mainly drug handling that is affected rather than intrinsic drug actions.

The most relevant factors include:

- Large increase in circulating volume (40–50%)
- Concomitant large increased in renal blood flow and consequent GFR

- Increased third space availability (amniotic fluid and peripheral oedema)
- Relatively increased fat content due to laying down of maternal fat reserves
- Reduced albumin and other binding proteins due to the overall plasma dilution effect
- Progressive insulin resistance affecting medication for diabetes

This results in:

- Increased clearance of most drugs reducing serum concentrations and sometimes efficacy. There are certain clinical conditions in pregnancy where this may require close drug monitoring and usually increases in drug doses over the course of pregnancy:
  - Anticonvulsants such as carbamazepine, phenytoin, valproate, lamotrigine and gabapentin especially where fit frequency is closely related to serum levels.
  - Mood stabilisers such as lithium where stable mood is vital and toxicity is particularly significant.
  - Common endocrine disorders in young women such as hypothyroidism – thyroxine inevitably need to be increased to keep thyroid function normal.
- Pregnancy is characterised by progressive insulin resistance – women with pre-existing diabetes invariably need large increases in diabetic medication, especially insulin, as pregnancy advances.

TABLE 26.1 **Examples of drugs with agonistic and antagonistic actions on receptors**

Drug name	Receptor
Agonists	
Salbutamol	β1 and β2 adrenergic
Methyldopa	α2 adrenergic
Phenylephrine	α1 adrenergic
Pilocarpine	Muscarinic
Diazepam	GABA
Morphine	μ-opioid
Cabergoline	Dopamine
Antagonists	
Atenolol	β1 adrenergic
Labetolol	α1, β1 adrenergic
Doxazocin	α1 adrenergic
Tolterodine	Muscarinic
Ranitidine	Histamine (H2)
Cyproterone acetate	Testosterone
Metoclopramide	Dopamine

TABLE 26.2 **Examples of drugs that act by inhibiting enzymes**

Drug name	Enzyme
Diclofenac	Cyclo-oxygenase (COX) inhibition
Ramipril	Angiotensin-converting enzyme (ACE) inhibition
Neostigmine	Anti-cholinesterase inhibition
Zidovudine	Reverse transcriptase inhibition
Acyclovir	HSV-specific thymidine kinase inhibition
Warfarin	Vitamin K epoxide reductase inhibition
Methotrexate	Dihydrofolate reductase inhibition

FIGURE 26.2 **Muscarinic receptors as a signaling molecule act via G-protein coupled receptors to influence intracellular events. An antagonist will block the receptor and hence its action**

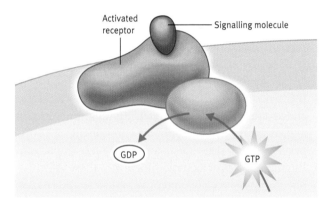

The signalling molecule acts via a G-protein-coupled receptor to influence intracellular events. An antagonist will block the receptor and hence the signalling molecule's action. | GDP = Guanosine diphosphate | GTP = Guanosine-5'-triphosphate

- While most drugs have reduced levels due to altered Pk, the effect may be less marked for:
  - Highly protein bound drugs as the free, active concentration is less affected due to the reduction in albumin levels e.g. warfarin
  - Fat soluble drugs due to the increased fat reservoir e.g. chloroquine. The drug can be stored in fat reservoirs increasing the time scale of available drug.

Pharmacodynamics

Describe what the drug does to the body i.e. the drug effect. There are generally four major drug effects:

- Receptors – tend to be metabotropic or ionotropic
  - Ionotropic receptors directly open or close an ion-pore in a membrane
  - Metabotropic receptors are indirectly linked to ion channels in plasma membranes via signal transduction by secondary messengers, usually G-coupled proteins.

Drugs can be **agonists, antagonists** or occasionally have a **mixed** effect on receptors. Table 26.1 gives some examples of drugs and their target receptors.

- Enzyme interaction – the majority of licensed drugs that influence enzymatic reactions tend to inhibit them (Table 26.2 and Figure 26.3)

396

- Membrane ion channels – most licensed drugs are generally designed to block ion channels (Table 26.3 and Figure 26.4)
- Metabolic processes e.g. antibiotics and ribosome / DNA synthesis (Table 26.4 and Figure 26.5)

Drug interactions

These occur when one drug has an effect on the pharmacokinetics +/or dynamics of another used at the same time. The more drugs a person takes the more likely there is to be an interaction. These can occur by:

- **Enzyme induction** - Phenytoin is a potent inducer of cytochrome p450 enzyme complex activity and leads to reduced levels of many drugs metabolised in the liver and indeed reduced efficacy e.g. COCP, warfarin. Other examples of enzyme inducers are: rifampicin, griseofulvin and spironolactone
- **Enzyme inhibition** - Sulphonamides inhibit hepatic metabolism and therefore increase plasma levels increasing the risk of toxicity and side effects e.g. phenytoin.

FIGURE 26.3 **The enzyme block due to warfarin**

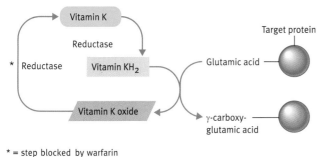

* = step blocked by warfarin

TABLE 26.3 **Examples of drugs acting on membrane ion channels and their effect**

Drug name	Ion channel
Nifedipine	Calcium blocker
Diltiazem	Calcium blocker
Verapamil	Calcium blocker
Lignocaine	Sodium blocker
Amiloride	Sodium blocker

FIGURE 26.4 **Ligands which may be drugs can bind directly to ion channels and open or close them. Nifedipine blocks the calcium influx seen here**

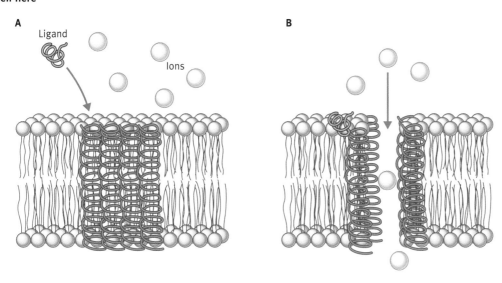

Ligands, which may be drugs, can bind directly to ion channels and **A** close or block them or **B** open them

TABLE 26.4 **Examples of antibiotics that affect metabolic processes**

Drug name	Process
Gentamicin	Inhibition of ribosome synthesis
Erythromycin	Inhibition of protein translocation
Doxycycline	Inhibition of protein translation
Carboplatin	DNA alkylating agent
Paclitaxel	Cellular microtubule function
Vincristine	Spindle poison

FIGURE 26.5 **Various actions of antibiotics on metabolic processes**

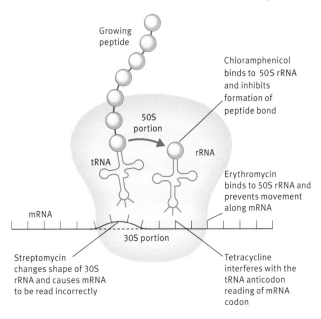

- **Individual effects** - Ampicillin alters the bacterial gut flora and thus leads to a reduced entero-hepatic re-circulation of oestrogens thus potentially impairing the efficacy of the COCP.

These effects may be potentiated in the very young and very old and where there is altered renal and hepatic function

Drugs in relation to pregnancy

General principles to consider:

- Remember all women of reproductive age might be pregnant

- Always question the need for drug therapy
- Avoid drugs in the first trimester if possible
- The benefits to the mother should outweigh the risks to the fetus (fetal therapy is sometimes a notable exception here)
- Do not stop a useful drug without careful risk-benefit analysis – drugs for epilepsy, asthma and thrombo-embolic disease are good examples
- Most drugs cross the placenta; few have been shown to be teratogenic
- Pre-pregnancy counselling for chronic medical conditions is the gold standard to optimise, alter or stop treatment to reduce the risk of harm
- Consider screening if exposure has occurred

When you need to prescribe:

- Use the smallest effective dose for the shortest possible time
- Choose a drug of which there is extensive experience in human pregnancy wherever possible
- Avoid poly-pharmacy where possible – the risk of teratogenesis with anti-epileptics increases each time another agent is introduced

Teratogenesis

Teratogenesis due to prescribed drugs would not exist if pregnant women never took medication. So, can we avoid drugs in pregnancy? Facts to consider:

- 35% of women take prescribed drug therapy at least once in pregnancy
- This is increasing as ever more women with medical problems becoming pregnant
- 6% of women take prescribed drug therapy in the first trimester (excluding iron and folic acid)
- 90% of women take something!

The reality is that prescribing is common in pregnancy as many medical problems arise (e.g. hyperemesis gravidarum) or pre-exist and can be exacerbated by pregnancy (e.g. heart disease). There are also times when it is considered safer to prescribe known teratogens, or drugs where safety is unknown, as the risk to the mother outweighs the risk of teratogenesis. Two good examples of this are for potentially life threatening conditions where pregnancy has a big effect on disease occurrence and potentially prognosis; epilepsy and malaria. Withholding or withdrawing treatment because of fetal concerns puts the mother at unacceptable risk.

The background incidence of congenital abnormalities is approximately 2–3%. So, what proportion of these is likely to be caused by drugs? It is calculated that up to 1% may be due to prescription drugs. However, a recent UK review looking at two of the most commonly studied drugs in pregnancy, Anti-Epileptic Drugs (AEDs) and anti-depressants (especially SSRIs), was clear that the true risks to the fetus remain unknown [1].

There are lots of problems with known data:

- Pregnant women are excluded from drug trials – teratogenic risk is therefore not assessed
- Retrospective cohort studies comparing exposed with non-exposed women are difficult to interpret because:
  o Congenital abnormalities are relatively common (2–3%)
  o Detection of a significant drug effect is therefore very difficult as it would need to be a large effect
  o Retrospective data is highly prone to recall bias – pregnancies affected by congenital anomaly are much more likely to remember taking a drug if asked
- Most drugs do reach the fetus to some extent, but teratogenesis remains difficult to predict e.g. warfarin, as a known teratogen has an exposure risk estimated at around 5%; therefore 95% of exposed pregnancies are unaffected
- Animal studies are idiosyncratic; many risks are likely to be dose and/or species specific.
- Negative animal study results therefore provide information but do not guarantee that a drug is safe

Drugs that do NOT cross the placenta:

- Heparin (unfractionated or LMWH)
- Tubocurarine
- Insulin

Teratogenic categorisation

The Food and Drug Administration (FDA) in the USA has a categorisation of drugs as per below (other categorisation systems exist in Germany and Australia, with slight variation but essentially the same message), see Table 26.5

When and where do drugs have an effect?

- **Pre-embryonic up to day 17** – as the conceptus consists of totipotent cells there is an "all or nothing effect" i.e. death and resorption or survival. Therefore, if there is drug exposure at this specific time and the pregnancy continues, then a woman can be reassured.
- **CAUTION**: As well as drugs taken during this time, caution is required with certain drugs taken previously e.g. retinoids can be present for up to two years, methotrexate for up to three months.
- **Embryonic from day 18 to 55 (Organogenesis weeks 2–8)**
  o Here is the biggest potential for structural damage and major anatomical defects due to irreparable tissue damage
  o The earlier the exposure the more marked the effect is likely to be
  o Every individual organ or system has a period of maximum sensitivity
  o Some systems (e.g. external genital tract) are not complete till well after the embryonic period and are therefore at risk much later e.g. cyproterone acetate having an anti-androgenic effect on male genitalia
  o Below are some examples of timings for some of the more common defects:
- **Post-embryonic from eight weeks to term** – the effects may be:
  o On fetal growth and development leading to Intra-Uterine Growth Restriction (IUGR) e.g. β blockers
  o Continued differentiation and maturation in organs such as the brain and kidney e.g. ACE inhibitors reducing fetal renal function

TABLE 26.5 **FDA drug categorisation**

Pregnancy Category	Description
A	**No risk in controlled human studies:** Adequate and well-controlled human studies have failed to demonstrate a risk to the fetus in the first trimester of pregnancy (and there is no evidence of risk in later trimesters).
B	**No risk in other studies:** Animal reproduction studies have failed to demonstrate a risk to the fetus and there are no adequate and well-controlled studies in pregnant women OR animal studies have shown an adverse effect, but adequate and well-controlled studies in pregnant women have failed to demonstrate a risk to the fetus in any trimester.
C	**Risk not ruled out:** Animal reproduction studies have shown an adverse effect on the fetus and there are no adequate and well-controlled studies in humans, but potential benefits may warrant use of the drug in pregnant women despite potential risks.
D	**Positive evidence of risk:** There is positive evidence of human fetal risk based on adverse reaction data from investigational or marketing experience or studies in humans, but potential benefits may warrant use of the drug in pregnant women despite potential risks.
X	**Contraindicated in pregnancy:** Studies in animals or humans have demonstrated fetal abnormalities and/or there is positive evidence of human fetal risk based on adverse reaction data from investigational or marketing experience, and the risks involved in use of the drug in pregnant women clearly outweigh potential benefits.
N	FDA has not yet classified the drug into a specified pregnancy category.

- o Shortly before term and labour e.g. pethidine immediately before delivery leading to neonatal respiratory depression,
- o Potential late effects such as sub-fertility and/or carcinogenesis e.g. chemotherapy exposure in utero

TABLE 26.6 **Types of defect arising as a result of a drug effect during the first 84 days of gestation**

Days	Defect
12–40	Limb reduction defects
24	Anencephaly
34	Transposition of great vessels
36	Cleft lip
42	VSD Syndactyly
84	Hypospadias

Further sources of information available:

- ■ Appendix 4 of the BNF in pre-version 70. In versions 70 onwards the risks are with each drug
- ■ National Teratology Information service 0191 232 1525
- ■ www.nyrdtc.nhs.uk/Services/teratology/teratology .html

Known teratogens

Particular teratogenic drugs to consider – Remember: "**All the A's**"

- ■ Anticonvulsants
- ■ Antibiotics
- ■ Anticoagulants
- ■ Antimetabolites
- ■ Antipsychotics
- ■ Androgens
- ■ Acne drugs ("A-Vitamin")
- ■ Alcohol

Certain drugs that may result in miscarriage

- ■ Ergotamine
- ■ Misoprostol
- ■ Mifepristone
- ■ Thrombolytics

The following highlight some of the issues with the more commonly known teratogens in pregnancy:

Anticonvulsants

- 90% of women with epilepsy have a normal pregnancy
- The risk is slightly increased regardless of anti-epileptic therapy (2.4% no therapy, 3- 4% single agent carbamazepine or phenytoin, 6% valproate, 3% lamotrigine [2])
- The risk increases with polypharmacy
- Valproate repeatedly been shown to have the highest risks
- Valproate also appears to have a dose-related effect on verbal IQ [3]
- Current data on lamotrigine suggests no extra risk above baseline
- Topiramate, Gabapentin, Levetiracetam currently have no firm information in pregnancy to guide risk assessment

Phenytoin is associated with malformations mainly due to alterations in folate metabolism. The fetal anticonvulsant syndrome is:

- Cleft lip/palate
- Microcephaly
- Cardiac abnormalities
- Mental retardation

Carbamazepine

- Similar effects to phenytion
- Plus neural tube defects

Valproate

- Neural tube defects also

Risk reduction appears to be possible if:

- Pre-conceptual folic acid 5mg once daily is taken for at least three months
- Polypharmacy is avoided wherever possible
- The lowest dose required for fit control is used (this may require level monitoring)
- Vitamin K is routinely given to mothers from 36 weeks and IM to babies to reduce the risk of post-partum haemorrhage and neonatal haemorrhage (evidence for a significant effect is however lacking)

Antibiotics

Antibiotics are one of the commonest classes of drugs prescribed in pregnancy as infective morbidity is relatively common.

Antibiotics to avoid are:

- Tetracyclines
  - Animal and human teratogenicity has been demonstrated
  - They cause permanent discolouration of teeth and impaired bone growth in-utero and up to age seven as they chelate calcium
- Sulphonamides
  - They inhibit folate metabolism - benzoic acid to folate (sulphonamides) and folate to tetrahydrofolate (trimethoprim)
  - Sulphonamides displace bilirubin from protein and may cause kernicterus in the neonate
  - Sulphasalazine, used for inflammatory bowel disease is probably safe

Caution is required and safer alternatives are preferred if possible with the following:

- Aminoglycosides (usually used for uro-sepsis and/or severe general sepsis):
  - They are nephrotoxic causing tubular destruction
  - They cause VIIIth nerve damage (the vestibular component)
  - Use only if essential and levels need to be monitored
- Quinolones
  - There appears to be a risk of permanent arthropathy in animals – data too limited in humans
  - Better alternatives are usually available
- Nitrofurantoin
  - Has been associated with neonatal haemolysis
- Chloramphenicol
  - May cause cardiovascular collapse (Grey baby syndrome) if given close to term. Local eye treatment with chloramphenicol eye drops is safe as the systemic absorption is minimal

The following antibiotics have the most experience in their use in pregnancy and appear to be safe:

- Penicillins
  - 70% of maternal serum levels are present in the fetus so can also treat fetal infection, e.g. syphilis
  - There is a theoretical risk of allergic sensitisation of the fetus, though this appears to be very rare
- Cephalosporins appear safe and are often first line
- Macrolides e.g. erythromycin appear safe
  - There is a small risk of neonatal cholestatic jaundice

Anticoagulants

- Heparin
  - Both unfractionated + LMW Heparins are very large and do not cross the placenta – they are extensively used in pregnancy for prophylaxis and treatment of thrombo-embolic disease. They have no teratogenic risks but like all drugs have some maternal side effects:
  - Haemorrhage
  - Heparin-induced thrombocytopaenia
  - Local skin reaction and bruising
- Warfarin is contra-indicated between 6-12 weeks gestation as a recognised teratogen unless the thrombo-embolic risk is so high that it needs to be continued e.g. metallic heart valves. They are not teratogenic after 12 weeks and may be used between 12 – 36 weeks if absolutely necessary, but as they cross the placenta they cause anti-coagulation in the fetus – there is no relationship between maternal INR measurements and fetal ones and as such there is a risk of fetal intracranial haemorrhage, especially if taken close to delivery.
  - They are teratogenic between 6-12 weeks gestation – risk appears to be around 5% if exposed
  - They are causally associated with multiple cranio-facial and skeletal abnormalities (Conradi-Hunnerman syndrome)

Antimetabolites

- Most anti-neoplastics have been shown to be teratogenic at some stage

- However information is based on mainly animal studies (relatively small numbers of humans), most fetuses have multi-agent exposure and the longer term effects are not yet known
- They are contraindicated in the first trimester and breastfeeding
- They should be avoided within 2–3 weeks of delivery to allow marrow suppression to recover in the mother
- Most agents have actually been safely used in the second and third trimester[4]

Drugs in relation to lactation

- Most drugs enter breast milk – therefore all the principles of prescribing in pregnancy are equally applicable to lactation
- Drugs in breast milk may:
  - Be harmful e.g. lithium
  - Have no effect e.g. digoxin
  - Potentially cause hypersensitivity in the neonate e.g. penicillin
  - Suppress lactation e.g. bromocriptine and cabergoline
  - Reduce suckling due to neonatal sedation e.g. phenobarbitone
- The likelihood of a problem in the neonate is determined by a number of factors:
  - The concentration of drug in the milk
  - The transfer of drugs depends on molecule size and lipid solubility – the smaller and more lipid soluble they are the more likely they are to cross into breast milk
  - The volume of milk taken (hind-milk has a higher fat concentration than fore-milk so longer, deeper suckling will contain more drug if it is lipid soluble)
  - The Pk of the drug in the infant – the ability of the infant to absorb and then clear any given drug will determine its serum concentration
  - The inherent toxicity of the drug – some drugs matter and some do not!
- If a drug is deemed necessary post-natally and known to be harmful to the neonate then invariably the best advice is to bottle feed

- Below are drugs which are contra-indicated in breast feeding mothers:
  - Cytotoxics
  - Mood stabilisers - lithium
  - Sedatives - Benzodiazepines, barbiturates
  - Amiodarone
  - Antibiotics – tetracyclines, metronidazole, chloramphenicol
  - COCP (reduced milk)
  - Theophylline (irritability)
  - Aspirin (Reyes syndrome)

Further sources of information available:

Appendix 5 of the BNF in pre-version 70. In versions 70 onwards the risks are with each drug.

Fetal pharmaco-therapy

Drugs that cross the placenta are deliberately administered via the mother to treat fetal conditions. They have the potential for maternal harm due to side effects and can present a clinical and ethical dilemma. Examples in use are:

- Betamethasone - proven to reduce RDS and IVH between 26–32 weeks
- Corticosteroids to prevent masculinisation of female fetuses in CAH
- Flecainide for fetal tachycardia
- Amiodarone for resistant fetal tachycardia
- Salbutamol for hydrops fetalis due to congenital heart block
- Penicillin for the treatment of congenital syphilis

REFERENCES:

1. CHAN M, WONG ICK, SUTCLIFFE AG. Prescription drug use in pregnancy: more evidence of safety is needed. *The Obstetrician & Gynaecologist* 2012;14:87–92.

2. TOMSON T, HIILESMAA V. Epilepsy in pregnancy. *BMJ* 2007;335:769–773.

3. ADAB N, KINI U, VINTEN J, AYRES J, BAKER G, CLAYTON-SMITH J, COYLE H *et al*. The longer term outcome of children born to mothers with epilepsy. *J Neurol Neurosurg Psychiatry* 2004;75:1575–1583.

4. CARDONICK E, IACOBUCCI A. Use of chemotherapy during human pregnancy. Lancet Oncol. 2004 May;5(5):283–91.

CHAPTER 27

Non-Hormonal Therapy in obstetrics and gynaecology

Kevin Hayes

Many conditions in pregnancy require prescribed medication and increasing numbers of women are on regular drugs for pre-existing medical conditions. This chapter reviews the common drugs used in obstetric patients and looks at their mechanisms of action, side effects and evidence of efficacy.

Drugs in common use in pregnancy

ANTI-HYPERTENSIVES

Hypertension and pre-eclampsia (PET) affect approximately 10% and 3% of all pregnancies respectively and are amongst the commonest medical problems in pregnancy. Whilst the benefits of treatment are clear for a minority with severe hypertension, much controversy exists over the benefit of treatment in mild and moderate hypertension. The purpose of treatment is to reduce the risk of acute intra-cerebral events in the mother.

The only clear indications for treatment are:

Persistent BP >/= 160/100
Acute severe hypertension
Fulminating PET
Eclampsia

Treatment from 140/90 – 160/110 is debatable but most obstetricians pragmatically medicate from 150/100 upwards.

- β blocker labetolol is considered safe and has been used extensively in human pregnancy – it is generally considered as first line treatment

  ○ It has non-specific α + β blockade
  ○ It may be also be used for acute hypertension as a first line IV infusion

Side effects:

  ○ It may cause IUGR (even after controlling for BP) with prolonged use
  ○ Neonatal hypoglycaemia + bradycardia have rarely been reported

The safety of other β-blockers, atenolol in particular, in the early and late stages of pregnancy is unresolved; their use is therefore generally contraindicated according to several guidelines [1].

- Methyldopa is considered safe and has been used extensively in human pregnancy - it is now generally considered as second line treatment as an add on to labetolol but may be used first line instead

  ○ It is centrally acting and is metabolised to α-methylnoradrenaline (it's active component)
  ○ It works as a post-synaptic α2 agonist reducing central sympathetic outflow

Side effects include:

  ○ Rebound hypertension
  ○ Depressed mood (with long term use)
  ○ Flattened CTG variability
  ○ Autoimmune haemolytic anaemia (rare)
  ○ Raised prolactin (outside of pregnancy)
  ○ Hepatitis

■ Nifedipine – nifedipine is not licensed in pregnancy but is a commonly used second line treatment – a modified release (MR) preparation is recommended due to the potential acute hypotensive effect it can have [2].
   ○ It is a member of the dihydropyridine group and blocks inward flux of calcium through voltage gated calcium channels
   ○ It has a preferential effect on vessels as a vasodilator rather than the myocardium
   ○ It can also be used for acute hypertension
   ○ It has no anti-arrhythmic activity
   ○ It also has a known effect on the myometrium – it may inhibit premature labour (unlicensed use) and has been used as a tocolytic agent

Side effects include:

○ Acute hypotension if given sub-lingually
○ Peripheral oedema
○ Headache + flushing

■ Hydralazine IV is used for acute hypertension
   ○ It needs to be given slowly over a minimum of 5 minutes IV
   ○ It can be repeated IV every 15 minutes if needed
   ○ It is a potent vasodilator with a poorly understood mechanism of action
   ○ It is metabolised by acetylation in the liver (fast and slow acetylators are genetically determined)

Side effects include:

○ Acute hypotension if given too fast or too often
○ There is a recognised idiosyncratic adverse event (AE) of a lupus like syndrome rarely in slow acetylators

■ MgSO4 is proven to be the best prevention and best treatment of fits in severe PET / Eclampsia. The landmark MAGPIE trial showed that it halved the risk of eclampsia and probably reduced the risk of maternal death. There did not appear to be any substantive harmful effects to mother or baby in the short term [3]. It's mechanism of action:
   ○ It acts as a membrane stabiliser
   ○ It has a rapid onset of action – maintained for 24 hours post delivery / fit
   ○ It does require Mg level monitoring only usually if the patient is oliguric

Side effects in toxicity:

○ Hyporeflexia presents in advance of more serious effects
○ Respiratory depression
○ Cardio-respiratory arrest

Drugs to avoid for hypertension

■ ACE-Inhibitors are contra-indicated in pregnancy. They are associated with:
   ○ Congenital malformations – especially CVS
   ○ Skull defects
   ○ Oligohydramnios + impaired fetal renal function
■ Thiazides diuretics - diuretic-associated harmful effects on maternal and fetal outcomes are controversial: their use is discouraged in pregnancy[1].
   ○ neonatal thrombocytopaenia has been reported with bendromethafluazide

Tocolytic agents

Tocolytic agents are used to abolish unwanted uterine activity most commonly for preterm labour (PTL) but also for acute hyperstimualtion and external cephalic version.

Preterm labour (PTL)

There is little evidence of benefit to overall outcome for the fetus with blanket tocolysis for PTL and not using it is reasonable. Currently the two clinical uses are:

■ To achieve 24 hour steroid latency < 34 weeks
■ Where in-utero transfer is necessary for neonatal care

The following drugs have been and are used. The recent NICE guidelines [4] recommend nifedipine as first line if used reserving Atosiban if there is a contra-indication to nifedipine:

■ Nifedipine (unlicensed use) – it is at least comparable with the below agents and appears to have a better side effect profile
■ Atosiban (oxytocin antagonist) – has less side effects than most other tocolytics but the Cochrane review suggests no overall benefit.
■ Side effects: nausea, tachycardia, hypotension. Appears to cause no fetal/neonatal harm

- Beta-sympathomimetics (salbutamol, ritodrine, terbutaline). These are historically the most used tocolytic agents, however their use is limited by significant side effects: tachycardia, hypotension, pulmonary oedema, hypokalaemia, hyperglycaemia. Current NICE guidelines advise avoiding using them
- Mg SO$_4$ – more commonly used in USA. This now recommended for neuroprotection from 24–30 weeks gestation and possibly 30–34 weeks.
- GTN patches – no evidence of benefit over ritodrine, but side effects are relatively reduced.
- Side effects: headache, rarely hypotension
- NSAIDS have been used historically but are currently not recommended

External cephalic version

Terbutaline s/c prior to ECV has some evidence of increased procedural success in primigravidae and should only be used for this group. It is a one off dose so the only common side effect is usually a transient maternal tachycardia and tremor.

Emergency tocolysis

Terbutaline IV has been shown to improve fetal heart rate patterns and fetal pH in the presence of hyperstimulation (usually with oxytocin) and possibly even without hyperstimulation. Side effects are as above for Beta-sympathomimetics.

Analgesia

Analgesics are arguably the most commonly prescribed drugs in pregnancy and gynaecological care.

PARACETAMOL

Paracetamol has both analgesic and anti-pyretic effects. It is considered safe in pregnancy for mild pain relief and simple analgesia and is thus the first line analgesic recommended. It has very few side effects in recommended doses but in excess can cause irreparable liver damage (usually seen with deliberate overdose).

NON-STEROIDAL ANTI-INFLAMMATORY DRUGS (NSAIDS)

Aspirin has been studied extensively in low doses (75mg), principally as a method of preventing pre-eclampsia and IUGR. It should not be used liberally in low risk women. Currently advice is that women at high risk of pre-eclampsia take 75 mg of aspirin daily from 12 weeks until 36 weeks gestation. Women at high risk are those with any of the following [2]:

- hypertensive disease during a previous pregnancy
- chronic kidney disease
- autoimmune disease such as SLE or antiphospholipid syndrome
- type 1 or type 2 diabetes
- chronic hypertension.

Aspirin in low doses appears to have few adverse effects though it is recommend that it is stopped within 2–3 weeks of delivery due to the theoretical risks of neonatal haemorrhage at delivery due to its anti-platelet effect.

Other NSAIDs have been used for the prevention and treatment of pre-term labour, as above, as well as their analgesic properties. They are controversial but current evidence suggest that they are associated with:

- A possible increase in miscarriage [5]
- Fetal renal impairment and oligohydramnios
- Increased risks of premature closure of the ductus arteriosus – the evidence for this is actually poor
- Potential small increased risk in necrotising enterocolitis (NEC)
- They can also cause maternal upper GI symptoms and renal impairment over prolonged periods

As an analgesic they are essentially contra-indicated and alternative drugs should be used in pregnant patients.

OPIOIDS

Codeine phosphate and Dihydrocodeine are commonly used for moderate pain relief and belong to the opioid family. They work by activating μ opioid receptors reducing cerebral appreciation of pain. They are also often given with paracetamol in the combined proprietary compounds Co-codamol® and Co-dydramol®.

Dextropropophene is a more potent oral opioid reserved for more severe pain – it is used more sparingly therefore.

They are considered safe in pregnancy in recommended doses and there is a large experience of human pregnancy exposure.

Side effects include:

- Sedation
- Nausea and vomiting
- Constipation
- In large quantities (invariably as drugs of abuse) they may cause a neonatal withdrawal syndrome

Drugs used as pain relief in labour

- ENTONOX – 50/50 nitrous oxide / O_2 mix. This is safe, stable and has a very rapid onset and offset. It is widely used and highly effective for many.
- Side effects: nausea, "feeling drunk"
- Pethidine IM is widely used despite little evidence of effective pain relief. It has a rapid onset and short half life.
- Side effects: nausea and vomiting, narcosis, respiratory depression in the neonate if within 2 hours of delivery.
- Morphine though less widely used appears to be more effective and as safe. Both pethidine and morphine are μ–opioid receptor agonists.
- Combinations of bupivicaine (local anaesthetic) and fentanyl (opiate) in epidural administration provide highly effective pain relief.
- Side effects: hypotension, loss of mobility, higher chance of assisted delivery and rarely complications associated with insertion (dural tap, haematoma, high blockade).

Drugs used in the third stage of labour

Active management of the third stage has been shown to reduce the rate of PPH by around 50%. Most women receive drugs for their third stage as recommended routine practice. Drugs commonly used are:

- Syntometrine® (Ergometrine 500mcg / Sytocinon 5IU) IM. Ergometrine causes prolonged vasoconstriction.

- Side effects include: nausea and vomiting, hypertension.
- It is contraindicated in hypertensive pregnancies.
- Syntocinon is synthetic oxytocin and causes short term uterine contraction.
- Syntocinon (infusion of 40IU in saline) and ergometrine can also be used singly for the treatment of PPH
- Misoprostol 800mcg (PGE_1 analogue) taken orally / vaginally / rectally is highly effective in treating and preventing PPH. Stable and cheap and does not need refrigeration. Side effects: commonly diarrhoea and nausea/vomiting
- Carboprost® ($PGF_{2\alpha}$ analogue) is effective IM or intra-myometrial as second line treatment of PPH. Caution required in hypertension and to be avoided in asthmatics

Anti-emetics

Nausea and vomiting, particularly in the first trimester are common. Hyperemesis gravidarum affects up to 1–2% of pregnancies throughout the first trimester and can be highly debilitating necessitating hospital admission, often on multiple occasions. As well as hydration, anti-emetics are used liberally to try and reduce nausea and vomiting. The evidence for their efficacy is relatively weak.

Common agents used: Promethazine (from the Phenothiazine family) is the current first line recommended drug as a long established anti-emetic with extensive experience in human pregnancy. It works principally by its antagonist action on H1 (Histamine) receptors but does have a weaker anti-muscarinic effect. Side effects include: sedation and more rarely extra-pyrimidal neurological effects such as tardive dyskinesia.

Second line agents: Metoclopromide is another drug where there appears to be no recognized fetal harm. It is a dopamine (D2) antagonist and a 5-HT3 antagonist and has its anti-emetic effect centrally as well as increasing gastric emptying. Side effects include akathisia (restlessness) and tardive dyskinesia.

Prochlorperazine (also from the Phenothiazine family) is another potent D2 antagonist used extensively in pregnancy without demonstrable harm. Side effects are as per promethazine.

Third line agents: Ondansetron and related compounds are potent 5-HT3 antagonists. They are not licensed in pregnancy and are only used once the above first and second line agents have failed. They appear to be safe in pregnancy. Side effects include headache, diarrhoea and sedation.

Fourth line; Corticosteroids (either methylprednisolone or hydrocortisone) are used in resistant cases once everything else has been tried. They have some evidence of efficacy, though large trials are not available [6]. They have not been shown to be teratogenic though most women are post-embryonic at commencement and treatment duration is usually kept to short duration.

Anti-acids

Reflux and "heartburn" are very common due to the reduced lower oesphageal sphincter tone induced by progesterone. Most pregnant women will get this to some degree. These agents are basic and work by neutralizing gastric acid. They do not affect its production. The commonest used in the UK is Gaviscon® which contains sodium alginate, calcium carbonate and sodium bicarbonate. Maalox® is an aluminium and magnesium hydroxide containing alternative. They appear safe in pregnancy and are used extensively.

Drugs used commonly in gynaecological practice

DRUGS FOR MENORRHAGIA

Mefanamic acid is a NSAID widely used for the treatment of dysmenorrhea and menorrhagia. As a prostaglandin production inhibitor they are highly effective for menstrual pain taken at the time of menstruation. They have been shown to reduce average menstrual blood loss by up to 30% in dysfunctional uterine bleeding and are therefore highly effective for managing menorrhagia. Side effects are as for other NSAIDs used for analgesia

Tranexamic acid is an anti-fibrinolytic drug which works by blocking the conversion of plasminogen to plasmin and reducing fibrinolysis. It has been shown to be a highly effective treatment for menorrhagia reducing mean blood loss by 40–50%. Side effect include mild GI upset and caution is needed in women with pre-existing heart disease.

Urogynaecological agents

Urge incontinence is commonly treated by drugs with anti-muscarinic properties

Tolterodine and Oxybutynin are both muscarinic antagonists (particularly the M3 receptor; there are 5 sub-types of muscarinic receptor M1 – M5; oxybutynin is somewhat less selective). Both are effective in reducing symptoms of detrusor over-activity. Improvements in incontinence and irritative symptoms such as urgency and frequency are seen in up to 60–70%. The side effects are predictable with their anti-muscarinic action: dry mouth, dry eyes, constipation and dizziness. These unwanted effects can limit their use but usually habituate over time. The use of modified release products also seems to reduce side effects.

- Imipramine is often used second line but may be effective due to its anti-muscarinic effect
- Trospium chloride, propiverine and desmopressin are also effective for some women

Stress Urinary Incontinence

Duloxetine is a balanced serotonin and noradrenaline reuptake inhibitor (SNRI). It increases urinary sphincter tone and has been shown to reduce (but not cure) stress incontinence by about 50%, with improvements in quality of life. Side effects of nausea, dizziness, insomnia occur in 10–20% of patients.

Chemotherapeutic drugs in gynaecological oncology

Chemotherapeutic agents (usually given as an out-patient) interfere with cell division by acting on a specific phase of the cell cycle (e.g. taxanes are active against cells in the G2/M phases) or non-specifically (e.g. alkylating agents which exert their effects throughout the cell cycle). As chemotherapy has a propensity for actively proliferating cells, cancer cells are more vulnerable than normal cells. However they do act on normal cells so side effects are not unusual. Chemotherapy has a narrow therapeutic index and close monitoring whilst on treatment is essential under oncological guidance.

Some classes of cytotoxic agents:

- **Antimetabolites** - interfere with DNA and RNA synthesis e.g. 5-FU, methotrexate (folate antagonist)
- **Alkylating agents** - form covalent bonds with DNA bases e.g. cyclophosphamide, isofosfamide
- **Intercalating agents** - bind to DNA, thus inhibiting its replication e.g. cisplatin, carboplatin
- **Anti-tumour antibiotics** - complex mechanisms leading to inhibition of DNA synthesis e.g. bleomycin, doxorubicin, etoposide
- **Drugs directed against spindle microtubules inhibiting mitosis** e.g. paclitaxel, vincristine

Common regimens:

- **Ovarian cancer** – they are usually sensitive to platinum-based regimens. Response rates around 70% are seen in clinical practice. Carboplatin +/- paclitaxel may be used neoadjuvantly, adjuvantly or palliatively. More than 50% of patients will relapse and require further treatment usually due to advanced stage of disease at diagnosis. If more than six months have elapsed since initial chemotherapy, the tumour is more likely to be sensitive to carboplatin and is often given again.
- **Endometrial cancer** - chemotherapy has a more limited role and is usually reserved for recurrent or metastatic disease: carboplatin +/- paclitaxel or doxorubicin and cisplatin are the most commonly used combinations.
- **Cervical cancer** - cisplatin combined with radiotherapy has been shown to reduce the risk of relapse for those undergoing radiotherapy after surgery. Cisplatin and methotrexate may be used for metastatic disease though the reported response rate is low.
- **Vulval cancer** - 5-FluUracil (5-FU) +/- cisplatin is used in combination with radiotherapy for patients unfit for surgery or as sole therapy for symptom control in metastatic disease.
- **Trophoblastic disease** - chemotherapy alone is highly curative. Methotrexate for simple trophoblastic disease. EMA-CO (Etoposide, Methotrexate, Dactimomycin, Cyclophosphamide, Vincristine) for high risk trophoblastic disease. Both have cure rates of around 99%.

Side effects of chemotherapy

- **Haematological** - bone marrow suppression which eventually recovers; cellular nadir is around 7-14 days resulting in neutropenia, anaemia and thrombocytopenia.
- **Gastrointestinal** - side effects are due to loss of epithelial cells:
  o Nausea and vomiting are very common with most agents and are actively prevented with anti-emetics.
  o Mucositis: (esp. methotrexate) resulting in ulcers in mucous membranes especially oral – these usually resolve spontaneously.
  o Diarrhoea is less common and usually transient.
- **Alopecia** - Taxanes (e.g. paclitaxel), doxorubicin and etoposide commonly cause temporary hair loss. This is seen less commonly with carboplatin and cisplatin.
- **Neurological** – usually dose-related and improve on dose reduction or stopping:
  o Peripheral neuropathy is commonly seen with paclitaxel and cisplatin
  o Tinnitus is associated with cisplatin
- **Constitutional** - tend to have cumulative effects but resolve on cessation.
  o Lethargy
  o Anorexia

REFERENCES:

1. Al Khaja KA, Sequeira RP, Alkhaja AK *et al.* Drug treatment of hypertension in pregnancy: a critical review of adult guideline recommendations. *J Hypertens.* 2014;**32**(3):454–63.

2. Hypertension in pregnancy. NICE guideline 2015.

3. Altman D, Carroli G, Duley L *et al.* Do women with pre-eclampsia, and their babies, benefit from magnesium sulphate? The Magpie Trial: a randomised placebo-controlled trial. *Lancet.* 2002 Jun 1;**359**(9321):1877–90.

4. Pre-term labour and birth. NICE guideline 2015.

5. Nakhai-Pour H, Broy P, Sheehy O *et al.* Use of non-aspirin nonsteroidal anti-inflammatory drugs during pregnancy and the risk of spontaneous abortion. *CMAJ* 2011: doi: 10.1503/cmaj.110454.

6. Wegrzyniak L, Repke J, Ural S. Treatment of hyperemesis gravidarum. Rev Obstet Gynecol. 2012; **5**(2): 78–84.

CHAPTER 28

Hormonal treatment in nonmalignant gynaecological conditions

Michael Marsh

Pharmacology of hormones used in gynaecological treatment

ESTROGENS AND PROGESTOGENS

Natural or synthetic estrogens are compounds that bind to estrogen receptors and exert biological effects characteristic of endogenous estradiol. Progestogens are synthetic versions of progesterone and bind to progesterone receptors, resulting in effects similar to endogenous progesterone.

Female sex hormones have a long history of therapeutic applications. In combination, estrogens and progestogens are used for contraception, menstrual regulation, treatment of endometriosis and postmenopausal hormone replacement therapy (HRT).

Exogenous estrogen used alone, unopposed by progestogen therapy, is of limited use because of its proliferative effects on the uterine endometrium, leading to irregular menstrual bleeding when used in premenopausal women and to endometrial hyperplasia when used alone as HRT.[1] Thus, estrogen-only therapy in gynaecology is restricted to HRT use in women who have undergone hysterectomy. In contrast, progestogens used alone have widespread applications and are used in contraception, menstrual regulation in women suffering from dysfunctional uterine bleeding and menorrhagia and treatment of endometriosis and endometrial hyperplasia. Exogenous progesterone is used in assisted reproduction to provide support for embryo implantation in the luteal phase.

ENDOGENOUS ESTROGENS

In the reproductive years, the most potent endogenous estrogen is 17-beta-estradiol (E_2), followed by estrone (E_1). In young women, both are secreted by the ovaries, with a production rate of E_2 ranging from 100–600 micrograms/ day, varying during the menstrual cycle. Small amounts of E_1 derive from aromatisation of androstenedione from the adrenal glands and ovaries. Estriol (E_3) is the least potent physiological estrogen and is not a secretory product of the ovary. It is formed by irreversible metabolism of E_1.

After the menopause, E_1 is the predominant estrogen as ovarian secretion of all estrogens ceases. The residual production of E_2 and E_1 after the menopause originates from the peripheral aromatisation of circulating androstenedione and E_2 and E_1 are found in the range of 15 and 45 micrograms/day, respectively. As this aromatisation process occurs in adipose tissue, women who are obese may produce twice as much E_2 and E_1 as women who are not obese.

The estrogen receptor

Estrogens, through binding to their specific receptor in the target cell, promote development of secondary sexual characteristics in women and stimulate endometrial proliferation, thickening of the vaginal mucosa and maintenance of urogenital tissues. Estrogen receptors are present in many organ systems and demonstrate actions that are not directly related to reproduction, such as maintenance of bone strength, initiation and termination of the pubertal growth spurt and pigmentation of the nipples and genitals.

The estrogen receptor belongs to the steroid receptor superfamily, which comprises the glucocorticoids, vitamin D, thyroid hormone, androgen and retinoid receptors. Estrogen acts through two receptors, alpha and beta. The alpha estrogen receptor is found in endometrium, bone, breast cancer cells, ovarian stroma cells and in the hypothalamus. The expression of the beta estrogen receptor protein has been documented in kidney, brain, bone, heart, lungs, intestinal mucosa, prostate and endothelial cells. The presence of the receptor in a tissue does not predict its role in mediating estrogenic effects. For example, alpha receptors appear to be the chief mediator of estrogen's actions on the skeleton. Osteoblasts express beta receptor but the actions of beta receptor agonists on bone are less clear. Some reports suggest that the effects of estrogen signalling through alpha and beta receptors are in opposition, while other studies suggest that activation of these receptors have similar effects on bone.

Different ligands may differ in their affinity for alpha and beta isoforms of the estrogen receptor. E_2 appears to bind equally well to both receptors, whereas E_1 and raloxifene bind preferentially to the alpha receptor and E_3 and genistein bind preferentially to the beta receptor.

Estrogen metabolism

Circulating estrogens are metabolised primarily in the liver by conjugation and hydroxylation. Conjugation is catalysed by glucuronyl transferases and by sulphotransferases, whereas hydroxylation is catalysed by the enzymes of the cytochrome P450 complex. The residence time of E_2 is prolonged by conversion to E_1 and by enterohepatic recirculation of estrogen conjugates excreted in the bile. E_2 is rapidly cleared from the circulation with a mean half-life of 1.7 hours. The half-life for E_1 and E_1 sulphate is about four times longer.

Effects of estrogen

The physiological effects of estrogens are influenced by sex hormone-binding globulin (SHBG) and albumin production. E_2 bound to SHBG is not biologically active. Thyroxine and E_2 itself promote SHBG production, while androgens, insulin, corticoids, progestogens and growth hormone suppress hepatic SHBG production.

Pharmacological estrogens

Orally administered natural estrogens are inactivated in the gut and the residual small amount that is absorbed undergoes considerable metabolism in the liver before reaching the circulation. In 1938, it was realised that the addition of an ethinyl group to E_2 prevented inactivation and enabled efficient gut absorption. However, the first-pass hepatic effect was still present. Currently, most oral contraceptives contain ethinyl estradiol as the estrogenic component.

Natural estrogen preparations are derived from plant or animal sources and are widely used in HRT. They do not have potent enough effects on the E_2 receptor to control the endometrium and menstrual cycle in premenopausal women and are therefore not used in the contraceptive pill. Conjugated equine estrogens contain the sodium salts of the sulphate ester forms of various naturally occurring estrogens derived from the urine of pregnant mares. Micronised estradiol is manufactured by the formation of extremely small particles of drug with a relatively high surface area to improve gastric absorption. E_2 valerate, piperazine E_1 sulphate and E_2 cypionate are conjugated forms that have been modified for better absorption in the gastrointestinal system and are also used in HRT.

Selective estrogen receptor modulators

Selective estrogen receptor modulators are compounds that interact with estrogen receptors. Selective estrogen receptor modulators were originally thought to be anti-estrogens. However, it is now clear that they contain an admixture of agonist and antagonist activities.

The first selective estrogen receptor modulator, clomiphene citrate, a triphenylethylene, was synthesised in 1956 and is used widely in the treatment of polycystic disease and for ovulation induction. It acts centrally to block the negative feedback of estrogen and to induce a follicle-stimulating hormone surge of anterior pituitary gonadotrophs through positive feedback. In 1984, it was observed that clomiphene citrate attenuated bone loss in the oophorectomised rat, suggesting that it had estrogenic agonist activities on the bone. Clomiphene is a combination of two geometric isomers. The *trans* isomer, enclomiphene, is a partial estrogen whereas the *cis* isomer, zuclomiphene, is a pure estrogen.

Another triphenylethylene, tamoxifen, was subsequently shown to prevent bone loss in the oophorectomised rat. Tamoxifen acts as an estrogen antagonist in the breast but as an agonist in the skeleton and the cardiovascular system. Tamoxifen was not further developed as a bone-sparing agent as it causes endometrial stimulation and endometrial hyperplasia and adenocarcinoma in some women. Tamoxifen is widely used in the management of estrogen receptor positive breast cancer.

Raloxifene is a nonsteroidal benzothiophene that inhibits bone mineral density loss but does not stimulate the endometrium and is an estrogen antagonist for breast tissue. Raloxifene is not a steroid and hence not technically an estrogen but it possesses a phenolic ring – similar to the A ring of estradiol – necessary to obtain lodgement in the ligand-binding cavity of the estrogen receptor. There is no evidence that raloxifene decreases the incidence of nonvertebral fractures, so although raloxifene can be used for the prevention of vertebral fractures in women with osteopenia/osteoporosis, its use is probably not appropriate for women who are at high risk of nonvertebral fractures.

ENDOGENOUS PROGESTERONE

Outside of pregnancy, progesterone is chiefly produced by the corpus luteum, with very small amounts produced by the adrenal cortex and the glial cells of the central nervous system. The production rate of progesterone in the preovulatory phase is less than 1 mg/day, which increases to 20–30 mg/day during the luteal phase. Progesterone is responsible for induction of secretory activity and decidual development in the endometrium in the estrogen-primed uterus. If pregnancy does not occur, withdrawal of progesterone results in menstrual sloughing of the endometrium. Progesterone is needed

for the implantation of the fertilised ovum and maintenance of pregnancy. It increases viscosity of cervical mucus, promotes glandular development of the breast and increases basal body temperature. During pregnancy, the placenta eventually becomes the major source of progesterone and this placental progesterone is believed to inhibit uterine contractions, allowing for the maintenance of the gestation until the start of labour.

Effects of progestogens

Progestogens and progesterone, have a well-established anti-estrogenic effect on the endometrium. In an estrogen-primed endometrium, progestogens downregulate nuclear E_2 receptors by inhibiting receptor synthesis and accelerating their turnover, and downregulate the genes required for epithelial growth, leading to reduced epidermal growth factor production. Progestogens promote differentiation of glands and stroma, decidualisation and secretory activity of the endometrium, increase blood vessel volume and stimulate secretion of insulin-like growth factor binding protein-1. Progestogens also stimulate 17-hydroxysteroid dehydrogenase production, which converts E_2 to the weaker estrogen, E_1 sulphate, and induce endometrial sloughing and uterine bleeding.

Progesterone and progestogen metabolism

Progesterone and progestogens are metabolised primarily by the liver, largely to pregnanetriols and pregnanediols, which are then conjugated in the liver to glucoronides and sulphates. These metabolites are excreted in the bile and may be deconjugated and further metabolised in the gut. There is no significant enterohepatic circulation of progesterone.

Pharmacological properties of progesterone and progestogens

When first produced pharmaceutically, progesterone was ineffective when given orally, as it is metabolised extensively in the gastrointestinal tract by microorganisms and digestive enzymes. Although micronised progesterone results in more efficient absorption from the gastrointestinal tract, large doses need to be given often to obtain therapeutic serum levels. However, natural progesterone is also available in transvaginal or transrectal suppositories and absorption is sufficient for it to be used as the progestogenic component of HRT regimens.

Progestogens are synthetic preparations with progesterone action that were developed to be orally effective. These are divided into the 21-carbon steroids derived from 17-alpha-hydroxyprogesterone and the 19-carbon steroids derived from nortestosterone.

The 21-carbon steroids (for example, medroxyprogesterone acetate and dydrogesterone) simulate the profile of progesterone more closely, especially in their effects on the hypothalamic–pituitary system and on carbohydrate and lipid metabolism. Medroxyprogesterone acetate is probably the most widely used compound in this group. It is used in depot preparations for contraception and in oral form for postmenopausal hormone replacement and treatment of endometriosis and menorrhagia.

Progestogens derived from 19-nortestosterone are subdivided into compounds related to norethisterone (estranes) or to levonorgestrel (gonanes). Norethisterone is widely used in oral contraceptives and has androgenic properties and potent progestational activity. Many related progestogens have since been developed, including norethisterone acetate and etynodiol diacetate. However, all are converted *in vivo* to norethisterone before they are active. The gonanes are all derived from norgestrol, made from the addition of a methyl group to norethisterone. Norgestimate is a prodrug, which is metabolised in two steps to the active levonorgestrel. Gestodene and desogestrel are closely related gonanes developed for use in the contraceptive pill and in HRT. An active intermediate metabolite of this conversion, levonorgestrel oxime, is a component of the weekly contraceptive patch. Drospirenone, a new progestogen for oral contraception, is chemically related to spironolactone and demonstrates potent progestational activity, together with antimineral corticoid and antiandrogenic properties.

Routes of administration of progestogens

A progestogen-containing intrauterine device (the intrauterine system containing levonorgestrel), subcutaneous pellets, transdermal cream, transdermal patch, vaginal suppositories and intramuscular injection of progesterone are all delivery systems in use, although oral administration remains the most common mode of delivery. For HRT, progestogens are added in either a cyclic or continuous fashion to prevent endometrial hyperplasia and endometrial cancer. This is usually accomplished using the oral route, the transdermal patch or the progestogen-containing intrauterine system.

Adverse effects of progestogens

Common symptoms of progestogens include weight gain, acne, fluid retention, headaches and breast tenderness. Sedation and mood changes reflect progestogenic effects on the central nervous system and may be related to progestogen binding to a membrane receptor of gamma aminobutyric acid in the central nervous system, which is the same receptor site for benzodiazepines and barbiturates.

Many progestogens (particularly 19-carbon compounds) when used alone cause androgenic effects such as acne and hirsutism owing to their similarity to testosterone. However, when combined with ethinyl estradiol in oral contraceptives, the suppression of ovarian androgens and the beneficial effect on SHBG induces an overall antiandrogenic effect in most women. Drospirenone, given its similarity to spironolactone, may be associated with less bloating and weight gain.

Danazol

Danazol, an isoxazole derivative of ethinyl testosterone, is an orally active, pituitary-gonadotrophin inhibitory agent with androgenic effects but minimal estrogenic and progestational activity. It has the inhibitory effect on the synthesis and/or release of pituitary–gonadotrophic hormones by an effect on the pituitary. Androgen-like effects limit use and include weight gain, acne and seborrhoea. Mild hirsutism, oedema, hair loss and voice change, which may take the form of hoarseness, sore throat or instability or deepening of pitch, may occur and have been reported to persist after cessation of therapy. Clitoral hypertrophy is rare. Flushing, sweating, vaginal dryness and irritation and reduction in breast size occasionally occur and reflect gonadotrophin suppression.

GONADOTROPHIN-RELEASING HORMONE ANALOGUES

Hypothalamic gonadotrophin-releasing hormone (GnRH) is a decapeptide that is synthesised and released in a pulsatile manner from hypothalamic neurosecretory cells. It stimulates pituitary synthesis and secretion of gonadotrophins and therefore causes increased secretion of gonadal hormones. Synthetic GnRH antagonists inhibit the endogenous hormone from binding to its receptor, inducing a pharmacological hypophysectomy. Nonpulsatile administration of GnRH agonist results in downregulation of GnRH receptors. The exact mechanism of suppression is unclear. Such agonists are used widely for the treatment of endometriosis and other gynaecological conditions when estrogen suppression is required (for example, for the shrinking of fibroids prior to surgery). Use of GnRH agonists is accompanied by an initial gonadotrophin and gonadal hormone surge known as the 'flare' and women will experience a temporary worsening of symptoms in the first 2 weeks of treatment.

GnRH agonists may be given by 3-monthly injection, monthly injection, daily injection and nasal spray. Common adverse effects when GnRH anologues are used without estrogen add-back therapy are the symptoms associated with the menopause, such as hot flushes, night sweats, insomnia, decreased libido, headaches, mood swings, vaginal dryness, change in breast size, acne, muscle pains and poor mood. These symptoms usually disappear soon after treatment ceases.

As in the menopause, bone density falls when GnRH analogues are used without estrogen add-back therapy. The decrease in bone density is about 4–6% during a 6-month course of treatment. Most of the bone lost during treatment regenerates within 6 months of completing treatment. Most lost bone will probably have been regained 18–24 months after completing treatment.

The management of specific gynaecological conditions with hormonal therapy

PROGESTOGENS USED ALONE FOR MENORRHAGIA

A variety of cyclical regimens of both 19-carbon and 21-carbon progestogens have been widely used for the treatment of menorrhagia. A Cochrane meta-analysis in 1998 concluded that progestogens administered from day 15 or 19 to day 26 of the cycle offer no advantage over other medical therapies such as danazol, tranexamic acid, nonsteroidal anti-inflammatory drugs and the intrauterine system in the treatment of menorrhagia in women with ovulatory cycles.[2] However, progestogen therapy for 21 days of the cycle results in a significant reduction in menstrual blood loss, although women found the treatment less acceptable than intrauterine levonorgestrel. The 21-day regimen of progestogen may have a role in the short-term treatment of menorrhagia. Progestogenic adverse effects may limit their use. In one randomised controlled trial within the Cochrane meta-analysis, 56% of women taking oral progestogens did not feel 'well' or 'very well' and only 22% elected to continue treatment with oral progestogens after the 3 months of the study.

THE COMBINED CONTRACEPTIVE PILL AND MENORRHAGIA

The combined contraceptive pill has been widely used for the treatment of menorrhagia for many years and anecdotally appears effective. Surprisingly, a Cochrane analysis in 1997 found only one satisfactory small study, which found no significant difference between groups treated with the combined contraceptive pill, mefenamic acid, low-dose danazol or naproxen.[3] They concluded that the evidence from the one study was not sufficient to adequately assess the effectiveness of the combined contraceptive pill.

THE INTRAUTERINE SYSTEM AND MENORRHAGIA

The levonorgestrel-releasing intrauterine system (LNG-IUS) appears to be more effective than 21-day cyclical norethisterone as a treatment for heavy menstrual bleeding.[4] Women with an LNG-IUS are more satisfied and willing to continue with treatment but experience more adverse effects, such as intermenstrual bleeding and breast tenderness. The LNG-IUS treatment costs less than hysterectomy but there is no evidence of a difference in quality of life measures between these groups.

DANAZOL AND MENORRHAGIA

Danazol appears to be an effective treatment for heavy menstrual bleeding compared to other medical treatments. However, the use of danazol is limited by its adverse effects, its acceptability to women and the need for long-term treatment. A meta-analysis in 2002 concluded that danazol was more effective than placebo, progestogens, nonsteroidal anti-inflammatory drugs (NSAIDs) and the combined contraceptive pill at reducing menstrual blood loss.[5] Treatment with danazol caused more adverse events than NSAIDs and progestogens. Danazol was also shown to significantly lower the duration of menses when compared with NSAIDs and a progestogen-releasing intrauterine device.

COMBINED CONTRACEPTIVE PILL AND DYSMENORRHOEA

A recent Cohrane review concluded that there is limited evidence for pain improvement with the use of the oral contraceptive pill (both low- and medium-dose estrogen) in women with dysmenorrhoea. There is no evidence of a difference between different oral contraceptive pill preparations.[6]

HORMONAL TREATMENT OF ENDOMETRIOSIS

Ovarian hormones are required for the establishment or continued presence of endometriosis and it is clear that estrogen is needed to support the growth of ectopic endometrial tissue. The disorder occurs only after the onset of puberty and normally disappears after menopause. Medical therapy for endometriosis aims to relieve pain and bleeding. It is very seldom offered to women wishing pregnancy because treatment may compromise fertility. Long-term or repeated courses of treatment are often required.

Oral estrogens and progestogens

The contraceptive pill is widely used for treating endometriosis-related pain, but the clinical trial evidence for its use is poor.[7] A recent Cochrane review concluded that the limited data available suggest that there is no evidence for a difference in outcomes between the oral

contraceptive pill studied and GnRH analogue. The oral contraceptive pill was as effective as a GnRH analogue in treating for endometriosis-associated pain.[7] Long cycle use (using the combined pill for 3 months in a row with a week break every 3 months) of the combined contraceptive is common for the relief of pain.

Progestogens have been used for the therapy of endometriosis worldwide for 50 years. Progestogenic adverse effects and irregular bleeding limit their use.

The mechanism of action and the morphological changes induced by progestogens remain unclear, although high-dosage regimens are likely to act by menstrual-cycle suppression. Progesterone receptors in endometriotic foci are present in a very low concentration or are even absent, and enzyme systems differ widely in eutopic and ectopic endometrial tissue. Progestogens reduce the synthesis of their own receptors, resulting in diminished sensitivity of the implants during long-term treatment.[8]

Levonorgestrel-releasing intrauterine system

The steady low-level release of levonorgestrel from the coil is likely to have a direct effect on endometriotic deposits through peritoneal fluid, possibly via a haematogenous spread. Three studies, two of which were controlled studies, have shown reduction in pain.

Danazol

Danazol has been shown to be effective in some studies of mild and moderate endometriosis in the short term. However, the rate of recurrence of endometriosis is high and danazol causes marked weight gain and androgenic adverse effects in up to 25% of women, so its use is now uncommon in the medical management of endometriosis. Although it is still licensed for treatment of endometriosis, there remains insufficient evidence to recommend usage over other treatment methods.

Gonadotrophin-releasing hormone analogues and add-back therapy

There is good evidence that inducing a medical menopause with nonpulsatile GnRH analogues to downregulate the pituitary will reduce endometriotic deposits and symptoms, but the induced bone loss and climacteric symptoms limit their use alone. Add-back therapy, with either estrogens and progestogens or tibolone, appears to prevent climacteric symptoms and reduce the degree of bone loss without apparent reduction in efficacy.[9]

HORMONE REPLACEMENT THERAPY

The chief role of HRT at present is for the prevention or treatment of climacteric symptoms around the time of the menopause. There is overwhelming evidence that HRT provides the most effective method of treating climacteric hot flushes, night sweats and vaginal dryness. When hormonal treatment of the menopause was first introduced, estrogen was used alone, but it became clear in the 1970s and 1980s that unopposed estrogen may stimulate endometrial growth and lead to endometrial hyperplasia and a high risk of developing endometrial carcinoma. As a result, progestogens were added to HRT regimes, initially cyclically and later continually in continuous combined regimens, in which progestogens are added to estrogens every day.

Endometrial cancer and unopposed estrogen use

The relationship between unopposed estrogen use in HRT and endometrial cancer has been clearly established since the 1970s by numerous experimental and epidemiological studies.[10–13] The estimated increase in relative risk for users compared with non-users from a 1995 meta-analysis was reported as 2.3 (95% CI 2.1–2.5), with a greater relative risk associated with prolonged duration of use (9.5 for 10 or more years).[14] Unopposed estrogen is associated with an increased risk of endometrial hyperplasia at all doses and durations of therapy between 1 and 3 years.[12]

Estrogen and progestogen use

Histological changes produced by progestogens are dose- and duration-dependent. In a 28-day estrogen regimen, progestogen supplementation for less than 10 days/month is associated with increased risk of endometrial abnormalities compared to non-users, while the use of a progestogen for 10–12 days or more day/month, depending on its potency and half-life, removes the excess risk. The currently recommended duration of progestogens to protect the endometrium is 12–14 days each month.

Long-cycle HRT regimens, in which progestogens are added to continuous estrogens every 2 or 3 months, have been shown to be associated with an increased risk of endometrial hyperplasia. Such regimens should be used with caution and the endometrium should be carefully monitored during treatment. It is not known whether long-cycle therapy elevates the risk of endometrial carcinoma after treatment is stopped, as occurs with unopposed estrogen.

It is probable that most commercially available sequential HRT preparations do not cause any clinically significant rise in the risk of endometrial carcinoma.[15] However, many studies are not placebo controlled and are of short duration. Longer-term studies of sequential HRT using endometrial cancer as the endpoint have produced conflicting results. Some do not demonstrate an increase in risk whereas others show an increase in risk after 5 years of use.[16] In contrast to the studies of sequential therapy, where current data suggest no effect on endometrial cancer risk, or a very slight increase, continuous combined HRT in which estrogens and progestogens are both given daily appears to reduce the risk.[17]

Estrogen therapy: routes of administration and dosage

Exogenous estrogens can be prescribed orally or parenterally. Currently available parenteral methods of delivery include transdermal patches, vaginal creams, pessaries or rings and subcutaneous implantation.

Estradiol transdermal patches contain E_2 either dissolved in alcohol within a thin, clear, circular multilayered patch with an outer impermeable membrane or within a solid matrix. The latter form of patch adheres best and is now most commonly used. Patches are available that must be changed twice or once a week. The most troublesome problem is skin reactions, which lead to discontinuation of this method in approximately 5% of women. A transdermal method of delivery for progestogen in a solid matrix patch is available.

Crystalline implants containing E_2 in a cholesterol base are inserted into the subcutaneous fat of the abdominal wall or buttock under local anaesthesia, a procedure that causes little discomfort and that takes approximately 5 minutes. Implants need to be repeated every 3–6 months. This form of administration of estrogens is no longer widely commercially available in the UK. There is significant tachyphylaxis in some women, leading to women requesting further implantation at ever-decreasing intervals. There is also concern about the long-lasting effects of E_2 implants on the endometrium after implant therapy has been withdrawn and about the effect of ceasing implant treatment on symptoms. The duration of endometrial stimulation after the last implantation can be prolonged up to 43 months. Therefore, cyclical progestogens should be given until withdrawal bleeding has not occurred for 3 consecutive months.

Long-term risks and benefits

Postmenopausal women who use exogenous estrogens are at an increased risk for venous thromboembolism, partly through a reduction in antithrombin III.[18] HRT has also been associated with an increased risk of gallbladder disease, stroke and breast cancer, particularly with long-term therapy.[19] The actual risk of these conditions for an individual is small.[17, 20]

HRT is a well-established method for the treatment and prevention of osteoporosis whose effects, beneficial or not, have been widely studied. However, HRT use for the treatment or prevention of osteoporosis has declined as a result of women's concern about breast cancer and following the publication of studies that failed to show an effect of HRT on cardiovascular disease risk.[17, 20]

The use of progestogens alone

Progestogens are effective in the treatment of hot flushes and an efficacy better than placebo has been noted using oral norethisterone, intramuscular or oral medroxyprogesterone acetate and oral megestrol acetate. There is no consistent evidence of an effect of progestogens on other symptoms of the menopause, nor of significant metabolism to estrogenic substances. Some data suggest that certain progestogens (for example, norethisterone 5–10 mg/day) may preserve bone density.

Tibolone

Tibolone is a synthetic steroid that has estrogenic, progestogenic and androgenic properties and is used orally as an alternative to estrogen/progestogen HRT. Structurally it is related to 19-nortestosterone. Tibolone is metabolised predominantly to three other steroid molecules; a delta-4-isomer, 3-alpha-hydroxymetabolite and 3-beta-hydroxymetabolite. In the endometrium, the delta-4-isomer predominates and, because it has a progestogenic effect, the endometrium atrophies. As there is no stimulation of the endometrium, there is no withdrawal bleeding. Tibolone is therefore a suitable alternative to continuous combined HRT and it has many comparable effects to HRT in the relief of menopausal symptoms and prevention of bone loss.[21]

Adverse effects reflect the androgenic and progestogenic activity of the molecule and include weight change, ankle swelling, dizziness, headache, vaginal bleeding, gastrointestinal symptoms, some increased facial hair, depression and joint pains.

REFERENCES

1. WHITEHEAD M I, TOWNSEND P T, PRYSE-DAVIES J, RYDER TA, KING RJB. Effects of estrogens and progestins on the biochemistry and morphology of the postmenopausal endometrium. *New Engl J Med* 1981;305:1599–605.

2. LETHABY A, IRVINE G, CAMERON I. Cyclical progestogens for heavy menstrual bleeding. *Cochrane Database Syst Rev* 2008;(4): C D 001016.pub2.

3. FARQUHAR C, BROWN J. Oral contraceptive pills for heavy menstrual bleeding. *Cochrane Database Syst Rev* 2009;(3):C D 000154.pub2.

4. LETHABY A E, COOKE I, REES M. Progesterone or progestogen-releasing intrauterine systems for heavy menstrual bleeding. *Cochrane Database Syst Rev* 2005;(2):C D 002126.pub2.

5. BEAUMONT H, AUGOOD C, DUCKITT K, LETHABY A. Danazol for heavy menstrual bleeding. *Cochrane Database Syst Rev* 2007;(2):C D 001017.pub2.

6. WONG C L, FARQUHAR C, ROBERTS, H, PROCTOR M. Oral contraceptive pill for primary dysmenorrhoea. *Cochrane Database Syst Rev* 2009(4):C D 002120.pub3.

7. DAVIS L, KENNEDY S S, MOORE J, PRENTICE A. Oral contraceptives for pain associated with endometriosis. *Cochrane Database Syst Rev* 2007;(3):C D 001019.pub2.

8. SCHWEPPE K W. Drug treatment of endometriosis. *Contemporary Clinical Gynecology and Obstetrics* 2001;2:167–77.

9. FARMER J E, PRENTICE A, BREEZE A, *et al.* Gonadotrophin-releasing hormone analogues for endometriosis: bone mineral density. *Cochrane Database Syst Rev* 2003;(4):C D 001297.

10. BERAL V, BANKS E, REEVES G. Evidence from randomised trials on the long-term effects of hormone replacement therapy. *Lancet* 2002;360:942–4.

11. BERAL V, BANKS E, REEVES G, APPLEBY P. Use of H R T and the subsequent risk of cancer. *J Epidemiol Biostat* 1999;4:191–210.

12. FURNESS S, ROBERTS H, MAJORIBANKS J, LETHABY A. Hormone therapy in postmenopausal women and risk of endometrial hyperplasia. *Cochrane Database Syst Rev* 2012;(2): C D 000402.pub4.

13. BRINTON L A, HOOVER R N. Estrogen replacement therapy and endometrial cancer risk: unresolved issues. The Endometrial Cancer Collaborative Group. *Obstet Gynecol* 1993;81:265–71.

14. GRADY D, GEBRETSADIK T, KERLIKOWSKE K, ERNSTER V, PETITTI D. Hormone replacement therapy and endometrial cancer risk: a meta-analysis. *Obstet Gynecol* 1995;85:304–13.

15. The Writing Group for the P E P I Trial. Effects of hormone replacement therapy on endometrial histology in postmenopausal women. The Postmenopausal Estrogen/Progestin Interventions (P E P I) Trial. *J A M A* 1996;275:370–5.

16. BERESFORD S A, WEISS N S, VOIGT L F, MCKNIGHT B. Risk of endometrial cancer in relation to use of oestrogen combined with cyclic progestagen therapy in postmenopausal women. *Lancet* 1997;349:458–61.

17. ROSSOUW J E, ANDERSON G L, PRENTICE R L, LACROIX A Z, KOOPERBERG C, STEFANICK M L, *et al.* Risks and benefits of estrogen plus progestin in healthy postmenopausal women: principal results from the Women's Health Initiative randomized controlled trial. *J A M A* 2002;288:321–33.

18. DALY E, VESSEY M P, HAWKINS M M, CARSON J L, GOUGH P, MARSH S. Risk of venous thromboembolism in users of hormone replacement therapy. *Lancet* 1996;348:977–80.

19. COLDITZ G A, HANKINSON S E, HUNTER D J, *et al.* The use of estrogens and progestins and the risk of breast cancer in postmenopausal women. *New Engl J Med* 1995;332:1589–93.

20. ANDERSON G L, LIMACHER M, ASSAF A R, BASSFORD T, BERESFORD S A, BLACK H, *et al.* Effects of conjugated equine estrogen in postmenopausal women with hysterectomy: the Women's Health Initiative randomized controlled trial. *J A M A* 2004;291:1701–12.

21. RYMER J, CHAPMAN M G, FOGELMAN I. Effect of tibolone on postmenopausal bone loss. *Osteoporosis Int* 1994;4:314–17.

Physiology

CHAPTER 29

Female reproductive physiology

Helen Mason

Introduction

The structure of the female reproductive organs and the cycles that control adult reproductive function are designed to bring about a number of important processes that permit fertility. These range from storage of sufficient ova for the lifetime, sequential follicular growth and regular spontaneous ovulation, to fertilisation, preparation of the endometrium of the uterus and support of the fertilised oocyte by the corpus luteum prior to implantation.

Storage of sufficient ova for a lifetime

During embryonic life, the primordial germ cells migrate from the hindgut into the tissue that will develop into the gonad. In the absence of the *SRY* gene, the gonad develops into an ovary and the germ cells become oogonia. The small number of oogonia that initially populate the ovary is increased dramatically by rapid mitosis until several million oogonia are present. Each oogonium is surrounded by cells that differentiate from the surrounding stroma to become granulosa cells and the whole structure is now a primordial follicle. The oocyte enters the first meiotic division at this time but does not complete it. These follicles are stored in the outer cortical layer of the ovary and many are lost through atresia from the second trimester onwards. By puberty, the numbers are reduced to less than one million.

Sequential growth of follicles

Following pubertal activation of the hypothalamus and pituitary, the follicles in the ovary become activated. It is clear that follicle-stimulating hormone (FSH) is not required for the very earliest stages of follicle growth as women who have inactivating defects in the FSH receptor are still able to grow small follicles. The primordial follicles grow by divisions of the granulosa cells such that the oocyte is contained within a ball of growing cells. These cells then produce a noncellular barrier around their outsides, a basal lamina, which subsequently acts as a protective layer for the oocyte. External to this, a second layer of cells differentiates from the stroma and becomes the theca layer. It is within the theca layer that the capillaries, which will provide nutrients for the growing follicle, reside. The theca layer is the only layer that is vascular; the inner granulosa layer remains avascular.

It is thought that follicles grow for approximately 80 days until they reach the size at which they can release the oocyte (Figure 29.1). There is continual loss of follicles by death during this process so that only a few follicles reach the size at which they can respond to the hormonal changes in the menstrual cycle. Once initiated, follicles take approximately 65 days to reach the size at which they can be recruited into a menstrual cycle. Follicle diameter increases by 1000-fold, from approximately 0.02 mm to 20–50 mm, by the time the single selected follicle is at the pre-ovulatory stage. The follicle reaches the antral phase (Figure 29.2), the oocyte

FIGURE 29.1 **The main stages of follicle growth**

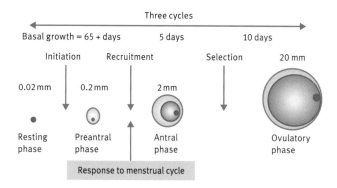

FIGURE 29.2 **Cross-section through an antral, or Graafian, follicle**

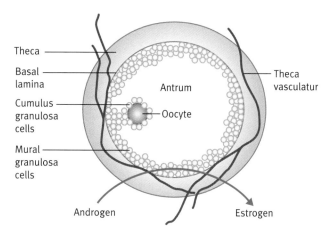

is displaced to one side and the granulosa cells surround a fluid-filled central cavity called the antrum. A subset of granulosa cells differentiates and surrounds the oocyte. These cells are called cumulus cells and their role is protective and nourishing. The granulosa cells against the follicle wall, the basal lamina, are called mural cells.

Selection of a single follicle and oocyte

Folliculogenesis is defined as growth of the follicles from the earliest resting phases through to ovulation. Only the latter stages of this process are dependent on the hormonal changes of the menstrual cycle. The granulosa cells develop receptors for FSH and the theca cells develop receptors for luteinising hormone (LH). Once follicles develop an antrum, they are dependent on FSH for further growth.

FIGURE 29.3 **Ovarian steroid production**

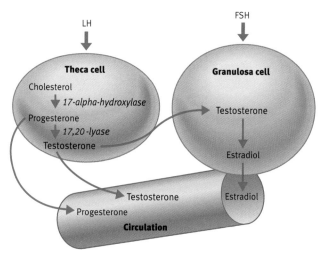

FSH = follicle-stimulating hormone | LH = luteinising hormone

The ovarian steroids are produced in the follicle by sequential loss of carbon atoms from cholesterol (Figure 29.3). LH drives the conversion of cholesterol to androgen by the theca layer. Androgens act as the precursor for estradiol synthesis and FSH primarily drives the conversion of androgen diffusing across the basement membrane to estradiol, a reaction that is catalysed by the enzyme aromatase in the granulosa cells. Both theca and granulosa cells can convert cholesterol into progesterone but only theca cells express *CYP 17*, which encodes for the enzymes necessary for androgen production, 17-alpha-hydroxylase and 17, 20-lyase, and only granulosa cells contain aromatase. Therefore, both cell types are essential for the production of all steroids. This is known as the two-cell two-gonadotrophin theory. It is the cyclical changes in the peptide hormones and the steroids subsequently produced by the follicles that bring about the menstrual cycle and permit selection of a single ovulatory follicle.

Assuming that pregnancy did not occur in the previous cycle, the cells in the corpus luteum will die 14 days after ovulation. Death of the cells results in a fall in progesterone and estrogen and subsequent shedding of the endometrium (Figure 29.4). At the beginning of the cycle (day 1) there are from four to six antral follicles of size 2–4mm in the ovary. As the corpus luteum dies, the fall in steroids results in removal of negative feedback at the hypothalamus and pituitary and this causes a specific

FIGURE 29.4 **Changes in principal hormones during the menstrual cycle and the accompanying changes in the follicle**

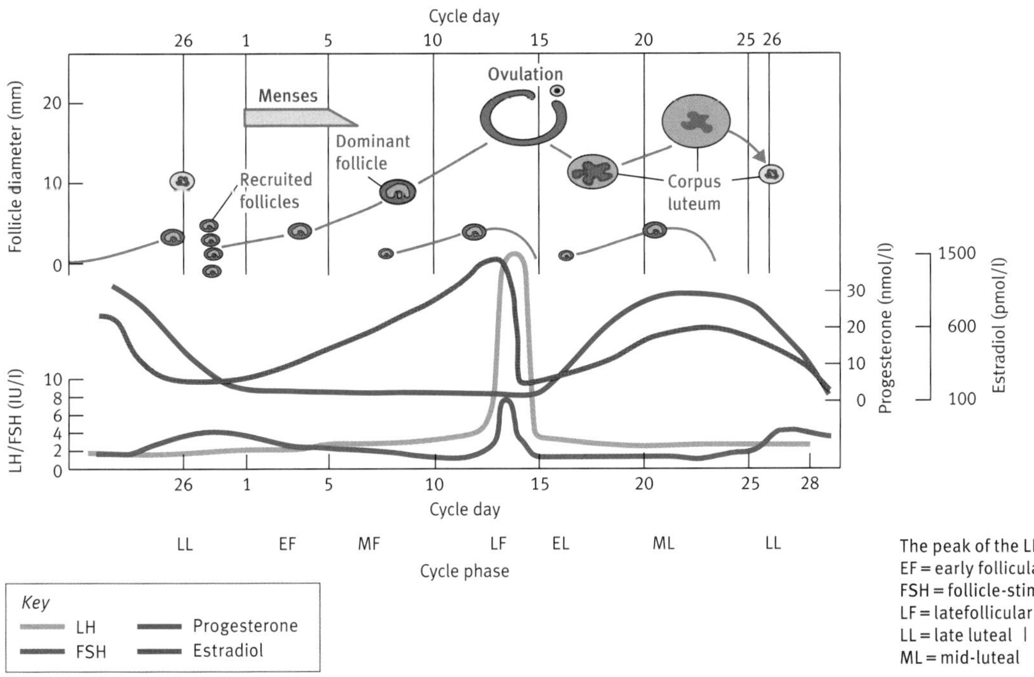

The peak of the LH surge is >50 iu/l.
EF = early follicular | EL = early luteal |
FSH = follicle-stimulating hormone |
LF = late follicular | LH = luteinising hormone |
LL = late luteal | MF = mid-follicular |
ML = mid-luteal

rise in FSH (Figure 29.5A). Although both LH and FSH are produced by the pituitary gonadotrophs, it is only FSH that rises at this time. FSH levels remain elevated for approximately 3 days: this is known as the intercycle rise in FSH. It is this rise in FSH that is primarily responsible for selection of the dominant follicle. One follicle has the correct qualities, because of FSH receptor numbers, intracellular cyclic adenosine monophosphate levels or granulosa cell number, and this follicle rapidly increases in size in response. As the number of granulosa cells in the follicle increases exponentially, their products, namely inhibin and estradiol, rise in the serum. This reinstates the negative feedback and FSH levels fall (Figures 29.4 and 29.5B).

The action of FSH on the dominant or selected follicle induces LH receptors on the granulosa cells at this time. No other follicle acquires granulosa cell LH receptors. This means that this follicle can survive the fall in FSH, whereas the other small follicles in the cohort, which are FSH dependent, will die by atresia.

Across the follicular phase, the level of LH gradually increases. The dominant follicle grows from 4 mm to 20 mm with an accompanying considerable increase in

granulosa cell number. As each cell is converting androgen from the theca cells into estrogen by the action of aromatase, the serum concentration of estradiol increases rapidly. Once the level has been above 300 nmol/l for 2–3 days, the negative feedback switches to positive.

This causes a rapid and massive release of LH from the pituitary, known as the LH surge (Figures 29.4 and 29.5C).

Regular spontaneous ovulation

The LH surge is responsible for the cascade of events leading to ovulation. The capillaries in the theca become leaky, leading to increased fluid pressure in the antrum. The pressure helps to assist the follicle in protruding from the surface of the ovary at the apex and the follicle wall becomes thin by stretching. Finally, a cascade of locally made enzymes breaks down the follicle wall and the oocyte and its surrounding cumulus cells are extruded because of the intrafollicular pressure.

The oocyte–cell complex is collected by the fimbrial end of the uterine tube, which is mobile and able to detect

FIGURE 29.5 **Hypothalamic–pituitary–ovarian feedback through the menstrual cycle**

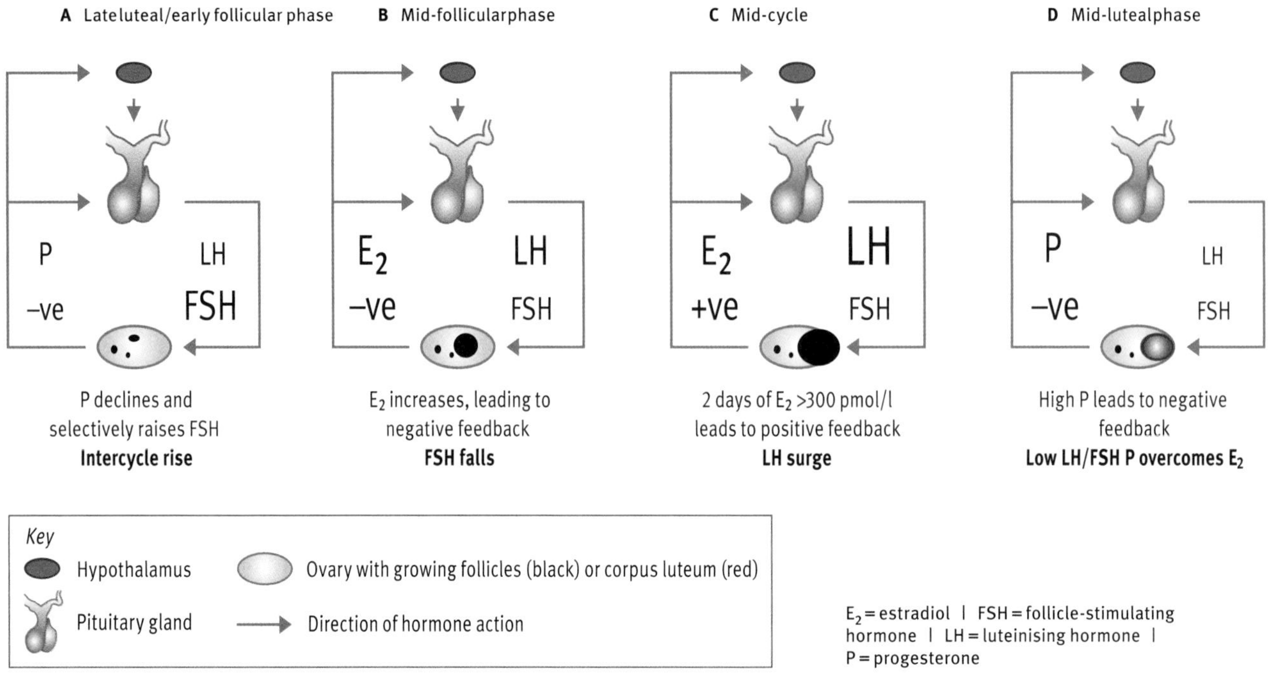

A Late luteal/early follicular phase   **B** Mid-follicular phase   **C** Mid-cycle   **D** Mid-luteal phase

P −ve   LH   FSH

E_2 −ve   LH   FSH

E_2 +ve   LH   FSH

P −ve   LH   FSH

P declines and selectively raises FSH
Intercycle rise

E_2 increases, leading to negative feedback
FSH falls

2 days of E_2 >300 pmol/l leads to positive feedback
LH surge

High P leads to negative feedback
Low LH/FSH P overcomes E_2

Key

⬤ Hypothalamus   ⬭ Ovary with growing follicles (black) or corpus luteum (red)

Pituitary gland   ⟶ Direction of hormone action

E_2 = estradiol | FSH = follicle-stimulating hormone | LH = luteinising hormone | P = progesterone

the oocyte, probably by a process of chemoattraction. The follicle that is left behind collapses, the basal lamina breaks down and the blood vessels invade the centre of the follicle to form a clot. The theca and granulosa layers are disrupted and there is a dramatic fall in steroid production directly after the release of the oocyte. The corpus luteum then forms from the involuted layers of the follicle and steroid production resumes in earnest, with estradiol and progesterone reaching a peak approximately 1 week after ovulation (Figures 29.4 and 29.5D). The corpus luteum is the only source of significant levels of progesterone during the cycle, making this the ideal marker of ovulation.

Correct number of chromosomes in the oocyte

In addition to its effects on the follicle, the LH surge also has an important effect on the oocyte in that it causes the oocyte to complete the first meiotic division. This would normally result in the production of two cells but the oocyte needs to remain as a large cell, as it has to provide for the early divisions of the blastocyst. To retain maximum cytoplasm, the second set of chromosomes produced at this time is parcelled into a package known as the first polar body. These chromosomes take no further part in the function of the oocyte. The second meiotic division is commenced and, like the first meiotic division, is not completed.

Transport of oocyte to uterus

The oocyte is passed along the tube by the combined action of peristalsis and cilia. The cells lining the tubes are of two types and are steroid sensitive. In response to estradiol production by the dominant follicle, the ciliated cells produce the cilia on the surface and the glandular cells secrete products that are designed to support the oocyte and provide an environment for sperm capacitation. Fertilisation normally occurs in the ampulla of the tube. Once the oocyte has passed into the uterus, the level of progesterone increases and this causes the cilia to retract and the glandular cells to shorten. This means that, even if a second oocyte were to be released, it would be unable to pass along the tube.

Fertilisation

Fertilisation causes a number of changes in the oocyte. The penetrating spermatozoon causes the oocyte to complete the second meiotic division. The second set of chromosomes is packaged into the second polar body. This leaves a haploid cell, which can combine with the nucleus of the sperm head. Penetration of the sperm head results in the movement of a specialised set of cellular contents, cortical granules, within the oocyte cytoplasm. The cortical granules migrate to the outer edge of the oocyte and release their contents. This results in a hardening of the oocyte membrane that precludes entry by a second spermatozoon and prevents polyspermy. Soon after fertilisation, the fertilised oocyte undergoes mitotic cell division to produce the blastocyst. Cells in the blastocyst then begin to produce human chorionic gonadotrophin, which acts on the LH receptors of the corpus luteum and prevents its demise.

Cyclical changes in the uterus, vagina and cervix

Production of ovarian steroids is not only vital for the growing follicle, but is also necessary to bring about cyclical changes in the uterus, vagina and cervix, all of which are designed to facilitate transport and implantation of the dividing blastocyst.

UTERUS

The myometrium of the uterus is covered by a layer of endometrial cells. Within this endometrial layer there are also glandular cells and vessels supplied by the uterine and, subsequently, the radial arteries. Following menstruation, the myometrium is covered by a basal layer of the endometrium. Under the stimulation of estrogen, these cells divide rapidly; this is known as the proliferative phase and corresponds to the follicular phase of the ovary. At the same time as the endometrial cells are undergoing rapid divisions, the glandular cells grow and expand to make glands and there is new growth of blood vessels. The actions of estrogen induce progesterone receptors on the endometrial cells so that after ovulation the cells can respond to the rising levels

of progesterone being made by the corpus luteum. Two or three days after ovulation, progesterone causes the rapid rate of cell division to reduce and, although the thickness of the endometrium continues to increase, this occurs mainly by oedema. Contributing to this oedema are the increased number of vessels, which become spiral, to accommodate maximum vascularity in a minimum space, and which become increasingly permeable. At the same time, the glands distend and increase in tortuosity to give the maximum surface area on which to produce their product (glycoproteins), which are secreted on to the surface. For this reason, this is known as the secretory phase, corresponding to the luteal phase in the ovary. The endometrium will now have reached approximately 6 mm in thickness. It is the responsiveness to steroids, estrogen in particular, that makes measurement of endometrial thickness a good indicator of the degree of estrogenisation of a woman.

Progesterone also has an effect on the myometrial wall of the uterus. This undergoes continual small contractions in response to estrogen and, during the luteal phase, these are suppressed by progesterone, presumably to increase the chances of implantation. If fertilisation does not occur, the corpus luteum will die and the level of steroids will fall. In response to steroid withdrawal, prosta-glandins are released by the endometrial cells. These cause a temporary constriction of the spiral arterioles, which later dilate and begin to bleed. The ensuing hypoxia in the surrounding tissues causes necrosis and as the cells break down they release proteolytic enzymes, which accelerate this process. The outer layer of the endometrium is thus shed with 50% being lost within the first 24 hours. Normal menstrual flow is difficult to measure in practice but is considered to be anything up to 80 ml. All but the basal layer is shed and this layer recommences division in response to rising estradiol in the next cycle.

VAGINA AND CERVIX

The vagina is lined by stratified, nonkeratinised squamous epithelium. The layers divide continually and are shed creating a downward movement of cells. This downflow is added to by cervical secretions and transudation from the vaginal epithelium. It is designed to decrease the chances of opportunistic infection. The secretions in the vagina change with the cycle and are generally acidic, thus providing an antimicrobial action.

During the follicular phase, there is an increase in vascularity of the cervix, which results in oedema. The mucus becomes watery as a result and the composition changes such that the glycoproteins contained within it align to form microscopic channels. These channels are designed to facilitate the passage of spermatozoa through the cervix. After ovulation, under the influence of progesterone, the oedema reduces, the mucus becomes thicker and the glycoproteins now form a mesh. This acts as a potential barrier to spermatozoa and is one of the mechanisms of action of the progesterone-only oral contraceptive.

CHAPTER 30

Male reproductive physiology and the fertilisation process

Helen Mason

Introduction

In terms of reproduction, the main requirement for the male is to deliver a package of chromosomes to the oocyte. The male reproductive tract is designed to facilitate every step of this process.

Gross anatomy

The gross anatomy of the male reproductive tract is shown in Figure 30.1. The structure is designed to have a combined outlet for the ureter and vas deferens through the urethra and to provide a site for sperm production that is protective and yet in close proximity to this outlet. The glands contribute to seminal fluid, which is important for preservation and transport of the spermatozoa.

The internal structure of the testes

The testes are oval structures of 3.3–5.5 cm in length and 2–3 cm wide giving a normal volume of 15–30 ml. Testicular volume is important as any reduction in the mass of tissue producing spermatozoa may result in a reduced sperm count. The volume is measured by means of an orchidometer. The testes lie in the scrotal sac outside the body cavity. The reason for this is that spermatogenesis requires a temperature that is 1.5–2 degrees C below core body temperature in order to proceed. It is common to find reduced sperm counts in men whose testes are overheated for significant periods of the day (for example, long-distance lorry drivers). The testes are very vascular and well innervated.

One of the main adaptations to improve the chances of fertilisation is to produce spermatozoa in very large numbers and much of the structure of the testes is designed to facilitate this. Internally, the testes are divided into a number of lobules, each of which is filled with coiled seminiferous tubules: these tubules make up 90% of the internal structure. The seminiferous tubule is the site of sperm production and the immense coiling permits the largest surface area to be contained in the smallest volume. The tubules lead to an area on one side called the rete. Here, the contents of many tubules are mixed and the number of tubes gradually reduces as they join together in the rete to become a single tube in the epididymis. The epididymis acts as a storage and maturation area and leads to the outlet to the penis, the vas deferens.

The tubules are lined with columnar endothelial Sertoli cells between which spermatogenesis takes place. The space between adjacent tubules is filled with blood and lymphatic vessels, Leydig cells and interstitial fluid. On the basement membrane between each pair of adjacent cells lie the gamete progenitor cells, the spermatogonia, which are equivalent to the oogonia in the ovary. Similarly to the oogonia, the spermatogonia are laid down during fetal life; however, in contrast to the oogonia, new progenitor cells will be made throughout reproductive life to give an inexhaustible supply.

FIGURE 30.1 **Anatomy of the male reproductive tract and fine structure of the rete, epididymis and vas deferens**

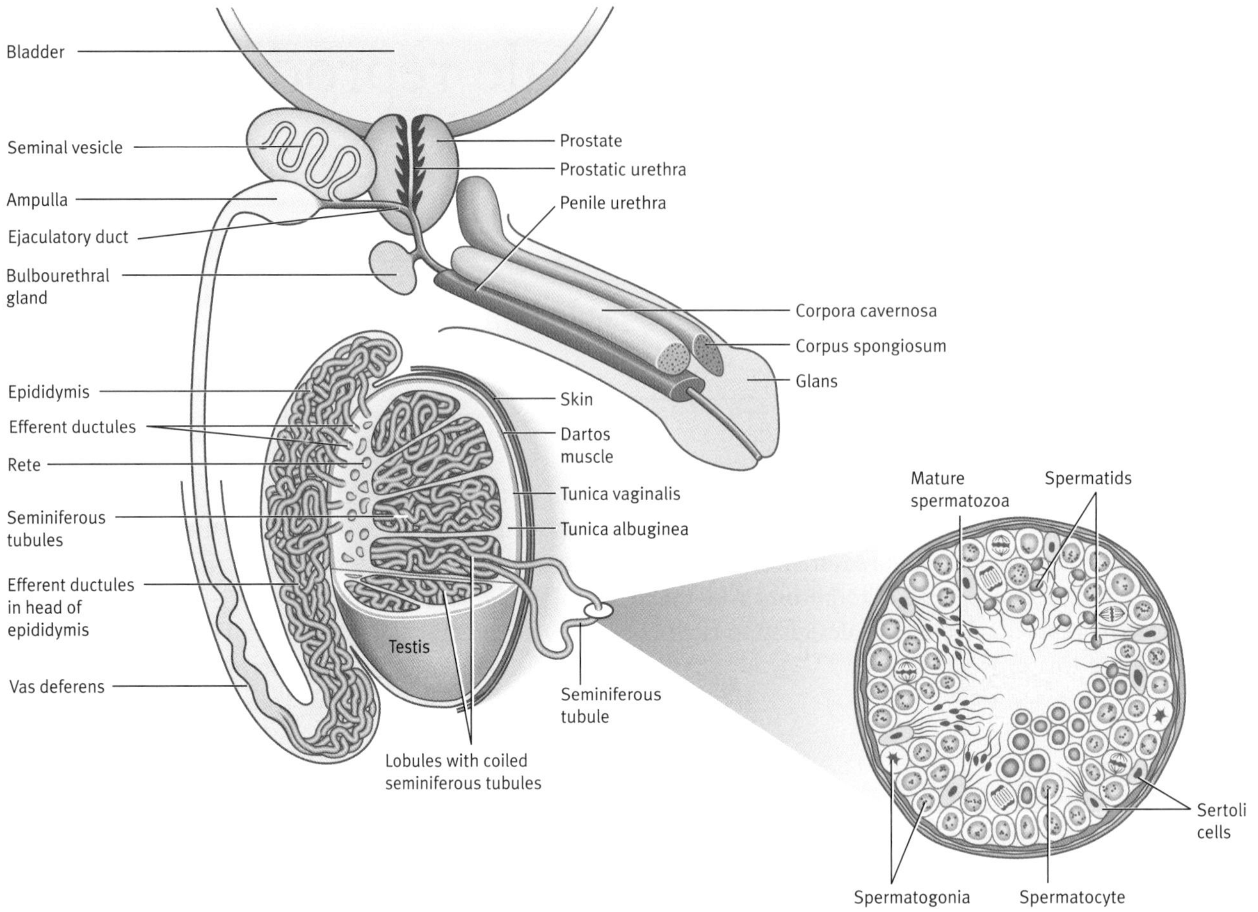

As in the ovary, the basement membrane provides protection from blood-borne contaminants and encloses an avascular region. The passage of hormones and nutrients necessary for the energy-demanding process of spermatogenesis, therefore, all occurs via the interstitial fluid. The volume of interstitial fluid within the testes is very high; such a volume would be considered oedemic in any other tissue. In addition to the basal lamina, there is also a second protective barrier in the testes, called the tight junction.

Spermatogenesis

The changes in cell morphology during the development of spermatogonia into a mature spermatozoon are illustrated in Figure 30.2A. Spermatogonia lie on the basement membrane of the seminiferous epithelium. Following puberty, as gonadotrophins rise, every 16 days there is a wave of mitotic division of the spermatogonia into primary spermatocytes or daughter spermatogonia. The daughter spermatogonia remain on the basal lamina and keep the pool replenished, whereas the primary spermatocytes are committed to starting development into spermatozoa. The primary spermatocytes still possess a diploid number of chromosomes. These cells must divide meiotically to form secondary spermatocytes possessing 23 chromosomes. Just before meiosis, the tight junction between the Sertoli cells parts and allows the spermatocytes to move from the basal (outside) to the adluminal (inside) compartment, then closes again. These tight junctions prevent molecules and cells passing into the intercellular spaces. This means that all molecules passing to the spermatocytes must pass

FIGURE 30.2 **Spermatogenesis and spermiogenesis**

A The cell stages of spermatogenesis

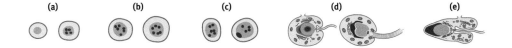

(a) Spermatogonia | **(b)** primary spermatocytes | **(c)** secondary spermatocytes | **(d)** spermatids | **(e)** spermatozoon

B Spermiogenesis

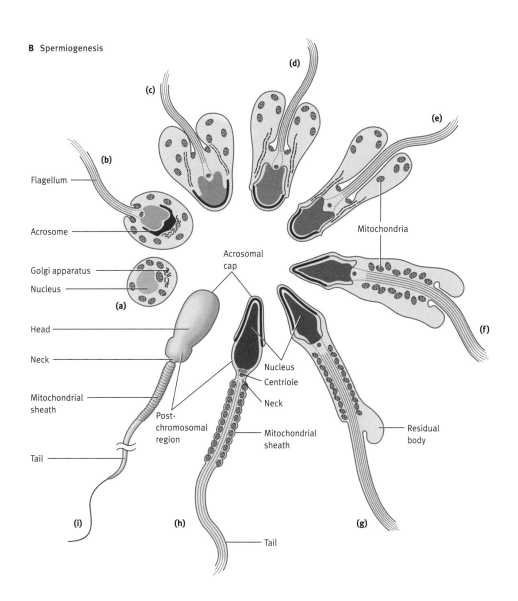

(a) Round secondary; **(b)** the flagellum starts to grow; **(c)**, **(d)** and **(e)** at the spermatid stage, the acrosome moves to the head of the cell, the cellular contents move behind the nucleus and the cell elongates; **(f)** mitochondria align with the mid-piece; **(g)** remaining cellular content enters the residual body, which is reabsorbed into Sertoli cells; **(h)** and **(i)** fully formed spermatozoa in section and in three dimensions, respectively.

through the blood–testes barrier or be secreted into the adluminal space by the Sertoli cells. Note that once meiosis has taken place, the haploid germ cells are 'foreign', so the blood–testes barrier isolates the germ cells from the rest of the body (including circulation) and protects them from attack by the immune system. In addition, it allows the haploid germ cell to exist within the adluminal compartment in a different and unique ionic microenvironment, with especially high levels of certain amino acids, peptides, steroids and sugars that are required for germ cell production.

Two meiotic divisions occur with doubling of the chromosomes in between to give first two secondary spermatocytes and then four spermatids, each containing 23Y or 23X. This results in a great reduction in cytoplasmic volume and each spermatozoon containing half of the DNA of its parent. At this point, the genetic constitution of each spermatozoon will also be different, as crossing over has occurred during meiosis. In order to retain access to all DNA for all cells, the new secondary spermatocytes and spermatids remain connected by a syncytium, a membrane that encompasses the four spermatozoa. This breaks when the spermatozoa leave the space between the Sertoli cells.

At this point, the spermatozoon is still a rounded cell and it must undergo the most remarkable cellular transformation to give the elongated spermatozoon. This process is known as spermiogenesis and it involves the elongation of the head, production of a tail and midpiece and the removal of the vast majority of the remaining cytoplasm, which is absorbed into the Sertoli cells (Figure 30.2B). All of these processes occur within the seminiferous epithelium, in the spaces between the Sertoli cells. After each division, the germ cells move toward the lumen of the tubule, so that eventually the spermatids are embedded in the apical region of the Sertoli cells, from where they are extruded into the lumen. This cyclical process is completed in 64 days. In addition, there are waves of development occurring every 16 days, longitudinally along the tubule, so that at a given site there are more mature stages in front and less mature stages behind. This ensures a continual supply of spermatozoa leaving the tubules and entering the rete. At each stage, the germ cells need different agents for their maintenance and development. These factors are all produced by Sertoli cells.

The spermatozoa, having reached the lumen of the seminiferous tubules, pass into a common area (the rete), where all the tubules open out. From there they pass into the ductus epididymis. The epididymis is a tube of 5 m in length, again highly coiled. Passage of spermatozoa through the epididymis takes 8–14 days. Its structure can be divided into three parts: caput, corpus and cauda (head, body and tail). In the epididymis, fluid is reduced, motility gained and maturation advanced. The spermatozoa become progressively motile; this means they can move forward. This is the final stage of maturation of the spermatozoa. In addition to gaining motility, it is possible that other maturational processes occur in the epididymis. It is for this reason that, in men with a blockage in the vas deferens, it is the preferred site of aspiration of spermatozoa to be used for intracytoplasmic sperm injection. Round spermatids aspirated from the seminiferous tubule have, however, also been shown to be capable of fertilisation by this method.

The spermatozoa are mainly stored in the epididymis, but also in the ampulla of the vas deferens. The spermatozoa are stored in epididymal fluid but, at ejaculation, secretions from the accessory sex glands are added to form seminal fluid and the latter make up a large percentage of the total volume. These secretory glands are the seminal vesicles, the prostate and the bulbourethral gland.

Steroidogenesis

The two functions of the testes, spermatogenesis and steroidogenesis, are controlled by luteinising hormone (LH) and follicle-stimulating hormone (FSH) released in a pulsatile manner from the anterior pituitary as for the female. Only the feedback mechanism differs between the male and female, in that progesterone and estradiol act alternately and cyclically in the female and testosterone and estradiol provide constant feedback in the male.

ANDROGEN SYNTHESIS

This occurs mainly in the interstitial Leydig cells and is predominantly under the control of LH. All of the steroids in these synthetic pathways leak out in small amounts into the circulation but the main circulating

FIGURE 30.3 **Testicular steroidogenesis**

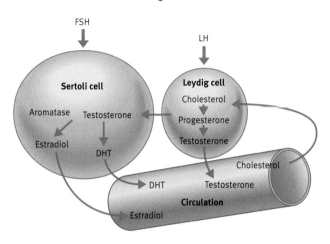

DHT = dihydrotestosterone | FSH = follicle-stimulating hormone | LH = luteinising hormone

androgen is testosterone. Once in the circulation, the testosterone can be either aromatised to estrone and estradiol in skin and adipose tissue or reduced by 5-alpha-reductase in peripheral target tissues to the more active dihydrotestosterone.

Within the testes, testosterone is aromatised to estradiol by the Sertoli cells under the control of FSH. In this sense, Leydig cells are equivalent to theca cells and Sertoli cells are equivalent to granulosa cells. LH acts on the Leydig cells to stimulate the production of testosterone via cyclic adenosine monophosphate. FSH can only act on Sertoli cells. The Sertoli cells produce over 50 protein substances, which are required for spermatogenesis and secreted into the intercellular gap. Testicular steroidogenesis is outlined in Figure 30.3.

Testosterone secretion by the Leydig cells in the fetal testes is under the control of human chorionic gonadotrophin (hCG) in early pregnancy and extends over the period of sexual differentiation when fetal testosterone levels are at their highest *in utero*. hCG is LH-like in action and acts on LH receptors present on the Leydig cells in the fetal testes. The level of testosterone then falls until adrenarche and puberty.

Hormonal control of spermatogenesis

Normal spermatogenesis requires the presence of testosterone and FSH, which act together synergistically.

There are androgen and FSH receptors on Sertoli cells. The situation can be compared to the two-cell two-gonadotrophin system in the ovarian follicle. Sertoli cells are the site of conversion of testosterone to estradiol by aromatase: estradiol is important for the negative feedback control of the gonadotrophins and has an inhibitory modulating effect on testosterone production by Leydig cells; there are estrogen receptors present on Leydig cells. Sertoli cells also make androgen-binding protein, which acts to concentrate testosterone within the seminal tubules and thus increase its availability at the time and site where it is required. No such protein is present in the follicle. Spermatogenesis cannot proceed without FSH and testosterone, and testosterone is also essential for maintenance of the prostate, seminal vesicles, ampulla and bulbourethral glands.

Control of gonadotrophin secretion in the male

LH and FSH release are controlled separately, which is not seen so clearly in the female. Testosterone and dihydrotestosterone exert a negative feedback effect on LH release at the hypothalamic level by inhibiting gonadotrophin-releasing hormone (GnRH) release. They also act at the pituitary level, reducing its sensitivity toward GnRH. Testosterone also inhibits FSH release but is five times less effective than on LH. Estrogen exerts a negative feedback effect on FSH release at both the hypothalamic level and also at the pituitary level, decreasing the pituitary gland's sensitivity towards GnRH. Estrogen also inhibits LH release but less potently than its effect on FSH release.

Transport of spermatozoa

The comparative distance that must be travelled by the mature spermatozoa collecting in the epididymis to reach the oocyte in the uterine tube is great and it is a journey that very few will survive. Mature spermatozoa are a few micrometres in length (10^{-6} m) and they must pass through the combined length of the male and female reproductive tract (30–40 cm). Emission of spermatozoa requires erection and ejaculation. Somatic and autonomic efferents to the genitalia can be stimulated psychogenically or by tactile stimulation. The afferent limb of the reflex is carried by the internal pudendal nerves and three efferent outflows influence erection: the parasympathetic pelvic nerve (stimulatory), the sympathetic hypogastric nerve (inhibitory and some stimulatory fibres) and the somatic pudendal nerve (stimulatory). Erection occurs owing to an inflow of blood primarily into the corpus cavernosum under the influence of vasodilator agents such as vasoactive intestinal peptide and nitric oxide. Blood is prevented from leaving, thus causing increased pressure. The pressure in the corpus spongiosum does not increase as much so as to prevent occlusion of the urethra.

Ejaculation consists of coordinated contractions of the vas deferens, the seminal vesicles and the prostate and bulbourethral glands. The ejaculated semen is made up of spermatozoa and seminal plasma. Movement of the spermatozoa into the pelvic urethra, expulsion of the glandular secretions making seminal plasma into the pelvic urethra and ejaculation are controlled by the sympathetic system together with a striated muscle component. Movement of semen into the bladder is prevented by contraction of the urethral sphincter. Ejaculation is partially fractionated, in that most of the spermatozoa are ejaculated in the first half of the fluid.

Three hundred million spermatozoa are produced each day and there are 40–100 million/ml in the ejaculate, of which 99.9% are lost. Thus, in a normal ejaculate volume of 3–5 ml, of the 120 million spermatozoa present, only 120 000 will have a chance of fertilising the oocyte. A sperm count of less than 20 million/ml is considered oligozoospermic and, in these cases, the quality is often poor also. Teratozoospermia is the condition where more than 70% of spermatozoa are abnormal in form.

The ejaculate coagulates within 1 minute of entry into the vagina and then gradually reliquifies after about 20 minutes. This forms a temporary reservoir of spermatozoa and also prevents loss from the vagina. The pH of vaginal secretions is between pH 3 and 4 and the motility of spermatozoa is inhibited by an acidic pH. The ejaculate raises the pH to 7.2; this is one of the functions of seminal fluid.

The cervix, with a narrow lumen and convoluted folds in its walls, is a barrier to spermatozoa. In addition, it is normally occluded by viscous impenetrable mucus. At the time of ovulation, however, under the influence of estrogen, the mucus becomes thinner as the water content rises and the protein content is reduced. Glycoprotein molecules within the mucus arrange themselves in parallel micelles (aggregations) and spermatozoa can swim along the channels formed between them. The micelles vibrate and help to propel the spermatozoa along, especially those whose tail-beat frequency coincides with the micelle vibration frequency; this will favour the healthy motile spermatozoa. Many of the spermatozoa are not orientated correctly to pass along the channels and so form a reservoir, protected from the phagocytosis that can occur in the uterine lumen. Many of the spermatozoa are destroyed in their passage along the uterus by leucocytes. The uterotubal junction is another site of accumulation of spermatozoa and is therefore another reservoir. Entry occurs spasmodically and only motile spermatozoa can pass into the tubes. By having these barrier-forming reservoirs, a continuous supply of small numbers of spermatozoa can be ensured over a period of time, which maximises the chance of an oocyte being fertilised.

Spermatozoa appear in the oviducts a few minutes after ejaculation; since spermatozoa travel at less than 8 mm/minute, the movement must be mainly due to propulsive contractions of the female tract. At the same time, pressure in the uterus falls sharply on female orgasm and therefore 'suction' of the spermatozoa from the vagina into the uterus may occur.

The events that occur during fertilisation can be divided into a number of distinct steps. Capacitation involves biochemical alteration of the sperm plasma membrane that initiates hyperactivated motility known as 'whiplash movement'. Capacitation occurs in the presence of uterine or uterine tube fluid and before contact with the oocyte. The factor that induces capacitation is unknown. It is the whiplash movement of the tail that endows the spermatozoa with the velocity required to reach the oocyte. This usually occurs in the ampulla of the tube. Capacitation alters the surface of the sperm head and makes it more responsive to signals in the immediate area of the oocyte.

Fertilisation and establishment of early pregnancy

The fertilisation process, from when a spermatozoon starts to respond to the oocyte's signal to when

FIGURE 30.4 **The fertilisation process**

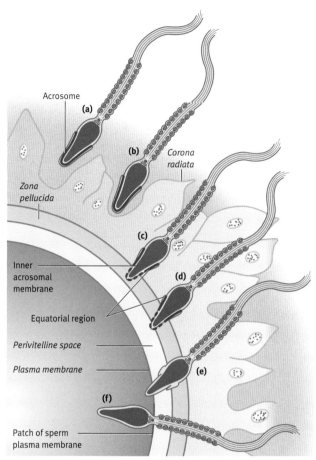

Acrosome
(a)
(b)
Corona radiata
Zona pellucida
(c)
Inner acrosomal membrane
(d)
Equatorial region
Perivitelline space
Plasma membrane
(e)
(f)
Patch of sperm plasma membrane

(a) Attraction to the oocyte; **(b)** Penetration of the corona radiata; **(c)** Binding to the zona pellucida; **(d)** Proteolysis of the zona pellucida; **(e)** Fusion with the oocyte's plasma membrane; **(f)** Entry of the spermatozoon. | Female elements in italics

spermatozoon–oocyte fusion occurs, is shown in Figure 30.4. Once the spermatozoon has undergone capacitation and penetrated the outer layer of remaining cumulus cells, it reaches the zona pellucida, a noncellular barrier secreted by the oocyte early in folliculogenesis. The spermatozoon is attracted to the oocyte by a combination of chemotactic agents and an increasing temperature gradient and passes between the cells of the corona radiata, which is composed of differentiated cumulus cells (Figure 30.4A and B). The equatorial region of the sperm head binds to the zona pellucida and the acrosome reaction is initiated, which fuses the outer acrosomal membrane and the plasma membrane

of the sperm head beneath it and forms pores through which hydrolytic enzymes are released. Eventually, the porous membrane breaks away and exposes the inner acrosomal membrane (Figure 30.4C and D). The hyperactivated motility generates the forward thrust necessary to penetrate the zona pellucida, and the spermatozoon moves into the perivitelline space (the space around the oocyte) by a process of proteolysis and forms a slit (Figure 30.4E). The spermatozoon fuses with the oocyte's plasma membrane, causing a series of calcium waves within the oocyte that lead to completion of the oocyte's second meiotic division and the second set of chromosomes is packaged into the extruded second polar body within the oocyte. The sperm head is taken up into the oocyte's cytoplasm by a process similar to phagocytosis, leaving the majority of the tail behind (Figure 30.4F).

The calcium waves arising from the fusion also cause migration of the cortical granules to the periphery of the oocyte. These fuse with the zona pellucida and release their contents, changing the nature of the plasma membrane of the oocyte and making it impenetrable to other spermatozoa, thus preventing polyspermy. The spermatozoon's and oocyte's nuclei come together, the nuclear membranes break down and the chromosomes mingle and come together on a common spindle, thus recreating a diploid cell. Fertilisation is only complete when there is a mitotic division and two cells are formed. The spermatozoon contributes only DNA and some of the cellular machinery required for cell division; the oocyte contributes the cytoplasm and, hence, the organelles, including mitochondria and the cell membrane. The fertilised oocyte is now called a zygote.

The zygote remains in the tube for a few days and then passes through the isthmus into the uterus aided by uterine-tube cilia. The initial cell divisions result in a reduction in the volume of each cell or blastomere. At around the 8–16-cell stage, the blastocyst begins to change its morphology and become a morula. At this stage, the cell mass becomes polarised and two distinctive cell types become visible: the outer trophoblast cells and the inner cell mass. The trophoblast cells will develop into the chorion, which contributes the fetal part of the placenta, and the inner cell mass develops into the embryo. It is important at this time for the conceptus to signal its presence and to prevent the demise of the corpus luteum, which would result in the shedding of the endometrium. This is achieved by production of beta-hCG by the syncytiotrophoblast; beta-hCG interacts with LH receptors on the corpus luteum and prevents luteolysis. At this time, the conceptus establishes attachment to the uterine wall and begins the process of implantation. During the next few weeks, the cells differentiate and the body plan is laid down. The conceptus signals its presence through the epithelial cells of the endometrium to the underlying stromal tissue and begins the process of decidualisation and production of the placenta.

Physiology of pregnancy

Asma Khalil

Introduction

In pregnancy, changes occur that are designed to meet the demands of the mother and the developing fetus and the birth process. The study of these changes, which may occur at different stages in pregnancy, is elemental in understanding normal and high-risk pregnancy.

Cardiovascular system

Cardiac output increases by approximately 40% in pregnancy, from 4.5 l/minute to approximately 6 l/minute. This rise starts early in pregnancy but reaches a plateau by 24–30 weeks. Early in pregnancy, this extra output goes mainly to the skin and breasts, but at term the extra 1.5 l/minute is distributed as follows: uterus (400 ml/minute), kidneys (300 ml/minute), skin (500 ml/minute) and the gastrointestinal tract, breasts and other organs (300 ml/minute). After delivery, cardiac output falls; most of this fall occurs in the first 6 weeks but it may take several months before prepregnancy levels are reached again. The changes in blood volumes in pregnancy are illustrated in Figure 31.1 and the cardiovascular changes are summarised in Table 31.1 and Figure 31.2, with the normal range of arterial blood gases summarized in Table 31.2. Stroke volume increases in pregnancy. Heart rate also increases (by approximately 10%, from 80 to 90 bpm). Peripheral vascular resistance is reduced in pregnancy, probably as a result of the relaxant effect of progesterone on arterial smooth muscle. Several other factors, such as an increase in nitric oxide, prostaglandin-I_2 and a

decline in asymmetrical dimethylarginine may also play a role in the vasodilation of pregnancy.

Overall, from 8 to 36 weeks, systolic blood pressure falls by approximately 5 mmHg and diastolic blood pressure by around 10 mmHg. Blood pressure reaches its nadir at approximately 24 weeks, rising again as term approaches, often reaching nonpregnant values by 40 weeks. If a pregnant woman in the third trimester lies supine, the gravid uterus may compress the inferior vena cava against her spine, impeding venous return and leading to a fall in cardiac output. She may

FIGURE 31.1 **Maternal intravascular volume changes**

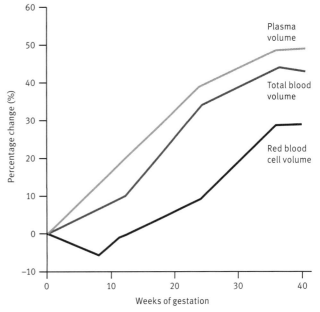

Anaesthesia UK, www.frca.co.uk

TABLE 31.1 **Cardiovascular changes in pregnancy**

Parameter	Change in pregnancy
Blood volume	30% increase
Plasma volume	45% increase
Red blood cell volume	20–30% increase
Cardiac output	40% increase
Stroke volume	30% increase
Heart rate	10% increase
Systolic blood pressure	5 mmHg decrease
Diastolic blood pressure	10 mmHg decrease
Peripheral resistance	Decrease
Oxygen consumption	30–50 ml/minute increase
PCO_2	Decrease to 4.1 kPa31

TABLE 31.2 **Normal range of arterial blood gases**

pH	7.35–7.45
PaO_2	9.3–13.3 kPa (80–100 mmHg)
$PaCO_2$	4.7–6.0 kPa (35–45 mmHg)
HCO_3^-	22–26 mmol/l
Base excess	−3 to +3 mmol/l

FIGURE 31.2 **Maternal cardiovascular changes**

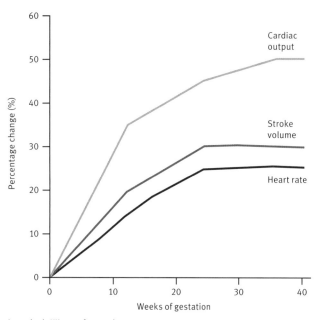

Anaesthesia UK, www.frca.co.uk

experience a marked fall in blood pressure and may feel faint, dizzy and nauseous. This is known as supine hypotensive syndrome; it is quickly relieved if the woman moves to the lateral position. Supine hypotensive syndrome reduces the uterine blood supply, which might cause fetal distress.

ELECTROCARDIOGRAPHIC CHANGES

The increase in cardiac output in pregnancy causes hypertrophy and dilation of the left ventricle and atrium. However, there is no change in contractility. As a result of the upward displacement of the diaphragm by the enlarging uterus, the axis of the heart is shifted anteriorly and to the left. These changes explain the typical features of the electrocardiogram in pregnancy: heart rate 10–15% faster than normal; left axis deviation by approximately 15 degrees; inverted T wave in lead III; a Q wave in leads III and aVF.

Respiratory system

Ventilation increases by approximately 40% owing to stimulation of the respiratory centre by progesterone both directly and indirectly (by increasing the sensitivity of the respiratory centre to carbon dioxide). This rise begins in the first trimester and the increased ventilation results in a mild fall in PCO_2 to 4.1 kPa and increase in PCO_2 to 14 kPa during the third trimester. Towards term, PCO_2 falls a little again to 13.5 kPa, as the increased cardiac output is unable to compensate for the increase in oxygen consumption. The mild decrease in PCO_2 leads to a slightly alkaline pH. In response, there is an increase in bicarbonate excretion by the kidney, leading to a fall in bicarbonate levels to approximately 19–20 mEq/l. This is associated with a fall in sodium levels and in osmolarity (by 10 mmol/l). The changes in maternal respiration are illustrated in Figures 31.3–31.5.

Progesterone also relaxes bronchial smooth muscle; the calibre of the tracheobronchial tree increases and resistance falls. During pregnancy, breathing is more diaphragmatic than thoracic. Tidal volume increases

FIGURE 31.3 **Maternal respiratory changes**

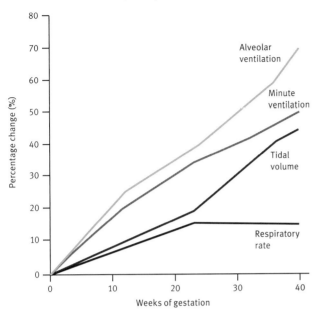

FIGURE 31.5 **Differences in lung volumes between pregnant and nonpregnant women**

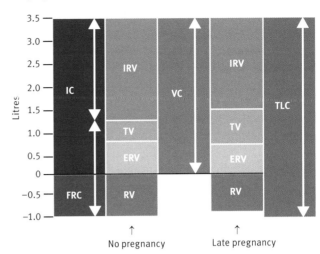

ERV = expiratory reserve volume | FRC = functional reserve capacity | IC = inspiratory capacity | IRV = inspiratory reserve volume | RV = residual volume | TLC = total lung capacity | TV = tidal volume | VC = vital capacity

FIGURE 31.4 **Lung volumes and capacities**

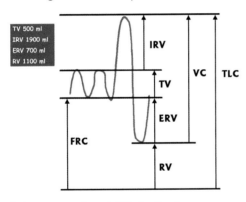

ERV = expiratory reserve volume | FRC = functional residual capacity | IRV = inspiratory reserve volume | RV = residual volume | TV = tidal volume | vital capacity

Vital capacity (the volume of gas that can be inhaled from forced expiration to forced inspiration) is unchanged at about 3.5 litres as the reduction in the expiratory reserve and inspiratory volumes are compensated for by the increase in tidal volume. Lung compliance is unaffected, but chest compliance is reduced, especially if the woman is in the lithotomy position. Seventy percent of pregnant women experience subjective dyspnoea. Oxygen consumption increases by 50 ml/minute at term. This increased demand comes from the fetus (20 ml/minute), increased cardiac output (6 ml/minute), increase in renal work (6 ml/minute) and increase in metabolic rate (18 ml/minute). During pregnancy, the increase in ventilation is greater than the increase in oxygen consumption. In pregnancy, there is also an increased risk of pulmonary embolism (see below).

by approximately 40%, but there is no change in the respiratory rate. The residual volume (the volume of gas that remains at the end of forced expiration, which is normally 1500 ml in the nonpregnant state) decreases by 200 ml, leading to a reduction in expiratory reserve volume and inspiratory reserve volume. Total lung capacity (5 litres in the nonpregnant individual) decreases by 200 ml. However, there is no change in the forced expiratory volume or peak flow rate.

Urinary system

In pregnancy, the kidneys increase in size by approximately 1 cm. The ureters dilate, partly from the effect of progesterone on the smooth muscle in their walls and partly from obstruction caused by pressure from the growing uterus. As a result, women are more prone to urinary tract infections in pregnancy and, if they have a urinary tract infection, are more likely to develop pyelonephritis. Both renal blood flow and glomerular filtration rate increase in pregnancy. These rises start in the first trimester and, by term, both are 50–60% higher than before pregnancy, the glomerular filtration rate reaching 140–170 ml/minute.

As a result of these changes, the urea level in pregnancy falls from 4.3 to 3.1 mmol/l and serum creatinine falls from 73 to 47 micromol/l. Urate and bicarbonate levels also fall. In pregnancy, there is mild glycosuria and proteinuria. Plasma osmolality decreases because of the combined effect of increased progesterone and changes in the renin–angiotensin–aldosterone pathway.

Gastrointestinal tract

The nausea and vomiting that commonly occur in early pregnancy are largely explained by increasing levels of human chorionic gonadotrophin and/or progesterone. Gastrointestinal tone and motility are reduced by the high levels of progesterone, leading to delayed gastric emptying, particularly during labour. Progesterone also relaxes the oesophageal sphincter, which means that acid reflux is common; at term, 81% of pregnant women complain of heartburn. More importantly, these changes make pregnant women more prone to aspiration of gastric contents, particularly during induction of general anaesthesia. Furthermore, because gastric contents are more acidic in pregnancy, if aspiration occurs, the resulting pneumonitis (Mendelson syndrome) may be severe and even fatal. Some of the dyspepsia in pregnancy can also be explained by reduced motility of the gallbladder, again most likely due to the effects of progesterone.

Small and large bowel motility is decreased. Stools become firmer as transit time is longer, allowing more time in the colon for reabsorption of water. Consequently, constipation is a common problem in pregnancy.

CHANGES AFFECTING THE LIVER

In pregnancy, plasma alkaline phosphatase increases up to three times the normal level, because it is also produced by the placenta. Gallbladder contractility decreases as cholecystokinin secretion falls. As a result, pregnant women are more prone to develop gallstones during pregnancy.

Obstetric cholestasis is a pregnancy-specific hepatic condition, characterised by itching in pregnancy and accompanied by raised liver transaminases and bile acids. This condition is associated with an increased risk of intrauterine fetal death and fetal distress in labour. One hypothesis proposes that obstetric cholestasis is caused by an interaction between inherited and acquired abnormalities in bile acid transport. Women who experience obstetric cholestasis in pregnancy may have a similar reaction to the combined oral contraceptive pill.

Haematological system

In pregnancy, plasma volume expands by around 45% (from 2600 ml to 3800 ml). This expansion begins early in pregnancy (around 6–8 weeks of gestation) and reaches a peak at 32 weeks. Red cell mass increases steadily until term (from 1400 ml to 1700 ml), reaching a maximum of 20–30% above nonpregnant levels. This increase in erythro-poiesis is probably mainly explained by an increase in erythropoietin and, to a lesser extent, by an increase in human placental lactogen. Because the rise in plasma volume is proportionately greater than the rise in red cell mass, haemoglobin concentration and haematocrit fall, averaging approximately 11.5 g/100 ml and 34%, respectively, by 30 weeks. This dilution of haemoglobin and haematocrit levels in pregnancy is known as 'physiological anaemia' and is most marked at 32 weeks of gestation. The definition of anaemia must therefore be changed during pregnancy.

Other permanent elements in the blood are changed to a lesser extent in pregnancy. There is a modest rise in leucocyte count, although in the weeks after delivery the count may reach as high as 25 000 leucocytes/mm^3. This rise is primarily in neutrophils.

The effect of pregnancy on the platelet count is debated, but in some women there may be a modest decline by term, perhaps by as much as 25%. This fall is believed to be due to increased destruction of platelets not caused by immune factors and is termed gestational thrombocytopenia. Platelet size increases, indicating less mature platelets in the circulation.

IRON METABOLISM

Iron demand increases in pregnancy; the total extra requirement is around 1000 mg (500 mg for the increased red cell mass, 300 mg to meet the needs of the fetus and placenta and 200 mg to cover the obligatory excretion of iron). The extra requirement comes to approximately 4 mg/day (increased from 2.8 mg/day in a nonpregnant woman to 6.6 mg/day by the end of pregnancy).

In pregnancy, iron absorption is increased, owing to erythroid hyperplasia. Absorption is dependent on iron stores (represented by ferritin levels and iron binding saturation) and the amount of iron in the diet (including any supplements), but only 10–20% of ingested iron is absorbed. Absorption increases in the second and third trimesters, when the need is greatest, but may still not meet the needs of pregnancy and the puerperium. Consequently, iron deficiency anaemia is the most common haematological problem in pregnancy, with symptoms of dyspnoea, tiredness and occasionally faintness. Investigations usually reveal serum iron below 12 mmol/l and saturation of the total iron-binding capacity less than 15%. Thalassaemia trait may have a similar presentation to iron deficiency anaemia, so this possibility must be considered and excluded. Fortunately, maternal iron deficiency does not appear to reduce iron transport to the fetus.

HAEMOSTASIS IN PREGNANCY

Pregnancy is known to be a hypercoagulable state. This is due to an increase in coagulation factors and a decrease in fibrinolytic activity, changes that can be demonstrated from the third month of pregnancy. The concentrations of most of the coagulation factors (VII, VIII, X) increase in pregnancy, but factors XI and XIII do not. The rise in fibrinogen levels leads to an accelerated erythrocyte sedimentation rate, which, in late pregnancy, reaches double nonpregnant levels.

Routine coagulation screening in pregnancy is essentially normal; the activated partial thromboplastin time is unchanged or slightly shortened and the bleeding and clotting times are unaffected. Levels of antithrombin III (the main physiological inhibitor of thrombin and factor Xa) change little although, as plasma volume expands, production is increased to maintain this normal concentration. The activity of the fibrinolytic system remains low in pregnancy and labour, but returns to normal within one hour of delivery of the placenta. During the third stage of labour, myometrial contraction and increased coagulability of the blood combine to stop bleeding after delivery of the placenta.

Implications of maternal physiological changes on therapeutic drug administration

Absorption of drugs from the gastrointestinal tract may be impaired by gastric stasis, poor gut motility and, for some drugs, lower gastric pH. The increase in plasma volume means that the volume of distribution of the drug increases, so concentrations may be lower than expected. This is particularly important in women taking anticonvulsant drugs or thyroxine. Because of the increased glomerular filtration rate, excretion of drugs that are mainly excreted by the kidneys will be accelerated. These changes often require doses of a drug given during pregnancy to be adjusted.

Physiology of lactation

Development of human breasts takes place around the time of puberty (that is, prior to pregnancy). From then on, the adult breasts require surprisingly little hormonal stimulation to begin milk secretion: 14 days' exposure to estrogen followed by stimulation of prolactin secretion may be enough to establish milk production; this has been used to encourage lactation in women who wish to breastfeed an adopted baby. Prolactin is a long-chain polypeptide hormone and is essential for successful lactation. In early pregnancy, there is hyperplasia of the alveolar cells and lactiferous ducts, which is followed in later pregnancy by alveolar cell hypertrophy and the initiation of secretion. These changes are stimulated by the increased levels of prolactin and human placental lactogen. During pregnancy, the high levels of estrogen and progesterone hold this process in check and full milk production is achieved only after delivery, when progesterone and estrogen levels fall rapidly. Similarly, women who take estrogen while breastfeeding (for example, in the combined oral contraceptive pill) will find that milk production is decreased.

After delivery, the colostrum (or early milk) has a high concentration of protein relative to the concentration of lactose. However, over the following three days or so, the concentration of lactose increases sharply and the concentration of protein falls. However, the main reason for this fall in protein concentration is actually dilution. In order to maintain ionic equilibrium, water is drawn into the breast, causing an increase in milk volume while the total amount of protein in the milk remains unchanged.

Milk production averages 500–1000 ml/day and is highly dependent on continued suckling, which causes release of both prolactin and oxytocin. In women who do not suckle, milk production gradually falls and may persist for 3–4 weeks postpartum. In breastfeeding mothers, equilibrium is reached after around three weeks whereby milk production is tailored to the amount taken by the baby. Interestingly, mothers who are breastfeeding twins produce twice as much milk. A breastfeeding woman requires 2950 kcal/day. The recommended daily calorie intake is 2700 kcal (2200 kcal for the nonlactating nonpregnant requirement plus 500 kcal towards the energy requirement of the milk); an extra 250 kcal/day required for milk should come from maternal fat stores laid down during pregnancy.

The suckling stimulus sends afferent impulses to the hypothalamus that lead to a surge of prolactin release. This surge reaches a peak around 30 minutes after the baby is put to the breast and gradually declines to basal levels by 120 minutes. The control of prolactin release from the anterior pituitary is primarily via prolactin inhibitory factors from the hypothalamus that are secreted into the pituitary portal blood system. The most important prolactin inhibitory factor is dopamine. In fact, dopamine agonists, such as bromocriptine and cabergoline, can be used in the early puerperium to suppress milk production in women who do not wish to breastfeed. Conversely, dopamine antagonists such as metoclopramide increase prolactin levels and are sometimes used in breastfeeding women to stimulate milk production. Thyrotrophin-releasing hormone may also play a role in stimulating prolactin production. After the

sixth week postpartum, both basal prolactin levels and the peak level following suckling gradually decline; the greater the frequency and duration of suckling, the slower the decline.

Suckling also stimulates oxytocin release. The afferent impulses trigger the synthesis of this octapeptide hormone from specialised neurons in the supraoptic and paraventricular nuclei of the hypothalamus and its release from the posterior pituitary gland. This neuroendocrine reflex can also be initiated by the mother hearing her baby cry or even thinking about breastfeeding. In this way, the release of oxytocin, which typically occurs in short one-minute bursts, may begin even before the baby is put to the breast. Oxytocin binds to specific receptors on the myoepithelial cells, which surround the alveolar (milk-producing) cells in the breasts and are longitudinally arranged in the walls of the milk ducts. Contraction of the myoepithelial cells forces the milk into the ducts; contraction of the longitudinally arranged cells in the duct walls causes the ducts to dilate and allows milk to flow more easily towards the nipple. Both prolactin and oxytocin are necessary for successful breastfeeding; in general terms, prolactin stimulates the production of milk, while oxytocin stimulates its ejection (or let down).

Table 31.3 shows the typical composition of breast milk. The composition varies from woman to woman, over time in an individual woman and even differs between the beginning and end of the same feed. The

TABLE 31.3 **Constituents of breast milk**

Constituent	Content/100 ml
ENERGY	75 kcal
PROTEIN	1.1 g
Casein	40 (% of protein)
Whey protein	60 (% of protein)
LACTOSE	6.8 g
FAT	4.5 g
SODIUM	7 mmol
CHLORIDE	11 mmol

Source: This table was published in Lactation. Howie P. In *Turnbull's Obstetrics*. 3rd ed. Edinburgh: Churchill Livingstone. Copyright Elsevier; 2001.

TABLE 31.4 **Daily vitamin requirements in nonpregnant, pregnant and lactating women**

Vitamin	Nonpregnant	Pregnant	Lactating
A (microgram)	800	1000	1200
B$_1$ (mg)	1	1.3	1.3
B$_2$ (mg)	1.5	1.8	2
Niacin (mg)	15	20	20
Pantothenic acid (mg)	5	10	10
B$_6$ (mg)	2	2.5	2.5
Folic acid (microgram)	200	500	400
B$_{12}$ (mg)	2	3	3
C (mg)	30	60	80
D (microgram)	10	10	10
E (mg)	10	12	11
K	90mg	90mg	90mg

FIGURE 31.6 **Micronutrient supplements for pregnant women**

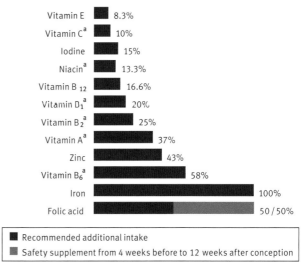

Vitamin E — 8.3%
Vitamin C[a] — 10%
Iodine — 15%
Niacin[a] — 13.3%
Vitamin B$_{12}$ — 16.6%
Vitamin D$_1$[a] — 20%
Vitamin B$_2$[a] — 25%
Vitamin A[a] — 37%
Zinc — 43%
Vitamin B$_6$[a] — 58%
Iron — 100%
Folic acid — 50 / 50%

■ Recommended additional intake
■ Safety supplement from 4 weeks before to 12 weeks after conception

[a] Vitamins to be taken from 4 months of pregnancy onwards.

Schwarz Pharma, www.ferro-info.com.

most important factor, however, is the time since the birth, suggesting that the milk is adapted in a very sensitive way to the changing needs of the baby. Thus, any statements about the composition of human breast milk are averages; these are the basis for the composition of artificial feeds.

The main carbohydrate in human milk is lactose. In the baby's intestine, it is broken down by the enzyme lactase into galactose and glucose. Of the protein in human milk, 40% is casein, compared with 80% of cow's milk. Other proteins include immunoglobulins and lactoferrin. Triglycerides are the main fat found in milk and are its most variable component, which means that the estimated energy content of 75 kcal/100 ml is only an approximation. Fat also carries the fat-soluble vitamins A, D, E and K. Vitamin D deficiency can lead to rickets, while vitamin K deficiency can lead to haemorrhagic disease of the newborn. A comparison of the daily vitamin requirements in nonpregnant, pregnant and lactating women is shown in Table 31.4 and the micronutrient supplementation regimen is illustrated in Figure 31.6.

Compared with cow's milk, human milk has approximately one-third the concentrations of sodium and chloride. This is advantageous in babies with diarrhoea

because a high solute load can exacerbate diarrhoea. There is little iron in breast milk.

IMMUNITY GAINED FROM BREAST MILK

The major immunoglobulin (Ig) in breast milk is IgA, with smaller amounts of IgM and IgG. The IgA in breast milk is poorly absorbed so most stays in the baby's intestinal tract, where it protects against infection. This is obviously particularly important in areas where there is poor access to clean water: in many developing countries, diarrhoea is one of the major causes of infant mortality. When a mother encounters a specific pathogen in her own gastrointestinal tract, plasma cells migrate from her gut to her breast where they release a specific IgA against that pathogen into the milk, thus protecting her baby. Clearly, the presence of immunoglobulin, as well as other anti-infective agents such as lysozyme and lactoferrin, is a major advantage of breast milk over artificial formula feed.

CONTRACEPTIVE EFFECT OF BREASTFEEDING

If a woman conceives during lactation, the rapidly rising levels of estrogen and progesterone will suppress milk production, despite the effects of the baby's suckling.

High prolactin levels during breastfeeding tend to suppress ovulation and therefore cause amenorrhoea. However, this is not a reliable form of contraception; at the end of a year of exclusive breastfeeding, 10% of women who do not use another form of contraception will have fallen pregnant. Nevertheless, it is estimated that, in developing countries, breastfeeding prevents more pregnancies than all other forms of contraception combined.

The onset of labour, myometrial contractility and cervical dilatation

The precise mechanism of the onset and maintenance of labour is still poorly understood. During pregnancy, myometrial quiescence is maintained by pro-pregnancy factors, the most important of which is probably progesterone. The fact that this quiescence is maintained despite the extreme stretching of the myometrial fibres and their tendency to contract when stretched is remarkable. Progesterone suppresses the formation of myometrial gap junctions and the effect of interleukin 8 (which causes cervical ripening). It also decreases uterine sensitivity to oxytocin. Antiprogesterones such as mifepristone cause cervical ripening and increase myometrial contractility. Catecholamines and relaxin may also play a role in the maintenance of uterine quiescence.

During the third trimester, maternal estrogen and corticotrophin-releasing hormone (CRH) gradually rise. Estradiol increases the concentration of oxytocin receptors in the myometrium and also increases oxytocin synthesis in the uterus. CRH increases prostaglandin synthesis and may stimulate myometrial contractility. The concentration of myometrial gap junctions increases as labour approaches; these are small communicating channels between adjacent myometrial cells that allow the transmission of electrical and chemical signals, thus promoting coordinated contraction. Estrogen promotes the formation of gap junctions. CRH also promotes an inflammatory-type mechanism by increasing the expression of inflammatory cytokines, such as interleukin 1β and interleukin 8, and cyclooxygenase type II (COX-2).

These gradual changes accumulate during the third trimester but it is not clear what event actually triggers the onset of labour. In some species (such as sheep),

an abrupt withdrawal of progesterone immediately precedes the onset of labour. For many years, investigators were convinced that the same must be true in humans, but it now seems certain that this is not the case. It is possible that there is a 'functional withdrawal' of progesterone, perhaps because it happens only locally within the fetal membranes or perhaps because, close to term, the dominant progesterone receptor within the uterus changes from type 1 to type 2.

Nitric oxide does not seem to play a significant role in the onset of labour. Neither does oxytocin; there is no significant rise in maternal oxytocin concentration immediately prior to labour (or indeed during labour). However, there is a marked increase in oxytocin receptors in the myometrium as term approaches so it seems certain that oxytocin plays an important role in labour, probably in combination with prostaglandins. Nevertheless, it does not seem to be the trigger for its onset. The fetus also secretes some oxytocin (the concentration in the umbilical artery is twice that in the umbilical vein) but it is not certain if this plays a role in labour. It is possible that the fetus triggers labour through increased cortisol release, which can stimulate placental CRH synthesis.

There is a rapid rise in the activity of COX-2 and other inflammatory cytokines at the onset of labour, leading some to compare labour to an inflammatory process. Increased COX-2 activity leads to an increase in prostaglandin synthesis; the amnion and chorion secrete primarily prostaglandin-E_2, while the decidua favours prostaglandin-$F_{2\alpha}$. Prostaglandin synthase inhibitors such as indometacin may thus be used in the management of preterm labour.

Prostaglandins act on the myometrium in the uterine body to cause contractions. Towards the end of pregnancy and in early labour, under the influence of prostaglandins and interleukin 8 (and perhaps in combination with relaxin and estrogen), neutrophils are attracted into the cervix where they release collagenase. This leads to gradual proteolysis of the collagen fibres in the cervix, making it softer and more stretchy; this process is known as cervical ripening.

Contraction of the myometrium results from the interaction of actin and myosin. This interaction is controlled by a calcium-modulated protein kinase.

FIGURE 31.7 **Physiology of labour**

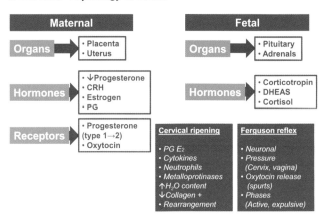

CRH = corticotrophin-releasing hormone | DHEAS = dehydroepiandrosterone sulphate | PG = prostaglandin

FIGURE 31.8 **Maternal–fetal interaction in the mechanism of onset of labour**

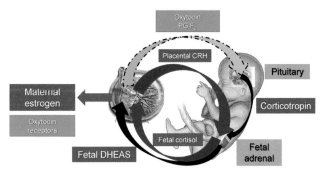

CRH = corticotrophin-releasing hormone | DHEAS = dehydroepiandrosterone sulphate | PG = prostaglandin

Communication between myometrial cells through gap junctions facilitates coordinated contraction of the uterus. Drugs that reduce available calcium, such as beta agonists (for example, ritodrine, salbutamol), thus cause uterine relaxation. Similarly, magnesium sulphate, which inhibits calcium influx into myometrial cells, inhibits the action of myosin-light-chain kinase, thus causing uterine relaxation. Calcium channel blockers also inhibit calcium influx through the cell membrane and are used for tocolysis. It seems that, once labour has started, there are multiple feedback mechanisms that further increase prostaglandin and cytokine activity; this process is currently poorly understood (Figures 31.7 and 31.8).

The third stage of labour

The third stage of labour is the time from delivery of the baby until delivery of the placenta and membranes. Soon after delivery of the baby, the uterus has a strong and sustained contraction. This reduces the surface area of the placental bed, thus shearing off the placenta. The placenta and membranes are usually delivered soon after. This contraction also helps to control bleeding from the vessels of the placental bed. It is likely that

prostaglan-dins such as prostaglandin-$F_{2\alpha}$ play a major role here; certainly, oxytocin levels do not change significantly during this time. This effect can be mimicked by the administration of synthetic prostaglandins (carboprost or misoprostol) to control postpartum haemorrhage.

Uterine involution

Immediately after delivery of the placenta, the uterus weighs around 900 g. By 7 days postpartum, it will weigh half that and by 6 weeks it will have almost returned to its prepregnancy size and weight of around 100 g. Uterine water, weight, muscle, protein and collagen all decrease in the same proportions during this time; these changes are likely to result from the rapid withdrawal of placental hormones after delivery.

Three days postpartum, the superficial layer of the decidua becomes necrotic and is shed with the lochia. Within 1 week, the uterine cavity has a new endometrial layer, with the exception of the placental bed; this takes around 3 weeks to establish an endometrial cover. The lochia gradually decreases over 3–6 weeks, changing in turn from red (lochia rubra) to pink (lochia serosa) to yellowish white (lochia alba).

FURTHER READING

BURROW G, FERRIS T. *Medical Complications During Pregnancy*. 4th ed. Philadelphia: Saunders; 1984.

CHAMBERLAIN G, PIPKIN F B. *Clinical Physiology in Obstetrics*. 3rd ed. Oxford: Blackwell Science; 1998.

COUSTAN D R. Maternal physiology. In: COUSTAN D R, HANING R V, SINGER D B, editors. *Human Reproduction: Growth and Development*. Boston: Little, Brown; 1995. p.161–81.

CRUIKSHANK D P, HAYS P M. Maternal physiology in pregnancy. In: GABBE S G, NIEBYL J R, SIMPSON J L, editors. *Obstetrics: Normal and Problem Pregnancies*. 2nd ed. New York: Churchill Livingstone; 1991. p.125–46.

CUNNINGHAM F G, MacDONALD P C, GANT N F, LEVENO K J, GILSTRAP L C. Maternal adaptations to pregnancy. In: *Williams Obstetrics*. 19th ed. Norwalk: Appleton and Lange; 1989. p.209–46.

DE SWIET M. *Medical Disorders in Obstetric Practice*. 4th ed. Oxford: Blackwell Publishing; 2002.

DE SWIET M, POSTON L, WILLIAMS D. Physiology. In: DE SWIET M, CHAMBERLAIN G, BENNETT P, editors. *Basic Science in Obstetrics and Gynaecology, A textbook for M R C O G part 1*. 3rd ed. Edinburgh: Churchill Livingstone; 2002. p.173–231.

HUNTER S, ROBSON S C. Adaptation of the maternal heart in pregnancy. *Br Heart J* 1992;68:540–3.

NELSON-PIERCY C. *Obstetric Medicine*. 3rd ed. Abingdon: Informa Healthcare U K; 2006.

OUZOUNIAN JG, ELKAYAM U. Physiologic changes during normal pregnancy and delivery. *Cardiol Clin* 2012;30(3): 317–29.

SAVU O, JURCUȚ R, GIUȘCĂ S, *et al*. Morphological and functional adaptation of the maternal heart during pregnancy. *Circ Cardiovasc Imaging* 2012;5(3):289–97.

WILLIAMS D J. Physiology of healthy pregnancy. In: WARRELL D A, COX T M, FIRTH J D, editors. *Oxford Textbook of Medicine*. 4th ed. Oxford: Oxford University Press; 2003. p.383–5.

CHAPTER 32

Fetal physiology

Aris T Papageorghiou

Fetal cardiovascular physiology

The fetal cardiovascular system develops early in fetal life, with blood circulation established by week 4. In this section, the heart and vessels are considered separately, but it is important to realise that development of these structures is synchronous.

THE FETAL HEART

Cardiac output

In the adult circulation, the circulatory system is in series and there are no shunts. Therefore, stroke volume of the right ventricle equals that of the left ventricle and cardiac output can be defined in terms of the volume of blood ejected by one ventricle (by convention the left) in 1 minute. This can be described by the equation:

Cardiac output = Stroke volume × Heart rate

In the fetus, there is shunting of blood through the ductus venosus, foramen ovale and ductus arteriosus (see fetal circulation below). As a result, the stroke volume of the fetal right ventricle is not equal to the stroke volume of the left ventricle: in fact about two-thirds of blood returns to the right ventricle and one-third to the left ventricle. Therefore, cardiac output in the fetus is measured as the total output of both ventricles, termed the combined ventricular output.

Myocardial function

The myocardium grows by cell division (hyperplasia) until birth and by cell enlargement (hypertrophy) after birth. Fetal heart myocytes have a much smaller amount of contractile tissue (30%) than in the adult (60%). Furthermore, fetal myofibrils are fewer in number and not arranged as parallel fibres but more randomly. Finally the fetal heart is less compliant (more stiff) than in the adult owing to the constraining effects of the lungs and chest wall in the absence of air. Owing to these factors, the fetal stroke volume is maximal with little functional reserve. The fetal heart has limited capacity to increase stroke volume. The principal way that cardiac output in the fetus is increased is, therefore, by an increase in heart rate.

Cardiac metabolism

In the adult heart, long-chain fatty acids are the main source of fuel, with glucose and lactate being minor fuels that are usually only used during hypoxia. In contrast, the fetal heart lacks the enzyme responsible for transport of fatty acids into mitochondria, which means that lactate and carbohydrates are the primary fuel.

Fetal heart rate

The fetal heart rate (FHR) is determined by depolarisation of the sinoatrial node, which is under sympathetic influence and inhibited by vagal (parasympathetic) stimulation. Vagal tone exerts the major influence, causing a fall in heart rate while sympathetic activity causes a rise in heart rate and myocardial contractility. Other factors influencing the heart rate include hormonal factors (epinephrine and norepinephrine released from the adrenal medulla), drugs and temperature. Finally, baroreceptors in the aortic arch and chemoreceptors are sensitive to changes in blood pressure and partial oxygen pressures, respectively, and mediate heart rate via the autonomic nervous system (Figure 32.1).

FIGURE 32.1 **Fetal heart rate modulators**

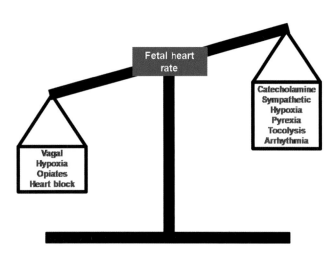

The FHR decreases with advancing gestation, a reflection of the maturing parasympathetic nervous system. The parasympathetic control also influences beat-to-beat variability via its interaction with the sympathetic system (a constant 'push and pull') and also changing vagal impulses. As these FHR patterns are controlled by the para-sympathetic and sympathetic nervous systems, the FHR is a reflection of the status of the fetal brain stem's medulla oblongata. Pathological events, such as fetal hypoxia, that affect these nerve fibre impulses can therefore be observed in FHR patterns. Other influences, such as the fetal sleep and wake states and drugs may also have effects.

Baseline FHR

After the early first trimester, the normal baseline FHR decreases with gestational age. At term, the normal FHR is 110–150 beats/minute.

Fetal tachycardia (at least 160 beats per minute for 10 minutes) can be normal at earlier gestation. Depending on the cause, it is usually mediated via catecholamine release, sympathetic nervous system stimulation or lack of parasympathetic stimulation. Common causes are fetal hypoxia (where it is accompanied by an evolving picture of loss of beat-to-beat variability and late decelerations), maternal pyrexia, chorioamnionitis, tocolysis using beta-sympathomimetic drugs or fetal heart rhythm abnormalities.

Bradycardia is defined as a heart rate of less than 110 beats/minute lasting 10 minutes or longer. Occasionally this can be the normal heart rate of the fetus, when it is an isolated abnormality with normal beat-to-beat variability and accelerations. If the bradycardia occurs with previously normal heart rate, it is usually the response to fetal hypoxia, in particular if the heart rate is below 100 beats/minute. Possible causes include cord compression, placental abruption, maternal hypotension or uterine hyperstimulation. Fetal heart block is a rare cause of persistent fetal bradycardia.

Beat-to-beat variability

The interval between successive fetal heart beats varies in normal circumstances. This beat-to-beat variability is defined as fluctuation in the FHR of at least two cycles per minute and it increases with gestational age. Beat-to-beat variability is divided into long-term variability (LTV) and short-term variability (STV). In clinical interpretation these two are usually reported together, but computerised cardiotocography (CTG) and fetal electrocardiogram (ECG) can measure LTV and STV separately. The LTV measures the oscillations or fluctuations of the heart rate within its baseline range (excluding accelerations or decelerations) and it is measured in cycles/minute. STV is measured in milliseconds and measures the R–R interval between two consecutive QRS complexes on the fetal ECG. Although modern external ultrasound devices use standard CTG to give a close approximation, STV can only be correctly measured using a scalp electrode. The STV therefore reflects the change in the FHR from one beat to the next and is the cause of the rapidly changing display in FHR when using fetal scalp electrode monitoring.

In the absence of any input from the autonomic nervous system, the fetal heart will beat at 110–150 beats/minute without variability. It is the constant modulation of this basal heart rate by the autonomic nervous system that produces the characteristic pattern of beat-to-beat variability. This is usually ascribed to the opposing actions of the sympathetic nervous system causing an increase and the parasympathetic causing a decrease in the FHR, but it may also be caused by repeated, short-lived parasympathetic impulses. Absent or reduced variability may simply be due to preterm gestation, but other causes include the fetal sleep cycle, fetal metabolic acidosis, drugs (central nervous system depressants such as magnesium sulphate, morphine or alcohol) or pre-existing neurologic abnormality.

Fetal heart accelerations

Fetal heart accelerations are defined as an increase of 15 beats/minute for at least 15 seconds. Accelerations are rarely seen in the presence of fetal hypoxia. Conversely, the absence of accelerations for more than 80 minutes correlates with increased neonatal morbidity. Accelerations are usually caused by fetal movements or stimulation (for example, vibroacoustic). Accelerations are thought to occur from direct sympathetic stimulation; repeated accelerations during uterine contractions may be due to mild umbilical vein compression leading to systemic hypotension, which triggers acceleration of FHR.

Fetal heart decelerations

Fetal heart decelerations are defined as a decrease of 15 beats/minute for at least 15 seconds. Decelerations are subclassified into early, variable and late decelerations. Early decelerations occur during uterine contractions. Fetal head compression leads to a transient reduction in fetal cerebral blood flow, hypoxia, hypercapna and hypertension. Triggering of baroreceptors causes parasympathetic stimulation, resulting in a reduction in heart rate.

Variable decelerations occur without a regular pattern in terms of relation with uterine contractions, duration and depth. They are thought to be caused by umbilical cord compression or stretching. The differential compression of umbilical vein and artery may be responsible for the variable appearance of the decelerations. Umbilical vein compression causes a transient reduction of venous return to the heart and reduction in blood pressure. Carotid body baroreceptors are triggered and stimulation of the sympathetic nervous system causes fetal tachycardia. Umbilical artery compression causes an increase in systemic vascular resistance and a rise in blood pressure, and baroreceptor-mediated parasympathetic stimulation causes fetal bradycardia. The frequently observed picture of an FHR deceleration with acceleration before and after its occurrence can be explained by the gradual compression of umbilical vein and then umbilical vein and artery, followed by a gradual release in reverse order. As the depth of variable decelerations is a reflection of baroreceptor stimulation rather than hypoxaemia, fetal wellbeing should be assessed based on the baseline rate, variability and presence of accelerations.

Late decelerations usually begin before the peak of the contraction and are defined as decelerations where the nadir of the deceleration is after the peak of the contraction. They usually have a slow recovery phase. During uterine contractions, the blood supply in the placental intervillous spaces temporarily stops. This means that gas exchange also ceases temporarily and, if there is reduced fetal reserve or uterine overactivity, this leads to a reduction in oxygen absorption (leading to hypoxaemia) and accumulation of lactic acid and carbon dioxide (and therefore acidosis). Hypoxaemia causes chemoreceptor stimulation and results in parasympathetic slowing of FHR. In addition, fetal myocardial hypoxia leads to inability of the myocardium to respond and to further bradycardia. This inability of the fetal heart to respond to autonomic nervous system stimulation often leads to a concomitant reduction in variability.

TRANSITIONAL EVENTS AT BIRTH

After birth, there is loss of the placental circulation and shunts between the pulmonary and systemic circulations. The cardiac output can then be measured as in the adult. There is a rapid change in the function of the myocardium, with an increase in myocardial contractility. During the first weeks, there is a preferential increase in left rather than right ventricular mass. In the myocardium, there is a switch from lactate and carbohydrate metabolism to using free fatty acids as the preferred fuel.

Fetal circulation

An important prerequisite for the understanding of fetal cardiovascular function is the fetal circulation and the differences with postnatal function. Unlike the adult heart, the four chambers of the fetal heart are arranged as a parallel system where the output of the right and left ventricles mix. This is due to shunts that normally close at birth. There are three such shunts, which are illustrated in Figures 32.2 and 32.3:

- ductus venosus: directs blood to the inferior vena cava
- foramen ovale: allows blood to pass from the right to the left atrium
- ductus arteriosus: connects the pulmonary artery to the aorta. It carries the output of the right ventricle owing to the higher pressure of the pulmonary compared with the systemic circulation.

Before birth, the pulmonary circuit is at high resistance, mainly becasue of compression of the pulmonary capillaries by the collapsed lung, the smooth muscle layer of the pulmonary arteries and the vasoconstrictive effects of low fetal partial pressure of oxygen (PO_2). At the same time, the systemic circulation is at low resistance to blood flow, owing to the large placental bed. The presence of shunts, high pulmonary resistance and low systemic resistance allows blood to be diverted from the lungs to the placenta.

FIGURE 32.2 **Main characteristics of the fetal circulation showing the fetal shunts**

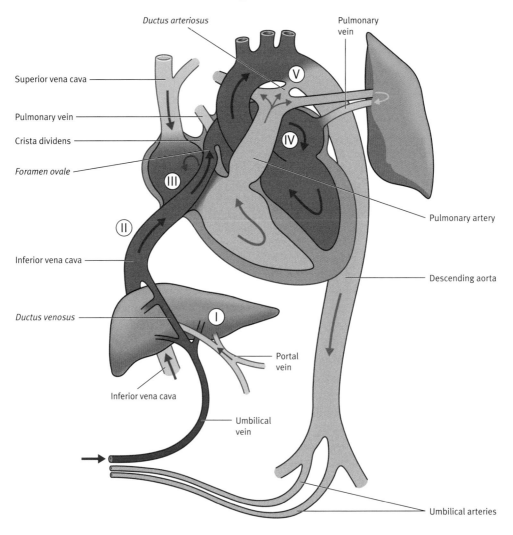

Red = fully oxygenated blood | blue = deoxygenated blood | red/blue = mixed blood | Shunts in italic

Source: Murphy PJ. The fetal circulation. *Continuing Education in Anaesthesia, Critical Care & Pain* 2005;5:107–12.

FIGURE 32.3 **Comparison of fetal and adult circulatory systems**

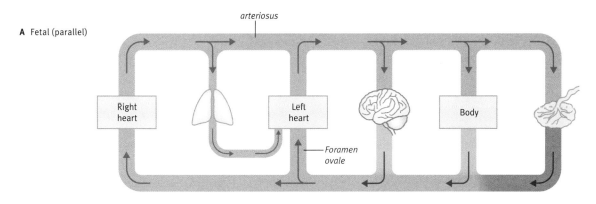

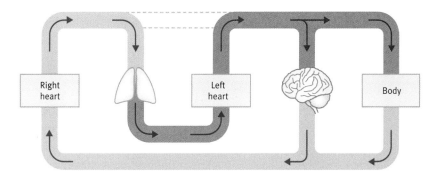

Adapted with permission from: Blackburn ST. *Maternal, Fetal and Neonatal Physiology.* 2nd ed. St Louis: Saunders; 2003.

An important feature of the fetal circulation is that, although there is mixing of oxygenated and deoxygenated blood, this does not result in homogenous semioxygenated blood. Rather, preferential streaming of oxygenated blood occurs from the umbilical vein via the ductus venosus and foramen ovale into the left ventricle and proximal aorta, allowing highly oxygenated blood to reach the coronary and carotid arteries. Deoxygenated blood enters the right atrium from the inferior and superior vena cava, through the tricuspid valve into the right ventricle, pulmonary trunk and ductus arteriosus, entering the descending aorta and the umbilical arteries. The physiology of the three fetal shunts allows this preferential streaming of blood.

DUCTUS VENOSUS

The ductus venosus connects the umbilical vein to the inferior vena cava (IVC) at the inlet to the heart. The ductus venosus has a small diameter (0.5 mm at midgestation to about 2 mm at later gestation) and this narrowing causes an acceleration in blood velocity. This high-velocity blood flow allows preferential streaming of the oxygenated blood coming from the ductus venosus and via the IVC by exerting pressure on the flap-valve of the foramen ovale. About 30% of the umbilical blood is shunted through the ductus venosus at midgestation and this drops to about 20% at 30–40 weeks. This is likely to be because of the development of the fetal liver at later gestations requiring a larger proportion of the umbilical venous blood.

FORAMEN OVALE

The foramen ovale is a communication between right and left atria and is formed by the overlap of the septum secundum over the septum primum, producing a flap-valve. The higher pressure in the right atrium ensures that the valve is maintained open and allows a right-to-left flow of blood. Blood enters the right atrium from the IVC. Within the IVC, blood flow is not uniform, with the highly oxygenated blood that originated from the umbilical vein flowing anteriorly and to the left within the IVC. As blood enters the atrium from the IVC, it is divided into two streams by the free edge of the atrial septum (the crista dividens). The high-velocity oxygenated blood is shunted towards the left, through the foramen ovale and into the left atrium. The lower velocity, less oxygenated blood is shunted towards the right, mixing with blood from the superior vena cava and coronary sinus.

The net result of this is that blood in the left ventricle is more highly oxygenated than in the right ventricle. The highly oxygenated blood in the left ventricle is pumped into the ascending aorta and 90% of it flows into the coronary arteries, left carotid and subclavian arteries; the remaining 10% flows via the aortic arch and into the descending aorta, mixing with blood from the ductus arteriosus.

DUCTUS ARTERIOSUS

The ductus arteriosus connects the pulmonary trunk to the descending aorta. This allows blood to bypass the immature lungs. After right ventricular contraction, blood flows mainly through this vessel and into the descending aorta, with about 13% of the combined cardiac output entering the pulmonary circulation, to support lung development. After 30 weeks, the proportion of blood flow to the lungs increases to about 20% of the combined cardiac output. The patency of the ductus arteriosus is maintained by the vasodilator effects of prostaglandins (PGE_1 and PGE_2) and prostacyclin (PGI_2) and reduced fetal oxygen tension.

FETOPLACENTAL CIRCULATION

Blood flow from the fetus to the placenta is via the umbilical arteries and this represents about 33% of the combined ventricular output at 20 weeks of gestation and about 20% after 32 weeks. With increasing fetal growth, the absolute volume of umbilical blood flow increases throughout gestation, but it is lowest at

41 weeks if normalised for fetal weight. The resistance to blood flow through the placental vascular bed has no neural regulation and catecholamines have little effect.

CONTROL OF FETAL CIRCULATION

The control of the fetal circulation is complex and poorly understood. The peripheral circulation of the fetus is under a tonic adrenergic influence (predominantly vasoconstriction), probably mediated by circulating catecholamines and in particular by norepinephrine. Other factors such as arginine vasopressin, the renin–angiotensin system and prostaglandins also have a role. Baroreceptors in the aortic arch and carotid arteries are sensitive to changes in arterial blood pressure. Chemoreceptors that are sensitive to changes in the oxygen content ensure that, during hypoxaemia, the blood flow increases to the brain, myocardium and adrenals and decreases to the lungs and lower body. This phenomenon of arterial redistribution is used in clinical practice in the monitoring of fetal growth restriction.

MEETING FETAL OXYGEN NEEDS

The mixing of oxygenated and deoxygenated blood in the fetal circulation means that oxygen content is lower in the fetus than in postnatal life. The mechanisms to ensure adequate oxygen delivery are:

- preferential delivery of oxygen-rich blood to the myocardium and brain by presence of shunts
- preferential shunting of oxygen-poor blood to the placenta for oxygenation
- high heart rate
- fetal haemoglobin, which results in oxygen binding even at a low PO_2, which results in high saturation, even at low oxygen tensions.

TRANSITIONAL EVENTS AT BIRTH

Shortly after birth, the low-resistance placental circulation is lost. This loss of blood flow through the placenta means that the systemic resistance is approximately doubled and pressures in the aorta, left ventricle and left atrium increase. At the same time, with the first breath of air there is lung expansion, vasodilation in the pulmonary vascular bed due to higher oxygen tension and a fall in the pulmonary vascular resistance.

The changes in the relative pressures between pulmonary and systemic systems mean that there is a change from the parallel (fetal) system with placental respiration to a neonatal circulatory system in series with pulmonary respiration.

The fall in pulmonary and rise in systemic pressures cause a massive reduction in blood flow through the ductus arteriosus. The ductus arteriosus then closes spontaneously, on average 2 days after birth, most likely because of the increase in oxygen tension. Failure of the closure of the ductus arteriosus can lead to the common problem of 'patent ductus arteriosus' in the postnatal period and this is more common in premature infants or those with low oxygen tensions from continuing hypoxia. The ductus arteriosus is sensitive to the influence of prostaglandin E_2, which maintains the patency of the vessel. Administration of prostaglandin synthase inhibitors (such as indometacin) can be used postnatally in cases of patent ductus arteriosus for therapeutic purposes, but can cause severe constriction of the ductus arteriosus antenatally if administered during the third trimester.

The ductus venosus usually closes 1–3 weeks after birth in term infants. Unlike closure of the ductus arteriosus, it is thought that in the ductus venosus this is mechanical. Finally, there is functional closure of the flap-like opening of the foramen ovale due to the increase in left atrial pressure. Anatomical closure of the septum primum and septum secundum occurs in the majority of cases by the age of one year. Persistent

patent foramen ovale can lead to paradoxical embolic events in later life.

Fetal respiratory physiology

Normal fetal lung development depends on normal anatomical development, fetal breathing movements, absorption of lung fluid at birth and surfactant production.

ANATOMICAL DEVELOPMENT

Lung development occurs in five stages, which are described below and in Table 32.1.

The embryonic phase is characterised by an outpouching of the ventral wall of the foregut. This is separated from the oesophagus by a septum and the lung bud divides into the two main bronchi and subsequently subdivides into the tracheobronchial tree. Pulmonary arteries, which develop from the sixth aortic arches, develop alongside these airways.

During the pseudoglandular phase, there is continued branching of both airways and blood vessels. By 16–17 weeks of gestation, this branching is complete and the total number of pre-acinar airways will not change further.

During the canalicular stage, the acinar structures are formed. These will give rise to the gas-exchanging structures of the lung and contain the terminal bronchioles, alveolar ducts and primitive alveoli.

The saccular phase is characterised by enlargement of the peripheral airways and thinning of the airway walls

TABLE 32.1 **Stages of fetal lung development**

Stage	Time period	Developmental events
Embryonic	Conception to 7 weeks of gestation	Formation of main bronchi and bronchopulmonary segments
Pseudoglandular	7–17 weeks	Branching of airways and blood vessels, forming the conducting airways of the lung
Canalicular	17–27 weeks	Formation of the acini, the gas-exchanging parts of the lung
Saccular	28–36 weeks	Enlargement of peripheral airways, thinning of the airway walls to form terminal sacs
Alveolar	36 weeks of gestation to 2 years post-birth	Formation of definitive alveoli

to form a large number of terminal sacs. This allows a large increase in the surface area of the lung.

The formation of definitive alveoli marks the alveolar stage, which continues well into the postnatal period. About 1000 alveoli will form per acinus.

FETAL BREATHING MOVEMENTS

Fetal breathing movements occur from the end of the first trimester and increase in frequency and strength with gestation. It is thought that fetal breathing movements regulate lung growth by lung fluid regulation and lung cell growth. The importance of fetal breathing movements has been demonstrated in animal experiments, which have shown that ablation of the phrenic nerve, which innervates the diaphragm, leads to lung hypoplasia. Fetal breathing movements increase after a maternal meal, maternal glucose administration and conditions of acidosis. They are decreased by fetal hypoxia, maternal consumption of alcohol and sedative drugs.

LUNG FLUID

Lung fluid is mainly formed from secretions of alveolar epithelial cells and this begins at the canalicular stage of development. Fluid is swallowed or released into the amniotic fluid, but lung fluid only contributes a small amount to amniotic fluid volume. Lung fluid is essential for normal lung development and lung hypoplasia can result if lung fluid is decreased or there is an absence of amniotic fluid.

SURFACTANT

Surfactant is a lipoprotein produced by type II pneumocytes. About 90% is made of lipids, with two-thirds of this being dipalmitoylphosphatidylcholine (DPPC). The remaining 10% of surfactant is made of proteins, including surfactant proteins A–D. Surfactant has a major role in pulmonary function. Its main functions include reducing the surface tension part of elastic recoil, thus increasing pulmonary compliance and allowing normal inflation. The same mechanism prevents lung collapse at the end of expiration. The surface tension is mainly regulated by DPPC, with surfactant protein B and surfactant protein C allowing surfactant spread over the alveolar surfaces. Surfactant protein A and surfactant protein D have pathogen-recognising functions and aid innate immunity.

Glucocorticoids, such as betamethasone and dexamethasone, allow accelerated surfactant synthesis and lung maturation. Other factors that have been shown to stimulate lung maturity are thyroid hormones, prolactin and catecholamines. Delayed lung maturation is seen in maternal diabetes and it is unclear whether this is an effect of insulin administration or hyperglycaemia. Androgens also delay lung maturation, which may explain why male infants are more likely to develop respiratory distress than female infants of similar gestational age.

TRANSITIONAL EVENTS AT BIRTH

Even before the onset of labour, lung fluid secretion falls and reabsorption of fluid from the alveolar spaces begins. With the first breath of air into the lungs, an air/liquid interface is created and surfactant facilitates the formation of the alveolar lining. The pulmonary fluid continues to be replaced by air and most has been actively absorbed (across the alveolar wall into capillaries and lymphatics) within 2 hours of breathing. The transition from fetal breathing movements to normal ventilation is triggered by a series of tactile and thermal stimuli. The first breaths are important in inflating the fluid-filled lungs. These initial inflation breaths generate pressures that are 10–15 times greater than that needed for subsequent breathing. Once the alveoli are aerated, breathing requires minimal negative intrathoracic pressure to maintain a normal tidal volume and alveolar surface tension is stabilised by the surfactant released by distension and ventilation of the lungs.

Fetal haematology

Fetal haematopoiesis occurs in three overlapping periods:

- mesoblastic period: in the yolk sac, from 14 days to 12 weeks
- hepatic period: from 6 weeks and peaking from 10 to 18 weeks, when it is the main source of fetal haematopoiesis
- myeloid period: from 8 weeks through to the adult period. Blood cells develop from stem cells, which

first appear in the yolk sac but migrate to these fetal tissues where they give rise to primitive cells in the first instance, followed by definitive cells.

FORMATION OF FETAL BLOOD CELLS

Fetal red blood cell formation occurs independently of the mother and is controlled endogenously. While primitive cells contain embryonic haemoglobin, which is not controlled by erythropoietin (EPO), definitive red blood cells containing mainly fetal haemoglobin (HbF) are regulated by EPO. Fetal EPO, produced initially from the liver and then the kidneys, increases from 20 weeks onwards and increased EPO production occurs in hypoxic conditions such as placental insufficiency and severe maternal anaemia. Fetal white blood cell formation begins at 6 weeks in the liver, but they are also produced in the spleen, thymus and lymphatic system. Circulating granulocytes increase rapidly in the third trimester and at birth they are equal to or greater than found in adults. Platelet production begins in the yolk sac at 6 weeks and in the liver from 8 weeks.

FETAL HAEMOGLOBIN

Adult haemoglobin (Hb) is made of two alpha (or alpha-like) and two beta (or beta-like) globulin chains. During development, embryonic haemoglobins (HbGower 1, HbGower 2, HbPortland) are replaced from 10 weeks by HbF, which consists of two alpha and two gamma chains. This is the predominant haemoglobin from 10 weeks and peaks at over 90% of haemoglobin at 32 weeks, declines to 60–80% of haemoglobin at birth and is present until 3–6 months postnatally. Adult haemoglobin (HbA) is present from 10 weeks of gestation in small amounts and increases rapidly in the third trimester. The switch from HbF to HbA as the predominant haemoglobin occurs between birth and 12 weeks of postnatal life.

Oxygen affinity of fetal haemoglobin

All forms of haemoglobin bind oxygen, but the affinity with which this occurs varies. An important feature of HbF is that it binds oxygen with greater affinity than HbA. This is because HbA binds with 2,3-diphosphoglycerate

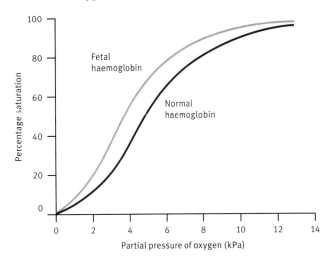

FIGURE 32.4 **Oxygen dissociation curves for fetal and adult blood**

(2,3-DPG) reducing its oxygen affinity, while HbF does not bind 2,3-DPG. The differences in affinity between HbA and HbF can be shown graphically using the oxygen saturation curve (Figure 32.4). The value of P_{50} is the partial pressure of oxygen at which Hb is 50% saturated: the lower the P_{50}, the greater the affinity for oxygen. The value of P_{50} for HbF is 3.6 kPa, whereas for HbA P_{50} is about 4.8 kPa. The oxygen saturation curve is therefore shifted to the left for HbF when compared with HbA. This greater affinity of HbF allows oxygen transfer across the placenta. Although this also reduces the ability to release oxygen to the tissues, fetal tissue acid–base balance aids oxygen delivery (Table 32.2).

Acid elution of fetal haemoglobin and the Kleihauer test

HbF is more resistant to alkali denaturation and acid elution than HbA and this forms the basis of the Kleihauer test. In this test, a maternal blood smear is prepared and an acid bath removes HbA. Staining of HbF allows pink-stained fetal cells to be seen on microscopy, while HbA-containing maternal cells appear as pale 'ghost cells'. A simple count allows estimation of the amount of fetal blood in the maternal circulation, as may occur after a fetal–maternal haemorrhage.

Persistence of maternally derived HbF in the maternal blood cells, as can occur in haemoglobinopathies, needs to be taken into account to avoid false interpretation.

TABLE 32.2 **Maternal–fetal PO_2 gradient**

	Maternal	Fetal
PO_2	80–100 mmHg 45 mmHg (placental pool)	Umbilical artery (20 mmHg) Umbilical vein (30 mmHg)
Hb	12 g/dl	17 g/dl
Blood O_2 content	15 ml/100 ml	25 ml/100 ml

Hb, haemoglobin O_2, oxygen, PO_2, partial pressure of oxygen

Postnatally the ability of the Kleihauer test to assess fetal red cells in the maternal circulation will depend on the persistence of the cells. If the mother and fetus are ABO, incompatible fetal red blood cells may be eliminated from the maternal bloodstream very quickly and a Kleihauer test should be performed as soon as possible in these circumstances.

FETAL IMMUNE DEVELOPMENT

Precursors of the immune system develop in the embryonic yolk sac and migrate to the liver, spleen, bone marrow and thymus. Lymphoid stem cells give rise to B lymphocytes (from the liver) and T cells (from the thymus). B cells appear in peripheral blood from 12 weeks and mature T cells from 14 weeks. Although immunoglobulin synthesis begins at 12 weeks of gestation, production remains low throughout fetal life and the rise in immunoglobulin (Ig) G seen in the second trimester is caused by placental transfer of maternal IgG. As IgM does not cross the placental barrier, any increase in IgM is fetal in origin and may be due to intrauterine infection. Although neutrophils and macrophages can be isolated from 14 weeks, their levels in fetal peripheral blood remain low until the last trimester. From 32 weeks, the function of the immune system rapidly approaches that of a term infant, whereas before this time the system is largely immature, an important aspect of care of the preterm infant.

TRANSITIONAL EVENTS AT BIRTH

The neonatal blood parameters change depending on the degree of placental transfusion. Late clamping of the cord and holding the newborn below the level of the

placenta results in a significant increase in blood volume and red blood cell mass. Whether this is of benefit is controversial. In preterm infants it has been suggested that hyperbilirubinaemia may result from excessive placental transfusion; however, hypovolaemia may result if immediate clamping occurs. Haemoglobin levels in newborns are usually around 16.5–17.5 g/dl with a haematocrit of around 53% and mean white blood cell counts are 15 000/mm^3. Red blood cell and white blood cell counts increase in the initial hours after birth before decreasing by day 4–7. Platelet counts are similar to adult values but increase throughout the first month of postnatal life. Platelet activity is reduced in the neonate and the risk of bleeding and coagulopathy is increased, particularly in preterm infants. This is compounded by the low levels of vitamin K-dependent clotting factors.

Fetal renal physiology

Functionally, urine production begins at 9–10 weeks and reabsorption in the loop of Henle begins by 12 weeks. Unlike the adult (where about 20% of cardiac output reaches the kidneys), only 2–3% of fetal cardiac output goes to the kidneys; fetal fluid and electrolyte balance is mainly under the control of the placenta rather than the kidney. Urine production is present and after 18 weeks fetal urine is the major contributor to amniotic fluid, while before 16 weeks most amniotic fluid is produced by the fetal skin and placenta. Therefore, reduced urine production from midgestation is an important cause of reduced amniotic fluid volume and can be seen in fetal growth restriction.

The fetal kidney has limited ability in concentrating urine and fetal urine is hypotonic. The ability to concentrate urine increases with fetal renal maturation and advancing gestation. Although the number of nephrons is similar to the adult from about 34 weeks of gestation, their functional maturity is not established until postnatal life. Preterm infants are therefore less able to maintain fluid and electrolyte balance.

TRANSITIONAL EVENTS AT BIRTH

After birth, there is a dramatic increase in renal blood flow to the kidney, increasing from 2–3% of combined ventricular output in the fetus to about 10% of cardiac output at age 4 days. With renal blood flow, glomerular filtration rate also increases at birth and this continues with a doubling by 2 weeks of neonatal life.

Gastrointestinal physiology

Although nutrition is provided by the placenta, functional development of the gut during fetal life begins early in gestation and swallowing movements are seen from 12 weeks. The rate of swallowing increases with age and reaches 250 ml/day at term, making swallowing an important aspect of amniotic fluid volume regulation. Intestinal villi start developing from 7 weeks of gestation and by 20 weeks these are well developed. Peristaltic motility develops gradually and is mature by the third trimester; intestinal absorptive processes are only partially available before 26 weeks of gestation. The fetal liver is mainly a haemopoietic organ during intra-uterine life and functionally it is the placenta that handles metabolic processes. Liver and pancreatic secretions develop early in gestation. Although the nutritional value of amniotic fluid and cells are in doubt, these enzymes are thought to play a role in preventing bowel obstruction due to cellular debris. Functional development of the gastrointestinal tract is summarised in Table 32.3.

MECONIUM

Meconium is composed of water (about 75%), intestinal secretions, squamous cells, lanugo hair, bile pigments (responsible for the green colour), pancreatic enzymes and blood. It appears from about 10–12 weeks of gestation and slowly moves into the colon by 16 weeks. Meconium passage is a normal developmental event and 98% of newborns pass meconium in the first 48 hours after birth.

Although the relationship between fetal hypoxia and increased intestinal peristalsis has been considered for many years, the precise mechanism of how stress or hypoxia results in meconium passage is unclear. The effects of meconium depend on the concentration of meconium, duration of exposure and the presence of

TABLE 32.3 **Functional development of the fetal gastrointestinal system**

Development	Gestational age (weeks)
SUCKING AND SWALLOWING	
Swallowing	10–14
Immature suck–swallow	33–36
STOMACH	
Motility and secretion	20
PANCREAS	
Zymogen granules	20
LIVER	
Bile metabolism	11
Bile secretion	22
SMALL INTESTINE	
Active transport of amino acids	14
Glucose transport	18
Fatty acid absorption	24

Adapted with permission from: Blackburn ST. *Maternal, Fetal and Neonatal Physiology*. 2nd ed. St Louis: Saunders; 2003.

associated stress factors (for example, hypoxia and infection).

Meconium-stained amniotic fluid is present in about 12% of all deliveries, but its incidence increases with gestational age and it is present in 30% of post-term pregnancies. Meconium aspiration syndrome occurs in about 5% of infants with meconium-stained amniotic fluid. It is dependent on the presence of both meconium and fetal hypoxia and is thought to be caused by gasping actions of the fetus causing aspiration of meconium into the lungs. This causes a combination of mechanical blockage of small airways and production of chemical pneumonitis by the inhaled meconium particles. In addition, meconium directly inhibits pulmonary function by displacing surfactant and inhibiting its function and promotes lung tissue inflammation by activating neutrophils and macrophages. If postnatal hypoxia continues, meconium contributes to pulmonary vasospasm, hypertrophy of the pulmonary musculature and pulmonary hypertension.

TRANSITIONAL EVENTS AT BIRTH

Gut maturation continues postnatally and is partly under the influence of gastrointestinal hormones and neuropeptides. A major stimulus for their release is commencement of enteral feeding and human milk, which is rich in trophic factors and antibodies, is the preferred feeding option.

Fetal skin physiology

Skin is permeable to water until midpregnancy, with a net loss of water across the skin by transudation. Initially, the water content of skin is close to 100% but this begins to decrease from 20 weeks owing to keratinisation in the epidermis and an increase in connective tissue and vernix caseosa. This thin fatty film forms from 17 weeks and is made up of sebaceous gland secretions and desquamated skin cells. Although this film prevents loss of water and electrolytes, the fetal skin continues to contribute to amniotic fluid production.

Fetal neurological system

The fetal central nervous system is one of the earliest systems to begin development but also the latest to mature. Lower level structures, including the basal ganglia, thalamus, midbrain and brainstem form first, while the cerebrum and cerebellum form later. Neuronal proliferation, migration, organisation and myelination are overlapping processes that continue throughout fetal life into the postnatal period: in particular, glial proliferation remains active throughout childhood.

Neurons proliferate from 8–20 weeks of gestation, with the most active period from 12–16 weeks. Neurons begin migration from the periventricular germinal areas from 8 weeks, in a radial fashion into areas where grey matter is established. By 20 weeks, the cortex has acquired the majority of neurons, while, in the cerebellum, proliferation and migration continue until 1 year postnatally. Organisation, including synapse formation, begins at 12 weeks of gestation and peaks in the last trimester of pregnancy. Alignment and orientation of cortical neurons continues well into the postnatal period.

Myelinisation begins in midgestation (around 24 weeks), peaks at birth and, especially in the corpus callosum, continues throughout childhood. Biochemical activity in the fetal brain is evident from 16 weeks. Spontaneous electroencephalographic activity appears at around 20 weeks and becomes synchronised at 26 weeks, while wake/sleep cycles are seen from 30 weeks.

PERIPHERAL NERVOUS SYSTEM

Derived from cells of the neural crest, ganglia appear at 4–5 weeks of gestation. Nerve fibres grow from the spinal plate and form the ventral root (motor fibres) and dorsal root (sensory fibres).

Motor movements depend not only on innervation but also intact muscle cells; body movements appear from 7 weeks and limb movements from 9 weeks of gestation. Motor movements become more coordinated as gestation advances and complex movements are seen in the third trimester. Maternal perception of movements occurs from around 16 weeks in multiparous women but may be as late as 24 weeks in the first pregnancy. There is a steady increase in movements, but a gradual reduction near term is common, most likely owing to reduced space within the uterus. A marked reduction in the quality or frequency of movements experienced by the mother can reflect fetal hypoxia (as in fetal growth restriction) or fetal anaemia (as in rhesus disease).

The earliest sensory abilities are touch sensation and afferent synapses develop from 10 weeks. However, spinothalamic connections do not occur until midgestation and myelination not until 30 weeks. The development of smell, taste, hearing and vision all begin at about 23–26 weeks.

FETAL PAIN

Although nociceptors first appear at 10 weeks of gestation in the fetus, their presence alone is not sufficient for the fetus to experience pain – electrical activity also has to be conducted from the nociceptors via the spinal cord to the brain.

Although the fetus may display a physiological stress response to painful stimuli (activation of the fetal hypothalamic–pituitary–adrenal axis) from around 19 weeks and the cortex is thought to be able to process sensory input from 24 weeks, controversy remains as to whether the fetus can perceive noxious stimuli at the cortical level as painful. Using activation of the hypothalamic pituitary–adrenal axis as a surrogate indicator of fetal pain has limitations. Pain perception during fetal (or indeed neonatal) development does not engage the same structures involved in pain processing as those used by human adults and this supports the argument that the fetus does not feel pain until late gestation.

TRANSITIONAL EVENTS

The main transitional event in nervous system activity is during the change from the intrauterine to the extrauterine environment. The nervous system continues to mature, but requires adaptation to independent breathing, oral nutrition, thermoregulation by the autonomic nervous system, movements against gravitational effects and adaptation to sensory stimuli by the motor and sensory systems.

Physiology of amniotic fluid

Amniotic fluid has protective, thermoregulatory and nutritive effects and allows movements and growth of the fetus. The amount of amniotic fluid is about 50 ml at 12 weeks and 150 ml at 16 weeks. It then increases by roughly 50 ml/week until 34 weeks (about 1000 ml) before a decrease to about 500 ml at term.

PRODUCTION AND REMOVAL

There are six areas where exchange of amniotic fluid occurs: the fetal renal system production, lung, skin, gastrointestinal tract, across the uterine wall and across the placenta/membranes and umbilical cord. Amniotic fluid production is initially from the amniotic membrane and transfer via the fetal skin occurs before keratinisation begins at 20 weeks. In the second trimester, the two primary sources of amniotic fluid are fetal urine and lung liquid. Fetal urine is the main contributor of amniotic fluid at this stage, with reduced production owing to urinary tract abnormalities leading to oligohydramnios, which is not usually evident before 16 weeks.

Amniotic fluid removal is caused by fetal swallowing and absorption into fetal blood across the surface of the placenta. Passive exchanges across the fetal skin and umbilical cord and via the transmembranous pathway (across the uterine wall) are not significant during the latter half of gestation (Figure 32.5).

FIGURE 32.5 **Summary of fluid flow in to and out of the amniotic space in late gestation**

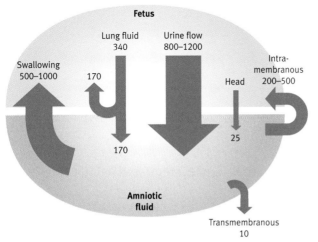

Arrow sizes are proportional to the flow rate | All measurements are in ml/day

FIGURE 32.6 **Composition of amniotic fluid**

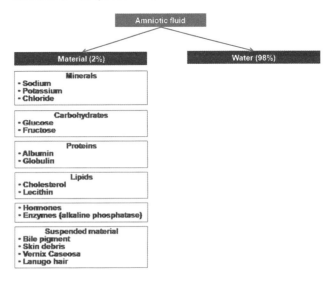

COMPOSITION

Over 98% of amniotic fluid is water. Minerals (mainly sodium, potassium, chloride), carbohydrates (glucose, fructose), proteins (albumin and globulins), lipids (chol-esterol, lecithin), hormones, enzymes (mainly alkaline phosphatase) and suspended materials (bile pigments, skin debris, vernix caseosa, lanugo hair) make up the remainder. The composition varies with gestational age; as fetal urine production begins to contribute

to amniotic fluid, the osmolarity decreases slightly compared with fetal blood. After keratinisation of the fetal skin, amniotic fluid osmolarity decreases further. The osmolarity of the amniotic fluid decreases with advancing gestation, owing to the contribution of hypotonic fetal urine, and sodium as well as chloride levels decrease with improving fetal kidney function. Amniotic fluid is thought to have antibacterial properties, mainly due to the presence of lysozymes and peroxidase (Figure 32.6).

FURTHER READING

BLACKBURN S T. *Maternal Fetal and Neonatal Physiology*, 3rd ed. St Louis: Saunders; 2007.

DU PLESSIS A J. Cerebral blood flow and metabolism in the developing fetus. *Clin Perinatol* 2009;36:531–48.

MARTIN C B. Normal fetal physiology and behavior, and adaptive responses with hypoxemia. *Semin Perinatol* 2008;32:239–42.

MOORE K L, PERSAUD T V N. *The Developing Human: Clinically Oriented Embryology*, 8th ed. St Louis: Saunders; 2007.

ROYAL COLLEGE OF OBSTETRICIANS AND GYNAECOLOGISTS. *Fetal Awareness – Review of Research and Recommendations for Practice. Report of a Working Party*. London: RCOG; 2010.

Statistics and epidemiology

CHAPTER 33

Basic statistics

Fiona Broughton Pipkin

Statistics are like bikinis – they give you an idea, but hide what is important. ANONYMOUS

Introduction

Statistics should be tools, not tyrants. This chapter sets out to describe, as simply as possible, the statistical concepts needed for the MRCOG Part 1 examination. This exam is designed to test understanding, not the ability to carry out complex mathematical procedures. There are a number of examples to try that, if answered correctly, will demonstrate a basic understanding of the concept.

Descriptive statistics

SCALES

Data can be described using three different kinds of scale:

- **Nominal:** a naming scale (for example, eye colour: blue, green, brown, black).
- **Ordinal:** an ordering scale (for example, winner: second, third, fourth).
- **Interval:** a scale in which the interval between any two neighbouring points is the same as that between any other two neighbouring points (for example, temperature, C: 1, 2, 3, 4, 5 or 5, 10, 15, 20). Values can be below zero.
- **Ratio:** an interval scale with a fixed zero (for example, height, weight).

Data measured on interval and ratio scales are sometimes called parametric data, while data expressed on nominal and ordinal scales are called nonparametric.

'Parametric' in this context means that the data set has a normal distribution.

CONCEPTS OF MEASUREMENT

There are four main points to bear in mind when making a measurement:

- **Accuracy:** a measurement is accurate if it matches exactly an accepted standard.
- **Precision:** a precise measurement is one that has a small random error of estimation.
- **Reliability:** a reliable measurement is one that can be repeated with minimal variation.
- **Validity:** a valid measurement gives genuine information about that which is being measured.

Summarising data

CENTRAL TENDENCY AND SCATTER

Most sets of data are samples from populations. Using descriptive statistics, the main measurable characteristics of a sample, in terms of its central tendency (mode or modal group, median, mean [average]) and the scatter in the sample (range, standard deviation, standard error of the mean) can be summarised.

Figure 33.1 is a frequency histogram of population data and shows that they approximate to what is called a normal (Gaussian) distribution. Normal distributions have a single peak, so are known as 'unimodal'. In a perfect normal distribution, there would be equal

FIGURE 33.1 **Frequency histogram of the data in Table 33.1**

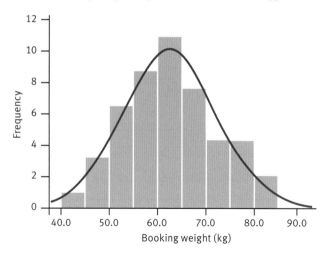

TABLE 33.1 **Ranked booking weights and weight groups for a random sample of 45 primigravidae**

Ranked data (kg)	Grouped data	
	Weight range (kg)	Number
42, 46, 46, 49, 50, 50, 51,	38–42	1
53, 54, 54, 55, 56, 56, 56,	43–47	2
57, 58, 59, 59, 60, 60, 61,		
61, 62, 62, 62, 63, 64, 64,	48–52	4
65, 66, 67, 67, 68, 68, 69,	53–57	8
70, 70, 72, 74, 75, 76, 77,	58–62	10
78, 80, 84	63–67	7
	68–72	6
	73–77	4
	78–82	2
	83–87	1

numbers of observations to the left and right of the midpoint of the horizontal axis and they would be symmetrical about the peak. Therefore, the mode, median and mean would be the same. The normal curve is characterised by its mean and standard deviation.

Assessing normality

An assumption that data are normally distributed underlies many of the commonly used statistical techniques. Therefore, statisticians need to be able to assess whether the data in a sample do indeed follow a normal distribution. Two common ways of doing this are the Shapiro–Wilk test and the Kolmogorov–Smirnov test. Running the Shapiro–Wilk test on the data set in Table 33.1 gives $P = 0.978$, (an explanation of P is given later in this chapter), showing that the data do not deviate significantly from a normal distribution.

Incidentally, it is possible for a distribution to be symmetrical but not normal; this can happen if the distribution is very widely distributed around the mean (i.e. flat) or very closely grouped around it, so the distribution is tall and thin. The 'peakedness' of distributions, both normal and non-normal, can be measured by calculating the kurtosis.

Range

Range is the spread of data in a sample. In Table 33.1, the range is 42–84 kg. The range is especially unhelpful when a data set is skewed.

Mode or modal group

The mode is the value that occurs most frequently in a data set. The modal group is the interval on a frequency histogram within which the greatest number of observations fall. In Figure 33.1, the modal group is 58–62 kg.

It is worth remembering that some data will have two or more peaks in their distribution. Always look critically at a frequency histogram to see whether there is evidence for a multimodal distribution.

Median

The median is the middle value in a ranked data set. The median is much less influenced by skewed data sets than the mean.

EXAMPLE 1

▷ Find the median of 5, 1, 8, 3, 4:

- First sort the measurements (put them in order): 1, 3, 4, 5, 8.
- The median is the $(n + 1)/2$th value in the set, where n is the number of observations.
- In this set, the median is the third value, i.e. 4 (not 3).

EXAMPLE 2

Where *n* is an even number, take the average of the two middle numbers.

▷ Find the median of 5, 1, 10, 8, 4, 3:

- First rank the measurements: 1, 3, 4, 5, 8, 10.
- The median is then the $(n + 1)/2$th value in the set, that is, the average of the third and fourth values, i.e. 4.5.

Mean

The mean is the statistician's term for an average $(\bar{x})$.

- Mean $(\bar{x}) = \frac{\sum x}{n}$
- where $\sum$ = 'the sum of', x = each individual observation and n = the number of observations.

EXAMPLE 3

▷ Consider a data set of six families with 4, 2, 1, 3, 2 and 3 children:

- $\bar{x} = \frac{\sum 4+2+1+3+2+3}{6} = 2.5$

QUANTIFYING VARIABILITY (SCATTER) IN A NORMAL DISTRIBUTION

Variance

By itself, variability is not very helpful in describing the 'average' family, as the same mean as for example 3 could have been arrived at if the families had had 2, 2, 2, 3, 3 and 3 children. To illustrate the differences in the data, an estimate of the scatter in the sample is needed. Variance is the average amount by which any individual measurement differs from the mean.

- Variance $(s^2) = \frac{\sum (x-\bar{x})^2}{(n-1)}$

Standard deviation

Standard deviation (*s* or SD) is the square root of the variance (in original units). It is used because some of the differences will be positive, and some negative and, if the squaring were not carried out when calculating the

FIGURE 33.2 **The normal distribution curve**

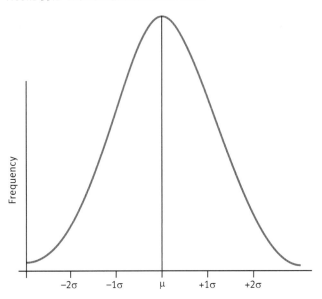

variance, some differences would cancel others out, which would be logically useless. The standard deviation gives information about the scatter in a sample.

Standard deviation $(s) = \sqrt{\text{variance}}$

Statisticians describe the population mean and standard deviation as μ and σ, respectively. This is different from the sample mean $(\bar{x})$ and standard deviation (s).

When data from a population can be described by a normal curve:

- The area covered by ± 1 σ from μ = 68%. This means that 32% of the area lies more than ± 1 σ away from the mean. Because the distribution is symmetrical, 16% lies to the left of μ and 16% to the right of it.
- The area covered by ± 2 σ from μ = 95%. Thus 5% lie outside this range, with 2.5% in each 'tail'.
- The area covered by ± 3 σ from μ = 99.8%. What proportion lies outside this range?

In a normally distributed sample with 30 or more observations $(n \geq 30)$, the same approximations can be used for the sample mean $(\bar{x})$ and standard deviation (s).

In Figure 33.2, any position on the *x* axis can be described by how many standard deviations (the distance) it is away from the mean, on either side. This distance is known as the normal (z) score or standard normal deviate. All statistical textbooks have tables of z scores.

Coefficient of variation

The coefficient of variation expresses the standard deviation as a percentage of the mean.

■ Coefficient of variation (COV) $= \frac{s}{\bar{x}} \times 100$

This is useful, for example, in quantifying the reliability of repeated measurements, since it puts the standard deviation in the context of the mean.

Standard error of the mean

The standard error of the mean (SEM) gives information on how close a sample mean is to the population mean. If several samples from a population were taken, each sample would have its own mean and variance and only by chance would the sample mean be the same as the population mean. In a normally distributed population, these sample means would themselves have a normal distribution. Calculating the mean of those sample means would usually give a better idea of the true population mean, so the variability of this distribution of sample means is assessed by calculating their standard deviation. This is known as the SEM. The smaller the SEM is, the closer the sample mean lies to the population mean. It is derived from the standard deviation (s) and the sample size (n).

■ SEM $= \frac{s}{\sqrt{n}}$ or SEM $= \sqrt{\frac{s^2}{n}}$

Arithmetically, these formulae are the same.

The SEM thus takes into account both the scatter and the sample size, thus allowing for the fact that the mean of a bigger sample will be more representative of the true population mean than will the mean of a smaller sample.

EXAMPLE 4

▷ Let the mean ($\bar{x}$) booking weight in a sample = 52 kg and the standard deviation (s) = 12 kg:

■ If $n = 9$, SEM = 12 /$\sqrt{9}$ = 12/3 = 4 kg.
■ If $n = 16$, SEM = 12 /$\sqrt{16}$ = 12/4 = 3 kg.
■ If $n = 100$, SEM = 12 /$\sqrt{100}$ = 12/10 = 1.2 kg.

Confidence intervals

For a normally distributed sample with 30 or more observations ($n \geq 30$), the same assumptions about the areas under the normal curve can be used for the sample mean, $\bar{x}$, and standard deviation, s, as for the population mean, μ, and standard deviation, σ. These allow the calculation of confidence intervals describing the distribution of data in the sample.

EXAMPLE 5

▷ Let the mean booking weight in a sample of $n = 36$ be 52 kg and the SEM be 3 kg:

■ 95% CI = 52 $\pm$ (2 $\times$ 3) = 52 $\pm$ 6 = 46–58 kg.

The practical interpretation of this is that, in this example, there is a 95% probability that the true population mean lies between 46 and 52 kg (or a 5% probability of the true population mean lying outside this range).

▷ If $n = 100$ and the SEM = 1.2 kg:

■ 95% CI = 52 $\pm$ (2 $\times$ 1.2) = 52 $\pm$ 2.4 = 49.6–54.4 kg.

SKEWED DATA

The distribution of positively skewed and negatively skewed samples are shown in Figures 33.3 and 33.4. The effect of the skewness is to make the mean less 'typical' than other measures that are less influenced by extreme values, such as the median. However, the SEM can still be used for confidence limits because, even with skewed data, the distribution of sample means approaches a normal distribution.

EXAMPLE 6

▷ Consider a sample of six women with different parities (number of pregnancies leading to a successful outcome after 20 weeks of gestation): para 4, para 2, para 1, para 3, para 2 and para 3:

■ Mean parity is 2.5.
■ Variance is 1.1.
■ s is 1.05.
■ SEM is 0.43.

FIGURE 33.3 **Frequency histogram of the data in example 7**

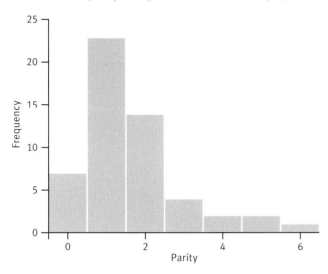

These data have a right-handed tail and are described as positively skewed. The modal group is para 1.

FIGURE 33.4 **Frequency histogram of parity from a sample of women in an area where large family size is the norm**

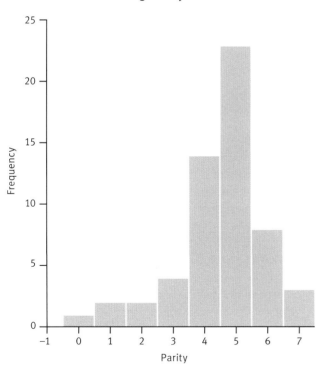

These data have a left-handed tail and are described as negatively skewed. The modal group is para 5.

▷ If a para 13 is now added to this group:

■ Mean parity becomes 4.0.
■ Variance becomes 16.67.
■ *s* becomes 4.08.
■ SEM is 1.54.

EXAMPLE 7

▷ In a larger sample of 53 women (Figure 33.3), 7 were para 0, 23 were para 1, 14 were para 2, 4 were para 3, 2 were para 4, 2 were para 5 and 1 was para 6:

■ Median parity is the $(53 + 1)/2$th value in the ranked set, i.e. the 27th value.
■ Since there are 7 para 0 and 23 para 1, the 27th value must be para 1.

Normalising skewed data

When data are not normally distributed, it may be possible to transform them to a normal distribution. This allows the correct use of the mean, standard deviation and standard error of the mean for each sample and thus the calculation of confidence intervals. It also allows the use of more powerful comparative statistics for hypothesis testing.

Endocrine data often follow a positively skewed distribution. This can be normalised by taking the logarithm of the data.

Other commonly used transformations are:

■ taking the square root $(\sqrt{x})$
■ squaring (x^2)
■ taking the reciprocal $(\frac{1}{x})$.

THE BINOMIAL DISTRIBUTION

The binomial distribution is the simplest form of distribution. It is used for data measured on a discontinuous dichotomous scale (for example, yes/no, alive/dead). With dichotomies, if the proportion (p) of subjects falling into one category is known, the proportion in the other, which is $(1 - p)$ or q, is automatically known.

When the number of observations is more than 30 $(n > 30)$, the binomial distribution approximates to the normal distribution, which is very useful. Under these circumstances, the standard deviation of p is given by $p \times (1 - p)$ and the standard error:

$$SEM = \sqrt{\frac{p * (1 - p)}{n}}$$

This can be used to establish confidence intervals for p.

EXAMPLE 8

▷ In a sample of 100 pregnant women, 20 admitted smoking; therefore $p = 0.2$ and $(1 - p) = 0.8$:

■ $SEM = \sqrt{\frac{0.2 * 0.8}{100}} = \sqrt{\frac{0.16}{100}} = 0.04$

▷ There is only 1 chance in 20 of the true population proportion of smokers lying outside the range:

■ 95% CI = $0.2 \pm (2 \times 0.04)$ = 0.12–0.28, or 12–28%.

▷ However, if only 30 women (the lowest acceptable) were sampled and 6 smoked, although the proportion is the same, the SEM is larger and the 95% CI is much wider:

■ $SEM = \sqrt{\frac{0.2 * 0.8}{30}} = \sqrt{\frac{0.16}{30}} = 0.073$
■ 95% CI = $0.2 \pm (2 \times 0.073)$ = 0.054–0.346, or 5.4–34.6%.

The Poisson distribution

This is another kind of distribution of discrete data, arising when the number of occurrences of an event per unit of time are counted. It therefore relates to integers (whole numbers). This type of distribution was first described by a Prussian army statistician (Figure 33.5). A modern example of the distribution could be the number of admissions to a gynaecological unit from the accident and emergency department each day. Over a period, an average number of admissions can be calculated, but the actual number of admissions each day will be randomly variable. The Poisson distribution allows the calculation of the probability of any specified number of admissions on a single day. Thus this is useful when considering random sums of rare events.

With a Poisson distribution, the distribution is skewed when the mean is close to zero, but the distribution approximates to normal as the mean increases. If

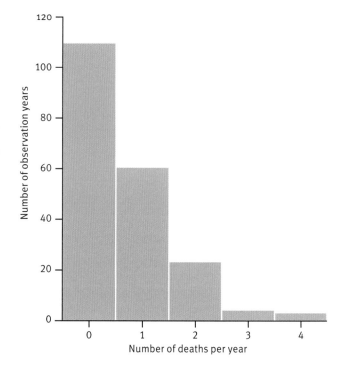

FIGURE 33.5 **Frequency histogram of the number of deaths/year in the Prussian Army caused by being kicked by a horse**

the mean number of events is around 9, then the normal approximation is reasonable.

The variance in a Poisson distribution is the same as the mean, so:

■ $s = \sqrt{mean}$

Probability

The probability of a specific outcome is the proportion of times that the outcome would occur if the observation or experiment was repeated a large number of times.

THE SHORTHAND OF PROBABILITY

Any probability has to vary between zero and one. A probability of zero means that something cannot happen; a probability of one means that it is certain to happen. For example:

■ the proposition that 'all men will die' could be written as $P = 1.0$

- a 50% chance of something happening could be written as $P = 0.5$
- less than one chance in 20 of something happening could be written as $P < 0.05$.

The inequality signs $<$ and $>$ simply mean 'less than' and 'more than'.

Comparative statistics and hypothesis testing

So far in this chapter, descriptive statistics have been considered. Another important branch of statistics is comparative statistics. These are used when comparing, for example, the effect of a fixed variable, such as gender on a disease or condition, or determining whether some intervention has an effect on a disease or condition. Under both circumstances, hypothesis testing works, by convention, from a null hypothesis (H0), which states that the variable is without effect, and then testing the null hypothesis.

The probability of any observed outcome arising if the null hypothesis is valid is calculated and used to support or reject the hypothesis. This probability is referred to as the P value and the smaller P is, the less can the null hypothesis be supported. The P value can be defined as the probability of having observed any specified outcome (or one more extreme) if the null hypothesis is valid.

By convention (and it is only by convention), H0 is usually rejected if $P < 0.05$. That is, an outcome causing rejection of H0 could occur less than one time in 20 even when the H0 was valid.

The use of P values is open to two main errors:

- alpha (α) or type 1 errors, when H0 is wrongly rejected (on average, once in 20 trials, if $P < 0.05$ is used)
- beta (β) or type 2 errors, when H0 is wrongly not rejected.

Always remember that statistical and biological significance need not be the same. Large studies can make very small differences statistically significant, while even large biological effects can be statistically nonsignificant in a small study. So do not rely too much on P values. The difference between $P = 0.053$ and $P = 0.047$ may technically be the difference between acceptance and rejection of the null hypothesis but should not constrain thinking about possible implications of erroneously stating that there is no effect.

SAMPLE SIZE DETERMINATION

When any study is being designed, the size of sample is very important. It must be big enough to give a high chance of any real difference being identified as statistically significant. This should be governed by taking both alpha and beta errors into account.

The power of a study is its ability to detect an effect of a specified size. It is expressed as $(1 - \beta)$ or $100(1 - \beta)\%$.

The sample size (n) is usually calculated to give a power of 0.8–0.9 (80–90%). For any hypothesis test, alpha is set in advance (usually 5%) so $P < 0.05$ supports rejection of H0.

TYPES OF TEST FOR HYPOTHESIS TESTING

The type of data that is collected will determine what forms of analysis it can be subjected to. Are the data nominal (categorical), ordinal, discrete (integers, for example, numbers of children) or continuous? Are they normally distributed? What is the null hypothesis? For example, are two or more groups being compared with each other or with the population? Is the investigation looking for evidence of association between variables? Is the investigation trying to describe or predict the effect of a change in one variable on another? Some of the most commonly used statistical tests are discussed here.

DISTRIBUTION-FREE (NONPARAMETRIC) ANALYSES

For nonparametric analysis, minimal assumptions are made about the underlying data distribution. That is, they can be used for data whether or not they are normally distributed.

For comparing groups, the following tests are available:

- sign test
- chi-square (χ^2) test, for 2×2 and larger contingency tables (be aware of the need for applying Yates' correction factor when the sample size is small)
- McNemar χ^2 test, for 'before' and 'after' categorical data
- Wilcoxon test, for paired data, for the same subject under different conditions

SECTION 13: STATISTICS AND EPIDEMIOLOGY

- Mann–Whitney U-test, for unpaired data
- Kruskal–Wallis analysis of variance.

The Wilcoxon, Mann–Whitney U and Kruskal–Wallis tests make no assumptions about the underlying data distribution and are the nonparametric equivalent of the Student's paired and unpaired t-tests and one-way analysis of variance.

For testing association between groups, the following test is available:

- Spearman's rho (ρ).

Again, Spearman's ρ makes no assumption about the underlying data distribution.

Normally distributed data

Tests for normally distributed data, properly speaking, should only be used when it has been formally confirmed that the data are indeed normally distributed, which may involve normalising skewed data.

For comparing groups, the following tests are available:

- Student's t-test, for paired and unpaired data (first check whether the variances differ significantly from each other using the Welch test)
- F test, to determine equality of variances
- analysis of variance (one-way, two or more way, repeated measures).

For testing association between groups, the following tests are available:

- Pearson's r
- linear regression analysis
- multiple regression analysis.

For both types of regression analysis, the response variable should be normally distributed; the independent variable need not be and it may have been fixed by the investigator.

SOME SPECIFIC TESTS

The chi-square test

In the simplest form of the very useful χ^2 test, the variable under investigation can be only one of two types.

EXAMPLE 9

▷ In an investigation concerning the common cold, a GP saw 900 people presenting consecutively at the surgery: 480 were men and 420 were women. Do these data conform to the null hypothesis that the incidence of the common cold is not gender related?

▷ If there were no gender difference, then the expectations (E) would be that 450 of the people are men and 450 are women. Instead the observations (O) are 480 men (an excess of 30) and 420 women (a deficit of 30).

- Now $\chi^2 = \sum \frac{(O-E)^2}{E}$
- so $\chi^2 = \frac{(480-450)^2}{450} + \frac{(430-450)^2}{450}$
- $= \frac{+30^2}{450} + \frac{-30^2}{450}$
- 4.0. Consulting a table of χ^2 shows this to be significant ($P < 0.05$).

▷ U But if the sample had been only of 90 people, 48 men and 42 women, although the proportions would have been the same, the outcome would be different:

- $\chi^2 = \frac{(48-45)^2}{45} + \frac{(43-45)^2}{45}$
- $= \frac{+3^2}{45} + \frac{-3^2}{45}$
- $= 0.4$, which is far from reaching significance.

From example 9, it can be seen that there are instances when χ^2 cannot be used:

- with proportions
- when any expected number of observations is less than 5
- when the total number of observations is less than 20.

The test can be expanded to develop contingency tables, where each cell of the table corresponds to a particular combination of characteristics relating to two or more classifications, which can be categorical.

EXAMPLE 10

▷ Table 33.2 is a 2 × 3 table. If the null hypothesis is valid and the two variables are unrelated, then the probability of an individual being in a particular row is independent of which column they are in:

- The proportion of married women is 2787/3438 = 81.1%.

TABLE 33.2 **Data relating to daily caffeine consumption and marital status from a sample of 3438 women**

		Caffeine consumption (mg/day)			
		0	1–150	151–300	Total
Marital status	Married	652	1537	598	2787
	Single	218	327	106	651
	Total	870	1864	704	3438

- The proportion of women who do not drink caffeine is 870/3438 = 25.3%.
- The expected proportion of married women who don't drink caffeine is 0.811 × 0.253 = 0.205.
- In terms of the whole sample, the expected number of married women who don't drink caffeine would be 0.205 × 3438 = 705 women.

▷ In fact, the observation was that only 652 married women drank no caffeine. Working through the table, calculating the observed and expected frequencies and then applying the formula for χ^2 will determine whether or not the data fitted the null hypothesis.

t-tests

t-tests are very commonly used to compare:

- the mean of a sample with a predicted value, often zero
- the means of two samples.

These can be paired or unpaired samples. Paired samples are those where a measurement(s) is made on the same person under two different conditions, such as the measurement of blood pressure in an antenatal booking clinic and again a month later. It is also sometimes possible to match two groups of subjects very carefully for variables perceived as being important confounders in their own right, such as age or smoking habit, so that each study individual has a matched control. Where observations are made on different groups of subjects without any such careful matching, the data are said to be unpaired.

In either case, the underlying population distribution must be normal.

Different types of t-test

EXAMPLE 11

▷ Diastolic blood pressure was measured in 29 women at booking and 3 weeks later and the results ($\bar{x} \pm s$) were as follows:

- booking: 60.5 ± 7.35; therefore SEM = 1.36 mmHg
- 3/52 later: 57.6 ± 7.97; therefore SEM = 1.48 mmHg
- change: –2.9 ± 6.80; therefore SEM = 1.26 mmHg.

▷ The H0 is that there is no difference (i.e. H0 = 0) between the diastolic blood pressure measured at these two visits. These are properly paired data, which can be compared using the paired *t*-test. This compares the mean difference between blood pressure measured at the first and second visits with (the hypothesised) zero, thus:

- *t* = (mean change – 0)/SEM of the mean difference
- *t* = 2.30; *P* = 0.03.

Confidence interval for the difference between two means

The confidence interval specifies a range of values within which the difference between the means of the two popu-lations (or samples) may lie. It contains all the values of ($\mu1 - \mu2$), or (sample mean 1 – sample mean 2), which would not be rejected in a two-tailed hypothesis test. If the confidence interval contains 0, there is no significant difference between the means of the two groups, at the specified level of confidence.

In example 11, the 95% CI of the difference is:

- –2.9 ± (1.26 × 1.96)
- = –2.9 ± 2.47
- = –0.43 to –5.37.

This does not include 0 (both values are negative), so the difference is statistically significant at the 5% level.

EXAMPLE 12

▷ Suppose now that data on diastolic blood pressure at booking in 30 women from one hospital have been obtained and are to be compared with those from 22 women at booking in another hospital. The results ($\bar{x} \pm s$) were as follows:

FIGURE 33.6 **Scatterplots**

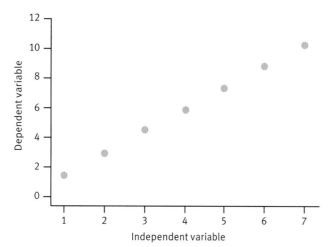

A Positive association

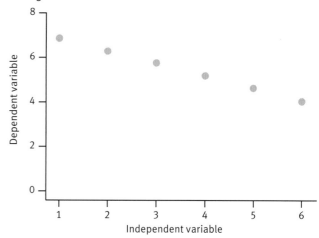

B Negative association

- hospital 1: 62.9 ± 8.44; therefore SEM = 1.54 mmHg
- hospital 2: 67.2 ± 7.96; therefore SEM = 1.70 mmHg.

▷ An unpaired t-test should be used to compare these two samples of booking diastolic blood pressures with respect to place of booking:

- $t = \dfrac{\bar{x}_1 - \bar{x}_2}{S\sqrt{\frac{1}{n_1} + \frac{1}{n_2}}}$

  where s is an estimate of the standard deviation for both samples
- the t statistic would be 1.857, which is not statistically significant ($P = 0.069$)
- the 95% CI for the difference would be −8.94 to 0.35, which includes 0.

▷ Therefore, there is no significant difference between the groups at the two hospitals.

Correlation

Investigators are often interested in whether two variables are associated, such that as one changes, it affects the other. When both variables are measured on a continuous scale and can be assumed to come from a random sample, correlation analysis is used. Pearson's correlation coefficient (r) tests the degree of association between two variables and is a measure of the scatter of the data around an underlying linear trend.

- $r = \dfrac{\Sigma(x-\bar{x})(y-\bar{y})}{\sqrt{\Sigma(x-\bar{x})^2(y-\bar{y})^2}}$

The data for at least one, and preferably both, of the observations should be normally distributed. If they are not, either try transforming the data or calculate the nonparametric measure of association, Spearman's ρ, which is a ranking test. In either case, tables of r or ρ can be consulted to show whether or not the correlation is statistically significant, although most statistical packages will provide this information automatically.

In Figure 33.6A, there is a perfect positive correlation between the independent (x) variable and the dependent (y) variable. Pearson's r would therefore be 1.0.

In Figure 33.6B, there is a perfect negative correlation between the independent and the dependent variables. The correlation coefficient, r, would therefore be −1.0.

A correlation coefficient of about zero means that there is no linear association between the two variables.

EXAMPLE 13

▷ In this example, a unit change in x is associated with an entirely predictable change in y. Nothing else influences y. To assess the amount of variability of y accounted for by x, simply square the correlation coefficient, r:

- If $r = 0.4$, $r^2 = 0.16$, or 16%.

FIGURE 33.7 **Scatterplot of booking systolic blood pressure in relation to body mass index**

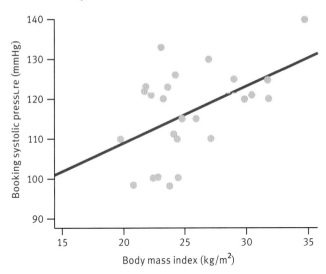

- In this case, 16% of the variability in y can be accounted for by change in x.

▷ In Figure 33.7, the correlation between the body mass index and booking systolic pressure in 26 women is statistically significant:

- Pearson's $r = 0.504$, $r^2 = 0.254$; $P = 0.009$.

▷ The line of best fit calculated from the regression equation has a slope of 0.254. Of the variation in the booking systolic blood pressure, 25.4% can be accounted for by variation in the body mass index.

Note for example 13 that if Spearman's ρ had been calculated for the same data, it would have been 0.365, which is not statistically significant ($P = 0.067$). There is considerable scatter around the line and the less sensitive nonparametric test did not therefore identify the association. On the other hand, Pearson's correlation is sensitive to outliers, so the rank correlation may have given a truer picture. An awareness of the characteristics of data sets is needed.

It should also never be assumed that, because an association is statistically significant, it is therefore causal. It is always possible that both variables are influenced by something else.

Another technique often used with data on two continuous variables is regression. This allows the value of one variable to be predicted, by knowing the value of the other. It is often possible to describe one as 'independent' and one as 'dependent' by thinking about it. For example, a child's height will be influenced by its age, but its age will not be influenced by its height. Age is therefore the independent variable, plotted, by convention, on the x (horizontal) axis, while height is the dependent variable, plotted on the y (vertical) axis.

Regression calculations allow a 'line of best fit', such as that shown in Figure 33.7, to be calculated, by calculating the slope and the point of intercept on the y axis where $x = 0$. The line of best fit can then be used to predict y for any given x.

Predictive tests

A good predictive test for a disease or condition must be sensitive and specific, with good positive and negative predictive values, which are defined as follows:

- **sensitivity:** the proportion of true positives that are correctly identified by the test
- **specificity:** the proportion of true negatives that are correctly identified by the test
- **positive predictive value:** the proportion of people with positive results who are correctly diagnosed
- **negative predictive value:** the proportion of people with negative results who are correctly diagnosed.

EXAMPLE 14

▷ Imagine a scenario in which the presence of an abnormal uterine artery resistance index (RI $\geq$ 0.58) at 24 weeks of gestation is used to predict pre-eclampsia in a group of 144 women:[1]

- 63 women had an RI $\geq$ 0.58 at 24 weeks; 28 went on to develop pre-eclampsia
- 81 women had an RI $<$ 0.58 at 24 weeks; 8 went on to develop pre-eclampsia.

▷ This would give the following values:

- true positives (a) = 28
- false positives (b) = 35
- false negatives (c) = 8
- true negatives (d) = 73.

▷ Therefore the sensitivity, specificity and positive and negative predictive values can be calculated:

- sensitivity = a/(a + c) = 28/(28 + 8) = 77.8%
- specificity = d/(b + d) = 73/(35 + 73) = 67.6%
- positive predictive value
  = a/(a + b) = 28/(28 + 35) = 44.4%
- negative predictive value
  = d/(c + d) = 73/(8 + 73) = 90.1%.

▷ A caveat is in order here. These formulae for positive and negative predictive values only apply if the proportion of women with pre-eclampsia in the sample accurately reflects the true prevalence of pre-eclampsia in the population. This will not in general be true with case–control type sampling as here.

Some useful concepts

INCIDENCE AND PREVALENCE

The incidence (I) of a disease is the rate at which new cases of the disease occur in a population previously free of it.

$$I = \frac{r}{N^* t}$$

where r = number of new cases, N = population size and t = time interval.

Incidence is often expressed per 1000 or 1 000 000 of the population, to avoid small decimals, and per year, to give the annual incidence rate. The incidence rate is thus the number of new cases per head of the population per unit time.

The prevalence (P) of a condition measures the frequency of existing disease at a given time.

$$P = \frac{R}{N}$$

where R = total number of cases at the given time and N = total population at that time.

- In a stable situation, incidence and prevalence are related by:

$$P = I \times D$$

where D is the average duration of the disease.

CRUDE AND STANDARDISED PROPORTIONS

A crude proportion is one expressed without making any allowance for factors that might influence it. Birth and death rates are crude rates. They are usually expressed per 10 000 or 100 000 of the population, to avoid small decimals.

A standardised proportion is one that has been corrected (standardised) for one or more factors such as smoking, gender, age or race.

When these proportions relate to all events occurring within a specified time, such as a year, they are known as crude and standardised rates.

EXAMPLE 15

▷ Table 33.3 presents data for a sample of 200 babies, in which 20 had birth weights at or below the 10th centile (fetal growth restriction; FGR):

- The crude proportion of FGR is thus 10%.

▷ Of the mothers, 35% smoked and 11 of these mothers had babies with FGR.

- Proportion of FGR in smokers = 11/70 = 15.7%
- Proportion of FGR in nonsmokers = 9/130 = 6.9%
- These are the proportions of FGR standardised for smoking.

Odds ratios

An odds ratio (OR) gives an estimate, for which a confidence interval can be calculated, for the association between two binary (for example, yes/no) variables and allows testing for the effects of other variables on that association (logistic regression). The odds of an event happening is the ratio of the probability that it does happen to the probability that it does not (for example if 5 in 50 people are 'yes', the odds is 5 in 45 or 1 in 9).

Table 33.4 shows data from the Genetics of Pre-eclampsia study.[2] For this retrospective analysis, the outcome of interest was delivery before 34 weeks of gestation, which is displayed in the rows, while the groups were defined on the basis of whether or not the mother had continued to smoke during pregnancy (the columns).

TABLE 33.3 **Data relating to maternal smoking in pregnancy and outcome (fetal growth restriction) from a sample of 200 pregnancies**

		Smoker		
		Yes	No	Total
Fetal growth restriction	Yes	11	9	20
	No	59	121	180
	Total	70	130	200

TABLE 33.4 **Data relating to maternal smoking in pregnancy and outcome (gestational age at delivery) from a sample of 926 pre-eclamptic pregnancies**

		Smoker		
		Yes	No	Total
Delivered before 34 weeks of gestation	Yes	31	178	209
	No	58	659	717
	Total	89	837	926

Source: Genetics of Preeclampsia Consortium.[2]

The odds that a woman who delivered before 34 weeks of gestation was also a smoker is calculated as 31/178 (17.42).

The odds that a woman who delivered at or after 34 weeks was also a smoker were 58/659 (8.80). The OR is thus 17.42/8.80, or 1.98. Statistical software will calculate the 95% confidence interval for this ratio, which is 1.24–3.16. The null hypothesis is that there is no difference between the two ORs, that is, that the OR is not significantly different from 1.0. However, in this example, the 95% confidence interval does not cross 1.0, so it can be inferred that continuing to smoke increases the risk of delivery before 34 weeks of gestation.

Relative risk

Relative risk (RR) compares the proportions with a particular outcome in two groups selected before the start of a study as differing in one or more features (for example, nulliparous compared with parous, normal build compared with obese). They are thus selected prospectively. This contrasts with OR, which can be calculated from a prospective or retrospective design.

To illustrate this, imagine that the data in Table 33.4 had come from a study designed to assess whether smoking is associated with very premature delivery. The proportions delivering prematurely are 31/89 (34.83%) in the smoking group and 178/837 (21.27%) in the nonsmokers. The relative risk of delivery before 34 weeks of gestation is thus 34.83/21.27, or 1.64. Statistical software will calculate the 95% confidence interval for this ratio, which is 1.20–2.24. The predicted value of the relative risk from H0 is again 1.0. However, in this example, the 95% confidence interval does not cross 1.0,

so it can be assumed that smoking is associated with a significantly greater risk of premature delivery.

Quantification of risk – the risk matrix

Clinical risk management is improved when there has been a clear assessment of the likelihood of a risk arising and the consequences if it does. The use of risk matrices such as that shown in Table 33.5 is one way of achieving this. The likelihood of a specified risk arising is shown horizontally and the consequences vertically. The likelihood will be defined from existing data, and there must be agreement as to what each term (Impossible, Unlikely, etc.) means in the context of the risk being assessed. The impact of each is also assigned a score, which should be arrived at as a consensus among experienced staff. Combining these scores, usually by multiplying, allows risks to be described as anything from no risk to high risk and colour coding is frequently used to alert the users to the overall risk level. An action plan must then be developed for each final risk score category. Another example of an NHS risk score matrix can be found in 'NHS 24 Risk Management Strategy 2009'.[4]

Levels of evidence

Evidence-based medicine has been described as 'the conscientious, explicit and judicious use of current best evidence in making decisions about the care of individual patients'.[5] To practise evidence-based medicine, the level of evidence needs to be assessed from the type of information that the particular study provides, which

TABLE 33.5 **Outline example of a risk matrix**

		Likelihood					
		Impossible (0)	Rare (1)	Unlikely (2)	Moderate (3)	Likely (4)	Certain (5)
Consequences	Negligible (0)	0	0	0	0	0	0
	Minor (1)	0	1	2	3	4	5
	Serious (2)	0	2	4	6	8	10
	Major (3)	0	3	6	9	12	15
	Fatal (4)	0	4	8	12	16	20

Risk levels: green = minor or negligible | yellow = moderate | orange = major | red = extreme

Source: Thompson PJ, Owen JH. (2005).[3]

may range from a systematic review to the purely anecdotal.

Level	Evidence
1 a	Systematic review and meta-analysis of randomised controlled trials
1 b	At least one randomised controlled trial
2 a	At least one well-designed controlled study, without randomisation
2 b	At least one other type of well-designed, quasi-experimental study
3	Well-designed descriptive studies
4	Expert committee reports or opinions and/or clinical experience of respected authorities.

These levels of evidence have been used by the Clinical Outcomes Group of the National Health Service Executive to develop a slightly simplified grading scheme:

- Grade A: requires at least one randomised controlled trial as part of a body of literature of overall good quality and consistency addressing the specific recommendation (evidence levels Ia Ib).
- Grade B: requires the availability of well-controlled clinical studies but no randomised clinical trials on the topic of recommendations (evidence levels IIa IIb III).

- Grade C: requires evidence obtained from expert committee reports or opinions and/or clinical experiences of respected authorities and indicates an absence of directly applicable clinical studies of good quality (evidence level IV).

Clinical trials

Clinical trials compare groups of people who differ only with respect to their treatment. In an open trial, both clinician and patient know what treatment the patient is receiving. Allocation to treatment may or may not be random.

It is, however, preferable if allocation to treatment groups is random (to avoid conscious and unconscious bias) and made by those otherwise unconnected with the trial so that neither the patient nor the clinician knows which treatment is being given (a double-blind study). Blinding is less important if the outcome is objective. If only the patient is unaware of the treatment being given, the study is a single-blind study.

However, the Consolidated Standards of Reporting Trials (CONSORT [www.consort-statement.org]) statement suggests that the widely used terms single-blinding and double-blinding should now be avoided as it is clearer to specify who is and who is not blinded.

Outcome measures should be defined before the trial starts. They are usually classified into primary and secondary study outcomes. It is best to concentrate on a single primary outcome, because this is more straight-forward to interpret.

CONTROLS

It is sometimes possible for a person to be their own control. This is optimal, as only one variable differs between 'before' and 'after' treatment or intervention. When this is not possible and allocation to treatment cannot be random and blinded, the control group should be matched for as many variables (for example, age, sex, body mass index, obstetric history) as possible with the treatment group. They should be studied at the same time as the treatment group. If time matching is really impossible, the controls become historical. This is much weaker, because so many underlying variables will have changed.

Final examples: maternal and neonatal mortality

Around 600 000 women per year die from pregnancy-related causes worldwide, the huge majority in low income countries. Investigators cannot know if mortality rates are falling without baseline data.

EXAMPLE 16

▷ In Figure 33.8A and B, note the very different scales on the *y* axes. These scatterplots illustrate the use of simple statistical methods to make numbers more easily assimilable. They show the same worrying trends in both countries. In Jamaica, the rise in indirect deaths is due to HIV/AIDS, cardiac disease and diabetes, while in the UK, the rise in indirect deaths is mainly attributed to cardiac and psychiatric disease.

EXAMPLE 17

▷ Table 33.6 shows a wide range of neonatal mortality rates across three geographically neighbouring local authorities. The rate in Bromsgrove is statistically significantly different from that in Birmingham because there is no overlap between the lower (5th) percentile for Birmingham and the upper (95th) percentile for Bromsgrove.

FIGURE 33.8 **Scatterplots of maternal mortality rates by triennia with their associated lines of best fit**

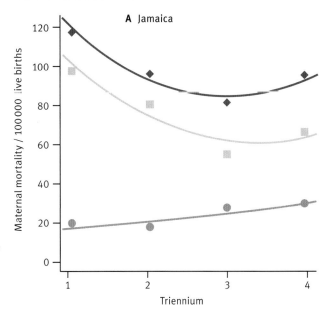

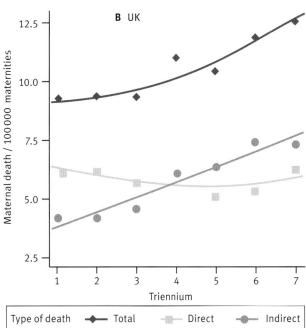

Triennium 1 = 1981–83; 2 = 1993–95; 3 = 1998–2000; 4 = 2001–03;
Triennium 1 = 1985–87; 2 = 1988–90; 3 = 1991–93; 4 = 1994–96;
5 = 1997–99; 6 = 2000–02; 7 = 2003–05.

Source: Saving Mothers' Lives.[6]

TABLE 33.6 **Neonatal mortality rates per 1000 live births (2000–02) in the West Midlands**

Local authority	Rate	95% confidence interval	
		Lower limit	Upper limit
Birmingham	9.19	8.31	10.13
Lichfield	6.29	3.60	10.19
Bromsgrove	2.45	0.90	5.32

Source: University of Birmingham. (2004).[7]

Don't forget that there will be many underlying factors affecting the neonatal mortality rates in example 17 and, if interpreted without knowledge of such factors, they could be seriously misinterpreted.

In a placebo-controlled trial of a drug, people are randomly allocated to receive either the active treatment or an apparently identical, but actually inactive, treatment, which may be combined with a standard treatment.

In a crossover trial, the same people are treated in (usually) two different ways (for example, both placebo and active treatment), with a 'washout' period between the two regimes. The order of administration of treatment should be randomised and double-blinded.

REFERENCES

1. PARRETTI E, MEALLI F, MAGRINI A, CIONI R, MECACCI F, LA TORRE P, *et al.* Cross-sectional and longitudinal evaluation of uterine artery Doppler velocimetry for the prediction of pre-eclampsia in normotensive women with specific risk factors. *Ultrasound Obstet Gynecol* 2003;22:160–5.

2. BROUGHTON PIPKIN F, The Genetics of Preeclampsia Consortium. Smoking in moderate/severe preeclampsia worsens pregnancy outcome, but smoking cessation limits the damage. *Hypertension* 2008;51:1042–6.

3. THOMPSON PJ, OWEN JH. Risk management in obstetrics; just another inspection or improving patient care? *Fetal Matern Med Rev* 2005;16:195–209.

4. National Health Service. *NHS 24 Risk Management Strategy 2009*. London: NHS; 2009. [www.nhs24.com/content/mediaassets/board/10.4a%20Risk%20Management%20Strategy.pdf].

5. STRAUSS S E, RICHARDSON W S, GLASZIOU P, HAYNES R B. *Evidence-based Medicine: How to Practice and Teach EBM*. 3rd edition. London: Churchill Livingstone; 2005.

6. LEWIS G, editor. The Confidential Enquiry into Maternal and Child Health. *Saving Mothers' Lives: reviewing maternal deaths to make motherhood safer– 2003–2005*. The Seventh Report on Confidential Enquiries into Maternal Deaths in the United Kingdom. London: CEMACH; 2007.

CHAPTER 34

Screening and trials statistics

Andrew H Shennan and Annette Briley

Introduction

All clinicians should have a fundamental understanding of statistics as they pertain to screening and clinical trials. Screening is a common phenomenon throughout medicine, but particularly in the reproductive sciences.

Research is an organised and systematic process of enquiry. Its aim is to develop concepts and theories and to be able to describe phenomena. It adds to the scientific body of knowledge.[1] Traditionally, knowledge has been gained by experience, but by applying research, one can expand and add to the knowledge far more quickly. Research takes the form of many assessments. Each assessment suits a different situation and its quality cannot always be judged by its size or method. For example, a case report may be extremely important in very rare diseases. Clinical trials involving a randomised design are generally viewed as a 'gold standard' for evaluating an intervention. There are a number of types of studies:

- retrospective studies
- systematic research
- qualitative research
- quantitative research
- surveys
- cohort studies
- case–control studies
- randomised control trials.

Statistics are required in clinical investigation to ascertain if events are by chance and to be able to quantify any risk determined.[2] Good clinical practice is now often determined by evidence-based medicine.

Although much of knowledge is still based on clinical judgement, increasing amounts of clinical care can be determined by research-acquired evidence. Good clinical care will always be a combination of applying experience with evidence-based knowledge. Whenever possible, clinicians should try to quantify what has previously been qualitative or intuitive decision making. This chapter will outline the principles involved in statistical analysis.

Determining the size of a study

To answer the research question it addresses, a study must have enough subjects. A study evaluating a single group should have a sample size large enough to give sufficient certainty to influence clinical practice; statistically, this is achieved by a suitably small standard error (SE) for the quantity estimated. When two groups are compared, then a power calculation can be used to give a reasonable certainty (generally 80 or 90%) of detecting a clinically important difference between two groups. It is wise to seek advice from a statistician before commencing any study.

A number of factors must be considered before a sample size can be calculated.

TYPE OF STUDY

This may range from a single sample study, such as a survey, or be a longitudinal study measuring endpoints at a number of times. When comparing two samples, this could be a case–control or a randomised clinical trial. Once the type of study is known, the sample size will be dependent on a number of other variables.

PRIMARY OUTCOME MEASURE

This is usually a proportion, that is, a categorical endpoint in a clinical trial (i.e. a yes/no answer). However, it may be the mean of a measurement or a summary score (based on the average of measurements at a number of time points or in different places).

Alternative endpoints may be an ordered scale (for example, worse, no change or better) or a survival time. The choice of endpoint will depend on the clinical situation and the research question. Often, far smaller sample sizes can be obtained from continuous variables (for example, gestational age) rather then categorical variables (for example, proportion of preterm birth). The same question can be answered using different methodology by considering alternative outcome measures, which can influence the feasibility of performing a trial. Equally, with very rare outcomes (for example, perinatal death), clinical trials may simply be impossible because of the inability to recruit sufficient patients; a composite endpoint may therefore be picked. If more than one endpoint is required (for example, if they are equally important or if both maternal and neonatal endpoints are required), then both (or more) can be powered for; *P*-values must take this into account and can be adjusted to account for this 'multiple hypothesis testing'. A secondary endpoint can be powered for, although rarely there is more than one 'primary outcome' – in effect, two or more studies are being performed.

THE EXPECTED LIKELY VALUES

In new research, pilot data are invaluable in determining likely proportions, or variation in continuous variables (standard deviation). If power is to be calculated from current literature, then, when standard errors are given, standard deviation is calculated as SE $\times \sqrt{n}$ for the standard error of a single mean, or as $SE/(1/\sqrt{n_1} + 1/\sqrt{n_2})$ for the difference between two means. When confidence intervals are given, the SE can be estimated as (upper limit – lower limit)/4 for 30 observations or more.

The difference should be both plausible and clinically important, although economic or scientific importance may be worthwhile, even if not clinically valuable.

When determining the power of a study, one must also determine the size of effect that is clinically important. Deciding the clinically important size of an effect cannot be done from statistical tables but must be a clinical judgement. The study should be able to determine a difference that is clinically important. There is no point in having a huge study that determines a tiny difference that does not matter. Sometimes it is not possible to carry out a study large enough to determine a clinically important difference and the design accepts that the study is underpowered but may add to new knowledge and possibly to future meta-analyses. It should be called a pilot study.

Significance level: alpha (*P*-values)

The size and design of a study will determine its ability to get to the truth. The power of the study is the probability that it will detect a difference if there is a real and important effect in reality. The significance level (or alpha) is the probability of falsely detecting a difference when there is in fact no effect. Alpha can be thought of as the target value of the significance test, which is compared with the observed value, also known as the *P*-value, which is found only at the end of the study. Alpha is usually fixed at 0.05 or 5%; so a *P*-value < 0.05 is taken as significant in most studies.

LIMITATIONS OF *P*-VALUES

The smaller the *P*-value, the stronger the evidence that there is something going on. (The *P*-value actually measures the chance of the observed result if there is in fact nothing going on.) By convention, a value of $P < 0.05$ (1 in 20) is generally taken as a significant difference. One in 20 is actually more likely than rolling a double 6 (one in 36); so it can and does happen by chance. So conventional cut-offs (to determine that something is significant), sometimes do get it wrong (that is, a *P*-value <0.05 when no real difference exists).

P-values are not magical or all-important. This should not come as a surprise. In all things in medicine, it is not always clear whether something is real or not (for example, a blood pressure of 88 mmHg does not guarantee that a patient does not have hypertension). Equally a *P*-value of 0.051 does not mean that a real difference does not exist. If there are multiple endpoints to a study, then the chance of one of them being significant when there is no real difference is higher than 5%. All these factors must be taken into account when interpreting *P*-values.

When determining the power of a study, a single primary endpoint is generally defined and powered for in the study design. This prevents the problem of multiple hypotheses testing.

Power of a study: beta values

At the same time as deciding the alpha value, we need to think about the chance of getting a significant result if there is a real and important effect (also known as the power of the study or beta). The beta value needs to be as high as possible. In an ideal world you would test every patient who had the disease but, in practice, one has to check a sample. The power therefore depends upon how big the sample is. A 90% power would have a 90% chance of finding a clinically important difference between groups. Studies are generally designed with a 90% power where possible, but sometimes 80% or less has to be accepted to make the trial or study feasible.

Type 1 and type 2 errors

Once results are published, it is clear that they may be misleading (that is, the truth cannot always be determined), depending upon whether a representative sample has been collected or whether you fall on the wrong side of an arbitrary standard by chance. These are known as type 1 or type 2 errors.

A type 1 error occurs when a correct hypothesis is rejected. In practice, a type 1 error means that a difference is found which is not real (for example, a study may be published that shows a drug reduces blood pressure when the truth is that the drug does not, but this study showed it by chance). This sometimes occurs because of publication bias (that is, many unpublished studies have been done on the drug but only the one that shows a significant difference is published whereas the others are not). The reason for type 1 errors is that the 5% arbitrary alpha value, determined by the *P*-value, will get it wrong in 1 in 20 times.

The other type of error, a type 2 error, is more common, which is when an incorrect hypothesis is accepted. It generally occurs because the sample size is too small (that is, there is a difference but it is not big enough to fall the right side of the *P*-value, for example, a drug affecting blood pressure is not found to do so). The difference in blood pressure may be 10 mmHg, which may be clinically important but, because of the small sample size, it does not have a *P*-value < 0.05 and therefore the study determines that the drug does not make the blood pressure fall.

Using correct power calculations will limit the chance of these errors.

Generalisability

When planning a study, one must consider if the sample is representative of the whole population. The larger the study, the more likely this will occur; however, in the rarefied environment of research one may select women who are not representative. For example, if you are doing a clinical trial on epidurals, the research team may be more likely to recruit women during the day who have different characteristics to women who present throughout the 24-hour period.

When evaluating the results of studies, one must consider whether those who entered the study were also likely to be from the general population. One way to determine this is to look at the event rates. For example, the normal vaginal delivery rate in women with epidurals may be higher in the general population than in the study. This suggests that women have been recruited who are different and therefore the generalisability, or the ability to apply the findings to all populations, of the results must be questioned.

Statistical packages are readily available to determine power. However, a basic understanding of the determinants of power (that is, the alpha or beta value) is required, together with the clinical factors.

Analysing the size of an effect: odds ratios and relative risks

A study or clinical trial may show a significant difference. Clinicians must be aware of the importance of this difference and how it applies to their patients or the population they are interested in.

Odds ratios are generally used to determine the difference between groups (for example, exposed to risk factors or not). Odds are calculated by dividing the number of times an event occurs by the number of times it does not. They are calculated by dividing the odds of being exposed to a risk factor with the odds in a controlled group. Therefore an odds ratio of 1 shows no difference between groups. An odds ratio of more or less than 1 demonstrates an increased or reduced effect, respectively. This may not be significant if the confidence limits cross 1.

Relative risk is similar but is calculated by dividing the risk in a treated or exposed group by a risk in a controlled or unexposed group. In a clinical trial, a relative risk reduction is therefore the proportion by which the intervention reduced the event rate. Relative risks are often given in preference to odds ratios when looking at an effect from a clinical trial. A relative risk reduction of 0.5, therefore, means the intervention will reduce the event by a half. The certainty to which this has occurred is determined by 95% confidence intervals. If the confidence intervals cross 1, then there is a higher possibility that the intervention does not work. Equally if the confidence intervals are wide and approach 1, then the effect may not be as certain. Confidence intervals therefore are the percentage of the time that the true value would fall within these limits. 95% is generally accepted as being appropriate and implies that 95% of the time the true effect is within the limits given.

As an example of how to calculate odds ratios and relative risk, imagine a new fertility drug is given to 100 women and in 1 year 12% conceive, whereas 4% conceive in 100 controls. The risk ratio or relative risk (of conceiving) is therefore:

- 12/4 = 3.

Odds ratios can also be used but usually are taken when an accurate denominator is unknown (for example, in a case–control study when the outcome is rare). For the same example as above, it is calculated by:

- 12/88 : 4/96 as a ratio.

In clinical trials, the denominator is known and therefore relative risks are generally used.

Screening

The National Screening Committee in 2001 described screening as 'a public health service in which members of a defined population, who do not perceive they are at risk of, or already affected by, a disease or its complications, are asked questions or offered a test to identify those individuals who are more likely to be helped than harmed by further tests or treatment to reduce the risks of disease or its complications'.[3]

The aim of all screening programmes is to detect an individual's predisposition for a disease, preferably at an early stage when the person is considered to be disease free and an intervention is possible. The efficacy of a screening test is assessed by the numbers of people screened who go on to develop the disease. It is impossible to determine absolute risk because of the inability to collect sufficient numbers, therefore screening is calculated using a mathematical formula. Because of the distribution of diseases, there is always a false positive rate. Currently, antenatal screening methods for chromosomal abnormalities mean that around 5% of women will be incorrectly identified to achieve approximately an 80% detection rate.[4] Women will also be incorrectly identified at low risk but will have an affected baby. Whether these risks are acceptable depends on the circumstances and higher or lower false detection rates can be accepted depending on the clinical scenario. For example, women will accept an unnecessary amniocentesis but would not want a Down syndrome baby 'missed', whereas a screening test for pre-eclampsia may not detect all cases of pre-eclampsia; this will be identified in most cases through antenatal screening, so it is not as important to detect all cases.

The prerequisites for screening tests are:[5]

- being simple, safe and acceptable
- having a high sensitivity and specificity with good predictor values
- being reproducible

- having limited overlap between affected and nonaffected individuals
- having defined cut-off levels
- being cost effective and therefore relatively inexpensive.

In addition, the condition to which the test is applied should have certain characteristics: it should be an important treatable health problem with established diagnostic strategies, which includes an acceptable test. The natural history of the disease should be defined, preferably with a latent stage, and there should be an agreed policy regarding who to treat.

To understand the statistics for screening, one must consider how useful a test is. A test can give a positive or negative result, both of which can be correct or incorrect (that is, there are four possibilities). To calculate the predictive statistics used in screening, one must consider whether the test result is a true or false positive or a true or false negative. The efficiency of a test can be determined by working out sensitivity and specificity or positive and negative predictive values. Other parameters such as relative risk and likelihood ratios can also be determined and will be described. Table 34.1 demonstrates how the clinical efficiency of a test can be calculated.

SENSITIVITY

Sensitivity is the proportion of all cases that have an abnormal test result. For example, if the detection of

TABLE 34.1 **Calculating the clinical efficiency of a test**

Measure	Formula
Sensitivity	TP/(TP + FP)
Specificity	TN/(FP + TN)
Predictive values (positive)	TP/(FP + TP)
Predictive values (negative)	TN/(TN + FN)
Relative risk	$\frac{TP/(TP + FP)}{FN/(FN + TN)}$
Likelihood ratio	$\frac{TP/(TP + FP)}{FP/TN + FP}$ or $\frac{Sensitivity}{Specificity}$
Odds ratio	Probability/(1 − probability)
Accuracy	(TP + TN)/total

T = true | F = false | P = positive | N = negative

umbilical artery notches has a 90% sensitivity to predict pre-eclampsia, it would imply that 90% of women with pre-eclampsia will have an abnormal uterine artery notch.

SPECIFICITY

Specificity is the proportion of cases that do not have a clinical abnormality with a normal test result. The equivalent statement would be that 90% of women without pre-eclampsia have a normal uterine artery Doppler result.

PREDICTIVE VALUES

Although sensitivity and specificity are useful for looking at the entire population, they do not give information about the individual. Predictive values are more applicable for an individual (that is, they give the percentage chance of that individual being affected or unaffected). These are useful to the clinician but are also highly dependent on the prevalence of the disease concerned. If a disease is rare, even a bad test will have a high negative prediction. A positive prediction is a proportion of cases with an abnormal test result that have the clinical abnormality. So, the positive prediction of an abnormal uterine artery Doppler result (where 1 in 5 get the disease) for prediction of pre-eclampsia would imply that 20% of women with an abnormal uterine artery Doppler result will get pre-eclampsia. Negative prediction is the proportion of cases with a normal test result that do not have the clinical abnormality. For example, 99% of women with a normal uterine artery Doppler result will not get pre-eclampsia.

LIKELIHOOD RATIOS

Other tests are sometimes used to look at the efficiency of a test. For example, a likelihood ratio is the effectiveness of a particular diagnostic test to confirm or exclude a particular diagnosis. The likelihood is a ratio of the event rate before and after the test, so therefore a likelihood ratio of 1 means that the patient is no more or less likely to have a condition once she has had the test. A good test will therefore have a high likelihood ratio. The advantage of using the likelihood ratio is that it can

FIGURE 34.1 **Receiver–operating characteristic curve**

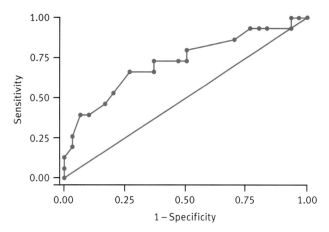

Area under ROC curve = 0.7289

be applied to different populations who are at lower and higher risk. Likelihood ratios generally stay the same in high and low risk populations although this cannot be guaranteed. For example, a fetal fibronectin test to predict preterm birth generally has a high likelihood ratio of approximately 10–15. This is similar in a high- and low-risk population, although the absolute risk (that is, the positive prediction) is very different depending on the risk status of the woman.

Receiver–operating characteristic curves

Figure 34.1 shows a receiver–operating characteristic (ROC) curve. This is a plot of the sensitivity against the false positive rate (also determined as 1 – specificity.) As the sensitivity of a test increases, there will be an inevitable increase in the false positive rate. If there is no discriminatory power, then a ROC curve will effectively be a straight line. This is equivalent to tossing a coin, but a good test will have a high sensitivity with only a small reduction in the false positive rate and therefore the ROC curve will head towards the top left-hand corner of the graph.

ROC curves are useful in determining the best cut-off. For example, a low blood pressure to diagnose pre-eclampsia would have a high sensitivity but clearly there would be a lot of false cases included. Equally, a high blood pressure, say a diastolic over 100 mmHg would ensure that there were very few false determinants of pre-eclampsia, but obviously some cases would be missed. A diastolic of 90 mmHg is at the highest point to the top left corner on a graph (that is, the optimal balance between sensitivity and false positive rates) and hence is used as a cut-off for determining risk when diagnosing hypertension in pregnancy. For some tests, sensitivity may be 'sacrificed' at the expense of improving false positive rates depending on the clinical significance. For example, in Down syndrome screening, one accepts very high false positive rates (as the test will be confirmed by amnio centesis) but sensitivity must be as high as possible because 'missed' cases are unacceptable to most women. Down syndrome screening is far from perfect.[6]

Conclusion

Statistical analysis is just another tool. All clinicians should understand the importance of asking the right question and understand the limitations of statistical analysis. Used correctly, statistics in clinical practice can augment our knowledge and benefit clinical care enormously. Clinicians do not have to be statisticians, but they must engage in the process to understand the best way to inform their practice.

REFERENCES

1. BOWLING A. *Research Methods in Health.* Buckingham, Philadelphia: Open University Press; 1997.

2. HARRIS M, TAYLOR G. *Medical Statistics Made Easy.* London: Taylor & Francis Group; 2004.

3. National Screening Committee. *Second Report of the UK National Screening Committee.* London: Department of Health; 2001.

4. WALD N J, KENNARD A, HACKSHAW A, MAGUIRE A. Antenatal screening for Down's syndrome. *Health Technol Assess* 1998;2:i–iv, 1–112.

5. CUCKLE HS, WALD NJ. Principles of Screening. In: *Antenatal and Neonatal Screening.* Oxford: Oxford University Press; 1984. p.1–22.

6. WHITTLE M. Down's syndrome screening: where to now? *BJOG* 2001;108:559–61.

USEFUL SOURCES OF INFORMATION

Centre of Research: Ethical Campaign [www.corec.org.uk].

EudraCT: [https://eudract.emea.europa.eu].

Institute of Clinical Research: e-mail: info@instituteofclinical research.com; Tel: 01628 899755; [www.instituteofclinical research.com].

Medicines and Healthcare products Regulatory Agency (MHRA): e-mail: info@mhra.gsi.gov.uk; Tel: 0207 084 2000; [http://www.mhra.gov.uk/].

RDDirect: e-mail: info@rddirect.org.uk; Tel: 0113 295 1122 (Monday to Friday 8.30 a.m. to 5.00 p.m.); [www.rddirect.org.uk].

CHAPTER 35

Epidemiology

Prathiba M De Silva and Arri Coomarasamy

An analytical clinical epidemiologist

Analyses of deaths due to puerperal fever by Ignaz Semmelweiss in Vienna in the early 19th century demonstrated the power of epidemiology. At the age of 28, Semmelweiss deduced that by not washing hands doctors caused or contributed to this deadly disease. In his maternity unit, 20% of the 3000 women who delivered died of puerperal fever. After he commanded that every doctor and nurse on his ward wash their hands with chlorine, the mortality rates from puerperal fever plummeted to about 1%! But doctors did not believe Semmelweiss's findings. Rather than being honoured, he was ridiculed and ultimately dismissed from his job.

A dismissed and desperate Semmelweiss stood next to the sink and scolded anyone who forgot to scrub their hands. He wrote to a fellow obstetrician: 'You, Herr Professor, have been a partner in this massacre.' Over time, he began to be considered a lunatic by his own staff. Practice only started to change two decades later when Lister published his seminal work on antisepsis in the medical journal *The Lancet*.

Introduction

The term 'epidemiology' was conceived to describe the study of epidemics, such as cholera and plague. The term has now acquired a wider meaning to include the study of the distribution of all varieties of diseases in various populations and the factors that influence the occurrence of these diseases. Epidemiology has numerous branches, including those discussed here.

OBSERVATIONAL EPIDEMIOLOGY

This branch relies on the surveillance of populations and subgroups, using various health statistics and resources. An example would be the study of maternal death rates categorised by age and cause of death. Data are often obtained from national or other registries and other administrative data sources. Analysis for trends, particularly over time, is often an important aspect of observational epidemiology. The Confidential Enquiry into Maternal Deaths (CEMD) reports represent an exercise in observational epidemiology.

ANALYTICAL OBSERVATIONAL EPIDEMIOLOGY

Addition of analytical methods to observational epidemiological studies can sometimes allow powerful inferences to be drawn about causation and associations. The main analytical methods are the case–control and the cohort study. Influential examples of this branch of epidemiology are again the CEMD reports, which use quantitative and qualitative methods.

EXPERIMENTAL EPIDEMIOLOGY

Experimental epidemiology includes studies in which the researcher investigates the effects of intentional intervention on the outcome of a disease. A study design that is often used in this branch of epidemiology is the randomised controlled trial (RCT), which employs random allocation of participants to alternative interventions, with the aim of reducing bias.

CLINICAL EPIDEMIOLOGY AND EVIDENCE-BASED MEDICINE

More recently, doctors and other healthcare professionals discovered the value of epidemiological methods in enhancing their clinical practice, particularly with regards to their diagnoses and therapies, primarily through meticulous attention to the nature and quality of the evidence on which clinical decisions are based. This discipline has now been given structure and form with the term 'evidence-based medicine' (EBM), which is the conscientious and judicious use of evidence in conjunction with clinical expertise and patients' preferences and values. EBM is now accepted as an essential tool to bring evidence to the bedside and it permeates right through from patient–clinician interaction to healthcare purchasing and policy making. EBM provides hierarchies of evidence to determine what constitutes best available evidence.

THE ORIGINS OF CLINICAL EPIDEMIOLOGY AND EVIDENCE-BASED MEDICINE

Ancient Greek and Roman philosophers considered healthcare and medicine to be a stochastic art. This means that it is an art with the peculiar characteristic of unpredictability between means and ends, such that from the outcome of patients it cannot be inferred that the correct principles of management were followed. Because of this unpredictability, healthcare practitioners cannot always infer what will happen to the individual patient before them without reliance on external evidence. The development of numerical methods in conducting patient-centred research (clinical epidemiology) has provided clinicians with the tools to deal with unpredictability.

The term EBM was coined in the 1980s to name the clinical strategy of asking questions, finding and appraising relevant data and harnessing this information for everyday clinical practice. Interestingly, it was not until 1992 that this clinical paradigm officially appeared in a peer-reviewed journal, the *Journal of the American Medical Association*. [1] The EBM paradigm

asserts that potential advances in healthcare must be tested and proven to do more good than harm before they are incorporated into practice.

Maternal, neonatal and perinatal mortality

DEFINITIONS

The International Classification of Diseases (ICD10) defines a maternal death as 'the death of a woman while pregnant or within 42 days of termination of pregnancy, from any cause related to or aggravated by the pregnancy or its management, but not from accidental or incidental causes'. [2] Maternal deaths can be subdivided into various groups, as given in Table 35.1. The definitions relating to fetal and neonatal deaths are summarised in Table 35.2.

MBRRACE-UK: MOTHERS AND BABIES: REDUCING RISK THROUGH AUDITS AND CONFIDENTIAL ENQUIRIES ACROSS THE UK

The UK national surveillance and Confidential Enquiry into Maternal Deaths (CEMD) was established in 1952 and its newborn and baby equivalent was founded much later, with the establishment of the Confidential Enquiry into Stillbirth and Deaths in Infancy (CESDI) in 1993. In 2003, these two enquiries fell under the newly commenced Centre for Maternal and Child Enquiries (CMACE). This organisation carried out confidential enquiries on a nationwide basis, with triennial reports and analyses on the health of mothers, babies and children.

In 2010, CMACE, together with its surgical, medical and mental health equivalents were put out for competitive tenders, collectively named Clinical Outcome Review Programmes (CORPs). After removing and reassigning the child health component of CMACE, it was rebranded as the Maternal, Newborn and Infant Clinical Outcomes Review Programme (MNI-CORP) by the National Patient Safety Agency (NPSA).

Since 2012, the MBRRACE-UK collaboration, led by the National Perinatal Epidemiology Unit (NPEU) at the University of Oxford, has been appointed by the Healthcare Quality Improvement Partnership (HQIP)

TABLE 35.1 **Definitions of maternal death**

Box 1.3. Definitions of maternal deaths (World Health Organization 2010)	
Maternal death	Death of a women while pregnant or within 42 days of the end of the pregnancy* from any cause related to or aggravated by the pregnancy or its management, but not from accidental or incidental causes.
Direct	Deaths resulting from obstetric complications of the pregnant state (pregnancy, labour and puerperium), from interventions, omissions, incorrect treatment or from a chain of events resulting from any of the above.
Indirect	Deaths resulting from previous existing disease, or disease that developed during pregnancy and which was not the result of direct obstetric causes, but which was aggravated by the physiological effects of pregnancy.
Late	Deaths occurring between 42 days and 1 year after the end of pregnancy* that are the result of Direct or Indirect maternal causes.
Coincidental[†]	Deaths from unrelated causes which happen to occur in pregnancy or the puerperium.

*Includes giving birth, ectopic pregnancy, miscarriage or termination of pregnancy.
[†]Termed "Fortuitous" in the International Classification of Diseases (ICD)

Reproduced from Saving Lives, Improving Mothers' Care: Lessons learned to inform future maternity care from the UK and Ireland, with permission from MBRRACE-UK (2014).

TABLE 35.2 **Definitions regarding perinatal deaths**

Late fetal loss	A baby delivered between 22^{+0} and 23^{+6} weeks gestational age showing no signs of life, irrespective of when the death occurred
Stillbirth	A baby delivered at or after 24^{+0} weeks gestational age showing no signs of life, irrespective of when the death occurred.
Antepartum stillbirth	A baby delivered at or after 24^{+0} weeks gestational age showing no signs of life and known to have died before the onset of care in labour.
Intrapartum stillbirth	A baby delivered at or after 24^{+0} weeks gestational age showing no signs of life and known to be alive at the onset of care in labour.
Neonatal death	A live born baby (born at 20^{+0} weeks gestational age or later, or with a birthweight of 400g or more where an accurate estimate of gestation is not available) who died *before* 28 completed days after birth.
Early neonatal death	live born baby (born at 20^{+0} weeks gestational age or later, or with a birthweight of 400g or more where an accurate estimate of gestation is not available) who died *before* 7 completed days after birth.
Late neonatal death	A live born baby (born at 20^{+0} weeks gestational age or later, or with a birthweight of 400g or more where an accurate estimate of gestation is not available) who died *from* 7 completed days but *before* 28 completed days after birth.
Perinatal death	A stillbirth or early neonatal death
Extended perinatal death	A stillbirth or neonatal death.
Post-neonatal death	A live born baby (born at 20^{+0} weeks gestational age or later, or with a birthweight of 400g or more where an accurate estimate of gestation was not available) who died *from* 28 completed days but *before* 1 year after birth.
Termination of pregnancy	The deliberate ending of a pregnancy, normally carried out before the embryo or fetus is capable of independent life.

Reproduced from Perinatal Mortality Surveillance Report: UK Perinatal Deaths for births from January to December 2013, with permission from MBRRACE-UK (2014).

TABLE 35.3 **Trends in maternal deaths in the UK**

3-year period	Total UK maternities	Direct deaths			Indirect deaths			Total Direct and Indirect deaths		
		n	Rate	95% CI	n	Rate	95% CI	n	Rate	95% CI
2003–05	2 114 004	132	6.24	5.26–7.41	163	7.71	6.61–8.99	295	13.95	12.45–15.64
2004–06	2 165 909	118	5.45	4.55–6.53	154	7.11	6.07–8.33	272	12.56	11.15–14.14
2005–07	2 220 979	113	5.09	4.23–6.12	146	6.57	5.59–7.73	259	11.66	10.32–13.17
2006–08	2 291 493	107	4.67	3.86–5.64	154	6.72	5.74–7.87	261	11.39	10.09–12.86
2007–09	2 331 835	101	4.33	3.53–5.26	153	6.56	5.56–7.69	254	10.89	9.59–12.32
2008–10	2 366 082	89	3.76	3.02–4.63	172	7.27	6.22–8.44	261	11.03	9.73–12.45
2009–11	2 379 014	83	3.49	2.78–4.32	170	7.15	6.11–8.30	253	10.63	9.36–12.03
2010–12	2 401 624	78	3.25	2.57–4.05	165	6.87	5.86–8.00	243	10.12	8.89–11.47

Source: CMACE, MBRRACE-UK, Office for National Statistics, National Records Scotland, Northern Ireland Statistics and Research Agency

Reproduced from Saving Lives, Improving Mothers' Care: Lessons learned to inform future maternity care form the UK and Ireland, with permission from MBRRACE-UK (2014).

to carry out the MNI-CORP on behalf of NHS England, NHS Wales, the Scottish Government Heath and Social Care Directorate, the Northern Ireland Department of Health, Social Services and Public Safety (DHSSPS), the States of Guernsey, the States of Jersey, and the Isle of Man Government. [2]

MATERNAL DEATHS IN THE UK

The most recent CEMD report, and the first by MBRRACE-UK, named *Saving Lives, Improving Mothers' Care*, was published in 2014, covering maternal deaths and serious morbidity from 2009 to 2012 [2]. For the first time, this report includes detailed information from the Republic of Ireland as well as the UK.

It also addresses the epidemiology of severe pregnancy-related complications, with the introduction of the Confidential Enquiries into Maternal Morbidity (CEMM). Here, topics are suggested by clinicians, policy-makers, third sector organisations and the public in an annual application process, and then chosen by the MBRRACE-UK Independent Advisory Group, where the focus of the 2014 report was maternal sepsis.

Between 2009 and 2012, 357 women died from conditions directly or indirectly related to pregnancy out of more than 2 million births in the UK, giving a maternal mortality rate of 10.12 per 100 000 live births, which represents a statistically significant decrease from previous figures. Whilst the rate of direct maternal deaths have halved over the last decade, there has been no significant change in the rate of indirect maternal deaths over this time period (Table 35.3). It is essential to action primary, secondary and mental health services as well as maternity care in order to identify and appropriately manage these women.

Despite multifaceted approaches over the years to reduce maternal mortality in the UK, there is an apparent lack of progress. The reasons for this are thought to be multifactorial, although the following issues have been highlighted to be contributory factors in the most recent report:

■ Age, socio-economic status and ethnicity: Older women, women living in deprived areas and women from specific ethnic groups are known to have higher maternal mortality rates than counterparts in other demographic groups. The number of migrant women in the UK has steadily risen and there are proportionately more deaths among these women. Many migrant women have poor obstetric histories, with complicated pregnancies or serious underlying medical conditions. Nearly three-quarters of women

TABLE 35.4 Causes and number and rates of direct and indirect deaths in the UK

Cause of death	Numbers									Rates per 100,000 maternities								
	1985–87	1988–90	1991–93	1994–96	1997–99	2000–02	2003–05	2006–08	2009–11	1985–87	1988–90	1991–93	1994–96	1997–99	2000–02	2003–05	2006–08	2009–11
All Direct and Indirect deaths	223	238	228	268	242	261	295	261	252	9.83	10.08	9.85	12.19	11.4	13.07	13.95	11.39	10.63
Direct deaths																		
Genital tract sepsis*	9	17	15	16	18	13	18	26	14	0.40	0.72	0.65	0.73	0.85	0.65	0.85	1.13	0.63
Pre-eclampsia and eclampsia	27	27	20	20	16	14	18	19	10	1.19	1.14	0.86	0.91	0.75	0.70	0.85	0.83	0.42
Thrombosis and thromboembolism	32	33	35	48	35	30	41	18	30	1.41	1.40	1.51	2.18	1.65	1.50	1.94	0.79	1.26
Amniotic fluid embolism	9	11	10	17	8	5	17	13	7	0.40	0.47	0.43	0.77	0.38	0.25	0.80	0.57	0.29
Early pregnancy deaths	16	24	17	15	17	15	14	11	4	0.71	1.02	0.73	0.68	0.80	0.75	0.66	0.48	0.17
Haemorrhage	10	22	15	12	7	17	14	9	14	0.44	0.93	0.65	0.55	0.33	0.85	0.66	0.39	0.59
Anaesthesia	6	4	8	1	3	6	6	7	3	0.26	0.17	0.35	0.05	0.14	0.30	0.28	0.31	0.12
Other Direct‡	27	17	14	7	7	8	4	4	0	1.19	0.72	0.60	0.32	0.33	0.40	0.19	0.17	–
All Direct	139	145	128	134	106	106	132	107	82	6.13	6.14	5.53	6.10	4.99	5.31	6.24	4.67	3.49
Indirect deaths																		
Cardiac disease	23	18	37	39	35	44	48	53	51	1.01	0.76	1.60	1.77	1.65	2.20	2.27	2.31	2.14
Other Indirect causes	43	45	38	39	41	50	50	49	72	1.90	1.91	1.64	1.77	1.93	2.50	2.37	2.14	3.03
Indirect neurological conditions	19	30	25	47	34	40	37	36	30	0.84	1.27	1.08	2.14	1.60	2.00	1.75	1.57	1.26
Psychiatric causes	↑	↑	↑	9	15	16	18	13	13	↑	↑	↑	0.41	0.71	0.80	0.85	0.57	0.55
Indirect malignancies	↑	↑	↑	↑	11	5	10	3	4	↑	↑	↑	↑	0.52	0.25	0.47	0.13	0.17
All Indirect	84	93	100	134	136	155	163	154	170	3.70	3.94	4.32	6.10	6.40	7.76	7.71	6.59	7.15
Coincidental	26	39	46	36	29	36	55	50	22	1.15	1.65	1.99	1.64	1.37	1.80	2.60	2.18	0.98

*Including early pregnancy deaths as a result of sepsis

‡Acute fatty liver and genital tract trauma; included with pre-edampsia and edampsia and haemorrhage respectively from 2009 onwards

†Deaths from these causes not included in reports from earlier years

Source: CMACE, MBRRACE-UK

Reproduced from Saving Lives, Improving Mothers' Care: Lessons learned to inform future maternity care from the UK and Ireland, with permission from MBRRACE-UK (2014).

who died were from Asia (primarily Pakistan, Bangladesh, India and Sri Lanka) and Africa (primarily Ghana, Nigeria and Somalia).

- Overweight and obesity: 49% of the pregnant women for whom body mass index was known were found to be overweight or obese in the report. Obesity is associated with a number of complications in pregnancy and childbirth, including cardiac disease, pre-eclampsia, gestational diabetes, thromboembolism, post-caesarean wound infection and postpartum haemorrhage.
- Access to antenatal care: More than two-thirds of women who died between 2009 and 2012 did not receive the recommended level of antenatal care as per NICE guidelines (booking up to 10 weeks and no routine antenatal visits missed) and a quarter of women did not receive the minimum level of care (booking at less than 13 weeks and less than four antenatal visits missed). [3]

Direct maternal deaths in the UK

Thrombosis and thromboembolism remain the greatest causes of direct maternal deaths (Table 35.4), exacerbated by the known association with maternal obesity; these deaths will be specifically reviewed in the upcoming 2015 report. Deaths from pre-eclampsia and eclampsia (including those from HELLP syndrome and acute fatty liver of pregnancy), are now lower than ever. Deaths from genital tract sepsis almost halved from 26 in 2006–8 to 14 in 2009-11, greatly helped by the international Surviving Sepsis Campaign and consequently updated management guidelines. [2]

Indirect maternal deaths in the UK

Following from previous reports, the greatest single cause of indirect and in fact all maternal deaths continues to be cardiac disease (Table 35.4).

Three-quarters of women who died had medical or mental health problems before they became pregnant. It is therefore important to consider how pre-pregnancy advice and joint specialist and maternity care could benefit such patients.

Maternal deaths from psychiatric causes also make a significant contribution to late maternal deaths, so

consideration is likewise warranted for how antenatal support systems could identify these cases.

Whilst it is encouraging to see that genital tract sepsis deaths have decreased significantly in recent years, more than three times as many women died from other infections and are hence classified as indirect deaths. The majority of these were due to influenza. Because as many as half of the influenza-associated deaths occurred after a vaccine became available, it must remain a public health priority to increase vaccination rates in pregnancy against seasonal influenza. [2]

KEY TOPIC-SPECIFIC MESSAGES FOR CARE

The authors of the latest CEMD report compiled a risk of key messages (Box 35.1) in order to move forward from the findings.

MATERNAL DEATHS – AN INTERNATIONAL PERSPECTIVE

The total number of maternal deaths, globally, decreased by 45% from 523,000 in 1990 to 289,000 in 2013 (Table 35.5). [4] Whilst this decrease is promising, 99% of these deaths remain in developing countries. For every woman who dies, it is estimated that 20 more mothers are left with serious injury or long-term illness. One-third of total global maternal deaths are in two countries: Nigeria and India. The lifetime risk of death from pregnancy and childbirth may be as high as 1 in 40 in Africa, compared with 1 in 3300 in Europe. [5] The maternal mortality rate is estimated to be about 510 per 100,000 live births in sub-Saharan Africa, compared with 16 per 100,000 live births in the developed world. [4] These figures represent the largest public health divergence in the world.

CAUSES OF MATERNAL DEATHS WORLDWIDE

A systematic review consisting of 417 datapoints (60,799 maternal deaths) found wide global regional variation in the causes of maternal deaths. [6] Some of the main findings are listed below:

- Nearly three-quarters (73%) of all maternal deaths between 2003 and 2009 were due to direct obstetric causes, whilst deaths due to indirect causes accounted for the remainder (Table 35.6).

494

TABLE 35.5 **Maternal mortality estimates by World Health Organization / United Nations Regions in 2013**

Region	MMR[a]	Range of MMR uncertainty		Number of maternal deaths[a]	Lifetime risk of maternal death[a] 1 in:
		Lower estimate	Upper estimate		
World	210	160	290	289 000	190
Developed regions[b]	16	12	23	2300	3700
Developing regions	230	180	320	286 000	160
Northern Africa[c]	69	47	110	2700	500
Sub-Saharan Africa[d]	510	380	730	179 000	38
Eastern Asia[e]	33	21	54	6400	1800
Eastern Asia excluding China	54	35	97	480	1200
Southern Asia[f]	190	130	280	69 000	200
Southern Asia excluding India	170	110	270	19 000	210
South-eastern Asia[g]	140	98	210	16 000	310
Western Asia[h]	74	50	120	3600	450
Caucasus and Central Asia[i]	39	31	53	690	940
Latin America and the Caribbean	85	66	120	9300	520
Latin America[j]	77	59	110	7900	570
Caribbean[k]	190	130	310	1400	220
Oceania[l]	190	100	380	510	140

[a] The MMFL, number of maternal deaths, and lifetime risk have been rounded according to the following scheme: <100, no rounding; 100–999, rounded to nearest 10; 1000–9999, rounded to nearest 100; and >10 000, rounded lo nearest 1000.

[b] Albania, Australia, Austria, Belarus, Belgium, Bosnia and Herzegovina, Bulgaria, Canada, Croatia, Cyprus, Czech Republic, Denmark, Estonia, Finland, France, Germany, Greece, Hungary, Iceland, Ireland, Israel, Italy, Japan, Latvia, Lithuania, Luxembourg, Malta, Montenegro, The Netherlands, New Zealand, Norway, Poland, Portugal, Republic of Moldova, Romania, Russian Federation, Serbia, Slovakia, Slovenia, Spain, Sweden, Switzerland, The former Yugoslav Republic of Macedonia, Ukraine, United Kingdom of Great Britain and Northern Ireland, United States of America.

[c] Algeria, Egypt, Libya, Morocco, Tunisia.

[d] Angola, Benin, Botswana, Burkina Faso, Burundi, Cameroon, Cabo Verde, Central African Republic, Chad, Comoros, Congo, Côte d'Ivoire, Democratic Republic of the Cooge, Djibouti, Equatorial Guinea, Eritrea, Ethiopia, Gabon, Gambia, Ghana, Guinea, Guinea-Bissau, Kenya, Lesotho, Liberia, Madagascar, Malawi, Mali, Mauritania, Mauritius, Mozambique, Namibia, Niger, Nigeria, Rwanda, Sao Tome and Principe, Senegal, Sierra Leone, Somalia, South Africa, South Sudan, Sudan, Swaziland, Togo, Uganda, United Republic of Tanzania, Zambia, Zimbabwe.

[e] China, Democratic People's Republic of Korea, Mongolia, Republic of Korea.

[f] Afghanistan, Bangladesh, Bhutan, India, Iran (Islamic Republic of), Maldives, Nepal, Pakistan, Sri Lanka.

[g] Brunei Darussalam, Cambodia, Indonesia, Lao People's Democratic Republic, Malaysia, Myanmar, The Philippines, Singapore, Thailand, Tlmor-Leste, Viet Nam.

[h] Bahrain, Iraq, Jordan, Kuwait, Lebanon, Occupied Palestinian Territory, Oman, Qatar, Saudi Arabia, Syrian Arab Republic, Turkey, United Arab Emirates, Yemen.

[i] Armenia, Azerbaijan, Georgia, Kazakhstan, Kyrgyzstan, Tajikistan, Turkmenistan, Uzbekistan.

[j] Argentina, Belize, Bolivia (Plurinational State of), Brazil, Chile, Colombia, Costa Rica, Ecuador, El Salvador, Guatemala, Guyana, Honduras, Mexico, Nicaragua, Panama, Paraguay, Peru, Suriname, Uruguay, Venezuela (Bolivarian Republic of).

[k] Bahamas, Barbados, Cuba, Dominican Republic, Grenada, Haiti, Jamaica, Puerto Rico, Saint Lucia, Saint Vincent and the Grenadines, Trinidad and Tobago.

[l] Fiji, Kiribati, Micronesia (Federated States of), Papua New Guinea, Samoa, Solomon Islands, Tonga, Vanuatu.

Reproduced from Trends in Maternal Mortality: 1990 to 2013 – estimates by WHO, UNICEF, UNFPA, the World Bank, and the United Nations population division with permission from WHO (2014).

BOX 35.1 **Key topic-specific messages for care**

THINK SEPSIS

- 'Think Sepsis' at an early stage when presented with an unwell pregnant or recently pregnant woman, take all appropriate observations and act on them.
- The key actions for diagnosis and management of sepsis are:
  - Timely recognition
  - Rapid administration of intravenous antibiotics
  - Quick involvement of experts – senior review is essential
- Repeated presentation to the general practitioner, or community midwife, or alternatively repeated self-referral to the obstetric triage or day assessment unit should be considered a 'red flag' and warrant a thorough assessment of the woman to investigate for signs of sepsis.
- Early advice from an infectious diseases physician or microbiologist should be sought; this is essential in instances where the woman fails to respond to the first choice antibiotic.
- To avoid preventable deaths, the benefits of influenza vaccination to pregnant women should be promoted and pregnant women at any stage of pregnancy should be offered vaccination.

PREVENTION AND TREATMENT OF HAEMORRHAGE

- Haemoglobin levels below the normal range for pregnancy should be investigated and iron supplementation considered if indicated to optimise haemoglobin before delivery.
- Stimulating or augmenting uterine contractions should be done in accordance with current guidance and paying particular attention to avoiding uterine tachysystole or hyperstimulation.
- Fluid resuscitation and blood transfusion should not be delayed because of false reassurance from a single haemoglobin result.
- Whilst significant haemorrhage may be apparent from observed physiological disturbances, young fit pregnant women compensate remarkably well. A tachycardia commonly develops but there can be a paradoxical bradycardia. Hypotension is always a very late sign, therefore ongoing bleeding should be acted on without delay.
- In a woman who is bleeding and is likely to develop a coagulopathy or has evidence of a coagulopathy, it is prudent to give blood components before coagulation indices deteriorate.
- Early recourse to hysterectomy is recommended if simpler medical and surgical interventions prove ineffective.

CARING FOR WOMEN WITH AMNIOTIC FLUID EMBOLISM

- Perimortem caesarean section should be carried out within five minutes or as soon as possible alter cardiac arrest and is carried out for the benefit of the woman; there is no need to confirm fetal viability, to do so wastes valuable time.

- It is prudent to trigger the massive obstetric haemorrhage protocol in an undelivered woman at the time the decision to proceed to perimortem caesarean section is made.
- The effectiveness of replacement and supportive therapy should be continuously monitored by the signs and symptoms of adequate oxygen delivery and tissue perfusion.

LESSONS FOR ANAESTHESIA

- Subdural haematoma and cerebral venous sinus thrombosis are well-recognised complications of dural puncture and pregnancy, respectively. Both should always be included in the differential diagnosis of persistent headache after dural tap or post dural puncture headache.
- Anaesthetists should practise drills for managing perioperative airway crises including severe bronchospasm, mechanical obstruction, and difficult intubation/oesophageal intubation.
- Pregnant or postpartum women recovering from anaesthesia require the same standard of postoperative monitoring, including documentation, as non-obstetric patients.
- Anaesthetists must be ready at all times to deal with the adverse effects of local anaesthetics including accidental intrathecal or intravenous injection, and minimise the use of strong concentrations as far as possible.
- All ambulance services should ensure their staff are trained in the relief of aortocaval compression during transfer of all pregnant women. How this was achieved must be routinely documented for each woman.

LEARNING FROM NEUROLOGICAL COMPLICATIONS

- Epilepsy remains a high-risk condition in pregnancy and should continue to be managed as such in antenatal and postnatal care. Services should be commissioned and organised to support joint obstetric and neurological care of women with epilepsy during pregnancy.
- Multi-agency evidence-based guidelines are urgently required to standardise and improve the care of pregnant and postpartum women with epilepsy.
- Pre-conception counselling for women with epilepsy is not always provided effectively and should be robustly delivered in all care settings on an opportunistic basis.
- Neurological examination including assessment for neck stiffness is mandatory in all new onset headaches or headache with atypical features, particularly focal symptoms.
- Pregnancy should not alter the standard of care for women with stroke. All women with stroke, pregnant or not, should be admitted to a Hyperacute Stroke Unit.
- Neither pregnancy, caesarean section delivery nor the immediate postpartum state are absolute contraindications to thrombolysis (intravenous or intra-arterial), dot retrieval or craniectomy.

CARING FOR WOMEN WITH OTHER MEDICAL AND SURGICAL COMPLICATIONS

- A single identified professional should be responsible for co-ordinating the care of women with pre-existing medical conditions.
- Appropriately trained senior physicians should be involved in the care of pregnant and postpartum women with new onset symptoms suggestive of or known underlying medical disorders.
- Routine advice for pregnant women with diabetes mellitus should include the increased risk of

hypoglycaemia and education of family members about optimal management of this condition.

- All women with proteinuria should have this quantified and further investigated if found to be significant.
- Senior surgical opinion is essential when dealing with surgical complications in pregnancy or postpartum and should not be delayed by team hierarchy. Early discussion between consultant obstetrician and consultant surgeon is vital.

Reproduced from Saving Lives, Improving Mothers' Care: Lessons learned to inform future maternity care from the UK and Ireland, with permission from MBRRACE-UK (2014).

- The global distribution of maternal mortality was dominated by sub-Saharan Africa and southern Asia, accounting for almost 84% of all maternal deaths.
- Haemorrhage was the leading direct cause of global maternal deaths, representing 27% of maternal deaths. Hypertension was the second most common direct cause worldwide (14%). Maternal mortality due to sepsis accounted for 11%, abortion accounted for 8%, and embolism and other direct causes accounted for the remaining 13% of global deaths.
- More than 70% of indirect causes were due to pre-existing medical conditions, including HIV, which when exacerbated by pregnancy, caused over 1 in 20 global maternal deaths.

  Figure 35.1 provides statistics of causes of maternal deaths by region. [7]

STILLBIRTHS AND NEONATAL DEATHS

The Perinatal Mortality Surveillance Report which provides information on all UK perinatal deaths, for births from January to December 2013, was the first report published by MBRRACE-UK. [8]

Stillbirths

In England, Wales and Northern Ireland, the stillbirth rate was 4.64 per 1000 total births (Table 35.7). The stillbirth rate has decreased over time, with 650 fewer stillbirths in 2013 compared to 2003, and the greatest reduction occurring from 2010.

MBRRACE-UK uses a CODAC classification system, adopting a three level hierarchical tree of coded causes of death, a full description of which can be found at http://codac-classification.org/. As many as 47% of stillbirths were classified as unknown causes but by use of the CODAC classification and close collaboration between MBRRACE-UK and Trusts and Health Boards, more detailed information will be available to help in the understanding of this type of death in the future.

Most stillbirths that had an identifiable cause were attributed to the placenta and the intrapartum phase (Table 35.8).

Neonatal deaths

In England, Wales and Northern Ireland, the neonatal mortality rate was 2.68 per 1000 total births in 2013. Congenital anomalies contributed to far more neonatal deaths compared to stillbirths. Like the stillbirth rate, the neonatal mortality rate has declined steadily between 2003 and 2013 (Table 35.7, Figure 35.2).

Extended perinatal deaths

In England, Wales and Northern Ireland, the extended perinatal mortality rate was 7.3 per 1000 total births in 2013. This figure has seen a steady decrease since 2003, as depicted in Table 35.7.

Multiple births

Multiple births accounted for only 3% of total births but were significantly associated with high rates of neonatal

TABLE 35.6 **Estimated distribution of maternal deaths by WHO Millennium Development Goal region**

	Abortion		Embolism		Haemorrhage		Hypertension		Sepsis		Other direct causes		Indirect causes	
	N	% (95% UI)	N	% (95% UI)	N	% (95% UI)	N	% (95% UI)	N	% (95% UI)	N	% (95% UI)	N	% (95% UI)
Worldwide	193 000	7·9% (4·7–13·2)	78 000	3·2% (1·8–5·5)	661 000	27·1% (19·9–36·2)	343 000	14·0% (11·1–17·4)	261 000	10·7% (5·9–18·6)	235 000	9·6% (6·5–14·3)	672 000	27·5% (19·7–37·5)
Developed regions	1100	7·5% (5·7–11·6)	2000	13·8% (10·1–22·0)	2400	16·3 (11·1–24·6)	1900	12·9% (10·0–16·8)	690	4·7% (2·4–11·1)	2900	20·0% (16·6–27·5)	3600	24·7% (19·5–33·9)
Developing regions	192 000	7·9% (4·7–13·2)	76 000	3·1% (1·7–5·4)	659 000	27·1% (19·9–36·4)	341 000	14·0% (11·1–17·4)	260 000	10·7% (5·9–18·7)	232 000	9·6% (6·4–14·3)	668 000	27·5% (19·7–37·6)
Northern Africa	490	2·2% (0·9–4·9)	720	3·2% (0·9–8·9)	8300	36·9% (24·1–51·6)	3800	16·9% (11·9–22·9)	1300	5·8% (2·3–12·9)	3800	17·1% (7·7–30·8)	4000	18·0% (9·5–30·2)
Sub-Saharan Africa	125 000	9·6% (5·1–17·2)	27 000	2·1% (0·8–4·5)	321 000	24·5% (16·9–34·1)	209 000	16·0% (11·7–21)	134 000	10·3% (5·5–18·5)	119 000	9·0% (5·1–15·7)	375 000	28·6% (19·9–40·3)
Eastern Asia	420	0·8% (0·2–2·0)	6500	11·5% (1·6–40·6)	20 000	35·8% (10·9–68·2)	5900	10·4% (3·9–20·2)	1500	2·6% (0·4–9·7)	8000	14·1% (2·0–51·3)	14 000	24·9% (6·4–58·8)
Southern Asia	47 000	5·9% (1·5–17·3)	17 000	2·2% (0·5–6·8)	238 000	30·3% (14·0–54·8)	80 000	10·3% (5·8–16·6)	107 000	13·7% (3·3–35·9)	65 000	8·3% (3·3–17·7)	229 000	29·3% (12·2–55·1)
South-eastern Asia	11 000	7·4% (2·8–18·4)	18 000	12·1% (3·2–33·4)	44 000	29·9% (15·2–51·3)	21 000	14·5% (8·4–22·7)	8100	5·5% (1·8–15·0)	20 000	13·8% (5·6–31·2)	25 000	16·8% (7·8–34·2)
Western Asia	860	3·0% (1·0–7·6)	2600	9·2% (3·3–22·6)	8900	30·7% (17·4–49·1)	3900	13·4% (7·5–21·2)	1400	4·8% (1·5–13·1)	4500	15·6% (6·6–33·7)	6700	23·4% (11·3–43·1)
Caucasus and central Asia	250	4·6% (2·7–8·2)	590	10·9% (6·2–18·2)	1200	22·8% (17·2–30·3)	790	14·7% (11·6–18·3)	460	8·5% (5·7–13·6)	910	16·8% (12·6–23·2)	1200	21·8% (16·2–29·9)
Latin American and Caribbean	6900	9·9% (8·1–13·0)	2300	3·2% (2·6–4·7)	16 000	23·1% (19·7–27·8)	15 000	22·1% (19·9–24·6)	5800	8·3% (5·6–12·5)	10 000	14·8% (11·7–19·4)	13 000	18·5% (15·6–22·6)
Oceania	290	7·1% (1·2–22·9)	610	14·8% (1·9–47·6)	1200	29·5 (8·5–61·7)	560	13·8% (4·9–25·8)	200	5·0% (0·6–18·5)	510	12·4% (2·3–38·7)	710	17·4% (4·7–44·3)

Data shown are the estimated proportion of cause of death (%) with 95% uncertainty interval (95% UI).
Table 1: Distribution of cause of deaths by Millennium Development Goal regions

Reproduced with permission from http://www.thelancet.com/pdfs/journals/langlo/PIIS2214-109X(14)70227-X.pdf.

FIGURE 35.1 **Causes of maternal death by geographic region between 1990 and 2013**

(a)

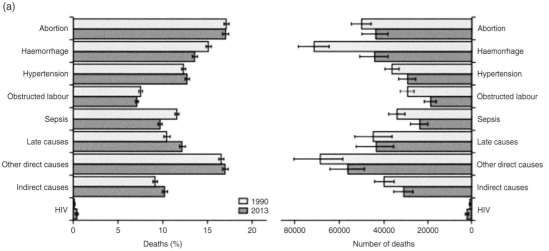

(b)

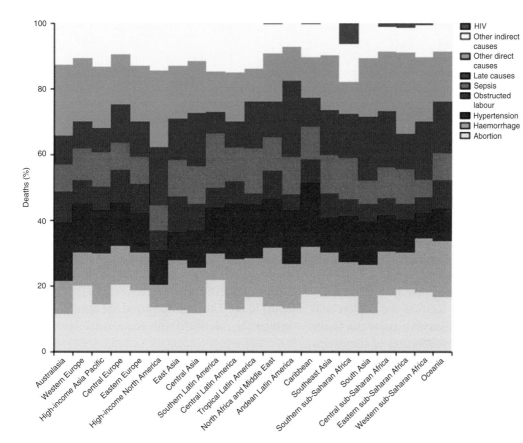

Reproduced with permission from http://www.thelancet.com/pdfs/journals/lancet/PIIS0140-6736(14)60696-6.pdf

TABLE 35.7 **Total stillbirth, neonatal extended perinatal mortality rates from statutory registrations by country: United Kingdom, 2003 to 2013**

Rate per 1,000 births	Country	Year of death										
		2003	2004	2005	2006	2007	2008	2009	2010	2011	2012	2013
Stillbirths[†]	UK	5.70	5.50	5.32	5.30	5.19	5.08	5.19	5.07	5.17	4.82	4.64
	England	5.74	5.47	5.35	5.35	5.18	5.07	5.17	5.08	5.23	4.81	4.65
	Scotland	5.61	5.84	5.34	5.29	5.63	5.38	5.34	4.93	5.08	4.70	4.16
	Wales	4.87	5.04	3.97	3.81	4.15	4.47	4.75	4.13	3.59	4.18	4.51
	Northern Ireland	5.07	5.51	5.34	5.09	4.94	4.61	5.13	5.26	4.67	5.11	4.51
Neonatal deaths[‡]	UK	3.64	3.43	3.50	3.46	3.26	3.18	3.12	2.96	2.95	2.78	2.68
	England	3.65	3.45	3.45	3.49	3.24	3.18	3.10	2.93	2.94	2.78	2.67
	Scotland	3.39	3.08	3.49	3.09	3.25	2.80	2.79	2.55	2.71	2.55	2.34
	Wales	3.94	3.72	4.97	3.87	3.31	3.71	3.89	4.58	3.48	2.77	3.38
	Northern Ireland	3.06	3.09	2.88	2.68	3.31	2.95	3.09	2.73	2.75	2.75	2.40
Extended perinatal deaths[†]	UK	9.32	8.92	8.80	8.74	8.43	8.24	8.30	8.01	8.11	7.59	7.30
	England	9.37	8.90	8.79	8.82	8.40	8.24	8.25	8.00	8.16	7.58	7.31
	Scotland	8.99	8.90	8.82	8.36	8.86	8.17	8.12	7.46	7.78	7.24	6.49
	Wales	8.80	8.74	8.92	7.66	7.45	8.16	8.63	8.69	7.06	6.94	7.87
	Northern Ireland	8.11	8.58	8.21	7.75	8.24	7.54	8.20	7.97	7.41	7.85	6.90

[†] per 1,000 total births
[‡] per 1,000 live births
Data sources: ONS. GRO, NISRA

Reproduced from Perinatal Mortality Surveillance Report: UK Perinatal Deaths for births from January to December 2013, with permission from MBRRACE-UK (2014).

mortality which showed an almost five-fold increase for twins, and over a twelve-fold increase for triplets and higher-order births. Preterm delivery is a major risk factor and accounts for a significant proportion of the excess mortality risk in such births.

Risk factors for stillbirths and neonatal deaths

The main factors associated with stillbirths and neonatal deaths are mother's age, obesity, social deprivation and ethnicity. Mothers aged less than 20 years and over 40 years had the highest rates of stillbirth, neonatal and perinatal deaths. One quarter of stillbirths in the UK were associated with a maternal body mass index (BMI) of greater than or equal to 30. The more deprived the quintile of society, the greater the risk of stillbirth or neonatal mortality.

Epidemiology of disorders leading to pregnancy failure

Miscarriages, recurrent miscarriages and ectopic pregnancy are associated with substantial psychological and physical burdens, including death. For instance, the most recent CEMD report reported 4 deaths from complications of early pregnancy between 2009 and 2011. [2]

TABLE 35.8 **Stillbirths, neonatal deaths and extended perinatal deaths by CODAC level 1 cause of death: United Kingdom and Crown Dependencies, for births in 2013**

CODAC cause of death: level 1	Stillbirths[§]		Neonatal deaths[§]		Extendex perinatal deaths[§]	
	Number	(%)	Number	(%)	Number	(%)
Infection	86	(2.6)	84	(5.8)	170	(3.6)
Neonatal	32	(1.0)	662	(46.1)	694	(14.7)
Intrapartum	289	(8.8)	93	(6.5)	382	(8.1)
Congenital anomaly	193	(5.9)	321	(22.4)	514	(10.9)
Fetal	100	(3.0)	78	(5.4)	178	(3.8)
Cord	129	(3.9)	1	(0.1)	130	(2.8)
Placenta	629	(19.1)	20	(1.4)	649	(13.7)
Maternal	112	(3.4)	9	(0.6)	121	(2.6)
Unknown	1,551	(47.2)	65	(4.5)	1,616	(34.2)
Missing	165	(5.0)	103	(7.2)	268	(5.7)

[§] excluding terminations of pregnancy and births $<24^{+0}$ weeks gestational age
Data sources: MBRRACE-UK

Reproduced from Perinatal Mortality Surveillance Report: UK Perinatal Deaths for births from January to December 2013, with permission from MBRRACE-UK (2014).

FIGURE 35.2 **Total stillbirth, neonatal and extended perinatal mortality rates from statutory registrations: United Kingdom, 2003 to 2013**

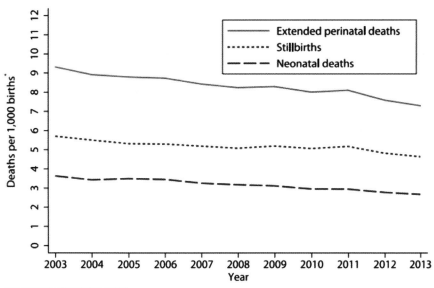

Data sources: ONS, GRO & NISRA

*stillbirth and extended perinatal deaths are per 1,000 total births, neonatal deaths are per 1,000 live births

Reproduced from Perinatal Mortality Surveillance Report: UK Perinatal Deaths for births from January to December 2013, with permission from MBRRACE-UK (2014)..

MISCARRIAGE

Miscarriage, defined as the spontaneous loss of an intra-uterine pregnancy before viability (that is, before 24 completed weeks), is the most common early pregnancy complication and is reported to occur in about 20% of all pregnancies, accounting for over 50 000 inpatient admissions every year in the UK [9]. This prevalence is likely to be an underestimation, as many miscarriages occur before or with the onset of menstruation and thus are not recognised as 'miscarriages'. The true rate of pregnancy loss after implantation is estimated to be over 50%. The definitions relating to miscarriage are given in Chapter 36, Table 36.6.

Risk factors and causes

The risk of miscarriage is known to decrease significantly after the first trimester. The factors associated with miscarriage are described below:

■ Age and chromosomal abnormalities: Chromosomal abnormalities (such as trisomy, XO and triploidy) are identified in more than 60% of embryos miscarried in the first 13 weeks. Most chromosomal problems are sporadic and are unlikely to recur. However, they are more likely to occur in older women, thus contributing to the increased rates of miscarriages observed in older women (Figure 35.3). Some chromosomal problems, such as balanced translocations in one of the parents, can result in an increased risk of recurrent miscarriages.
■ Thrombophilias: These include both acquired (antiphospholipid syndrome: lupus anticoagulant and anticardiolipin antibodies) and congenital cases (such as protein C or S deficiency, activated protein C resistance [factor V Leiden mutation] and antithrombin III deficiency).
■ Anatomic causes: These include uterine Müllerian anomaly, uterine septum (the anomaly most commonly associated with pregnancy loss), unicornuate uterus, diethylstilbestrol-linked conditions, acquired defects (for example, Asherman syndrome), cervical weakness, fibroids and uterine polyps.
■ Endocrine factors: These include polycystic ovary syndrome, diabetes mellitus (particularly if it is poorly

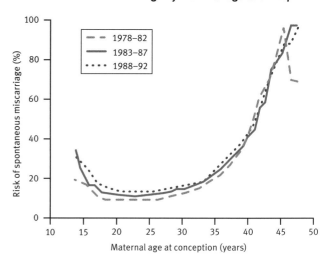

FIGURE 35.3 **Risk of miscarriage by maternal age at conception**

In this large prospective study, a total of 634272 women and 1 221 546 pregnancy outcomes were studied. Overall, 13.5% of the pregnancies intended to be carried to term ended with fetal loss. At age 42 years, more than 50% of such pregnancies resulted in fetal loss. The risk of a miscarriage was 8.9% in women aged 20–24 years and 74.7% in those aged 45 years or more.

Reproduced with permission from: Maternal age and fetal loss: population-based register linkage stude. Nybo Andersen AM, Wohlfahrt J, Christens P, Olsen J, Melbye M.*Br Med J* 2000; 320:1708–12.[7]

controlled), antithyroid antibodies (regardless of thyroid function test abnormalities) and luteal-phase deficiency (although the existence, definition, diagnosis and management of luteal phase deficiency have been and are likely to continue to be a matter of debate).
■ Infectious causes: These include rubella, cytomegalovirus, malaria, chlamydia, salmonella or any acute pyrexial illness, particularly when the infection involves peritonitis.
■ Smoking: Maternal and paternal smoking are both associated with miscarriage.
■ Excessive alcohol consumption and drugs: for example, cocaine and caffeine are associated with increased risk of miscarriage.
■ Multiple pregnancy: Higher-order multiples are associated with an increased risk of miscarriages and preterm births.

RECURRENT MISCARRIAGES

Recurrent miscarriage is defined as the loss of three consecutive pregnancies before viability. It affects approximately 1% of women. If the risk of sporadic miscarriage is about 15%, then the theoretical risk of having three consecutive miscarriages by chance is about 0.34% (15% × 15% × 15%), which is much less than the actual observed rate of 1% and suggests that some women have a predisposition to recurrent miscarriage. This is indeed the case.

Risk factors and causes

- Chromosomal abnormalities: 3–5% of screened parents have chromosomal abnormalities, most commonly a balanced reciprocal translocation and less commonly a Robertsonian translocation.
- Thrombophilias: In contrast to the 2% prevalence of antiphospholipid antibodies in the low-risk obstetric population, women with a history of recurrent miscarriages have a 15% risk of antiphospholipid syndrome (lupus anticoagulant in 9.1% and anticardiolipin antibodies in 5.5%). Women with antiphospholipid syndrome have a 90% risk of miscarriage, which can be reduced with aspirin and heparin therapy. See also section above.
- Anatomical causes: See section above.
- Endocrine causes: See section above.

The risk of live birth after three consecutive miscarriages is 40–70%. After five consecutive miscarriages, the risk falls to 20–50%.

ECTOPIC PREGNANCIES

The incidence of ectopic pregnancies (defined as the implantation of pregnancy outside the uterine cavity) can vary with the accuracy of the diagnostic tools, thoroughness of the work-up and the denominators used for the rates. Publications have used number of births, number of pregnancies or number of women of reproductive age as denominators. The number of women aged 15–44 years is commonly used as a denominator and the reported annual incidence rate varies between 100 and 175 in 100 000 women aged between 15 and 44 years in the UK (that is, 1 or 2 in 1000 women of reproductive age). The rate of ectopic

pregnancy is 11 per 1000 pregnancies, with a maternal mortality of 0.2 per 1000 estimated ectopic pregnancies. [9] Most (98%) ectopic pregnancies occur in the fallopian tubes, with the remainder occuring in the ovary, cervix or abdominal cavity.

Risk factors and causes

- Increasing age (see Figure 35.4).
- History of pelvic inflammatory disease.
- Previous ectopic pregnancies.
- History of infertility.
- Assisted conception (a heterotopic pregnancy): an intrauterine pregnancy and an extrauterine pregnancy at the same time can be found in up to 2% of in vitro fertilisation pregnancies.
- Pelvic surgery.
- Tubal surgery.
- Early age at intercourse.
- Failure of an intrauterine contraceptive device or progestogen-only oral contraceptive, including emergency contraception: the risk of a pregnancy being ectopic is greater than with other forms of contraception.

FIGURE 35.4 **Risk of ectopic pregnancy by maternal age at conception**

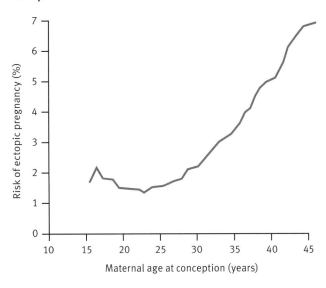

Reproduced with permission from: Maternal age and fetal loss: population-based register linkage stude. Nybo Andersen AM, Wohlfahrt J, Christens P, Olsen J, Melbye M. *Br Med J* 2000; 320:1708–12.[7]

Epidemiology of infertility

FERTILITY, INFERTILITY AND CAUSES

The National Institute for Health and Care Excellence (NICE) defines infertility as the inability to conceive despite regular unprotected intercourse after one year of trying to conceive. About 1 in 7 couples are infertile by this definition. It is therefore no surprise that infertility is the second most common reason for women aged 20–45 years to see their general practitioner, the most common reason being pregnancy itself.

TABLE 35.9 **Cumulative pregnancy rates over various periods of trying to conceive**

Time trying to conceive (months)	Cumulative pregnancy rates (%)
1	20–33
3	50
6	60–70
12	85
18	90
24	92–95

The highest conception rate per monthly cycle among couples with proven normal fertility occurs in the first month of trying and is reported to be 33%. The monthly rate (fecundability) then falls quickly over 6 months, to about 5% per month. The cumulative pregnancy rates over various periods of trying to conceive are given in Table 35.9.

The most common single reason for infertility is now recognised to be male factor (Figure 35.5), which includes men with semen volume <1.5ml, pH <7.2, sperm concentration <15 million spermatazoa/mL, total sperm number <39 million spermatazoa per ejaculate (azoospermia), total motility <40% (or progressive motility <32%), vitality of <58% live spermatazoa or normal sperm morphology of <4%. [10] The second most common reason is unexplained, where a recognised cause for infertility is not found (in about one in four couples).

TREATMENT AND SUCCESS

Although various specific therapeutic options may be available for specific causes of infertility, most couples with one or more of the main causes of infertility (male factor, unexplained, tubal factor and ovulatory) will ultimately have *in vitro* fertilisation (IVF) to

FIGURE 35.5 **Types of infertility treated by IVF and ICSI treatment cycles 2000–2007**

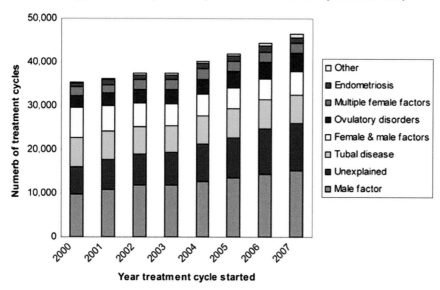

Reproduced from http://www.hfea.gov.uk/2585.html#3018 with permission from HFEA (2014).

504

attempt to achieve a pregnancy. It should therefore come as no surprise that about 2.2% of all births in the UK are now the result of IVF, although the NHS funds only about 41% of all IVF treatment. [11] In countries where the government provides liberal funding for IVF, as many as 5% of all births may be from IVF. The success rate for IVF depends on various factors, the two most important ones being the woman's age and the choice of clinic. The live birth rate for patients receiving IVF treatment in 2012 in the UK were:

- 32.8% for women aged 18–34 years
- 27.3% for women aged 35–37 years
- 20.7% for women aged 38–39 years
- 13.1% for women aged 40–42 years
- 4.4% for women aged 43 years and over

NICE recommends that in women aged under 40 who have not conceived after two years of regular unprotected intercourse, or after 12 cycles of artificial insemination (where six or more are by intrauterine insemination), three full cycles of IVF should be offered with, or without intracytoplasmic sperm injection

(micromanipulation to inject spermatozoa directly into the egg to aid fertilisation). [12]

Currently, more than 60,000 IVF cycles are carried out in the UK (Figure 35.6) in 78 clinics licensed by the Human Fertilisation and Embryology Authority. About 50% of IVF is conventional, with the other 50% representing IVF with intracytoplasmic sperm injection.

ASSISTED CONCEPTION AND MATERNAL MORTALITY

In the latest CEMD report (2009–2012), 10 women whose pregnancies were known to result from assisted reproductive technologies died, 4 from direct and 6 from indirect causes.

It should be appreciated that, beneath the iceberg of mortality, there is likely to be much greater morbidity. It is now widely accepted that the single most adverse effect from assisted reproduction is multiple pregnancy. Most embryo transfers in the UK are double embryo transfers, resulting in about 25% twin pregnancy rates in those who become pregnant. More women opting to

FIGURE 35.6 **Number of IVF cycles performed each year (1991–2013)**

Number of cycles

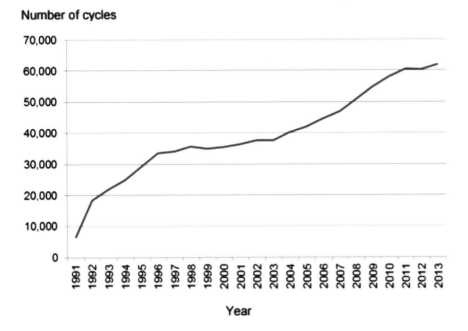

Reproduced from Fertility treatment in 2013: trends and figures, with permission from HFEA (2014)..

have only one embryo transferred at a time to reduce their risk of a multiple pregnancy and increasing numbers of embryo transfers at the blastocyst stage have resulted in a decrease in the multiple birth risk from one in four in 2008 to one in six in 2013. [11]

Epidemiology of cancers affecting women

The majority of cancer registries around the world belong to the International Association of Cancer Registries (IACR) and submit their data routinely to the International Agency for Research on Cancer (www.iarc.fr). Furthermore, as well as belonging to IACR, European cancer registries also belong to the European Network of Cancer Registries (www.encr .com.fr). The UK has its own network, the National Cancer Intelligence Network (NCIN), operated by Public Health England, which seeks to improve the prevention, standards of cancer care and outcomes for

cancer patients. These organisations act as rich resources of epidemiological data on cancers, including the four main cancers in gynaecology: ovarian, cervical, uterine and vulval cancers.

The most common female cancer worldwide is breast cancer. Gynaecological cancers as a group resulted in 7731 deaths in England and Wales in 2012. [13] The most common gynaecological cancer worldwide is cervical cancer, which is the fourth most common female cancer worldwide. The most common gynaecological cancer in the UK is endometrial cancer (of the uterus) as in Figure 35.7, where much of the increase has been since the early 1990s, due to lifestyle factors such as being overweight, obesity, lack of physical activity and hormone replacement therapy.

OVARIAN CANCER

In the UK, ovarian cancer is responsible for more deaths per year than all other gynaecological cancers combined,

FIGURE 35.7 **The 10 most common female cancers in the UK, 2011**

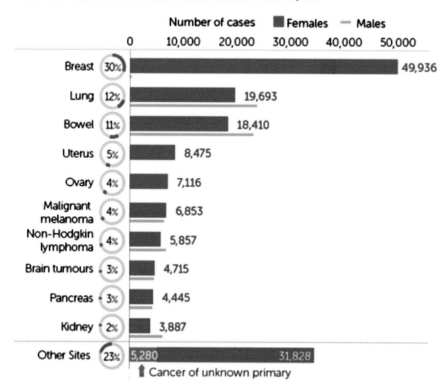

causing approximately 4300 deaths per year, ranking fifth after lung, breast, bowel and pancreatic cancer as one of the leading causes of cancer death in women [13]. There are 7000 new cases every year in the UK. The high mortality rate is largely a result of the late presentation of ovarian cancer; nearly 30% of women will have stage III disease at diagnosis and most will have lymphatic spread. The overall 5-year survival rate is 46%. The majority (85–90%) of malignant ovarian tumours will be serous, accounting for 32% of all cases in 2009. Nearly 50% of the women diagnosed with ovarian cancer were in their 60s or 70s, with over 80% of ovarian cancer deaths occurring in women aged 60 or over. Up to 5–10% of ovarian cancer is associated with genetic predisposition from one of three autosomally inherited gene classes: *BRCA1*, *BRCA2* and *HNPCC*.

ENDOMETRIAL CANCER

Endometrial cancer is the most common gynaecological cancer in women in the UK, with approximately 8500 cases per year [13]. Age-specific incidence rates peak in the 70–74 year age group, with the majority of women presenting in the postmenopausal period. The death rate also increases with age; nearly two-thirds of deaths occur in women aged 70 or over. Endometrial cancer commonly presents early in its natural history, with 67% of cases having stage I disease at the time of diagnosis. The most frequently found histological type of endometrial cancer is endometrioid carcinoma. Risk factors include obesity, nulliparity, late menopause, unopposed estrogen therapy, estrogen-secreting tumours, polycystic ovary syndrome and personal or family history of breast or bowel cancer.

CERVICAL CANCER

The incidence of cervical cancer in the UK decreased by nearly half between the late 1980s until the early 2000s, but the last decade has seen an increase in rates in younger women, to bring the total of new cases and deaths each year to approximately 3000 and 900 respectively [13]. A large proportion of the new cases are now diagnosed at an early stage in the disease. The distribution of the disease is bimodal, with peaks at 30–34 years and then again at 80–84 years. Worldwide, new cases are estimated to be around 527,000 each year, and cervical cancer is responsible for more deaths per year than any other gynaecological cancer. Two-thirds of cervical cancers are squamous cell and about 15% are adenocarcinomas. Risk factors include early onset of sexual activity, multiple sexual partners, low socio-economic class, cigarette smoking, use of the oral contraceptive pill, sexually transmitted infections (particularly human papilloma viruses 16 and 18), and immune suppression.

VULVAL CANCER

Vulval cancer is a rare gynaecological malignancy. It accounts for 6% of all gynaecological cancers diagnosed in the UK [13], with approximately 1000 new cases per year. Historically, this has been a cancer of the elderly, with 58% of women diagnosed in 2007–2009 aged over 70 years. However, there is an increasing incidence in younger women, with around 10% of all cases occuring in women under the age of 40 years. Over 90% of vulval cancer is squamous in origin. Risk factors include human papilloma virus, lichen sclerosus, vulval intraepithelial neoplasia, Paget's disease, melanoma, smoking, immune suppression, advanced age and history of cervical neoplasia.

REFERENCES

1. Evidence Based Medicine Working Group. *Evidenced based medicine: a new approach to teaching the practice of medicine. JAMA* 1992;268:2420

2. KNIGHT M, KENYON S, BROCKLEHURST P, NEILSON J, SHAKESPEARE J, KURINCZUK JJ (Eds.) on behalf of MBRRACE-UK. *Saving Lives, Improving Mothers' Care: Lessons learned to inform future maternity care from the UK and Ireland Confidential Enquiries into Maternal Deaths and Morbidity 2009-12.* Oxford:

National Perinatal Epidemiology Unit, University of Oxford, 2014. https://www.npeu.ox.ac.uk/downloads/files/mbrrace-uk/reports/Saving%20Lives%20Improving%20Mothers%20Care%20report%202014%20Full.pdf (accessed October 2015).

3. National Institute for Health and Care Excellence (NICE), 2008. *Antenatal care for uncomplicated pregnancies.* Clinical guideline 62. London: NICE. http://www.nice.org.uk/guidance/cg62/resources/antenatal-care-for-uncomplicated-pregnancies-975564597445 (accessed October 2015).

4. LEONTINE A, CHOU D, GEMMILL A, HOGAN D, MATHERS C, MILLS S, MOLLER A, SAY L, SUZUKI E. *Trends in Maternal Mortality: 1990 to 2013 – estimates by WHO, UNICEF, UNFPA, the World Bank, and the United Nations population division.* Geneva: World Health Organization, 2014. http://apps.who.int/iris/bitstream/10665/112682/2/9789241507226_eng.pdf?ua=1 (accessed October 2015).

5. LEONTINE A, CHOU D, GEMMILL A, HOGAN D, MATHERS C, MILLS S, MOLLER A, SAY L, SUZUKI E. *Trends in Maternal Mortality: 1990 to 2013 – estimates by WHO, UNICEF, UNFPA, the World Bank, and the United Nations population division – infographic: Saving Mothers' Lives.* Geneva: World Health Organization, 2014. http://www.who.int/reproductivehealth/publications/monitoring/infographic/en/ (accessed October 2015).

6. SAY L, CHOU D, GEMMILL A, TUNÇALP Ö, MOLLER A-B, DANIELS J, et al. *Global causes of maternal death: a WHO systematic analysis.* Lancet Global Health 2014;2(6):e323–33.

7. KASSEBAUM NJ, BERTOZZI-VILLA A, COGGESHALL MS, et al. *Global, regional, and national levels and causes of maternal mortality during 1990–2013: a systematic analysis for the Global Burden of Disease Study 2013.* Lancet 2014;384: 980–1004.

8. MANKTELOW BN, SMITH LK, EVANS TA, HYMAN-TAYLOR P, KURINCZUK JJ, FIELD DJ, SMITH PW, DRAPER ES on behalf of MBRRACE-UK. *Perinatal Mortality Surveillance Report: UK Perinatal Deaths for births from January to December 2013.* Oxford: National Perinatal Epidemiology Unit, University of Oxford, 2014. https://www.npeu.ox.ac.uk/downloads/files/mbrrace-uk/reports/MBRRACE-UK%20Perinatal%20Surveillance%20Report%202013.pdf (accessed October 2015).

9. National Institute for Health and Care Excellence (NICE), 2012. *Ectopic pregnancy and miscarriage: diagnosis and initial management.* Clinical guideline 154. London: NICE. http://www.nice.org.uk/guidance/cg154 (accessed October 2015).

10. World Health Organisation, 2010. *WHO laboratory manual for the examination and processing of human semen.* 5th Ed. Geneva: WHO. http://apps.who.int/iris/bitstream/10665/44261/1/9789241547789_eng.pdf (accessed October 2015).

11. Human Fertilisation Embryology Authority, 2014. *Fertility treatment in 2013: trends and figures.* HFEA. http://www.hfea.gov.uk/docs/HFEA_Fertility_Trends_and_Figures_2013.pdf (accessed October 2015).

12. National Institute for Health and Care Excellence (NICE), 2013. *Fertility: assessment and treatment.* Clinical guideline 156. London: NICE. http://www.nice.org.uk/guidance/cg156/resources/fertility-problems-assessment-and-treatment-35109634660549 (accessed October 2015).

13. Cancer research UK, 2011. http://www.cancerresearchuk.org/sites/default/files/cstream-node/cs_inc_10common_female.pdf (accessed October 2015).

Data interpretation

CHAPTER 36

Data interpretation

Andrew R Sizer

The Part 1 MRCOG domain of data interpretation was introduced with the revision of the syllabus in 2011, and the first questions appeared in the March 2012 exam diet.

Theoretically, questions could be derived from any aspect of the Part 1 syllabus, but questions tend to have an applied or clinical basis.

This chapter aims to give examples and advice on the type of data interpretation questions that may appear in Paper 2 of the Part 1 MRCOG and is organised by Modules according to the Part 1 blueprinting grid (https://www.rcog.org.uk/globalassets/documents/careers-and-training/mrcog-exam/part-1/ex-part-1-blueprinting-grid-new.pdf).

Module 1: clinical skills

Questions may surround results of blood tests with an accompanying clinical scenario.

For example:

SBA

A 45-year-old woman attends the gynaecology clinic with a 2-year history of heavy menstrual bleeding. She passes clots and bleeds for up to 10 days every cycle. She is feeling tired and lethargic. Clinical examination is unremarkable.

A full blood count is arranged with the following result (Figure 36.1).

How would you interpret this result?

A. Dilutional anaemia
B. Folate deficiency anaemia
C. Iron deficiency anaemia
D. Normal full blood count
E. Vitamin B$_{12}$ deficiency

Comment: The patient is not anaemic despite the clinical history. All parameters with the full blood count are normal.

When looking at a full blood count result, make sure to examine all the parameters given.

Other questions may surround electrolyte disturbance.

SBA

A 70-year-old woman who is taking bendroflumethazide for hypertension presents to the GP with muscle weakness, muscle cramps and constipation.

The GP arranges to check serum urea and electrolytes.

Which electrolyte disturbance is most likely to be present?

A. Hypercalcaemia
B. Hyperkalaemia
C. Hypernatraemia
D. Hypocalcaemia
E. Hypokalaemia

Comment: The symptoms are all features of hypokalaemia. The patient is taking a thiazide diuretic, a side effect of which is hypokalaemia.

It is important to have an understanding of all varieties of electrolyte disturbance, their causes and clinical manifestations (Table 36.1).

FIGURE 36.1

	Result	Unit	Range
WBC	8.8	10*9/L	(5.5 - 15.5)
Red blood cell (RBC) count	4.38	10*12/L	(4.20 - 5.40)
Haemoglobin estimation	121	g/L	(115 - 135)
Haematocrit	36.3	L/L	(34.0 - 40.0)
Mean corpuscular volume (MCV)	83.0	fL	(75.0 - 87.0)
Mean corpusc. haemoglobin(MCH)	27.6	pg	(27.0 - 31.0)
Red blood cell distribut width	13.5	%	
PLTS	386	10*9/L	(150 - 500)
Neuts ab	3.4	10*9/L	(1.5 - 8.5)
Lympho ab	4.2	10*9/L	(2.0 - 8.0)
Mono ab	0.8	10*9/L	(0.1 - 0.9)
Eos ab	0.3	10*9/L	(0.1 - 0.7)
Bas ab	0.1	10*9/L	(0.0 - 0.1)

FLUID BALANCE

Fluid balance is the state where the required amount of bodily water is present and correctly distributed amongst bodily compartments.

Total body water is 70% of lean body weight. Of this: One third is extracellular

- 25% as plasma
- 75% as interstitial fluid

and two thirds is intracellular.

Normal fluid intake is 2.5–3.0 litres per day.

Fluid loss has three main components:

Urine	1500 ml
Insensible loss (sweat, lungs)	850 ml
Faeces	100 ml

URINE OUTPUT

There are often questions about urine output after surgery, or after delivery.

For definitions of urine output, see Table 36.2.

MICROBIOLOGY

Regarding swabs, different organisms inhabit different sites, or different types of epithelium. It is therefore important to have the correct swab to identify the correct organism (Table 36.3).

Similarly, there may be results from the culture and sensitivity of a mid-stream specimen of urine where you are asked to make an interpretation.

Module 3: IT, clinical governance and research

There have been questions surrounding accuracy of tests in every paper since SBA questions were introduced in 2012. These questions are simple for examiners to write, and any mathematics will always be straightforward. If your calculation becomes very complex, then it is almost certainly wrong!

Make sure you have a firm understanding of the 2 × 2 table of diagnostic test and condition:

Sensitivity: the percentage of cases with the condition that are correctly identified by the test (TP/TP + FN) × 100.

		Condition	
		Present	Absent
Diagnostic test	Positive	True positives (TP)	False positives (FP)
	Negative	False negatives (FN)	True negatives (TN)

Specificity: the percentage of cases without the condition that have a negative test (TN/TN + FP) × 100.

Positive predictive value: the chance of having the condition with a positive test (TP/TP + FP).

TABLE 36.1 **The five most important electrolytes**

Electrolyte	Function	Distribution	Disturbance and causes
Sodium (Na)	Key role in fluid balance Contributes half the osmolarity of the extracellular fluid	Predominantly in extracellular fluid Regulated by antidiuretic hormone, aldosterone and atrial natriuretic peptide	Hyponatraemia: caused by insufficient intake (e.g. inadequate sodium in intravenous fluids), excessive water, diuretic therapy or hypoadrenalism Hypernatraemia: caused by excessive salt intake, excessive water depletion or hyperaldosteronism
Potassium (K)	Maintenance of intracellular fluid volume Regulation of pH Establishes resting membrane potential of cells	Predominantly in intracellular fluid Serum level regulated by aldosterone	Hypokalaemia: caused by dietary insufficiency, inadequate intravenous therapy, insulin therapy, beta agonists, vomiting, diarrhoea Hyperkalaemia: caused by excessive intravenous administration, blood transfusion, Addison's disease, potassium-sparing diuretics
Calcium (Ca)	Role in excitable cells, neurotransmitter release and blood clotting	Predominantly in bone Mainly extracellular Regulated by parathyroid hormone	Hypocalcaemia: caused by hypoparathyroidism, inadequate vitamin D intake and renal disease Hypercalcaemia: caused by malignancy or hyperparathyroidism
Chloride (CL)	Balances anions in all fluid compartments	Diffuses easily between extracellular fluid and intracellular fluid Levels linked to sodium concentration	Hypochloraemia: found in pyloric stenosis and respiratory alkalosis Hyperchloraemia: caused by excessive intravenous saline administration or severe dehydration
Bicarbonate (HCO$_3$)	Major buffer in plasma Helps maintain balance of anions and cations in all fluid compartments	Predominantly on extracellular fluid although small amounts also found in intracellular fluid Serum level controlled by kidneys	Deficit leads to metabolic acidosis; caused by use of carbonic anhydrase inhibitors, diarrhoea, fistulae Excess leads to metabolic alkalosis; caused by excessive bicarbonate administration, chronic vomiting, diuretic use

TABLE 36.2 **Definitions of urine output**

Urine output	Numerical definition	Comments
Anuria	<100 ml urine produced in 24 hours	–
Oliguria	<400 ml urine produced per day, but more than 100 ml/day	Many causes including drugs, dehydration, endocrine disturbance, abnormal renal function
Normal urine output	0.5–1.0 ml/kg/h (In infants 2 ml/kg/h)	Dependent upon age and renal function
Polyuria	>3 litres urine production per day	Many potential causes including diuretics, increased fluid intake, diabetes mellitus, diabetes insipidus, Addison's disease

TABLE 36.3 **Identifying different organisms using swabs**

Organism	Epithelium	Swab
Trichomonas vaginalis	Vaginal mucosa	High vaginal swab
Candida albicans	Vaginal mucosa	High vaginal swab
Neisseria gonorrhoeae	Columnar epithelium	Endocervical swab, urethral and rectal swabs
Chlamydia trachomatis	Columnar epithelium	Endocervical and urethral swabs
Bacterial vaginosis (*Coliforms*)	Vaginal mucosa	High vaginal swab

Negative predictive value: the chance of **not** having the condition with a negative test (TN/TN+ FN).

SBA

A specialty trainee undertakes a study of heavy menstrual bleeding. She surveys 200 women attending a gynaecology clinic and notes a history of passing clots vaginally during menstruation. She then takes a full blood count to look for the presence of anaemia. From the study, 110 women give a history of passing clots, and of these, 40 are shown to be anaemic. Sixty women are found to be anaemic in total.

What is the specificity of a history of passing clots for detecting the presence of anaemia?

1. 20%
2. 40%
3. 50%
4. 60%
5. 70%

Comment: The first thing to do here is to construct a 2 × 2 table:

There are 110 women with a history of clots, and 40 are anaemic:

		Anaemia	
		Present	Absent
History of passing clots	Positive		
	Negative		

There are 60 women that are anaemic in total, and the total number of women studied was 200:

		Anaemia	
		Present	Absent
History of passing clots	Positive	40	70
	Negative		

Specificity = TN/(TN + FP) = 70/(70 + 70) × 100 = 50%, so the answer is C.

		Anaemia		
		Present	Absent	Total
History of passing clots	Positive	40	70	110
	Negative	20	70	90
	Total	60	140	200

The questions may look complex, but actually the mathematics tends to be very straightforward if the 2 × 2 table is used correctly.

Module 5: core surgical skills

Questions in this area will tend to surround measurement of variables in relation to preoperative assessment, most commonly electrocardiogram and spirometry.

A 12-lead electrocardiogram may be supplied, with supplementary clinical information. For example:

SBA

A 65-year-old woman with a history of hypertension (treated with lisinopril) and hyperthyroidism (treated

FIGURE 36.2

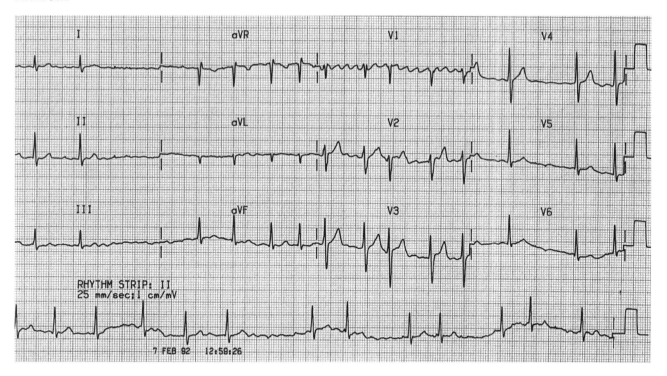

FIGURE 36.3

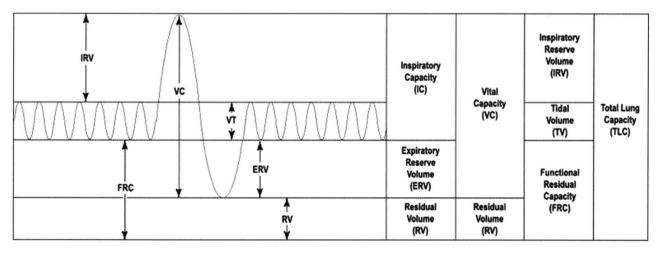

with carbimazole) presents to her GP with episodes of palpitations and fainting.

An ECG is arranged with the following result (Figure 36.2).

What is the diagnosis?

A. Atrial fibrillation
B. Atrial flutter
C. Ventricular fibrillation
D. Ventricular tachycardia
E. Wolff–Parkinson–White syndrome

Comment: The ECG shows absent P waves with an irregularly irregular rhythm. This is atrial fibrillation. Hypertension and hyperthyroidism are both risk factors for atrial fibrillation.

Concerning spirometry, it is important to have knowledge of lung volumes, especially since there are important physiological changes in pregnancy (see Figure 36.3).

Module 8: antenatal care

For more detailed information about evidence-based antenatal care in the UK, please see the National Institute of Health and Clinical Excellence (NICE) Clinical Guideline 62.

SCREENING TESTS

A variety of screening tests are undertaken during the antenatal period, and you may be asked to interpret data arising from these tests.

At the booking visit, blood is taken to screen for anaemia and antibodies. These tests are also repeated at 28 weeks of gestation. At each encounter with the midwife or doctor, the pregnant woman will have her blood pressure measured and a urine dipstick to check for proteinuria. These checks are aiming to screen for pre-eclampsia. Be aware of the normal physiological changes in blood pressure during pregnancy (see Chapter 31).

In certain ethnic groups, screening tests are offered for haemoglobinopathies.

SCREENING TESTS FOR DOWN SYNDROME

Trisomy 21 (Down syndrome) is the most common cause of mental retardation in the UK. The incidence of the condition in the fetus increases with maternal age (Table 36.4).

In the UK, the combined test (nuchal translucency on ultrasound, serum beta-human chorionic gonadotrohin

TABLE 36.4 **Incidence of trisomy 21 and maternal age**

Maternal age	Incidence of trisomy 21
30	1 in 1000
40	1 in 100
45	1 in 30

[β-hCG] and pregnancy-associated plasma protein A [PAPP-A]) is offered between 11 and 14 weeks of gestation. For women who book later, the serum screening test (quadruple test) can be offered from 15–20 weeks of gestation. From these tests, women are allocated to 'high' or 'low' risk groups (normally 1 in 150 being the cut-off point). Women who are deemed 'high risk' would then be offered invasive diagnostic tests. Remember that screening tests are not diagnostic, and only assign risk.

SBA

An anxious pregnant 40-year-old woman undergoes a combined test for Down syndrome screening. The risk comes back as 1 in 80. The result was delayed and she is now 17 weeks pregnant.

What is the appropriate course of action?

A. Advise that diagnostic tests are not indicated
B. Discuss amniocentesis
C. Discuss chorionic villus sampling (CVS)
D. Inform the woman that the baby does not have Down syndrome
E. Termination of pregnancy

Comment: This result indicates the fetus is in the high-risk group for Down syndrome. However, it is a screening test and not diagnostic. Although CVS can be undertaken at 17 weeks, it carries a higher risk of miscarriage than amniocentesis. If the woman wishes to have a diagnostic test, the correct option is amniocentesis.

DIAGNOSTIC TESTS FOR CHROMOSOMAL ABNORMALITIES

The conventional tests that are offered to obtain a diagnosis if a chromosomal abnormality is suspected, or a screening test is positive, are CVS and amniocentesis. The aim is to obtain tissue or cells that can be cultured in a genetics laboratory to obtain a karyotype. You may be given a karyotype to examine to provide a diagnosis. A recent development is the analysis of free-fetal DNA in maternal blood as a method of non-invasive diagnosis.

SCREENING FOR INFECTION

At the booking visit women are also offered screening tests for HIV, hepatitis B, rubella and syphilis. Screening for hepatitis C, cytomegalovirus and Group B Streptococcus is **not** offered in the UK.

MATERNAL MORTALITY STATISTICS

The maternal mortality ratio (MMR) is the most commonly derived statistic. This is defined as the number of maternal deaths per 100 000 live births in a particular time period (most commonly 1 year). This statistic is used to evaluate the effectiveness of maternal healthcare systems betweens countries or regions. Other statistics include maternal mortality rate (number of deaths per 1000 women of reproductive age) and lifetime risk of maternal death.

The MMR in the UK is 8.2 (2008). In most sub-Saharan African countries it is in excess of 500.

PERINATAL MORTALITY

The perinatal mortality rate (PNMR) is defined as the number of stillbirths and deaths in the first week of life per 1000 live births. The PNMR in the UK is approximately 8 per 1000 births.

Module 9: maternal medicine

DIABETES IN PREGNANCY

Up to 5% of pregnancies are complicated by some form of diabetes, although gestational diabetes is seen most commonly (Table 36.5). Certain groups of women will be screened for gestational diabetes using the 75g oral glucose tolerance test (see NICE Clinical Guideline 63 for further information). You may be asked to interpret the results of this test and provide a diagnosis.

Table 36.5 summarises the 2006 World Health Organization (WHO) recommendations for the diagnostic criteria for diabetes and intermediate hyperglycaemia.

TABLE 36.5 **Definition and diagnosis of diabetes mellitus and intermediate hyperglycaemia**

Diabetes	
Fasting plasma glucose 2–h plasma glucose[a]	≥7.0mmol/l (126mg/dl) or ≥11.1mmol/l (200mg/dl)
Impaired glucose tolerance (IGT)	
Fasting plasma glucose 2–h plasma glucose[a]	<7.0mmol/l (126mg/dl) and ≥7.8 and <11.1mmol/l (140mg/dl and 200mg/dl)
Impaired fasting glucose (IFG)	
Fasting plasma glucose 2–h plasma glucose[a]	6.1 to 6.9mmol/l (110mg/dl to 125mg/dl) and (if measured) <7.8mmol/l (140mg/dl)

[a] Venous plasma glucose 2–h after ingestion of 75g oral glucose load. If 2–h plasma glucose is not measured, status is uncertain as diabetes or IGT cannot be excluded

LIVER FUNCTION TESTS

Liver function tests change in pregnancy. Albumin levels tend to fall, due to dilutional effects of increased plasma volume and also increased permeability of the renal glomerulus. Remember that the placenta is also a source of the enzyme alkaline phosphatase, so serum levels can be more than three times higher in pregnancy. Obstetric cholestasis is a hepatic dysfunction particular to pregnancy. It is a diagnosis of exclusion, but can be suggested by elevated serum bile acids (although these would also be elevated in primary biliary cirrhosis).

THYROID FUNCTION TESTS

Thyroid function can also change in pregnancy. In early pregnancy there may be hyperthyroidism due to the effects of β-hCG on the thyroid-stimulating hormone (TSH) receptor. There is a fall in plasma iodide due to increased urinary excretion. Thyroid-binding globulin increases during pregnancy, meaning there are less free-thyroid hormones in the plasma. Women taking thyroxine often need to increase the dose to remain euthyroid in pregnancy.

THYROID AUTO-ANTIBODIES

Thyroid auto-antibodies may be elevated in certain conditions and can be diagnostic. In Graves disease, thyroid-receptor antibodies are present. These stimulate the TSH receptor and cause hyperthyroidism. In this condition serum TSH levels will be low. Hashimoto's thyroiditis is the most common cause of hypothyroidism, and this can be diagnosed by elevated levels of antibodies against the enzyme thyroid peroxidise. Here, TSH levels will be elevated.

SBA

A Caucasian woman with type II diabetes attends the obstetric endocrine clinic at 28 weeks of gestation complaining of lethargy, weight gain and constipation.

Thyroid function tests gave the following results:

TSH	4.5 mU/l
Free T_4	15 pmol/l
Thyroid peroxidase antibodies	Negative
Thyroid receptor antibodies	Negative

What is the most likely diagnosis?

A. Euthyroid
B. Iodine deficiency
C. Graves disease
D. Hashimotos thyroiditis
E. Previous treatment with radioactive iodine

Comments: normal ranges for TSH 0.4–5.5 mU/l and T_4 11–23 pmol/l. This patient is euthyroid and her antibody screen is negative. Physiological changes of pregnancy can present with similar symptoms to hypothyroidism.

Module 10: management of labour

CARDIOTOCOGRAPH

You may be given a cardiotocograph (CTG) to comment upon. The full spectrum of CTG interpretation is beyond this chapter, but it is recommended to either attend CTG training in your local hospital, or working through an online training package.

Normal values for a CTG are:

Baseline heart rate	110–160 bpm
Variability	>5 bpm

Absence of late or variable decelerations.
Early decelerations or accelerations may be present.

PARTOGRAM

You may be given a partogram to comment on the progress of labour, the frequency of contractions or other documented management.

FETAL BLOOD SAMPLING

If there are concerns about fetal wellbeing in labour, fetal scalp blood sampling can be performed. This is best undertaken in the left lateral position. Under direct vision, a shallow nick is made to the fetal scalp and the blood drawn into a tube by capillary action. The usual parameters then measured are pH and lactate.

The pH results should be interpreted as shown in Table 36.6.

Module 11: management of delivery

CORD BLOODS

You may be given paired cord blood samples taken after delivery to comment upon, especially regarding any derangement of acid–base balance. Remember that the base excess is a marker of the metabolic component of any acid–base disturbance.

SBA

A category 2 caesarean section is undertaken for failure to progress in the first stage of labour. Paired cord blood

TABLE 36.6 Interpreting pH results

pH	Action
>7.25	Normal result. But repeat sample in 30 min if CTG continues to be concerning
7.21–7.25	Borderline. Repeat sample in 30 min
<7.21	Abnormal. Delivery needs to be expedited

samples are taken for blood gas analysis and the results are as follows:

	Arterial	Venous
pH	7.28	7.35
Base excess	−6	−2

What type of acid–base disturbance is present?

A. Metabolic acidosis
B. Metabolic alkalosis
C. No disturbance
D. Respiratory acidosis
E. Respiratory alkalosis

Comment: These values are all within the normal range; therefore, there is no disturbance of acid–base balance.

APGAR SCORES

You may be given clinical information about a neonate after delivery and asked to calculate the APGAR score (Table 36.7).

Module 13: gynaecological problems

HORMONE LEVELS IN THE MENSTRUAL CYCLE

Ensure that you are totally conversant with the changes in hormone levels in the normal menstrual cycle (Figure 36.4).

For a fuller explanation see Chapter 29. Remember that there is a fall in the production of estrogens immediately after ovulation due to disruption of the follicle. This may be a cause of midcycle vaginal bleeding/spotting in some women as estrogen levels rise in the luteal phase due to production in the corpus luteum.

ULTRASOUND

You may be presented with some simple ultrasound images with corresponding clinical information and asked questions about diagnosis or simple clinical management.

Examples are (Figure 36.5A–D):

(A) A 25-year-old woman with a regular 28-day cycle presents with recurring midcycle pain. It is day 12 of her cycle. There is an anechoic structure in her left ovary measuring 18×17 mm. What is it most likely to be?

(B) A woman presents to the emergency department with marked right-sided pain. It is 3 weeks since her last menstrual period and she has a regular 30-day cycle. An ultrasound scan is performed. There is a cystic structure in the right ovary containing a fine reticular echo pattern. What is it most likely to be?

(C) A woman with a body mass index of 32 kg/m^2 presents to the gynaecology clinic with very infrequent periods. An ultrasound scan is performed with the attached appearance. What appearance is demonstrated?

(D) A woman presents to the gynaecology clinic with worsening left-sided pelvic pain and dysmenorrhoea. On questioning she also describes deep dyspareunia. An ultrasound is arranged with the following appearance. What is the structure identified in the left ovary?

TABLE 36.7 **APGAR scoring**

Parameter	Score		
	0	1	2
Pulse rate	Absent	<100/min	>100/min
Respiration, crying	Absent	Weak effort	Good cry
Muscle tone	Flaccid	Some flexion	Good flexion of arms and legs
Reflexes, irritability	No response	Grimace/feeble cry	Good cry/cough/sneeze
Colour	Blue/pale	Blue at extremities	Pink

FIGURE 36.4 **Hormone levels in the normal menstrual cycle**

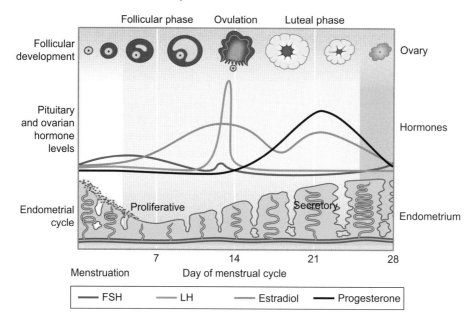

Answers

(A) This is most likely a preovulatory follicle. The patient is just before midcycle and the image appears to clearly represent a preovulatory follicle with the correct dimensions.

(B) This appears to be a haemorrhagic corpus luteum. The patient is in the luteal phase and the symptoms fit with a bleed into the corpus luteum. A fibrin clot within a cyst often has this lacy, reticular appearance.

(C) These ovaries have a clear polycystic morphology. In terms of diagnosis, this patient has polycystic ovarian syndrome since she also has oligomenorrhoea.

(D) This is an ovarian endometrioma. The symptoms the patient describes are also suggestive of endometriosis.

LAPAROSCOPY AND HYSTEROSCOPY IMAGES

Although laparoscopic and hysteroscopic images have not appeared in the exam to date, it is likely that they will in the future. It is possible that you would be asked to identify an anatomical or pathological structure. For example (Figure 36.6):

A woman with polycystic ovarian syndrome and infertility undergoes a laparoscopic ovarian drilling. The remainder of the pelvis appears normal. What is the structure identified by the arrows?

Answer – round ligament

A woman with heavy menstrual bleeding attends for a diagnostic hysteroscopy after an abnormal ultrasound scan which suggested thickened endometrium. The following view (Figure 36.7) is obtained. What (if any) pathological process is demonstrated?

Answer – this is a normal hysteroscopy with no evidence of polyp or fibroid

BIOPSIES

You may be given the clinical history of a patient with the results of a skin, endometrial or other biopsy and asked for a diagnosis.

SBA

A 68-year-old woman is referred to the gynaecology clinic by her GP. She has experienced intense vulval itching and on examination there is skin

FIGURE 36.5

(a)

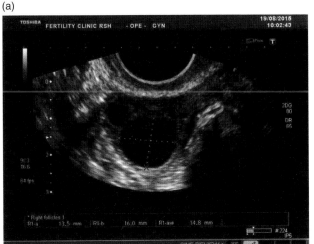

(b)

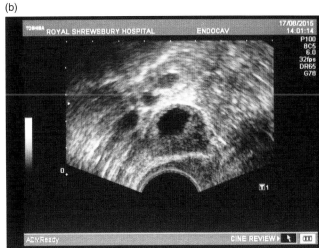

(c)

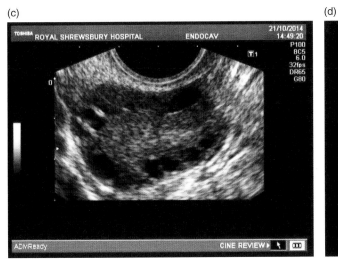

(d)

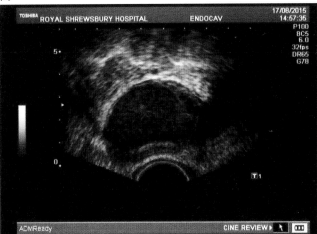

depigmentation around the introitus with atrophy of the labia. Two punch biopsies are taken in clinic.

Histology report

Two skin biopsies showing evidence of hyperkeratosis, epidermal atrophy and lymphocytic infiltration.

What is the most likely diagnosis?

A. Psoriasis
B. Eczema
C. Lichen sclerosus
D. Lichen planus
E. Vulval carcinoma

Comments: this is a textbook history of lichen sclerosus. The histology report also demonstrates all the features of this condition.

Module 14: subfertility

BLOOD TESTS

A variety of blood tests are undertaken as part of a fertility workup. Follicle-stimulating hormone (FSH)

FIGURE 36.6

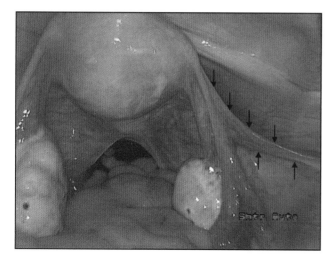

FIGURE 36.7

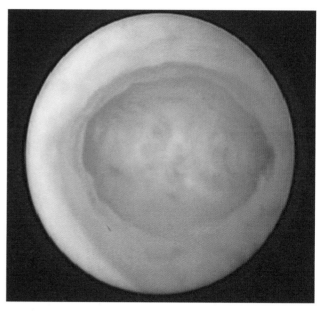

levels are measured early in the follicular phase because of variations throughout the cycle. Anti-Mullerian hormone (a measure of ovarian reserve) can be measured at any time as the levels are relatively constant with little variation within the cycle. A midluteal phase progesterone is a measure of ovulation, and is suggestive of ovulation if it exceeds 30 nmol/l. Remember the length of the luteal phase is fixed (14 days) so the progesterone level should always be measured 7 days before the expected day of menstruation. Chlamydial antibodies may also be measured as a surrogate marker of tubal damage.

TESTS OF TUBAL PATENCY

There are three main tests of tubal patency in current clinical use as shown in Table 36.8.

SEMEN ANALYSIS

There may be questions on the interpretation of a semen analysis on the basis of the most recent WHO manual (Table 36.9).

Module 15: sexual and reproductive health

ORGANISMS AND SWAB RESULTS

There may be questions with a clinical history and swab results (including Gram staining) for you to interpret and make a diagnosis. For example:

SBA

A 23-year-old woman attends the genitourinary medicine clinic with an offensive discharge.

Triple swabs are taken and the endocervical swab yields the following result:

Large numbers of Gram-negative diplococci identified

Which organism is most likely to be causing the infection?

A. *Neisseria gonorrhoeae*
B. *Chlamydia trachomatis*
C. *Trichomonas vaginalis*
D. *Candida albicans*
E. *Treponema pallidum*

Comment: *Neisseria gonorrhoea* is a Gram-negative diplococcus. It inhabits columnar epithelium which is found in the endocervix.

HEPATITIS B AND C

You may be given hepatitis serology results to interpret, particularly in terms of past or current infection, and whether or not the patient is currently infectious.

The interpretation of hepatitis B results can be complex. There are a variety of parameters to examine

TABLE 36.8 **Tests of tubal patency**

Test	Basis of test	Advantages	Disadvantages
Hystero-contrast-salpingography (HyCoSy)	Echo contrast agent is instilled through the tubes during an ultrasound scan	Simple outpatient test Inexpensive Uterus and ovaries can also be examined	In terms of verifying tubal patency it has good sensitivity, but poor specificity
Hysterosalpingogram (HSG)	A radio-opaque agent is instilled through the tubes during X-ray screening of the pelvis	Outpatient test Inexpensive	Exposure to X-ray radiation Ovaries not seen Tubes may go into spasm (the radio-opaque agent is quite viscous)
Laparoscopy and dye test	During a diagnostic laparoscopy, methylene blue due is instilled through the tubes using a transcervical catheter.	The whole of the pelvis can be examined 'Gold standard' test	Involves a general anaesthetic Operative risks

TABLE 36.9 **Lower reference limits (5th centiles and their 95% confidence intervals) for semen characteristics**

Parameter	Lower reference limit
Semen volume (ml)	1.5 (1.4–1.7)
Total sperm number (10^6 per ejaculate)	39 (33–46)
Sperm concentration (10^6 per ml)	15 (12–16)
Total motility (PR + NP,%)	40 (38–42)
Progressive motility (PR,%)	32 (31–34)
Vitality (live spermatozoa,%)	58 (55–63)
Sperm morphology (normal forms,%)	4 (3.0–4.0)

Source: WHO (2010) *WHO Laboratory Manual for the Examination and Processing of Human Semen*, 5th ed., p. 224.

which are the antigens from, and antibodies to various parts of the hepatitis B virus.

Therefore the antigens examined are core antigen (HBcAg), 'e' antigen (HBeAg) and surface antigen (HBsAg), and their corresponding antibodies (anti-HBc, anti-HBe and anti-HBs).

After an acute infection, the surface antigen (HBsAg) is the first to be detectable in the serum. This is followed by the core and 'e' antigens. Some individuals rapidly clear the infection, so the antigen levels may fall quickly, but during this time immunoglobulin (Ig) M antibodies to the core antigen (anti-HBc) will be detectable.

Ultimately once an infection has been cleared, IgG antibodies (anti-HBs, anti-HBc and anti-HBe) will all be present in the serum with no detectable antigen, and these would be the markers of previous infection.

For those individuals who have been vaccinated against hepatitis B, there will only be anti-HBs (ie no anti-HBe or c) since the vaccine is directed against the surface antigen (HBsAg).

Some individuals end up with a chronic hepatitis B infection, and their serology will show continued presence of both HBsAg and HBeAg. Those who continue to be HBeAg positive are generally considered to be the most infectious (although not all hepatitis B viruses produce an 'e' antigen)

In hepatitis C, initial testing looks for the presence of antibodies to the virus. If this is positive, a confirmatory test is performed, and the viral load determined by the presence of viral RNA. If the antibody test is positive, but the viral RNA undetectable, this indicates an infection that has either cleared spontaneously, or with treatment. If viral RNA is detected, this indicates ongoing acute or chronic infection.

SYPHILIS SEROLOGY

There are two main serological tests for syphilis in current clinical use. The VDRL test is a nontreponemal test, which is often used as an initial screen. Patients with syphilis produce anti-cardiolipin antibodies that react with diphosphatidyl glycerol and this produces a foaming or flocculation reaction. The test can be non-specific, and there are a number of false-positives.

Treponemal tests include the *Treponema pallidum* particle agglutination assay (TPPA) and the haemoagglutination assay (TPHA), which work in similar ways.

Module 16: Early Pregnancy care

HUMAN CHORIONIC GONADOTROPHIN LEVELS

In an early viable intrauterine pregnancy human chorionic gonadotrophin (hCG) levels tend to rise by at least 70% every 48 hours. In an ectopic or nonviable pregnancy, the rate of rise tends to be lower.

After a complete miscarriage, hCG levels tend to fall by at least 50% in 48 hours, but if there are retained products of conception the rate of fall may be lower or static.

SBA

A woman attends the Early Pregnancy Unit. It is 6 weeks since her last menstrual period and she had a positive pregnancy test 2 weeks ago.

She presents with a heavy PV bleed.

An ultrasound scan is arranged with the following report:

> *Normal size uterus with endometrial thickness 5 mm. No evidence of a gestational sac. Both ovaries appear normal. No free fluid.*

A serum β-hCG level is taken. Result: 1400 IU/l. This is repeated 48 hours later. Result: 600 IU/l.

What is the most likely diagnosis?

A. Complete miscarriage
B. Ectopic pregnancy
C. Incomplete miscarriage
D. Heterotopic pregnancy
E. Missed miscarriage

Comment: The history is suggestive of complete miscarriage. The ultrasound scan shows no worrying features, but no evidence of pregnancy either. The hCG levels have fallen by more than 50%. This is a complete miscarriage.

ULTRASOUND FINDINGS

Be aware of the ultrasound milestones in early pregnancy (Figures 36.8A–D).

Module 17: gynaecological oncology

RISK OF MALIGNANCY INDEX (OVARIAN CYSTS)

You may be given clinical information and results for a patient and asked to calculate the Risk of Malignancy Index (RMI). For more information on this topic, please look at the Green top guideline on the management of postmenopausal ovarian cysts.

Calculation of the RMI

RMI combines three presurgical features: serum CA-125, menopausal status (M) and ultrasound score (U). The RMI is a product of the ultrasound scan score, the menopausal status and the serum CA-125 level (IU/ml) as follows:

RMI = U × M × CA-125.

- The ultrasound result is scored 1 point for each of the following characteristics: multilocular cysts, solid areas, metastases, ascites and bilateral lesions.U = 0 (for an ultrasound score of 1), U = 3 (for an ultrasound score of 2–5)
- The menopausal can be defined as scored as 1 = premenopausal and 3 = postmenopausal.
- Postmenopausal can be defined as a woman who has had no period for more than one year, or a woman over the age of 50 who has had a hysterectomy.
- Serum CA-125 is measured in IU/ml and can vary between zero to hundreds or even thousands of units.[i]

---

[i] Text excerpt reproduced from: Royal College of Obstetricians and Gynaecologists/British Society for Gynaecological Endoscopy. *Management of Suspected Ovarian Masses in Premenopausal Women.* Green-top Guideline No. 62. London: RCOG; 2011, with the permission of the Royal College of Obstetricians and Gynaecologists.

FIGURE 36.8A **Five-week ultrasound**

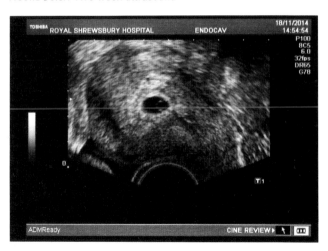

FIGURE 36.8B **Six-week ultrasound**

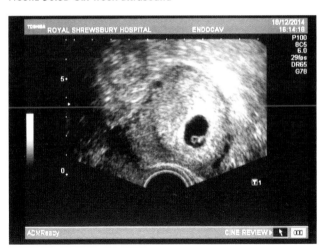

FIGURE 36.8C **Seven-week ultrasound**

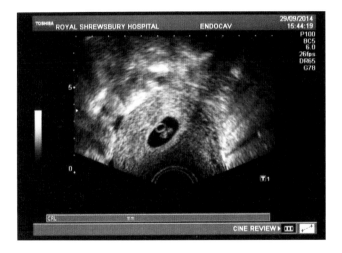

FIGURE 36.8D **Eight-week ultrasound**

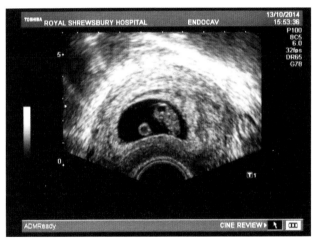

BIOPSY RESULTS

As in earlier examples, you may get information about a patient history and/or a clinical examination and be asked to interpret a biopsy or histopathology report.

Module 18: urogynaecology

URODYNAMICS

Although not explicitly mentioned in the syllabus, there have been questions on simple cystometry and urodynamics as this could be considered the measurement of a physiological variable. Questions will be straightforward and involve the simple interpretation of data showing overactive bladder (unprovoked contractions of the detrusor muscle) and urodynamic stress incontinence (leakage of urine when intra-abdominal pressure is raised).

Cystometry involves the placement of a catheter in the bladder which contains a pressure tranducer (both for filling of the bladder with fluid and for measuring intra-vesical pressure) and a second catheter in either the vagina or rectum to measure intra-abdominal pressure. The detrusor pressure can be obtained from subtracting intra-abdominal pressure from intravesical pressure. It is recommended that you attend a session of urodynamics, as this will clearly show the techniques in action.

FURTHER READING

NICE (2008) *Antenatal Care* (NICE Clinical Guideline 62) guidance. www.nice.org.uk/cg62

NICE (2008) *Diabetes in Pregnancy* (NICE Guideline 3) updated February 2015. www.nice.org.uk/guidance/ng3

NICE (2012) *Ectopic Pregnancy and Miscarriage* (NICE Clinical Guideline 154). guidance.nice.org.uk/cg154

NICE (2013) *Fertility: Assessment and treatment for people with fertility problems* (NICE Clinical Guideline 156). guidance.nice. org.uk/cg156

RCOG (2003) *Ovarian Cysts in Postmenopausal Women* (Green-top Guideline No. 34) https://www.rcog.org.uk/en/guidelines-research-services/guidelines/gtg34/

RCOG (2011) *Management of Suspected Ovarian Masses in Premenopausal Women* (Green-top Guideline No. 62) https://www.rcog.org.uk/globalassets/documents/guidelines/gtg62_021211_ovarianmasses.pdf

WHO (2006) *Definition and Diagnosis of Diabetes Mellitus and Intermediate Hyperglycemia.* http://whqlibdoc.who.int/publications/2006/9241594934_eng.pdf?ua=1

Index

diet
  in diabetes 258, 265
  in lactation 444
  lipids 115
  in phenylketonuria 123
  vitamins and minerals 92, 100, 445
DiGeorge syndrome 279
dipeptidyl peptidase 4 inhibitors 259
DNA
  analytical techniques 71–3, 287–9, 319
  fetal, in maternal blood 285
  replication 65, 68–9
  structure 68
docosahexaenoic acid (DHA) 124
donovanosis 369–70
dopamine 219, 236, 444
dopamine agonists 226, 228, 444
dopamine antagonists 444
Doppler ultrasound 135
dorsal nerve of the clitoris 38
dorsal sacroiliac ligament 11
Down syndrome (trisomy 21) 274–5,
  283–5, 516
doxycycline 338, 340
drospirenone 416
drug–drug interactions 397
dual energy X-ray absorptiometry (DEXA) 103,
  138–9
ductus arteriosus 197–9, 454–5
  patent 455
ductus venosus 196, 198, 453, 455
duloxetine 409
duodenum 175, 180–1, 183
dysmenorrhoea 418
dyspepsia 442

ECG (electrocardiography) 129–31, 440, 514–16
ectoderm 155–7, 174
ectopia cordis 194
ectopic pregnancy 208, 384
Edwards syndrome (trisomy 18) 274–5
efavirenz 374
eicosanoids 57–8
  see also prostaglandins
ejaculation 436
electrocardiography (ECG) 129–31, 440, 514–16
electrolytes 85, 210–11, 236, 511, 513
  Conn syndrome 239–40
electrosurgery (diathermy) 141–5
embolus 382
embryology 151–61, 203–4, 437–8
  see also individual organs or systems
endocardial cushion defects 194
endocrine signalling 55
endoderm 156, 159–60, 174
endometrial cancer 290, 388–9, 410, 419
endometrial changes during menstrual cycle 429
endometrial hyperplasia 389, 419
endometriosis 383–4, 418–19, 519

endometritis 364, 366, 374–6
endoplasmic reticulum 54, 59
endotoxins 320, 328
endpoints in clinical trials 478–9, 482
energy metabolism 107–24
eNOS (endothelial NO synthase) 58–9
Enterobacteriaceae 326–8
Entonox 408
eosinophils 294
epidemiology 476
  maternal deaths 479, 517
  miscarriage 384
  stillbirth / neonatal deaths 479–80, 517
epididymis 169, 431, 434
epigenetics
  histone modification 80
  imprinting 277–8, 282
epilepsy, maternal 401
epinephrine (adrenaline) 61, 114, 236–7
  phaeochromocytoma 240–1
epispadias 171
eplerenone 240
erection 435–6
ergometrine 408
erythrocytes see red blood cells
erythropoietin (EPO) 457
Escherichia coli 320, 327–8
estradiol 77–8, 413–14, 435, 446
estriol 78, 211–12, 413
estrogen receptors 79, 413–14
estrogens 413–14
  bone and 102, 414
  HRT 419–20
  lactation 443–4
  in the male 435
  menarche 221
  menstrual cycle 427, 429
  in pregnancy 211–12, 446
  SERMs 414–15
  synthesis 77–8, 212
estrone 77, 413
ethinyl estradiol 414
evidence-based medicine 477–8, 481
exomphalos 182
exons 70
exotoxins 61, 320
exstrophy of the bladder 166, 171
exstrophy of the cloaca 166
external cephalic version 406
external genitalia 170–2, 223
  in CAH 243–4
external oblique muscle 11–12
external-beam radiotherapy 147

falciform ligament 175
fallopian tubes see uterine (fallopian) tubes
Fallot's tetralogy 195
falx inguinalis (conjoint tendon) 12–13, 16
fascia lata 17

fat metabolism 111–17, 124, 217, 255
  in pregnancy 261
femoral hernia 17
femoral nerve 23–4
femoral sheath 17
femoral triangle 17
fertilisation 152–3, 429, 436–7
fetal blood sampling 518
fetal material in the maternal circulation
  DNA 285
  red blood cells 306, 311, 457–8
fetus
  acid–base balance 89
  calcium 100
  circulation 196–7, 451–4
  glucose metabolism 123–4, 210, 261–2
  growth
    macrosomia 118, 264
    restriction 264
  infections 326, 347–9, 351, 354–5
  maternal diabetes and 118, 218, 263–4
  maternal–fetal exchange 209–11, 310
  monitoring 450–1, 518
  oxygen 210, 454
    and HbF 457
    hypoxia 264, 450–1, 459
  pharmacotherapy 403
  physiology 196–7, 261–2, 449–62
  steroid production 76, 78, 211–12, 435
  thyroid hormones 251–2
  vitamin D 101
  see also prenatal screening and diagnosis
FHR (fetal heart rate) 449–51, 518
fibroblast growth factor 23: 93, 100
fibroids 389, 520
FISH (fluorescence in situ hybridisation) 287
Fitz-Hugh–Curtis syndrome 365
flucloxacillin 340
fludrocortisone acetate 242
fluid balance 512
  diabetes insipidus 227, 229
  fetal 458
  hormones and 220, 236
  in pregnancy 85, 210
fluorescence in situ hybridisation (FISH) 287
folic acid 264
follicle-stimulating hormone see FSH
folliculogenesis 152, 425–7
  pre-ovulatory follicle on US 519
foramen ovale 188, 199, 453–5
  patent 194, 455
foramen secundum ASD 194
foregut 173–81
FSH (follicle-stimulating hormone) 219–20,
  425–7
  infertility 231, 521
  in the male 435
  puberty 221
fulguration 144